Geriatrics Medicine: Assessment and Intervention

Geriatrics Medicine: Assessment and Intervention

Edited by Benjamin Thornberg

AMERICAN
MEDICAL PUBLISHERS
www.americanmedicalpublishers.com

American Medical Publishers,
41 Flatbush Avenue,
1st Floor, New York,
NY 11217, USA

Visit us on the World Wide Web at:
www.americanmedicalpublishers.com

ISBN: 978-1-63927-004-0

Cataloging-in-Publication Data

Geriatrics medicine : assessment and intervention / edited by Benjamin Thornberg.
p. cm.
Includes bibliographical references and index.
ISBN 978-1-63927-004-0
1. Geriatrics. 2. Older people--Diseases. 3. Geriatrics--Diagnosis. 4. Older people--Diseases--Treatment.
5. Older people--Health and hygiene. 6. Aging. I. Thornberg, Benjamin.
RC952 .G47 2022
618.97--dc23

Table of Contents

Preface

Geriatrics medicine is a branch of a medical specialty that focuses on the health and care of elderly people. It deals with treating and preventing diseases and disabilities in elderly people in order to promote their health. Geriatric medicine is different from standard adult medicine as it focuses on the unique needs of the older adult. Various sub-specialty such as cardiogeriatrics, geriatrics dentistry, geriatrics dermatology and geriatrics diagnostic imaging fall under this domain. Geriatricians distinguish between diseases and the effects of normal aging and focus on the treatment accordingly. For example, renal impairment may be a part of aging, but renal failure and urinary incontinence are not. Geriatric medicine aims to treat existing diseases and help in achieving healthy aging. This book unravels the recent studies in the field of geriatrics medicine. Different approaches, evaluations, methodologies and advanced studies on geriatrics medicine have been included herein. This book is a complete source of knowledge on the present status of this important field.

Various studies have approached the subject by analyzing it with a single perspective, but the present book provides diverse methodologies and techniques to address this field. This book contains theories and applications needed for understanding the subject from different perspectives. The aim is to keep the readers informed about the progresses in the field; therefore, the contributions were carefully examined to compile novel researches by specialists from across the globe.

Indeed, the job of the editor is the most crucial and challenging in compiling all chapters into a single book. In the end, I would extend my sincere thanks to the chapter authors for their profound work. I am also thankful for the support provided by my family and colleagues during the compilation of this book.

Editor

Preface

1

Sarcopenia is Associated with High Pulse Pressure in Older Women

**Hélio José Coelho Júnior,[1,2] Samuel da Silva Aguiar,[2,3]
Ivan de Oliveira Gonçalves,[4] Ricardo Aurélio Carvalho Sampaio,[1] Marco Carlos Uchida,[1]
Milton Rocha Moraes,[3] and Ricardo Yukio Asano[2,5]**

[1]*School of Physical Education, State University of Campinas, 130883851 Campinas, Brazil*
[2]*Center of Health Sciences, University of Mogi das Cruzes, 08770-490 Mogi das Cruzes, Brazil*
[3]*Graduate Program on Physical Education, Catholic University of Brasilia, 71966-700 Brasilia, Brazil*
[4]*Community Center for Older People of Poá, Poá, Brazil*
[5]*School of Sciences and Letters of Bragança Paulista, SP, Brazil*

Correspondence should be addressed to Hélio José Coelho Júnior; coelhojunior@hotmail.com.br

Academic Editor: Guido Iaccarino

Introduction. Sarcopenia is a geriatric syndrome associated with impairment of muscle function, metabolism, and cognition in older women. Recent studies have shown a relationship between changes in muscle mass and the cardiovascular system. However, this relationship has not been fully elucidated. *Methods.* One hundred and thirty community-dwelling Brazilian older women (65.4 ± 6.3 years) were recruited to participate in this study. Data on body composition (via bioelectrical impedance measurements), cardiovascular parameters (using an automatic and noninvasive monitor), and muscle function (using a 3-meter gait speed test) were measured. *Results.* Sarcopenic older women (n = 43) presented higher levels of pulse pressure (PP) (60.3 ± 2.6 mmHg) and lower muscle function (0.5 ± 0.0 m/s) compared with nonsarcopenic subjects (n = 87) (53.7 ± 1.5 mmHg; 0.9 ± 0.0 m/s) ($P < 0.05$). Linear regression analysis demonstrated a significantly negative association between skeletal muscle index (SMI) and PP levels ($\beta = -226$, $P < 0.05$). Furthermore, sarcopenic older women showed a 3.1-fold increased risk of having higher PP levels compared with nonsarcopenic women (IC = 1.323–7.506) ($P < 0.05$). *Conclusion.* Sarcopenic older women showed lower muscle function and higher cardiovascular risk due to increased PP levels compared with nonsarcopenic subjects.

1. Introduction

Sarcopenia is a geriatric syndrome primarily characterized by progressive and generalized loss of skeletal muscle mass. In addition, it is strongly associated with the aging process and can be exacerbated in the presence of pathological conditions (e.g., diabetes mellitus type II) [1–5]. Sarcopenia negatively affects the autonomy and quality of life of older adults in different ways (e.g., by decreasing muscle strength and muscle power and increasing the risk of falls) [6]. In this respect, sarcopenia is associated with increased risk of falls and bone fractures, cognitive and muscle impairment, frailty, impaired performance of activities of daily living, loss of independency, and early death [1–5].

With regard to metabolic processes, older adults with lower skeletal muscle index (SMI) can present hyperinsulinemia, dyslipidemia, high levels of glycosylated hemoglobin, and predisposition to prediabetic and metabolic syndrome conditions, particularly if SMI is associated with obesity [7, 8]. Moreover, sarcopenic and nonsarcopenic older adults showed higher levels of insulin resistance and fasting glucose compared with nonsarcopenic older adults [4].

Although some studies demonstrated the relationship between morphofunctional and metabolic alterations due to sarcopenia, the effects of the decrease in skeletal muscle mass on the cardiovascular system are still inconclusive. Recent studies have reported that alterations in the SMI and increased arterial stiffness can negatively affect the cardiovascular system [9–11]. Ochi and colleagues [9] indicated that older adults with lower thigh muscle cross-sectional area presented higher levels of risk factors for cardiovascular disease, including increased intima-media thickness and increased pulse-wave velocity. Similarly, Abbatecola and colleagues [10] observed higher pulse-wave velocity in American older adults with lower SMI.

Pulse pressure (PP) is a simple and inexpensive measurement of arterial stiffness and is closely related to pulse-wave velocity [12, 13]. Furthermore, meta-analysis data indicate that increased PP is a good predictor of cardiovascular death and death from other causes in older people [14].

Therefore, in addition to the impairment of muscle function, autonomy, and metabolism caused by sarcopenia in older adults, recent studies showed a possible negative effect of sarcopenia on the cardiovascular system [4, 9]. Therefore, the aim of the present study was to evaluate the relationship between the sarcopenia index and hemodynamic dysfunctions in older women. The proposed hypothesis is that high levels of sarcopenia can negatively influence hemodynamic variables.

2. Methods

2.1. Study Design. This cross-sectional study evaluated 130 community-dwelling older women living in Brazil. All volunteers were recruited from two specialized healthcare centers for older women: (I) a community center for older adults and (II) Institute Reborn for seniors. In both centers, volunteers developed activities that involved predominantly the physical and cognitive domains. The physical activities offered were (1) a multimodal exercise program, which stimulates some physical capabilities (i.e., muscle strength, muscle power, and cardiorespiratory fitness) in the same session of exercise; these sessions lasted approximately 40 minutes and were performed in low-moderate intensity; (2) water aerobics; (3) folk dance; and (4) yoga. Painting was the only activity that involved predominantly the cognitive domain. After registration, older adults were automatically enrolled in all activities. However, they were not required to participate in or perform activities every day.

Participation in the present study involved the completion of all measurements after signing the informed consent form. This study was approved by the Research Ethics Committee of the Universidade de Mogi das Cruzes (UMC) under protocol number 621-614. This study was developed in accordance with the Declaration of Helsinki and according to Resolution 196/96 of the National Health Council.

2.2. Participants. All older women were ≥60 years of age. The exclusion criteria were use of hormone replacement and/or psychotropic drugs, cardiovascular disease (e.g., acute myocardial infarction, stroke, peripheral arterial disease, and transient ischemic disease), pulmonary disease, neurological or psychiatric disease (e.g., Parkinson's or Alzheimer's disease), musculoskeletal disorders, and comorbidities associated with greater risk of falls. All clinical information (i.e., disease status, age, and drug therapy) was obtained by reviewing the medical records of each subject.

All subjects were instructed to refrain from physical exercise for 96 hours before the tests and to refrain from eating or drinking (including water) for 8 hours before the tests. All tests were conducted between 07:00 am and 10:00 am under a controlled temperature of 26°C.

2.3. Measurements

2.3.1. Assessment of Body Composition and Sarcopenia. A data acquisition system (Tanita InnerScan 50v, Tokyo, Japan) was used to measure the bioelectrical impedance. This system uses an electrical current to quantify the amount of intracellular and extracellular water in the body. The device has four electrodes: two are placed on the feet while the other two are placed on the hands of the volunteers. The device measures body mass index (BMI), total body mass, total muscle mass, and percentage of fat mass [15]. Sarcopenia was defined by the criterion of Janssen and colleagues [16]. In summary, the bioelectrical impedance test allows the normalization of absolute muscle mass (AMM) to height (AMM/height^2), which is denominated skeletal muscle mass index (SMI). Sarcopenia was classified into tertiles [11]. Older women classified into the first tertile (<15, 68 kg/m^2) were classified as sarcopenic.

2.3.2. Cardiovascular Parameters. All cardiovascular parameters were analyzed at rest. The procedures for the measurement of blood pressure were adapted from the VII Joint National Committee of High Blood Pressure (JNC7) [17]. In summary, older women remained in the sitting position in a comfortable chair for 15 minutes in a dark and quiet room. After this period, a cuff with the right size was placed approximately at the midpoint of the upper left arm (heart level). An automatic, noninvasive and validated [18] arterial blood pressure monitor (Microlife-BP 3BT0A, Microlife, Widnau, Switzerland) was used to measure systolic blood pressure (SBP), diastolic blood pressure (DBP), and heart rate (HR). The mean arterial pressure (MAP), rate pressure product (RPP), and pulse pressure (PP) were evaluated according to the following equations: $MAP = [SBP + (2 * DBP)]/3$; $RPP = SBP * HR$; $PP = SBP - DBP$ [12, 19]. The size of the arm cuff was selected after measuring the arm circumference (Sanny, São Paulo, Brazil).

2.3.3. Muscle. Muscle function was evaluated using the 3-meter walk speed test (WS) test. During the test, the volunteers were instructed to walk a distance of 5 meters at a normal cadence. To ensure this, the researcher requested the following: "Please, walk as you were going to a supermarket or bakehouse." Volunteers should remain with both feet on the starting line and counting started when one foot touched the 1-meter line and stopped when one foot touched the 4-meter line. After a 1-minute rest, a second attempt was made. The mean values were used in the analysis [15].

2.3.4. Pathological Conditions and Cofactors. Medical records were reviewed to obtain information of the health status of

TABLE 1: Comparison between the groups with regard to morphological and functional variables and health indicators.

	Healthy patients (n = 87)	Sarcopenic patients (n = 43)	P
Age (years)	64.1 ± 0.8	64.5 ± 0.5	ns
Body mass (kg)	66.2 ± 1.0	66.3 ± 2.5	ns
Height (cm)	155.9 ± 0.0	156.8 ± 0.0	ns
Body mass index (kg/m^2)	28.1 ± 0.4	24.3 ± 0.5	<0.05
Absolute muscle mass (kg)	41.5 ± 0.4	34.9 ± 1.3	<0.05
Skeletal muscle index (kg/m^2)	17.4 ± 0.1	14.6 ± 0.1	<0.05
Fat mass (%)	34.8 ± 0.8	36.4 ± 1.7	ns
SBP (mmHg)	138.8 ± 0.0	144 ± 0.1	ns
DBP (mmHg)	84.3 ± 1.1	83.4 ± 2.1	ns
MAP (mmHg)	102.6 ± 1.3	103.7 ± 2.1	ns
HR (bpm)	75.7 ± 1.2	74.9 ± 1.7	ns
RPP (mmHg·bpm)	10530 ± 256.7	10750 ± 303.9	ns
PP (mmHg)	53.7 ± 1.5	60.3 ± 2.6	<0.05
Functionality (m/s)	0.9 ± 0.0	0.5 ± 0.0	<0.05
Hypertension (%)	41.0	65.0	ns
Diabetes mellitus type II (%)	4.4	5.8	ns
Metabolic syndrome (%)	4.0	4.0	ns
Respiratory pathology (%)	4.0	1.0	ns
Mean of drugs	1.1 ± 0.1	1.7 ± 0.2	ns
Smoker (%)	5.0	5.0	ns

Data are presented as mean ± SE. SBP = systolic blood pressure; DBP = diastolic blood pressure; MAP = mean arterial pressure; HR = heart rate; RPP = rate pressure product; PP = pulse pressure.

each volunteer. The head physician recorded the pathological conditions but a specialist not affiliated to/outside the center made the pathologic diagnosis. The cofactors (the number of drugs used by older women (mean of drugs) and smoking status) were recorded by a head nurse after interviewing the participants. The medical records were updated every six months.

2.4. Statistical Analysis. The Shapiro-Wilk test was used to calculate data normality. Student's t-test was used to compare quantitative variables and χ^2 was used to compare qualitative variables. Pearson's correlations were conducted with and without adjusting for pathological conditions. After statistical analyses, it was verified that PP values were higher in the sarcopenic group and were significantly associated with SMI; subsequently, the correlation between SMI and PP was investigated. Stepwise linear regression was conducted to predict the best model to evaluate the association between SMI and PP. Multiple linear regression analysis was used to assess the significance of the proposed model. To assess whether the IMM was a risk factor for PP, logistic regression was conducted. Differences were considered statistically significant at $P < 0.05$. Sample size was determined on the basis of a population of 112.481 individuals and a confidence level of 95%. All analyses were conducted using the Statistical Package for the Social Sciences (SPSS; IBM, Chicago, IL, USA) software version 20.0.

3. Results

Subjects were dichotomized in two groups according to the SMI cutoff. Table 1 presents the characteristics of the study group. Sarcopenic older women presented lower values of BMI, SMI, and AMM and lower muscle function but higher PP values compared with normal older women.

Pearson's correlation was performed to assess possible associations between the cardiovascular variables and SMI. Our results showed a significantly negative association between SMI and PP (−0.25; P = 0.03). Moreover, adjustment for pathological conditions alone or in combination did not change the significance of the association (hypertension (−0.25; P = 0.05); diabetes mellitus type II (−0.25; P = 0.05); metabolic syndrome (−0.25; P = 0.04); respiratory pathology (−0.25; P = 0.05); and metabolic syndrome together with respiratory pathology (−0.25; P = 0.04)).

Table 2 shows data on linear and multiple linear regression. The findings on linear regression showed a significant R^2 (0.49) for IMM in relation to PP. However, multiple regression did not show significant results for any of the proposed models from stepwise linear regression.

The odds ratio results indicate that older women with sarcopenia have three times increased risk (3.151) of having increased PP values compared with nonsarcopenic volunteers (1.323–7.506 (95% confidence interval), $P < 0.05$).

4. Discussion

The results of the present study indicate that sarcopenic older women have lower muscle function and higher PP levels compared with nonsarcopenic older women. These results were confirmed by using multilinear and linear regression and indicate a significantly negative association between SMI and PP. Furthermore, sarcopenic volunteers had a three times

TABLE 2: Linear and multilinear regression considering pulse pressure as the dependent variable.

Variable(s)	R^2	β	P
SMI	0.49	−0.226	<0.05
Model 1	0.94	0.157	ns
Model 2	0.136	0.104	ns
Model 3	0.174	0.98	ns

SMI = skeletal muscle index; Model 1 = SMI plus age; Model 2 = Model 1 plus metabolic syndrome, smoking status, hypertension, and diabetes mellitus type II; Model 3 = Model 2 plus height and functionality.

higher risk of having increased PP values compared with nonsarcopenic individuals.

These findings are in accordance with those of other studies, which demonstrated a relationship between the sarcopenia index and cardiovascular alterations in older adults [4, 9–11, 20]. Recently, Han and colleagues [4] evaluated a large sample of older Koreans (n = 4.846) and observed a higher prevalence of hypertension in sarcopenic older adults compared with nonsarcopenic adults, regardless of the obesity level. In addition, nonobese sarcopenic older adults had a 1.5 times higher risk of presenting with hypertension compared with nonsarcopenic subjects.

Furthermore, other experiments have investigated whether sarcopenia could be associated with increased arterial stiffness, which can promote the development of hypertension as well as other cardiovascular and cerebrovascular diseases [12, 21–23]. It has also been demonstrated that increased PP levels are an important risk factor for coronary heart disease [18].

Similar to the results of the present study, other studies demonstrated an association between the degree of sarcopenia and arterial stiffness. These experiments observed that increase in sarcopenia was associated with increase in brachial-ankle pulse-wave velocity in Japanese [7, 11, 20] and American older adults [10]. Furthermore, Srikanthan and Karlamangla [7] observed that the sarcopenia index was negatively associated with carotid intima-media thickness, suggesting a possible correlation with the formation of atherosclerotic plaques.

In the present study, older women with lower SMI showed higher odds ratio for higher PP levels compared with nonsarcopenic women. Higher levels of brachial PP are associated with increased pulse-wave velocity, which is mainly due to the decrease large-vessel compliance [12]. Complications associated with higher PP values have been previously studied [21–23]. In normotensive and hypertensive populations, higher PP was the most important determinant of the risk of death (mainly due to cardiovascular complications) [21, 22]. For this reason, the possibility of using PP as a better predictor of cardiovascular death compared with other hemodynamic measurements (e.g., SBP and DBP) has been recently considered [23].

One of the limitations of the present study was the failure to assess the influence of pathological conditions on the association between SMI and PP. However, no changes were observed in our results using Pearson's correlation and multilinear regression after adjusting for morbidities. Diabetes type II (DMTII) seems to enhance the loss of muscle mass primarily in individuals with uncontrolled glycemia [5–24]. Furthermore, patients with low SMI with and without DMTII demonstrated increased insulin resistance, hyperinsulinemia, and glycosylated hemoglobin levels compared with individuals with higher SMI [7]. Recent evidence suggests a potential correlation between sarcopenia and dyslipidemia, which leads to hyperglycemia and ultimately metabolic syndrome [8]. However, these data were not confirmed in the present study.

It is possible that the number of volunteers with pathologies was insufficient to evaluate the impact of each condition on the parameters evaluated. However, an advantage of the limited number of older people with illnesses is that, even in healthy older women, decreased muscle mass can impair the cardiovascular system.

A possible mechanism that could explain the association between SMI and higher PP levels in the sarcopenic group is increased chronic inflammation due to decreased muscle function, which can lead to physical inactivity. Decreased muscle function resulted in higher levels of inflammatory markers in the blood of older adults [25]. Chronic low-grade inflammation is characterized by an increase in blood levels and gene expression of proinflammatory cytokines, which can—via paracrine and autocrine mechanisms—decrease the bioavailability of nitric oxide, increase arterial stiffness, increase the formation of atherosclerotic plaques, and promote endothelial dysfunction, which, in turn, can promote an increase in PP levels [26–28].

On the other hand, the increase in muscle activity has been suggested as a mechanism that can inhibit chronic low-grade inflammation [29]. It is known that bioactive proteins known as myokines (e.g., IL-6) are produced by muscle fibers from muscle contraction [30, 31]. Myokines can inhibit the activity of proinflammatory cytokines (e.g., TNF-α), thereby avoiding the deleterious effect of cytokines on the human body [25, 27]. Animal experiments showed that the increase in muscle activity by physical exercise could decrease the activity of TNF-α in mice that overexpress this protein [32]. In addition, the cytokine levels of volunteers who practiced physical exercise in the same day and who were stimulated to produce TNF-α did not increase. However, the group that did not practice physical exercise had increased TNF-α concentrations [33]. In the present study, nonsarcopenic older women with improved muscle function possibly performed more muscle contractions, which led to the increased production of myokines, which in turn acted as a protective factor against chronic low-grade inflammation.

Insulin resistance can also explain the results of this study. Individuals with low SMI with and without diabetes demonstrated increased insulin resistance, hyperinsulinemia, and increased levels of glycosylated hemoglobin compared with individuals with higher SMI, which was probably caused by decreased insulin levels in the target organ [7]. Furthermore, hyperinsulinemia due to insulin resistance can activate NFκB, which is an important regulator of the production of proinflammatory cytokines [34]. Clearly, a synergistic effect of both mechanisms cannot be discarded and is probably the best explanation.

Interestingly, the cofactors identified in the present study (BMI, percentage of body fat, age, and muscle function) had no effect on the association between SMI and PP. Other factors that can influence vascular homeostasis, such as nitric oxide, cholesterol, and low- and high-density lipoproteins, can be used to create a better model to investigate the relationship between SMI and PP. Moreover, studies involving study groups with specific pathologic conditions, such as DMT2, hypertension, obesity, and metabolic syndrome, can help elucidate the impact of pathological conditions on muscle mass homeostasis and their effect on the cardiovascular system [5, 8].

Some of the limitations of the present study include (i) its cross-sectional design, which precluded the assessment of a time-effect relationship; (ii) the limited number of volunteers enrolled, which can be partially explained by sample homogeneity, which contributed to a better understanding of the effect of sarcopenia on older women; and (iii) the absence of biochemical measurements, which could have elucidated possible interacting mechanisms. However, to the best of our knowledge, this is the first study that addressed the relationship between low SMI and changes in the arterial stiffness index in Brazilian older women.

5. Conclusion

The present study showed that older women with higher SMI (which is predominantly influenced by an active lifestyle) presented lower PP levels and decreased cardiovascular risk whereas older women with a sarcopenic profile had a cardiovascular risk 3 times higher than that of nonsarcopenic women. Therefore, beneficial therapies, such as strength exercise, can help increase or maintain muscle mass and consequently improve the quality of life of older people.

Conflict of Interests

The authors declare that there is no conflict of interests regarding the publication of this paper.

Acknowledgments

The authors are grateful to the Conselho Nacional de Desenvolvimento Científico e Tecnológico (CNPq) and to FAPESP (2014/07667-3) for funding this research through study grants to Hélio José Coelho Júnior and Marco Carlos Uchida, respectively. They are also very grateful to Daisy dos Reis (Head Nurse) and Flávio Romano, Manager of the facility for older adults, for their support.

References

[1] S.-H. Kim, T.-H. Kim, and H.-J. Hwang, "The relationship of physical activity (PA) and walking with sarcopenia in Korean males aged 60 years and older using the Fourth Korean National Health and Nutrition Examination Survey (KNHANES IV-2, 3), 2008-2009," *Archives of Gerontology and Geriatrics*, vol. 56, no. 3, pp. 472–477, 2013.

[2] A. J. Cruz-Jentoft, J. P. Baeyens, J. M. Bauer et al., "Sarcopenia: European consensus on definition and diagnosis: report of the European working group on sarcopenia in older people," *Age and Ageing*, vol. 39, no. 4, pp. 412–423, 2010.

[3] W.-J. Lee, L.-K. Liu, L.-N. Peng, M.-H. Lin, and L.-K. Chen, "Comparisons of sarcopenia defined by IWGS and EWGSOP criteria among older people: results from the I-Lan longitudinal aging study," *Journal of the American Medical Directors Association*, vol. 14, no. 7, pp. 528.e1–528.e7, 2013.

[4] K. Han, Y.-M. Park, H.-S. Kwon et al., "Sarcopenia as a determinant of blood pressure in older Koreans: findings from the Korea National Health and Nutrition Examination Surveys (KNHANES) 2008–2010," *PLoS ONE*, vol. 9, no. 1, Article ID e86902, 2014.

[5] J. E. Morley, "Diabetes, sarcopenia, and frailty," *Clinics in Geriatric Medicine*, vol. 24, no. 3, pp. 455–469, 2008.

[6] C. Pongchaiyakul, P. Limpawattana, P. Kotruchin, and R. Rajatanavin, "Prevalence of sarcopenia and associated factors among Thai population," *Journal of Bone and Mineral Metabolism*, vol. 31, no. 3, pp. 346–350, 2013.

[7] P. Srikanthan and A. S. Karlamangla, "Relative muscle mass is inversely associated with insulin resistance and prediabetes. findings from the Third National Health and Nutrition Examination Survey," *Journal of Clinical Endocrinology & Metabolism*, vol. 96, no. 9, pp. 2898–2903, 2011.

[8] S. J. Baek, G. E. Nam, K. D. Han et al., "Sarcopenia and sarcopenic obesity and their association with dyslipidemia in Korean elderly men: the 2008–2010 Korea National Health and Nutrition Examination Survey," *Journal of Endocrinological Investigation*, vol. 37, no. 3, pp. 247–260, 2014.

[9] M. Ochi, K. Kohara, Y. Tabara et al., "Arterial stiffness is associated with low thigh muscle mass in middle-aged to elderly men," *Atherosclerosis*, vol. 212, no. 1, pp. 327–332, 2010.

[10] A. M. Abbatecola, P. Chiodini, C. Gallo et al., "Pulse wave velocity is associated with muscle mass decline: health ABC study," *Age*, vol. 34, no. 2, pp. 469–478, 2012.

[11] R. A. C. Sampaio, P. Y. Sewo Sampaio, M. Yamada et al., "Arterial stiffness is associated with low skeletal muscle mass in Japanese community-dwelling older adults," *Geriatrics & Gerontology International*, vol. 14, no. 1, pp. 109–114, 2014.

[12] A. M. Dart and B. A. Kingwell, "Pulse pressure—a review of mechanisms and clinical relevance," *Journal of the American College of Cardiology*, vol. 37, no. 4, pp. 975–984, 2001.

[13] G. Assmann, P. Cullen, T. Evers, D. Petzinna, and H. Schulte, "Importance of arterial pulse pressure as a predictor of coronary heart disease risk in PROCAM," *European Heart Journal*, vol. 26, no. 20, pp. 2120–2126, 2005.

[14] L. Zhao, Y. Song, P. Dong, Z. Li, X. Yang, and S. Wang, "Brachial pulse pressure and cardiovascular or all–cause mortality in the general population: a meta–analysis of prospective observational studies," *The Journal of Clinical Hypertension*, vol. 16, no. 9, pp. 678–685, 2014.

[15] M. Yamada, S. Nishiguchi, N. Fukutani et al., "Prevalence of sarcopenia in community-dwelling Japanese older adults," *Journal of the American Medical Directors Association*, vol. 14, no. 12, pp. 911–915, 2013.

[16] I. Janssen, R. N. Baumgartner, R. Ross, I. H. Rosenberg, and R. Roubenoff, "Skeletal muscle cutpoints associated with elevated physical disability risk in older men and women," *American Journal of Epidemiology*, vol. 159, no. 4, pp. 413–421, 2004.

[17] Joint National Committee on Prevention, Detection, Evaluation, and Treatment of High Blood Pressure, "The seventh report of the Joint National Committee on Prevention, Detection, Evaluation, and Treatment of High Blood Pressure (JNC7)," *Journal of the American Medical Association*, vol. 19, no. 289, pp. 2560–2572, 2003.

[18] A. C. Cuckson, A. Reinders, H. Shabeeh, and A. H. Shennan, "Validation of the Microlife BP 3BTO-A oscillometric blood pressure monitoring device according to a modified British Hypertension Society Protocol," *Blood Pressure Monitoring*, vol. 7, no. 6, pp. 319–324, 2002.

[19] D. U. Silverthorn, *Human Physiology: An Integrated Approach*, Pearson/Benjamin Cummings, 2009.

[20] K. Sanada, M. Miyachi, M. Tanimoto et al., "A cross-sectional study of sarcopenia in Japanese men and women: reference values and association with cardiovascular risk factors," *European Journal of Applied Physiology*, vol. 110, no. 1, pp. 57–65, 2010.

[21] S. S. Franklin, S. A. Khan, N. D. Wong, M. G. Larson, and D. Levy, "Is pulse pressure useful in predicting risk for coronary heart disease? The Framingham Heart Study," *Circulation*, vol. 100, no. 4, pp. 354–360, 1999.

[22] A. Benetos, "Pulse pressure and cardiovascular risk," *Journal of Hypertension, Supplement*, vol. 17, no. 5, pp. S21–S24, 1999.

[23] F. Thomas, J. Blacher, A. Benetos, M. E. Safar, and B. Pannier, "Cardiovascular risk as defined in the 2003 European blood pressure classification: the assessment of an additional predictive value of pulse pressure on mortality," *Journal of Hypertension*, vol. 26, no. 6, pp. 1072–1077, 2008.

[24] T. S. Akpinar, M. Tayfur, F. Tufan et al., "Uncomplicated diabetes does not accelerate age-related sarcopenia," *The Aging Male*, vol. 17, no. 4, pp. 205–210, 2014.

[25] S. G. Wannamethee, G. D. O. Lowe, P. H. Whincup, A. Rumley, M. Walker, and L. Lennon, "Physical activity and hemostatic and inflammatory variables in elderly men," *Circulation*, vol. 105, no. 15, pp. 1785–1790, 2002.

[26] M. El Assar, J. Angulo, and L. Rodríguez-Mañas, "Oxidative stress and vascular inflammation in aging," *Free Radical Biology and Medicine*, vol. 65, pp. 380–401, 2013.

[27] R. Y. Asano, M. M. Sales, J. M. Coelho et al., "Exercise, nitric oxide, and endothelial dysfunction: a brief review," *Journal of Exercise Physiology Online*, vol. 15, no. 1, pp. 76–86, 2012.

[28] R. Y. Asano, M. M. Sales, R. A. V. Browne et al., "Acute effects of physical exercise in type 2 diabetes: a review," *World Journal of Diabetes*, vol. 5, no. 5, article 659, 2014.

[29] A. M. W. Petersen and B. K. Pedersen, "The anti-inflammatory effect of exercise," *Journal of Applied Physiology*, vol. 98, no. 4, pp. 1154–1162, 2005.

[30] M. Penkowa, C. Keller, P. Keller, S. Jauffred, and B. K. Pedersen, "Immunohistochemical detection of interleukin-6 in human skeletal muscle fibers following exercise," *The FASEB Journal*, vol. 17, no. 14, pp. 2166–2168, 2003.

[31] B. K. Pedersen and M. Febbraio, "Muscle-derived interleukin-6—a possible link between skeletal muscle, adipose tissue, liver, and brain," *Brain, Behavior, and Immunity*, vol. 19, no. 5, pp. 371–376, 2005.

[32] C. Keller, P. Keller, M. Giralt, J. Hidalgo, and B. K. Pedersen, "Exercise normalises overexpression of TNF-α in knockout mice," *Biochemical and Biophysical Research Communications*, vol. 321, no. 1, pp. 179–182, 2004.

[33] R. Starkie, S. R. Ostrowski, S. Jauffred, M. Febbraio, and B. K. Pedersen, "Exercise and IL-6 infusion inhibit endotoxin-induced TNF-alpha production in humans," *The FASEB Journal*, vol. 17, no. 8, pp. 884–886, 2003.

[34] M. H. Park, D. H. Kim, E. K. Lee et al., "Age-related inflammation and insulin resistance: a review of their intricate interdependency," *Archives of Pharmacal Research*, vol. 37, no. 12, pp. 1507–1514, 2014.

2

Effect of Dementia on the Use of Drugs for Secondary Prevention of Ischemic Heart Disease

Nicole R. Fowler,[1] Amber E. Barnato,[1,2] Howard B. Degenholtz,[2,3] Angela M. Curcio,[4] James T. Becker,[5] Lewis H. Kuller,[6] and Oscar L. Lopez[7]

[1] *Division of General Internal Medicine, Department of Medicine, School of Medicine, University of Pittsburgh, Pittsburgh, PA 15213, USA*
[2] *Department of Health Policy and Management, Graduate School of Public Health, University of Pittsburgh, Pittsburgh, PA 15261, USA*
[3] *Center for Bioethics and Health Law, University of Pittsburgh, Pittsburgh, PA 15260, USA*
[4] *College of Medicine, Drexel University, Philadelphia, PA 19129, USA*
[5] *Department of Psychiatry, School of Medicine, University of Pittsburgh, Pittsburgh, PA 15213, USA*
[6] *Department of Epidemiology, Graduate School of Public Health, University of Pittsburgh, Pittsburgh, PA 15261, USA*
[7] *Department of Neurology, School of Medicine, University of Pittsburgh, Pittsburgh, PA 15213, USA*

Correspondence should be addressed to Nicole R. Fowler; fowlernr@upmc.edu

Academic Editor: F. Richard Ferraro

Background. Dementia and cardiovascular disease (CVD) are frequently comorbid. The presence of dementia may have an effect on how CVD is treated. *Objective*. To examine the effect of dementia on the use of four medications recommended for secondary prevention of ischemic heart disease (IHD): angiotensin-converting enzyme inhibitors, beta-blockers, lipid-lowering medications, and antiplatelet medications. *Design*. Retrospective analysis of data from the Cardiovascular Health Study: Cognition Study. *Setting and Subjects*. 1,087 older adults in four US states who had or developed IHD between 1989 and 1998. *Methods*. Generalized estimating equations to explore the association between dementia and the use of guideline-recommended medications for the secondary prevention of IHD. *Results*. The length of follow-up for the cohort was 8.7 years and 265 (24%) had or developed dementia during the study. Use of medications for the secondary prevention of IHD for patients with and without dementia increased during the study period. In models, subjects with dementia were not less likely to use any one particular class of medication but were less likely to use two or more classes of medications as a group (OR, 0.60; 95% CI, 0.36–0.99). *Conclusions*. Subjects with dementia used fewer guideline-recommended medications for the secondary prevention of IHD than those without dementia.

1. Introduction

Among medicare beneficiaries diagnosed with dementia, 30% also have a diagnosis of ischemic heart disease (IHD) [1], and as many as 54% have had a myocardial infarction at some point in their lives [2], making them candidates for the use of medications for the secondary prevention of IHD. There appears to be a link between cardiovascular disease (CVD) [3] and the development of clinical dementia, and the aggressive treatment of CVD may delay or reduce the risk of developing dementia [4–6]. For example, studies show an inverse relationship between statin use and risk for Alzheimer's disease, possibly due to the role that lipids may play in the development of this disease [7, 8].

Additionally, dementia in older adults has an effect on the management of comorbid cardiovascular disease: patients with myocardial infarction are half as likely to receive invasive cardiac procedures if they have dementia listed in their hospital chart [9]; community-dwelling patients with a diagnosis of dementia are less likely to use either cardiovascular medications [10] or a lipid-lowering medication [11], and even after controlling for IHD, use of cardiovascular medications is lower in nursing home residents with dementia, especially severe dementia [12].

While the presence of clinical dementia plays a role in decisions to use invasive procedures and medications for the management of CVD, no studies, to date, have examined and compared the use of medications recommended for the secondary prevention of IHD in a population with and without dementia over time. We used an epidemiologic cohort of subjects serially assessed for dementia and IHD to explore the relationship between dementia and the use of guideline-recommended medications for the secondary prevention of IHD between 1989-1998, a decade with substantial growth in the use of these medications. We hypothesized that use of these medications for the secondary prevention of IHD would be lower in individuals with dementia than in individuals without dementia.

2. Methods

2.1. Setting, Participants, and Study Design. We conducted a retrospective analysis of prospectively collected data from the Cognition Study within the Cardiovascular Health Study-Cognition Study (CHS-CS) [13, 14]. We used CHS-CS data concerning dementia, IHD, medication usage for the secondary prevention of IHD, and comorbidity status.

The CHS is a longitudinal, observational, community-based study of the onset, progression, and course of cardiovascular disease in 5,201 older men and women from four sites: Forsyth County, North Carolina; Sacramento, California; Washington County, Maryland; and Pittsburgh, Pennsylvania [14]. The CHS cohort was aged 65 and older at enrollment in 1989-1990 and was supplemented with 687 men and women during a minority participant recruitment effort at these same sites in 1992-1993.

Each year, the CHS-CS investigators captured data on the study participants' cognitive status by administering the Modified Mini-Mental State Examination (3MSE) [15] and the Digit Symbol Substitution Test [16]. To obtain additional information on the cognition of participants, the investigators administered the Informant Questionnaire on Cognitive Decline in the Elderly [17] and the Dementia Questionnaire [18] to proxies (e.g., spouses or children of participants). The CHS-CS protocol for the classification of dementia was previously reported [19].

The CHS investigators collected detailed diagnostic information about the study participants' cardiovascular health, including clinical, radiologic, and laboratory data. They defined prevalent cardiovascular disease as a history of myocardial infarction, angina, congestive heart failure, or stroke, as indicated by participant self-report and confirmed by a medical record review, the results of a baseline electrocardiogram, or both [20]. Incident cardiovascular disease is defined as the onset of any of these conditions after baseline assessment, subject to adjudication at the field sites with the use of information from treating physicians or from hospital discharge summaries. For this study, we defined prevalent IHD as history of myocardial infarction and angina (stable and unstable) indicated by CHS and incident IHD as the onset of either of these conditions after baseline assessment.

To ascertain information about the participants' use of prescription medications, members of the CHS team performed in-person (home or clinic) medication inventories each year [21]. In cases when the medication information could not be obtained from the participant (e.g., too cognitively impaired), a proxy provided the information for the medication inventory. The CHS-CS protocol did not include collecting data on prescriptions written by physicians. Details about the medication use assessment and validation of this method for estimating drug exposure were previously reported [21].

2.2. Independent Variables. For our primary analyses, the independent variable was dementia status (present/absent) of study participants with IHD for each year of longitudinal follow-up, as classified by the CHS-CS investigators. For participants with prevalent cases of dementia, we assigned their study baseline year as the year of onset. For participants with incident cases of dementia, we used the onset date determined by the CHS-CS investigators. If participants had mild cognitive impairment but did not convert to dementia during the study period, we considered them to be without dementia. Patients contributed multiple years of data with an average of 8.7 years of follow-up and could have been demented throughout or nondemented throughout or could have converted from non-demented to demented during the observation period.

As a sensitivity analysis, we explored an alternate specification of dementia, presence of dementia from the perspective of the subject or their proxy using any of the following items on the Dementia Questionnaire: a proxy report of memory or cognition problem, an indication that the participant had been told by a physician that they had memory or thinking problems, or a report that the participant had been prescribed a medication for memory. We used this variable because the CHS-CS cognitive diagnosis— a research-based assessment—may not have been known by the subject, proxy, or the community physician responsible for prescribing the medications, whereas the Dementia Questionnaire items directly measure proxy and/or physician recognition of impairment. The CHS study did not collect data on participants' treating physicians or the prescribing physician for medications.

2.3. Dependent Variables and Covariates. As dependent variables (main outcome measures) for our study, we used four classes of guideline-recommended cardiovascular medications: ACE inhibitors, beta-blockers, lipid-lowering medications, and antiplatelet medications. We selected these classes for two reasons: they had the strongest evidence of reducing mortality from IHD following a myocardial infarction at the time of the CHS, and they were included in clinical practice guidelines for the treatment and management of patients with IHD during all or some of the study period [22–25].

In unadjusted models, we compared medication use for two representative years: 1992 (study year 5 of original sample and baseline year for supplemented minority cohort) and 1998 (study year 11 and final study year for full sample). In our primary multivariable analyses, we determined whether participants used drugs from one or more of the four drug classes. To test for use separately and jointly, we dichotomized the variables as taking a drug from a particular class (yes/no) or taking drugs from two or more classes (yes/no) during each study year. Our models for ACE inhibitors, beta-blockers, and antiplatelet medications were from 1989 to 1998. Our model for lipid-lowering medications over time was restricted to the seven-year period from 1992 to 1998, since the use of these drugs was not standard practice until later in the study period.

Covariates tested for inclusion in each final model included age, sex, race, education level, income level, functional status (e.g., activities of daily living), clinically important factors (e.g., atrial fibrillation, congestive heart failure, stroke, depression, diabetes, hypertension, hyperlipidemia, and kidney disease), and study site.

2.4. Statistical Analyses. To characterize the study sample in terms of sociodemographic data and use of medications (ACE inhibitors, beta-blockers, lipid-lowering medications, antiplatelet medications, all other cardiac drugs, and total number of prescription medications), we used descriptive statistics. Chi-square tests for categorical variables and t-tests for continuous variables were used to compare the sociodemographic and medication data for participants with and without dementia, at different time points. Where non-parametric procedures were indicated, we used Fisher's exact tests for analysis. We examined the relationship between dementia status and use of medication for the secondary prevention of IHD by calculating the odds that individuals with dementia would be taking drugs from one or more classes of guideline-recommended medications (relative to those without dementia). To test differences in use of any drugs compared to no use, we created an "any use" variable for the four classes; we then modeled use of each drug individually and then use of any two classes together. Then, to better understand the specific role of certain covariates as confounders, we examined the unadjusted odds ratio for each covariate and the change in the ratio after adjusting for dementia status. In the final models, we included all demographic and clinical covariates that had clinical relevance or a strong association ($P \leq 0.10$) with the use of ACE inhibitors, beta-blockers, lipid-lowering medications, or antiplatelet medications.

To model the use of the four classes of drugs individually and as a group of two or more over time, we fitted a generalized estimating equation (GEE) with binomial distribution, logit link function, and autoregressive correlation structure. For the autoregressive correlation structure, we selected a lag period of 1 year, given that the likelihood of being treated with a particular drug was higher if the same drug was used the previous year. Because GEE models assume missing data completely at random, we created weights for each observation that were inversely proportional to the probability of missing. Only participants with a determination of IHD were included in the model, so participants with incident IHD were not included until their incident year.

We used Stata/SE version 12 (StataCorp, College Station, Texas) to perform all analyses and considered a P value of <0.05 as significant.

3. Results

3.1. Characteristics of the Study Sample. Our study sample consisted of the 1,087 CHS-CS participants who had IHD; 591 subjects had IHD at baseline, and 496 developed IHD during the study period. The average follow-up period for the cohort was 8.7 years. The mean age of the study sample at baseline was 76.6 years. Of the 1,087 participants, 567 (52%) were male, 928 (85%) were white, 617 (57%) had a high school education or less, 786 (72%) had an annual income of $34,999 or less, and 265 (24%) had dementia identified by the CHS-CS either at baseline or later during the study (Table 1). Among the 1,087, 118 (11%) had a family member or other proxy indicated on the Dementia Questionnaire that they were aware that the participant had a cognitive impairment or that they were taking a cognitive enhancement medication (i.e., Donepezil and Memantine—1996 and later).

3.2. Comparison of Groups. Table 1 compares sociodemographic characteristics and functional and comorbidity status of participants without dementia and participants with dementia in two representative years, 1992 (study year 5 of original sample and baseline year for supplemented minority cohort) and 1998 (study year 11 and final study year for full sample). In each year, partcipants with dementia were significantly older, were more likely to have a high school education or less, and have lower activities of daily living score. Participants with and without dementia differed regarding comorbidity status. In both year 5 and year 11, participants with dementia were significantly more likely to have a history of atrial fibrillation, congestive heart failure, kidney disease, depression, and stroke.

Table 2 compares medication use of participants in these same years. Overall, the use of guideline-recommended medications for the secondary prevention of IHD for patients with and without dementia increased over time but was lower for those with dementia compared to those without dementia. In contrast, the use of other cardiac medications did not show substantial secular growth and they were used at similar or higher rates among those with dementia compared to those without dementia. Table 3 shows results from the longitudinal multivariable models that adjusted for age, race, sex, hypertension, diabetes, atrial fibrillation, congestive heart failure, study site, interaction term for dementia and age, and study year. We found that participants with dementia were no more or less likely to use any one drug class, but they were significantly less likely to use two or more guideline-recommended medications (odds ratio (OR), 0.60; 95% confidence interval (CI), 0.35–0.99). Results for other covariates indicate that being nonwhite (OR, 2.26; 95% CI 1.34–3.86) and older (OR, 0.97; 95% CI 0.92–0.99) was also independently associated with less use of two or more guideline-recommended medications.

Table 1: Characteristics of study participants in 1992 and 1998, stratified by dementia status*.

Characteristic	1992 (study year 5)† Number (%)			1998 (study year 11)‡ Number (%)		
	Without dementia (n = 1,005)	With dementia (n = 82)	P value	Without dementia (n = 672)	With dementia (n = 190)	P value
Age, years			<0.0001			<0.0001
≤75	562 (55.9)	25 (31.0)		76 (11.3)	7 (3.7)	
76–85	408 (40.6)	44 (54.3)		447 (66.6)	89 (47.0)	
86–95	26 (2.6)	12 (14.8)		92 (13.7)	59 (31.1)	
≥96	9 (1.0)	0 (0)		56 (8.4)	35 (18.4)	
Sex			0.10			0.46
Male	517 (51.4)	50 (61.0)		337 (50.1)	101 (53.2)	
Female	488 (48.6)	32 (39.0)		335 (49.9)	89 (46.8)	
Race			<0.0001			0.0002
White	873 (87.9)	55 (67.1)		582 (86.6)	143 (75.3)	
Nonwhite	132 (13.1)	27 (32.9)		90 (13.4)	47 (24.7)	
Education level			0.006			0.004
≤High school	559 (55.7)	58 (71.6)		358 (53.4)	124 (65.3)	
>High school	444 (44.3)	23 (28.4)		313 (46.7)	66 (34.7)	
Annual income			0.49			0.02
≤$34,999	724 (72.0)	62 (75.6)		473 (70.4)	150 (79.0)	
>$35,000	281 (28.0)	20 (24.4)		199 (29.6)	40 (21.0)	
ADL score, mean (SD)	0.17 (0.6)	0.54 (1.1)	<0.0001	0.41 (0.9)	1.63 (2.0)	<0.0001
COPD	167 (16.8)	10 (12.5)	0.31	150 (22.3)	35 (18.4)	0.28
Depression§	270 (27.3)	40 (50.6)	<0.0001	166 (29.4)	52 (51.5)	<0.0001
Diabetes	167 (16.6)	15 (18.3)	0.70	161 (24.0)	44 (23.3)	0.83
Hyperlipidemia	592 (59.2)	54 (67.5)	0.15	408 (61)	124 (66.3)	0.18
Hypertension	470 (47.5)	41 (51.2)	0.51	336 (60.0)	72 (62.1)	0.68
Kidney disease	183 (18.2)	26 (31.7)	0.003	90 (13.4)	43 (22.6)	0.002
Stroke	79 (7.8)	24 (29.3)	<0.0001	138 (21.3)	60 (33.9)	<0.001
Comorbidity			0.002			0.02
<3 comorbid conditions	968 (96.3)	73 (89)		598 (89.0)	157 (82.6)	
≥3 comorbid conditions	37 (3.68)	9 (11)		74 (11.0)	33 (17.4)	
Died	0 (0)	1 (1.2)	0.08	28 (4.2)	29 (59.3)	<0.0001
Follow-up, years, mean (SD)	5.20 (1.81)	0.59 (0.06)	<0.0001	6.27 (0.63)	3.14 (1.34)	<0.0001

ADL: activities of daily living; CES-D: Center for Epidemiological Studies Depression Scale; COPD: chronic obstructive pulmonary disease; SD: standard deviation.

*Because of rounding, percentages may not total 100.

†Study year 5 for initial sample and baseline year for supplemented minority cohort.

‡Final study year for full sample.

§Depression indicated with a score of >7 on the CES-D.

3.3. Effects of Proxy-Recognized Dementia. In sensitivity analyses, we found that whether or not a participant's family member or an other proxy recognized the participant's cognitive impairment had no effect on the participant's use of guideline-recommended medications (results not shown).

4. Discussion

To our knowledge, this is the first study to examine the effect of dementia on the use of guideline-recommended medications for the secondary prevention of IHD. During the study period, the proportion of all patients with IHD who reported using a guideline-recommended mediation increased substantially; however, those with dementia were less likely than those without dementia to use these medications. In adjusted analyses, individuals with dementia identified by the CHS-CS were less likely than individuals without dementia to use guideline-recommended drugs from two or more classes. This was not driven by lower rates of using drugs from any particular class. Cognitive impairment

TABLE 2: Unadjusted use of guideline-recommended medications by study participants in 1992 and 1998, stratified by dementia status.

Medication	1992 (study year 5)* Number (%) Without dementia (n = 1,005)	With dementia (n = 82)	P value	1998 (study year 11)† Number (%) Without dementia (n = 672)	With dementia (n = 190)	P value
Medications for IHD						
ACE inhibitor	131 (13.2)	15 (18.3)	0.20	146 (24.4)	35 (25.0)	0.89
Beta-blocker	221 (22.3)	8 (9.8)	0.008	220 (36.8)	36 (25.7)	0.01
Lipid-lowering medication‡	102 (10.3)	3 (3.7)	0.05	184 (30.8)	22 (15.7)	<0.001
Antiplatelet medication§	511 (51.5)	37 (45.1)	0.27	360 (63.8)	69 (58.0)	0.23
Use of two or more medications for IHD	266 (26.8)	15 (18.3)	0.09	300 (50.1)	50 (35.5)	0.002
Use of other cardiac medications						
Calcium channel blocker	348 (35.1)	27 (32.9)	0.70	205 (34.3)	43 (30.7)	0.42
Diuretic	297 (30.0)	31 (37.8)	0.14	217 (36.3)	52 (37.1)	0.85
Digoxin	149 (15.0)	18 (22.0)	0.10	116 (19.4)	30 (21.4)	0.59
Nitrate	250 (25.2)	18 (22.0)	0.52	158 (26.4)	44 (31.4)	0.23
Class 1A antiarrhythmic agent	36 (3.6)	2 (2.4)	0.76	2 (0.33)	4 (2.9)	0.01
Total number of all prescription medications, mean (SD)	0.99 (0.9)	0.79 (0.7)	0.04	1.57 (1.0)	1.27 (1.0)	0.003

ACE: angiotensin-converting enzyme; IHD: ischemic heart disease; SD: standard deviation.
*Study year 5 for initial sample and baseline year for supplemented minority cohort.
†Final study year for full sample.
‡Lipid-lowering medications included statins (3-hydroxy-3-methylglutaryl-coenzyme A [HMG-CoA] reductase inhibitors) and nonstatins.
§Antiplatelet medications included cyclooxygenase inhibitors (e.g., aspirin) and adenosine diphosphate (ADP) receptor inhibitors.

acknowledged by proxy on the Dementia Questionnaire did not impact use of drugs from any particular class individually or as a group.

Our study did not examine why there were differences in the use of medications between individuals with and without dementia or differences in prescribing or adherence, but several related points about our study limitations and about physicians' knowledge of dementia and prescribing practices in general should be considered.

First, in our main study analyses, the dementia status was determined by a detailed CHS-CS protocol, yet the individuals in our study were being treated by their own community-based physicians. Research shows that impaired cognitive status goes unrecognized by primary care physicians in 30%–50% of cases, [26] so it is possible that the physicians who prescribed medications for IHD were not aware of their patients' dementia status [26, 27]. We should note, however, that in 1997-1998 (the same year the Dementia Questionnaire was administered to proxies) the CHS-CS investigators informed the participants' physicians if test results showed strong evidence of cognitive impairment.

Second, we were unable to measure who the prescribing physician(s) was for each of these medications and the reasons why a patient may have reported less use of a guideline-recommended medication (e.g., lack of an indication, never received a prescription, nonadherence, patient preferences, and poor prognosis) [28]. Therefore, we could not make any conclusions if the lower use was appropriate or inappropriate. Because the medications recommended for the secondary prevention of IHD are relatively low-cost and likely considered to be low-burden and low-risk, we might expect them to be considered for any patient with IHD. Yet, dementia is known to reduce life expectancy, and the progressive nature of this condition may reduce the priority placed on secondary prevention of IHD. It is possible that this reprioritization of care would include evidence-based management for comorbidities and the changing of treatment plans during the course of dementia to match patient life expectancy, preferences, and treatment goals.

Third, medications for the secondary prevention of IHD are generally recommended to continue indefinitely. Their use may be challenging for any patient who is already receiving multiple drugs or if a patient had been taken off of a drug due to side effects. It can be particularly challenging for patients with dementia or their caregivers to have prescriptions filled and to take medications as instructed.

Fourth, although physicians are more reluctant to stop prescribing a medication than they are to not prescribe it in the first place, guideline-recommended medications could ethically be withdrawn if necessary (e.g., if the patient were using the drug erratically) [29]. Nevertheless, some physicians may not feel comfortable stopping medications, either because of the risk of adverse events or because they believe that stopping the drugs might be seen as a sign of "giving up" or contradicting earlier advice. In a follow-up study using the same dataset, we will investigate the relationship of the timing of onset of both dementia and IHD to measure if those who develop IHD prior to dementia are

Table 3: Association between dementia and use of one or more classes of guideline-recommended medications for secondary prevention of ischemic heart disease by study participants, 1989 to 1998.

Variable	Odds ratio (95% confidence interval)				
	Use of an ACE inhibitor	Use of a beta-blocker	Use of a lipid-lowering medication*	Use of an antiplatelet medication†	Use of two or more classes of guideline-recommended medications
Dementia	1.19 (0.79–1.77)	0.97 (0.65–1.44)	0.76 (0.37–1.55)	0.74 (0.45–1.23)	0.60 (0.35–0.99)‡
Age	0.99 (0.94–1.03)	0.98 (0.94–1.02)	0.99 (0.93–1.05)	0.97 (0.94–0.99)‡	0.97 (0.92–0.99)‡
Age and dementia interaction	1.01 (0.92–1.10)	1.03 (0.98–1.07)	0.99 (0.92–1.07)	1.06 (0.99–1.14)	1.10 (1.03–1.19)‡
White race	1.93 (0.95–3.91)	0.91 (0.43–1.92)	2.28 (0.99–5.20)‡	2.66 (1.65–4.30)‡	2.26 (1.34–3.86)‡
Male sex	1.12 (0.69–1.82)	1.32 (0.78–2.23)	1.21 (0.58–2.54)	1.40 (1.00–1.94)	1.24 (0.80–1.90)
Atrial fibrillation	1.16 (0.71–1.90)	0.95 (0.53–1.70)	0.29 (0.15–0.56)‡	0.98 (0.70–1.38)	1.03 (0.66–1.61)
CHF	2.87 (1.33–6.55)‡	0.40 (0.11–1.28)	1.42 (0.37–5.50)	0.95 (0.49–1.84)	1.12 (0.50–2.53)
Hypertension	1.12 (1.00–1.23)	1.15 (1.08–1.24)‡	1.47 (1.00–2.15)‡	1.07 (0.96–1.19)	1.16 (1.05–1.30)‡
Diabetes	1.21 (1.00–1.46)‡	0.86 (0.78–0.96)‡	1.14 (0.96–1.37)	1.06 (0.91–1.23)	1.08 (0.94–1.23)

ACE: angiotensin-converting enzyme; CHF: congestive heart failure.

*Lipid-lowering medications included statins (3-hydroxy-3-methyglutaryl-coenzyme A [HMG-CoA] reductase inhibitors) and nonstatins. The model for these medications was restricted to data from 1992 to 1998.

†Antiplatelet medications included cyclooxygenase inhibitors (e.g., aspirin) and adenosine diphosphate (ADP) receptor inhibitors.

‡$P < 0.05$.

more likely to use these medications compared to those who develop IHD after dementia.

Fifth, the data used for this study are from 1989 to 1998, and use of these medications in current practice is higher. Also, we did not include use of angiotensin receptor blockers which have been shown in recent studies to reduce the risk of dementia [30]. Nonetheless, the objective of this study was to determine differences in use between those with and without dementia, not rates of use per se. Although the data used in these analyses are from 1989 to 1998, we believe our findings are relevant given the evidence regarding the aggressive treatment of CVD and a possible delay or reduction in the risk of developing dementia. Additionally, we believe our findings are valid because differences in the treatment and management of comorbidities among older adults with dementia persist and continue to be reported in the literature [31, 32] despite greater overall health care utilization for older adults with dementia. It would be important for future research to assess the magnitude and consequences of these disparities, as well as the source, and whether differences are a reflection of differences in patient goals of care or possible provider biases.

In summary, the dementia status of patients is associated with less use of drugs for secondary prevention of IHD. Further studies are needed to determine why this is true for these particular drugs and whether it is true for other prescription drugs. Additionally, future studies investigating prescription patterns and subsequent patient adherence as a function of cognitive status could inform sources of the disparity. This line of inquiry could prove valuable for heightening physicians' awareness of their patients' cognitive status and its role in the overall management of their health. Our study also provides preliminary information for efforts to develop interventions to improve how physicians present information about treatment options and outcomes to patients with dementia and other comorbidities. Based on our findings, we believe it is important that future studies investigate sources of variation in the use of medications and the possible factors that influence medical decision making for patients with dementia.

Conflict of Interests

Nicole Fowler, Amber Barnato, Howard Degenholtz, Angela Curcio, James Becker, Lewis Kuller, and Oscar Lopez declare that they have no conflict of interests.

Authors' Contribution

All authors were responsible for the study concept, design, acquisition of data, analysis and interpretation of data, and preparation of the paper.

Acknowledgments

The research reported in this paper was supported by contracts HHSN268201200036C, N01-HC-85239, N01-HC-85079 through N01-HC-85086, N01-HC-35129, N01 HC-15103, N01 HC-55222, N01-HC-75150, N01-HC-45133, and Grant HL080295 from the National Heart, Lung, and Blood Institute (NHLBI), with additional contribution from the National Institute of Neurological Disorders and Stroke (NINDS). Additional support was provided through AG-023629, AG-15928, AG-20098, and AG-027058 from the National Institute on Aging (NIA). A full list of principal CHS investigators and institutions can be found at http://www.chs-nhlbi.org/pi.htm. This work was also supported in part by a Comparative Effectiveness Career Development Award (K12HS019461-01) to Dr. Fowler from the Agency for Healthcare Research and Quality.

References

[1] K. Maslow, "Dementia and serious coexisting medical conditions: a double whammy," *Nursing Clinics of North America*, vol. 39, no. 3, pp. 561–579, 2004.

[2] D. J. Brauner, J. C. Muir, and G. A. Sachs, "Treating nondementia illnesses in patients with dementia," *The Journal of the American Medical Association*, vol. 283, no. 24, pp. 3230–3235, 2000.

[3] R. S. Tilvis, M. H. Kähönen-Väre, J. Jolkkonen, J. Valvanne, K. H. Pitkala, and T. E. Strandberg, "Predictors of cognitive decline and mortality of aged people over a 10-year period," *Journals of Gerontology A*, vol. 59, no. 3, pp. 268–274, 2004.

[4] T. J. Bunch, J. P. Weiss, B. G. Crandall et al., "Atrial fibrillation is independently associated with senile, vascular, and Alzheimer's dementia," *Heart Rhythm*, vol. 7, no. 4, pp. 433–437, 2010.

[5] A. Hofman, A. Ott, M. M. B. Breteler et al., "Atherosclerosis, apolipoprotein E, and prevalence of dementia and Alzheimer's disease in the Rotterdam Study," *The Lancet*, vol. 349, no. 9046, pp. 151–154, 1997.

[6] P. B. Rosenberg, M. M. Mielke, J. Tschanz et al., "Effects of cardiovascular medications on rate of functional decline in alzheimer disease," *American Journal of Geriatric Psychiatry*, vol. 16, no. 11, pp. 883–892, 2008.

[7] H. Jick, G. L. Zornberg, S. S. Jick, S. Seshadri, and D. A. Drachman, "Statins and the risk of dementia," *The Lancet*, vol. 356, no. 9242, pp. 1627–1631, 2000.

[8] E. Zamrini, G. McGwin, and J. M. Roseman, "Association between statin use and Alzheimer's disease," *Neuroepidemiology*, vol. 23, no. 1-2, pp. 94–98, 2004.

[9] F. A. Sloan, J. G. Trogdon, L. H. Curtis, and K. A. Schulman, "The effect of dementia on outcomes and process of care for medicare beneficiaries admitted with acute myocardial infarction," *Journal of the American Geriatrics Society*, vol. 52, no. 2, pp. 173–181, 2004.

[10] K. E. Schmader, J. T. Hanlon, G. G. Fillenbaum, M. Huber, C. Pieper, and R. Horner, "Medication use patterns among demented, cognitively impaired and cognitively intact community-dwelling elderly people," *Age and Ageing*, vol. 27, no. 4, pp. 493–501, 1998.

[11] E. G. Rodriguez, H. H. Dodge, M. A. Birzescu et al., "Use of lipid-lowering drugs in older adults with and without dementia: a community-based epidemiological study," *Journal of the American Geriatrics Society*, vol. 50, pp. 1852–1856, 2002.

[12] F. Landi, G. Gambassi, K. L. Lapane et al., "Comorbidity and drug use in cognitively impaired elderly living in long-term care," *Dementia and Geriatric Cognitive Disorders*, vol. 9, no. 6, pp. 347–356, 1998.

[13] L. P. Fried, N. O. Borhani, P. Enright et al., "The cardiovascular Health Study: design and rationale," *Annals of Epidemiology*, vol. 1, no. 3, pp. 263–276, 1991.

[14] O. L. Lopez, L. Kuller, A. L. Fitzpatrick, D. Ives, J. T. Becker, and N. Beauchamp, "Evaluation of dementia in the Cardiovascular Health Cognition Study," *Neuroepidemiology*, vol. 22, no. 1, pp. 1–12, 2003.

[15] M. F. Folstein, S. E. Folstein, and P. R. McHugh, "Mini-mental state: a practical method for grading the cognitive state of patients for the clinician," *Journal of Psychiatric Research* , vol. 12, pp. 189–198, 1975.

[16] D. Wechsler, *WAIS-R Manual*, Psychological Corporation, New York, NY, USA, 1981.

[17] A. F. Jorm and P. A. Jacomb, "The informant questionnaire on cognitive decline in the elderly (IQCODE): socio-demographic correlates, reliability, validity and some norms," *Psychological Medicine*, vol. 19, no. 4, pp. 1015–1022, 1989.

[18] C. Kawas, J. Segal, W. F. Stewart, M. Corrada, and L. J. Thal, "A validation study of the dementia questionnaire," *Archives of Neurology*, vol. 51, no. 9, pp. 901–906, 1994.

[19] A. L. Fitzpatrick, L. H. Kuller, D. G. Ives et al., "Incidence and prevalence of dementia in the Cardiovascular Health Study," *Journal of the American Geriatrics Society*, vol. 52, no. 2, pp. 195–204, 2004.

[20] B. M. Psaty, L. H. Kuller, D. Bild et al., "Methods of assessing prevalent cardiovascular disease in the cardiovascular health study," *Annals of Epidemiology*, vol. 5, no. 4, pp. 270–277, 1995.

[21] B. M. Psaty, M. Lee, P. J. Savage et al., "Assessing the use of medications in the elderly: methods and initial experience in the cardiovascular health study," *Journal of Clinical Epidemiology*, vol. 45, no. 6, pp. 683–692, 1992.

[22] C. V. Pollack Jr. and W. B. Gibler, "2000 ACC/AHA guidelines for the management of patients with unstable angina and non-ST-segment elevation myocardial infarction: a practical summary for emergency physicians," *Annals of Emergency Medicine*, vol. 38, no. 3, pp. 229–240, 2001.

[23] J. Smith S.C., S. N. Blair, R. O. Bonow et al., "AHA/ACC guidelines for preventing heart attack and death in patients with atherosclerotic cardiovascular disease: 2001 update: a statement for healthcare professionals from the american heart association and the american college of cardiology," *Circulation*, vol. 104, no. 13, pp. 1577–1579, 2001.

[24] T. J. Ryan, J. L. Anderson, E. M. Antman et al., "ACC/AHA guidelines for the management of patients with acute myocardial infarction. A report of the American College of Cardiology/American Heart Association Task Force on Practice Guidelines (Committee on Management of Acute Myocardial Infarction)," *Journal of the American College of Cardiology*, vol. 28, no. 5, pp. 1328–1428, 1996.

[25] S. A. Hunt, W. T. Abraham, M. H. Chin et al., "ACC/AHA guidelines for the diagnosis and management of chronic heart failure in the adult: a report of the American College of Cardiology/American Heart Association Task Force on Practice Guidelines (Committee on the Evaluation and Management of Heart Failure)," *Journal of the American College of Cardiology*, vol. 46, pp. 1116–1143, 2005.

[26] M. Boustani, B. Peterson, L. Hanson, R. Harris, and K. N. Lohr, "Screening for dementia in primary care: a summary of the evidence for the U.S. preventive services task force," *Annals of Internal Medicine*, vol. 138, no. 11, pp. 927–I60, 2003.

[27] C. M. Callahan, H. C. Hendrie, and W. M. Tierney, "Documentation and evaluation of cognitive impairment in elderly primary care patients," *Annals of Internal Medicine*, vol. 122, no. 6, pp. 422–429, 1995.

[28] N. Campbell, M. Boustani, E. N. Skopelja et al., "Medication adherence in older adults with cognitive impairment: a systematic evidence-based review," *American Journal of Geriatric Pharmacotherapy*, vol. 10, no. 3, p. 165177, 2012.

[29] J. A. Rhymes, L. B. McCullough, R. J. Luchi, T. A. Teasdale, and N. Wilson, "Withdrawing very low-burden interventions in chronically ill patients," *The Journal of the American Medical Association*, vol. 283, no. 8, pp. 1061–1063, 2000.

[30] N. Li, A. Lee, R. A. Whitmer et al., "Use of angiotensin receptor blockers and risk of dementia in a predominantly male population: prospective cohort analysis," *British Medical Journal*, vol. 340, Article ID b5465, 2010.

[31] C. T. Thorpe, J. M. Thorpe, A. J. Kind, C. M. Bartels, C. M. Everett, and M. A. Smith, "Receipt of monitoring of diabetes mellitus in older adults with comorbid dementia," *Journal of the American Geriatrics Society*, vol. 60, no. 4, pp. 644–651, 2012.

[32] R. A. Morrison and L. A. Siu, "A comparison of pain and its treatment in advanced dementia and cognitively intact patients with hip fracture," *Journal of Pain and Symptom Management*, vol. 19, no. 4, pp. 240–248, 2000.

3

Systemic Vascular Function Is Associated with Muscular Power in Older Adults

Kevin S. Heffernan,[1] Angela Chalé,[2] Cynthia Hau,[2] Gregory J. Cloutier,[2] Edward M. Phillips,[2] Patrick Warner,[3] Heather Nickerson,[3] Kieran F. Reid,[2] Jeffrey T. Kuvin,[3] and Roger A. Fielding[2]

[1] *Human Performance Laboratory, Department of Exercise Science, Syracuse University, Syracuse, NY 13244, USA*
[2] *Nutrition, Exercise Physiology and Sarcopenia Laboratory, Jean Mayer USDA Human Nutrition Research Center on Aging at Tufts University, Boston, MA 02111, USA*
[3] *The Vascular Function Study Group, Division of Cardiology and the Molecular Cardiology Research Institute, Tufts Medical Center, Boston, MA 02111, USA*

Correspondence should be addressed to Kevin S. Heffernan, ksheffer@syr.edu

Academic Editor: Karl Rosengren

Age-associated loss of muscular strength and muscular power is a critical determinant of loss of physical function and progression to disability in older adults. In this study, we examined the association of systemic vascular function and measures of muscle strength and power in older adults. Measures of vascular endothelial function included brachial artery flow-mediated dilation (FMD) and the pulse wave amplitude reactive hyperemia index (PWA-RHI). Augmentation index (AIx) was taken as a measure of systemic vascular function related to arterial stiffness and wave reflection. Measures of muscular strength included one repetition maximum (1RM) for a bilateral leg press. Peak muscular power was measured during 5 repetitions performed as fast as possible for bilateral leg press at 40% 1RM. Muscular power was associated with brachial FMD ($r = 0.43$, $P < 0.05$), PWA-RHI ($r = 0.42$, $P < 0.05$), and AIx ($r = -0.54$, $P < 0.05$). Muscular strength was not associated with any measure of vascular function. In conclusion, systemic vascular function is associated with lower-limb muscular power but not muscular strength in older adults. Whether loss of muscular power with aging contributes to systemic vascular deconditioning or vascular dysfunction contributes to decrements in muscular power remains to be determined.

1. Introduction

As life expectancy in the United States continues to rise, the maintenance of physical independence of older adults has also emerged as a major clinical and public health priority. A critical factor in an older person's ability to function independently is the ability to move without assistance. Older adults who lose mobility are less likely to remain in the community, have higher rates of mortality, and experience a poorer quality of life [1, 2]. Age-associated loss of muscular strength (the ability to generate maximal muscle force) and muscular power (the product of the force and velocity of muscle contraction) is an important determinant of this loss of physical function and progression to disability [3]. Interestingly, although muscular strength and power are associated, muscular power has been shown to be a stronger predictor of physical function than muscular strength in older adults [4, 5]. Poor muscular power is associated with a 3-fold greater risk for mobility impairment than poor muscle strength [6] and improving muscular power leads to improvements in physical function independent of changes in muscular strength [7].

Although numerous potential mechanisms have been put forth, no single common etiology is believed to be responsible for age-associated loss of muscular strength/power and progression to disability. In many cases, physical disability is directly caused or aggravated by cardiovascular disease (CVD) or chronic CVD-related conditions (heart failure, coronary heart disease, and diabetes) [8–10]. Vascular senescence is a phenotypic expression of human aging that contributes to increased CVD risk [11, 12]. With advancing age, there is pervasive macrovascular and microvascular dysfunction that manifests as stiffening of central elastic arteries, elevation of pressure from wave reflections, and peripheral endothelial dysfunction [11, 12]. An ever-growing literature now supports the notion that vascular function may affect physical function.

Several cross-sectional associations between metrics of vascular function and metrics of functional reserve have been noted [13–16]. Nitric oxide (NO) is a potent vasoactive metabolite released by endothelial cells that helps regulate vascular tonus. Age-associated reduction in NO contributes importantly to the development of endothelial dysfunction and vasomotor dysfunction [17]. This may affect physical function by reducing blood flow into the active capillary bed and curtailing efficient nutrient transport (e.g., oxygen, lactate, pyruvate) [18]. To date, most studies that have explored associations between vascular function and physical function have examined activities that are more aerobic in nature (long distance gait performance, exercise capacity/endurance, etc.). Few studies have explored the association between vascular function and measures of physical function that are of anaerobic origin. Separate from its effects on blood flow and tissue perfusion, NO also plays a crucial role in maintaining optimal skeletal muscle contractile function in vitro. NO enhances velocity of muscle fiber shortening, reduces twitch time-to-peak contraction, and increases rate of force development via modulation of mechanical and metabolic muscle fiber machinery [19]. Conversely, inhibition of NO significantly reduces skeletal muscle maximal force generating capacity and increases muscular fatigue [20]. Thus loss of NO bioavailability may impact skeletal muscle function (force and velocity), manifesting as reductions in muscular power and strength in vivo although this has yet to be explored.

The purpose of this study was to test the hypothesis that NO-mediated vascular reactivity (brachial artery flow-mediated dilation and digital pulse wave amplitude reactive hyperemia index) and systemic vascular function related to arterial stiffness/wave reflections (appraised via the augmentation index) is associated with muscular strength and muscular power in older adults with mobility limitations.

2. Methods

Twenty-four men and women ($n = 13$) between the ages of 70 and 85 years with mobility limitations were recruited from the greater Boston community to participate in this study. Individuals "at risk for mobility disability" were defined as scoring ≤10 on the Short Physical Performance Battery as previously described [21] and discussed below. Exclusion criteria were as follows: acute or terminal illness, myocardial infarction in the previous 6 months or other symptomatic coronary artery disease, upper or lower extremity fracture in the previous 6 months, uncontrolled hypertension (>150/90 mmHg), neuromuscular diseases and drugs which affect neuromuscular function, hormone replacement therapy, type 2 diabetes mellitus, renal disease (eGFR <60 mL/min/1.73 m^2), and body mass index (kg/m^2) <21 or >32.5. All participants gave written informed consent and this study was approved by the Tufts University Health Sciences Campus Institutional Review Board.

3. Study Design

All hemodynamic and vascular measures were carried out in the early morning with the participant in a fasted state (>12 postprandial). Participants on medication with known vasoactive properties were instructed to refrain from taking these medication(s) for 5 times the half-life of the agent (calculated individually per medication). Participants were required to rest quietly in a supine position for a minimum of 15 minutes in a dimly lit, climate control room prior to all measures. Blood pressure was measured in triplicate. This was followed by assessment of vascular function with ultrasound and concurrent measures of PAT. On a separate day prior to vascular assessment (within 3 days) physical mobility was assessed using the SPPB. Muscular strength and muscular power were determined using a pneumatic leg press machine. Finally, physical activity was assessed from 7-day accelerometry recordings.

3.1. Blood Pressure. Blood pressure was measured using a validated automated device (Dynamap, GE Healthcare, USA). Pulse pressure was calculated as systolic blood pressure (SBP)-diastolic blood pressure (DBP). Mean arterial pressure (MAP) was calculated as 1/3 SBP × 2/3 DBP. Following measurement of blood pressure, measures of vascular endothelial function were carried out.

3.2. Flow-Mediated Dilation. The brachial artery was longitudinally imaged 2 cm above the antecubital fossa using a 10 mHz linear array vascular ultrasound transducer and portable ultrasound unit (SonoSite Titan, Bothell, WA,USA) as previously validated by our group [22]. Diameters were measured during end diastole (gated with ECG R-waves) using ultrasonic calipers (the average of 5 evenly spaced measures along the lumen border) at baseline and 60 seconds after release of a blood pressure cuff around the upper arm (inflated to 200 mmHg for 5 minutes). Responses were calculated as percentage change in brachial artery diameter from baseline (flow mediated dilation, FMD). Mean intraobserver and interobserver variability of brachial reactivity measurements in our laboratory on normal volunteers were previously shown to be 1.9% and 2.8%, respectively [23]. Heart rate was computed from the aforementioned ECG recordings.

3.3. Reactive Hyperemia Index and Augmentation Index. Specially designed finger pneumatic sensors (EndoPAT, Itamar Medical Ltd, Israel) were used to continuously record pulsatile volume changes (measured as pulse wave amplitude) in the finger as previously validated by our group [24]. This was done before and during reactive hyperemia induced by brachial artery circulatory occlusion for 5 minutes as described previously. The pulse wave amplitude (PWA) reactive hyperemia index (RHI) is calculated as the ratio of the average PWA over a 1-minute epoch starting 60 seconds after 5 min of ischemia induced by brachial cuff inflation to a suprasystolic BP, divided by the average PWA of a 3.5-minute baseline epoch. A finger probe is also placed on the contralateral hand in order to capture any systemic changes that might occur during local reactive hyperemia. The signal is amplified, filtered, and stored in a computer for analysis. Diminution of PWA-RHI is suggestive of resistance vessel endothelial dysfunction.

From the digital pulse volume waveforms, peak volume and inflection points were identified using a 4th-order derivative computerized algorithm as previously described by Kelly et al. [25] and Takazawa et al. [26]. AIx was calculated as the ratio of the difference between the early and late systolic peaks of the waveform relative to the early peak expressed as a percentage. Previous studies have noted that the association of AIx derived from PAT and AIx derived from synthesized aortic pressure waves is comparable [27, 28]. Reproducibility of these techniques has previously been shown to be moderately high (ICC 0.5–0.8 with between day variability of approximately 11%) [29–31].

3.4. Physical Function. Participants completed the short physical performance battery (SPPB) which consists of the following tasks: timed short distance walk, repeated chair stands, and a balance test. Walking speed was assessed by asking the participants to walk at their usual pace over a 4 m course. Two trials were conducted and the faster of 2 used for subsequent analyses. The repeated chair stands test was performed by asking participants to first stand from a sitting position without using their arms. If they were able to perform the task, they were then asked to stand up and sit down 5 times, as quickly as possible. The time to complete the task was recorded. For the test of standing balance, participants were asked to maintain balance in 3 positions, characterized by a progressive narrowing of the base support: feet together (side by side position), the heel of one foot beside the big toe of the other foot (semi tandem position), and the heel of one foot in front of and touching the toes of the other foot (tandem position). For each of the 3 positions, participants were timed to a maximum of 10 sec. Each of the 3 performance measures was assigned a score ranging from 0 to 4, with 4 indicating the highest level of performance and 0 the inability to complete the test. A summary score ranging from 0 (worst performers) to 12 (best performers) was calculated by adding walking speed, chair stands, and balance scores. This scale has proven reliable [32] and valid for predicting institutionalization, hospital admission, mortality, and disability [33].

3.5. Muscular Strength and Power. One repetition maximum (1RM, greatest load that could be moved one time through the full range of motion using proper technique) was determined for a bilateral leg press using a pneumatic machine (K400, Keiser Sports Health Equipment Inc, Fresno, CA), designed to provide variable resistance via utilization of attached cylinders pressurized with air (i.e., compression of gas within affixed cylinder produces resistance). Range of motion was established by having the participant fully extend the dominant limb against minimal resistance. This position was recorded in real time. 1RM attempts were considered successful if the participant reached 90% of the established criterion limb position. Resistance was increased after each trial unless the participant failed to achieve 90% of maximal limb position, in which case the resistance was reduced by half of the previous increment. Testing continued until the participant failed two consecutive trials at a given level of resistance. Each trial was followed by 1 min of rest. Testing was carried out twice, separated by one week. The 1 RM was established as the best value from the two trials due to the well-established learning effect of this measure and this was typically attained within 6–8 trials. For the assessment of muscular power, all participants performed 5 repetitions as fast as possible for bilateral leg press at 40% 1RM. Five maximal effort trials were performed, with at least 30 s of rest between each trial. Software developed by the manufacturer calculates power during the concentric phase of each repetition by analyzing system pressure (force) and leg press platform displacement at a sampling frequency of 400 samples/second. The highest power output achieved during each of these 5 repetitions (data collected between 5% and 95% of the concentric phase in order to minimize signal noise) was taken as peak power/velocity. The reliability of these measurements in older subjects in our group is high (leg press ICC = 0.95) [34].

3.6. Physical Activity. Accelerometry allows objective measurement of physical activity by the use of a motion sensor which records both the number and magnitude of vertical accelerations generated by human movement and was performed using the Actigraph Model 7164 (Manufacturing Technology Inc., FL, USA). The Actigraph was worn superior to the iliac crest in a custom pouch, secured to the participant's belt by a Velcro fastening. Participants were instructed to wear the Actigraph for a 7-day period during waking hours and remove it for sleep and bathing only (confirmed with activity logs). Activity was recorded using 1 min epochs and a valid day of measurement was defined as >10 h of wear with <1 h of no accelerometer data (i.e., continuous zeros). Total daily movement counts were calculated by summing the minute-by-minute counts across each 24 h epoch and then averaging across valid days of measurement. Using this criterion, 4 participants did not have complete 7-day physical activity measures. All participants had 6 valid days of activity data; therefore daily activity was derived from 6 days.

3.7. Statistical Analysis. Normality of distribution was verified using Kolmogorov-Smirnov and Shapiro-Wilk tests. All data are reported as means ± standard error of the mean. A priori significance was set at $P < 0.05$. Pearson correlation coefficients were used to assess relationships between measures of physical function (1RM, peak power at 40% 1RM, physical activity counts, and SPPB score) and measures of vascular function (brachial FMD, PWA-RHI, and AIx). Given the potential confounding influence of sex,

BMI, mean arterial pressure, and heart rate on measures of muscular strength/power and vascular function, partial correlations were used to examine associations between measures of physical function and vascular function after adjusting for these potential confounders.

4. Results

Participant descriptive characteristics are presented in Table 1. Muscular strength and power were significantly higher in men versus women ($P < 0.05$). Groups did not differ in age, CVD risk factors or medication use. As seen in Table 2 and displayed in Figure 1, muscular power was associated with brachial FMD ($P < 0.05$), PWA-RHI ($P < 0.05$), and AIx ($P < 0.05$). Muscular strength was not associated with these parameters. After adjusting for sex, BMI, MAP, and HR, associations between measures of muscular power and vascular function remained (Table 3, $P < 0.05$). Associations between muscular power and FMD ($r = 0.59$, $P < 0.05$), PWA-RHI (0.58, $P < 0.05$), and AIx (−0.42, $P < 0.05$) remained after adjusting separately for strength.

5. Discussion

Muscle power has emerged as a critical determinant of impairment in older adults, independent of muscular strength. As such understanding factors that potentially limit muscle power and subsequently functional reserve in older adults have received considerable attention [35]. Vascular dysfunction with aging is associated with decreases in physical function and performance of activities of daily living [13, 36] alluding to the notion that the genesis and demise of muscular power may in part have a vascular basis. The novel findings from the present investigation were as follows. Our hypothesis was partially supported in that vascular endothelial function (appraised using two distinct techniques) and AIx were each associated with lower-limb muscular power in older adults. Contrary to our hypothesis, vascular function was not associated with lower-limb muscle strength.

To date, most studies that have explored associations between vascular function and physical function have examined activities that are more aerobic in nature (long distance gait performance, exercise capacity/endurance, etc.). With aging and disease, limitations in oxygen delivery may limit contractile work and age-associated impairment in endothelial-dependent vasodilation contributes to lower exercise hyperemia [37, 38]. During exercise, vasodilation occurs via an increase in several vasoactive agents including but not limited to nitric oxide (NO) [39, 40]. Resultant increases in blood flow ensure that oxygen delivery is closely matched to metabolic demand. Endothelium-dependent vasodilation increases circulatory time in the capillaries and allows for more effective oxygen and nutrient extraction in the tissues [41]. NO synthase inhibition reduces exercise blood flow to active skeletal muscle [40] and with aging the relative contribution of NO to exercise hyperemia is reduced by approximately 45% [37]. A reduction in flow to working skeletal muscle (i.e., reduced perfusion) may ultimately limit the ability to perform functional tasks. Indeed with aging there is a generalized reduction in limb blood flow and vascular conductance both at rest [42] and during exercise contributing to reduced exercise capacity [43, 44].

Recently, we and others have reported associations between vascular function and more anaerobic processes (i.e., muscular strength) [45, 46] and studies are emerging noting associations between measures of vascular function and skeletal muscle morphology and muscle fiber type in middle-aged [47] older adults [48, 49]. Endothelial-dependent (predominantly nitric oxide mediated) vasodilation of peripheral conduit vessels can be assessed in vivo by examining the change in brachial artery diameter in response to an increase in shear stress induced by regional occlusion (flow mediated dilation, FMD) [50, 51] whilst endothelial-dependent (predominantly nitric oxide mediated) vasodilation of peripheral resistance vessels can be quantified similarly by examining the change in digital pulse wave amplitude during reactive hyperemia (peripheral arterial tonometry reactive hyperemia index, PAT-RHI) [52]. Moreover, augmentation index (a measure of systemic vascular function related to arterial stiffness and pressure from wave reflections) can also be influenced substantially by NO [53]. Using these techniques, our findings extend previous observations and note that vascular function is also a correlate of muscle power in older adults.

Although the exact mechanism explaining preferential associations between vascular function and muscular power versus strength is not completely understood, we suggest that it may be related to loss of NO bioavailability. Age-associated loss of muscular power progresses at a faster rate then declines in muscular strength [54]. Selective loss of fast-twitch/type II fibers with aging may partially explain this observation as type II fibers have a peak power output 4 times that of type I fibers [55]. Of interest, NO has been shown to play a crucial role in satellite cell activation and subsequent hypertrophy of fast twitch fibers [56] and prevents muscle wasting in response to cachectic stimuli [57]. With aging, there appears to be redistribution of muscle blood flow during exercise from highly oxidative to highly glycolytic muscles and this is a nitric-oxide-mediated/endothelium-dependent process [58–60]. NO has been shown to play a pivotal role this phenotypic "slow-to-fast shift" [19]. Greater flow to fast-twitch glycolytic fibers may be a compensatory adaptation aimed at preserving contractile function concomitant with reduced fiber volume. Indeed recent studies note that, despite age-associated changes in muscle mass, single-fiber contractile properties of type II fibers are preserved [61, 62].

Type I oxidative fibers have severalfold greater blood flow than type II glycolytic fibers and NO inhibition drastically blunts blood flow to oxidative fibers [63, 64]. Thus flow to oxidative fibers also appears to be under endothelial control [60]. Although peak power development of type II fibers may not change with aging, peak power of type I fibers decreases [61]. NO has been shown to optimize shortening velocity of slower fibers without influencing faster fibers [65]. This is important as velocity (in addition to force) is a significant determinant of muscle power in older adults in vivo [35].

Table 1: Participant characteristics ($n = 24$).

Variable	All	Women ($n = 13$)	Men ($n = 11$)
Age, yrs	78 ± 1	77 ± 1	80 ± 1
Body mass index, kg/m^2	26 ± 1	26 ± 1	26 ± 1
Systolic blood pressure, mmHg	130 ± 3	130 ± 4	130 ± 4
Diastolic blood pressure, mmHg	74 ± 1	74 ± 3	75 ± 3
Mean arterial pressure, mmHg	93 ± 2	94 ± 2	93 ± 2
Heart rate, bpm	62 ± 2	63 ± 3	61 ± 2
Total cholesterol, mg/dL	177 ± 6	184 ± 8	163 ± 10
LDL cholesterol, mg/dL	105 ± 4	109 ± 6	100 ± 8
HDL cholesterol, mg/dL	54 ± 3	58 ± 3	46 ± 4*
Triglycerides, mg/dL	96 ± 9	107 ± 16	84 ± 5
Glucose, mg/dL	93 ± 2	94 ± 3	92 ± 3
White blood cell count	5.0 ± 0.3	5.2 ± 0.4	4.9 ± 0.3
Neutrophil/lymphocyte ratio	1.9 ± 0.1	1.8 ± 0.2	2.0 ± 0.2
Hyperlipidemia, %	33	31	36
Hypertension, %	50	38	62
Medications, %			
Aspirin	33	31	36
ACE inhibitor	26	15	36
Beta-blocker	25	18	31
Calcium channel blocker	17	8	27
Diuretic	25	23	27
Statin	33	31	36
Leg press 1 RM	1237 ± 77	1040 ± 76	1470 ± 107*
Leg press peak power 40% 1 RM	417 ± 30	351 ± 33	491 ± 46*
SPPB, score	8.5 ± 0.5	8.3 ± 0.4	8.9 ± 0.3
Physical activity, counts	93224 ± 14465	103072 ± 22766	81586 ± 17023
Brachial FMD, %	7.5 ± 0.8	8.8 ± 1.0	7.1 ± 1.0
PWA-RHI, %	2.1 ± 0.2	2.3 ± 0.1	1.8 ± 0.3
AIx, %	40 ± 3	46 ± 3	35 ± 3*

*Significant group difference, $P < 0.05$.

Table 2: Correlation matrix for measures of vascular function and muscle function.

	40% 1 RM	1 RM	SPPB	PA count	FMD	RHI
1 RM	0.69†					
SPPB	0.59†	0.47†				
PA Count	0.10	0.13	0.35†			
FMD	0.43†	0.11	0.37†	0.35†		
RHI	0.42†	0.08	0.13	0.11	0.27	
AIx	−0.54†	−0.32	−0.29	−0.12	−0.31	−0.28

†$P < 0.05$.

Table 3: Correlation matrix for measures of vascular function and muscle function adjusted for potential confounders*.

	40% 1 RM	1 RM	SPPB	PA count	FMD	RHI
1 RM	0.51†					
SPPB	0.58†	0.41†				
PA Count	0.38†	0.26	0.48†			
FMD	0.61†	0.16	0.38†	0.42†		
RHI	0.54†	0.12	0.11	0.11	0.34	
AIx	−0.43†	−0.29	−0.24	−0.08	−0.31	−0.32

*Sex, BMI, MAP, and HR adjusted.
†$P < 0.05$.

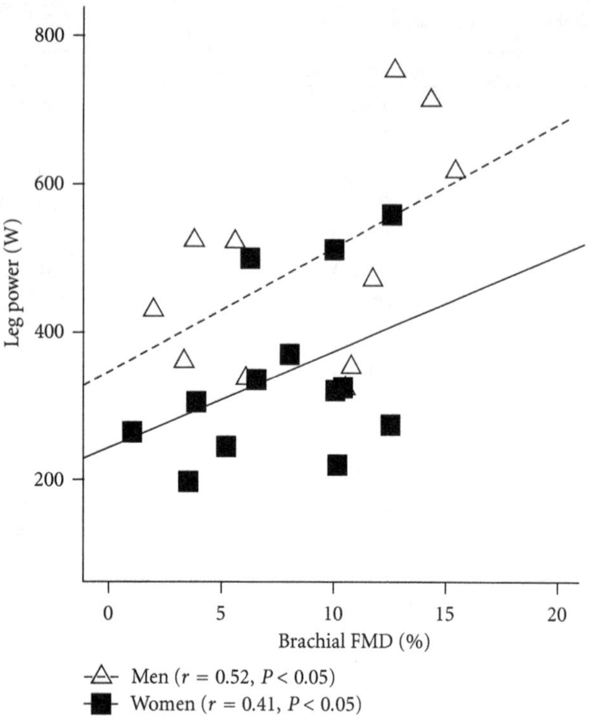

(a)

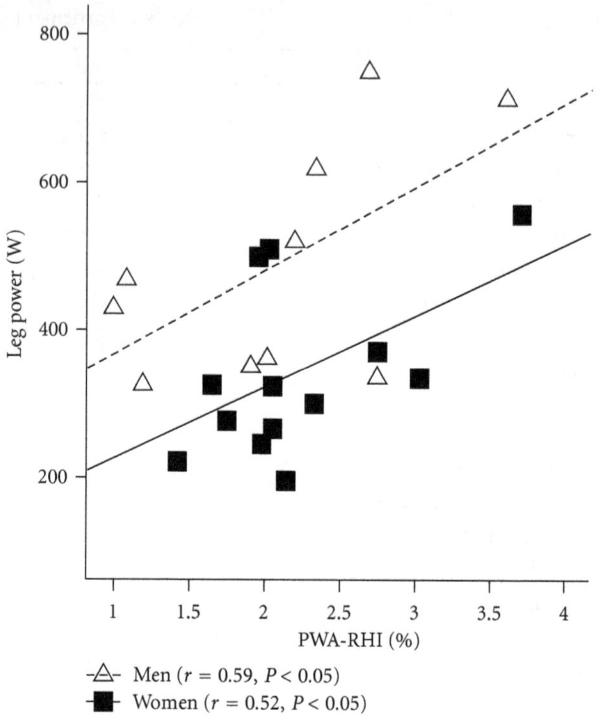

(b)

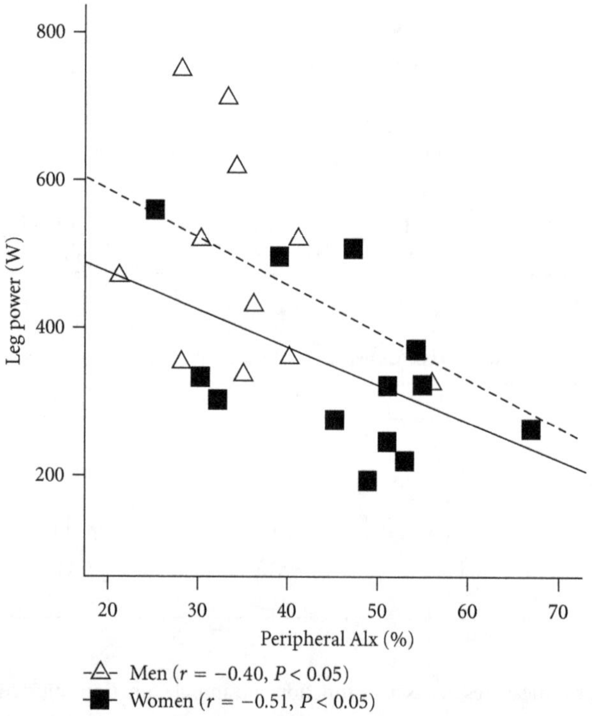

(c)

Figure 1: Association between leg power (assessed as 5 repetitions performed as fast as possible at 40% 1RM) and (a) brachial artery flow-mediated dilation (FMD); (b) pulse wave amplitude-reactive hyperemia index (PWA-RHI); (c) peripheral augmentation index (AIx). Open triangles with dashed line (men); closed squares with solid line (women).

With aging, there is increased oxidative stress which reduces NO bioavailability resulting in formation of peroxynitrite in vascular and skeletal muscle [66, 67]. Peroxynitrite has been shown to decrease contractile force in slow-twitch fibers with little effect on fast-twitch muscle fibers [68]. It is important to note that the size principle still prevails during maximal contractions. Thus initial recruitment of and perfusion to these type I fibers is an important component of the overall genesis of muscular power. NO has also been implicated in numerous aspects of excitation contraction uncoupling with aging (reduced sarcoplasmic reticulum calcium-ATPase activity, reduced ryanodine receptor-mediated calcium release, reduced calcium sensitivity) [67, 69, 70]. Endothelial dysfunction and loss of NO bioavailability may drastically reduce perfusion to type I fibers and directly impact fiber contractile characteristics of type II fibers, reducing overall force generating capacity and peak power development [19]. Taken together these findings suggest that NO is needed to maintain optimal contractile function (notably velocity) of both slow-twitch and fast-twitch fibers and this may explain preferential associations between NO-mediated measures of vascular reactivity and muscular power in vivo.

There is a bidirectional relationship between pressure from wave reflections (AIx) and NO bioavailability. Each cardiac contraction generates an outgoing pressure wave that traverses the systemic vasculature. Encountering areas of impedance both structural (i.e., bifurcations) and function (i.e., vasoconstricted vessel), these pressure waves are reflected back toward their origin. AIx assessed in the digital circulation is influenced by wave reflections originating in the hand microvasculature as well as the lower body [71]. NO blockade has been shown to increase AIx likely via altering vascular tone which may alter timing and magnitude of reflected pressure waves [53]. Pressure from peripheral wave reflections augment central pressure but subtract from flow. This reduces antegrade flow into the active vascular bed and increases retrograde flow in upstream conduit vessels which causes endothelial dysfunction and loss of NO bioavailability [72, 73]. Indeed retrograde flow increases with age and is associated with reduced physical function [36].

Given the cross-sectional nature of this study, direct causality cannot be determined, only inferred. Thus alternative interpretations should be considered. Mobility limitations perpetuate a sedentary lifestyle. This is important as physical inactivity is a CVD risk factor and a potent instigator of vascular maladaptation [74, 75]. Within 4-5 days of inactivity induced by bed rest there are reductions in limb blood flow [76] and signs of endothelial dysfunction [77]. As little as 2 weeks of limb immobilization has been shown to increase arterial stiffness [78]. Thus immobility in the elderly may perpetuate inactivity and reduce muscle power further promulgating a state of "extreme" vascular deconditioning.

A limitation to this study is the relatively small sample (i.e., examination of several correlations may increase chances of a type II statistical error). However, the observation that three *independent* measures of vascular function were each associated with muscular power lends support to the objectivity of overall findings. Although vascular measures have overlapping physiologic underpinnings, the direct association between techniques is nonexistent to weak at best [71, 79, 80]. Indeed recent large-scale studies note that each measure is associated with different measures of vascular risk and endothelial biology [81–83] suggesting that each provides slightly different insight into vascular physiology in vivo.

In conclusion, vascular function is associated with muscular power in older adults. This association remains after adjusting for important confounders such as sex, BMI, and muscular strength. Future research is needed to examine if improving vascular function and/or preserving NO bioavailability leads to concomitant improvements in muscular power and prevention of physical impairment in older adults.

Acknowledgments

This study was supported by funding from the American College of Sports Medicine Research Endowment Grant (to K. S. Heffernan) and the National Dairy Council (to R. A. Fielding). This research was also supported by the National Institute on Aging (AG-18844 to R. A. Fielding) and the Boston Claude D. Pepper Older Americans Independence Center (1P30AG031679). This material is based upon work supported by the US Department of Agriculture, under Agreement no. 58-1950-7-707.

References

[1] M. Hirvensalo, T. Rantanen, and E. Heikkinen, "Mobility difficulties and physical activity as predictors of mortality and loss of independence in the community-living older population," *Journal of the American Geriatrics Society*, vol. 48, no. 5, pp. 493–498, 2000.

[2] J. M. Guralnik, A. Z. LaCroix, L. G. Branch, S. V. Kasl, and R. B. Wallace, "Morbidity and disability in older persons in the years prior to death," *American Journal of Public Health*, vol. 81, no. 4, pp. 443–447, 1991.

[3] K. F. Reid and R. A. Fielding, "Skeletal muscle power: a critical determinant of physical functioning in older adults," *Exercise and Sport Sciences Reviews*, vol. 40, no. 1, pp. 4–12, 2012.

[4] D. A. Skelton, J. Kennedy, and O. M. Rutherford, "Explosive power and asymmetry in leg muscle function in frequent fallers and non-fallers aged over 65," *Age and Ageing*, vol. 31, no. 2, pp. 119–125, 2002.

[5] J. F. Bean, D. K. Kiely, S. Herman et al., "The relationship between leg power and physical performance in mobility-limited older people," *Journal of the American Geriatrics Society*, vol. 50, no. 3, pp. 461–467, 2002.

[6] J. F. Bean, S. G. Leveille, D. K. Kiely, S. Bandinelli, J. M. Guralnik, and L. Ferrucci, "A comparison of leg power and leg strength within the inCHIANTI study: which influences mobility more?" *Journals of Gerontology*, vol. 58, no. 8, pp. 728–733, 2003.

[7] J. F. Bean, D. K. Kiely, S. Larose, R. Goldstein, W. R. Frontera, and S. G. Leveille, "Are changes in leg power responsible for clinically meaningful improvements in mobility in older adults?" *Journal of the American Geriatrics Society*, vol. 58, no. 12, pp. 2363–2368, 2010.

[8] L. Ferrucci, J. M. Guralnik, M. Pahor, M. C. Corti, and R. J. Havlik, "Hospital diagnoses, Medicare charges, and nursing

home admissions in the year when older persons become severely disabled," *Journal of the American Medical Association*, vol. 277, no. 9, pp. 728–734, 1997.

[9] L. P. Fried, W. H. Ettinger, B. Lind, A. B. Newman, and J. Gardin, "Physical disability in older adults: a physiological approach. Cardiovascular Health Study Research Group," *Journal of Clinical Epidemiology*, vol. 47, no. 7, pp. 747–760, 1994.

[10] L. P. Fried and J. M. Guralnik, "Disability in older adults: evidence regarding significance, etiology, and risk," *Journal of the American Geriatrics Society*, vol. 45, no. 1, pp. 92–100, 1997.

[11] E. G. Lakatta and D. Levy, "Arterial and cardiac aging: major shareholders in cardiovascular disease enterprises: Part I: aging arteries: a "set up" for vascular disease," *Circulation*, vol. 107, no. 1, pp. 139–146, 2003.

[12] S. S. Najjar, A. Scuteri, and E. G. Lakatta, "Arterial aging: is it an immutable cardiovascular risk factor?" *Hypertension*, vol. 46, no. 3, pp. 454–462, 2005.

[13] M. A. Welsch, D. A. Dobrosielski, A. A. Arce-Esquivel et al., "The association between flow-mediated dilation and physical function in older men," *Medicine and Science in Sports and Exercise*, vol. 40, no. 7, pp. 1237–1243, 2008.

[14] A. R. Patel, J. T. Kuvin, D. DeNofrio et al., "Peripheral vascular endothelial function correlates with exercise capacity in cardiac transplant recipients," *American Journal of Cardiology*, vol. 91, no. 7, pp. 897–899, 2003.

[15] A. R. Patel, J. T. Kuvin, K. A. Sliney, W. M. Rand, N. G. Pandian, and R. H. Karas, "Peripheral vascular endothelial function correlates with exercise capacity in women," *Clinical Cardiology*, vol. 28, no. 9, pp. 433–436, 2005.

[16] K. S. Heffernan, R. H. Karas, E. A. Patvardhan, and J. T. Kuvin, "Endothelium-dependent vasodilation is associated with exercise capacity in smokers and non-smokers," *Vascular Medicine*, vol. 15, no. 2, pp. 119–125, 2010.

[17] J. E. Deanfield, J. P. Halcox, and T. J. Rabelink, "Endothelial function and dysfunction: testing and clinical relevance," *Circulation*, vol. 115, no. 10, pp. 1285–1295, 2007.

[18] D. N. Proctor and B. A. Parker, "Vasodilation and vascular control in contracting muscle of the aging human," *Microcirculation*, vol. 13, no. 4, pp. 315–337, 2006.

[19] G. Maréchal and P. Gailly, "Effects of nitric oxide on the contraction of skeletal muscle," *Cellular and Molecular Life Sciences*, vol. 55, no. 8-9, pp. 1088–1102, 1999.

[20] M. Y. Ibrahim and O. M. Ashour, "Changes in nitric oxide and free radical levels in rat gastrocnemius muscle during contraction and fatigue," *Clinical and Experimental Pharmacology and Physiology*, vol. 38, no. 12, pp. 791–795, 2011.

[21] J. M. Guralnik, E. M. Simonsick, L. Ferrucci et al., "A short physical performance battery assessing lower extremity function: association with self-reported disability and prediction of mortality and nursing home admission," *Journals of Gerontology*, vol. 49, no. 2, pp. M85–M94, 1994.

[22] A. A. Alsheikh-Ali, H. Z. Ouda, N. Pandian, R. H. Karas, and J. T. Kuvin, "Evaluation of peripheral vascular endothelial function with a portable ultrasound device," *Echocardiography*, vol. 23, no. 8, pp. 623–626, 2006.

[23] J. T. Kuvin, A. R. Patel, K. A. Sliney et al., "Peripheral vascular endothelial function testing as a noninvasive indicator of coronary artery disease," *Journal of the American College of Cardiology*, vol. 38, no. 7, pp. 1843–1849, 2001.

[24] J. T. Kuvin, A. Mammen, P. Mooney, A. A. Alsheikh-Ali, and R. H. Karas, "Assessment of peripheral vascular endothelial function in the ambulatory setting," *Vascular Medicine*, vol. 12, no. 1, pp. 13–16, 2007.

[25] R. Kelly, C. Hayward, A. Avolio, and M. O'Rourke, "Nonivasive determination of age-related changes in the human arterial pulse," *Circulation*, vol. 80, no. 6, pp. 1652–1659, 1989.

[26] K. Takazawa, N. Tanaka, K. Takeda, F. Kurosu, and C. Ibukiyama, "Underestimation of vasodilator effects of nitroglycerin by upper limb blood pressure," *Hypertension*, vol. 26, no. 3, pp. 520–523, 1995.

[27] M. J. Haller, J. H. Silverstein, and J. J. Shuster, "Correlation between radial artery tonometry- and fingertip tonometry-derived augmentation index in children with type 1 diabetes," *Diabetes and Vascular Disease Research*, vol. 4, no. 1, p. 66, 2007.

[28] M. Dhindsa, J. N. Barnes, A. E. DeVan, J. Sugawara, and H. Tanaka, "Comparison of augmentation index derived from multiple devices," *Artery Research*, vol. 5, pp. 112–114, 2011.

[29] Y. Reisner, R. Lusky, Y. Shay-El, R. Schnall, and S. Herscovici, "Reproducibility of endothelial function and arterial stiffness assessed using finger peripheral arterial tonometry," *European Heart Journal*, vol. 28, supplement, p. 484, 2007.

[30] J. Liu, J. Wang, Y. Jin, H. J. Roethig, and M. Unverdorben, "Variability of peripheral arterial tonometry in the measurement of endothelial function in healthy men," *Clinical Cardiology*, vol. 32, no. 12, pp. 700–704, 2009.

[31] S. Onkelinx, V. Cornelissen, K. Goetschalckx, T. Thomaes, P. Verhamme, and L. Vanhees, "Reproducibility of different methods to measure the endothelial function," *Vascular Medicine*, vol. 17, no. 2, pp. 79–84, 2012.

[32] G. V. Ostir, S. Volpato, L. P. Fried, P. Chaves, and J. M. Guralnik, "Reliability and sensitivity to change assessed for a summary measure of lower body function: results from the Women's Health and Aging Study," *Journal of Clinical Epidemiology*, vol. 55, no. 9, pp. 916–921, 2002.

[33] J. M. Guralnik, L. Ferrucci, E. M. Simonsick, M. E. Salive, and R. B. Wallace, "Lower-extremity function in persons over the age of 70 years as a predictor of subsequent disability," *New England Journal of Medicine*, vol. 332, no. 9, pp. 556–561, 1995.

[34] R. J. Carabello, K. F. Reid, D. J. Clark, E. M. Phillips, and R. A. Fielding, "Lower extremity strength and power asymmetry assessment in healthy and mobility-limited populations: reliability and association with physical functioning," *Aging*, vol. 22, no. 4, pp. 324–329, 2010.

[35] R. M. Pojednic, D. J. Clark, C. Patten, K. Reid, E. M. Phillips, and R. A. Fielding, "The specific contributions of force and velocity to muscle power in older adults," *Experimental Gerontology*, vol. 47, no. 8, pp. 608–613, 2012.

[36] D. P. Credeur, M. A. Welsch, D. A. Dobrosielski, and A. A. Arce-Esquivel, "Brachial artery retrograde flow increases with age: relationship to physical function," *European Journal of Applied Physiology*, vol. 107, no. 2, pp. 219–225, 2009.

[37] W. G. Schrage, J. H. Eisenach, and M. J. Joyner, "Ageing reduces nitric-oxide- and prostaglandin-mediated vasodilatation in exercising humans," *Journal of Physiology*, vol. 579, no. 1, pp. 227–236, 2007.

[38] B. S. Kirby, W. F. Voyles, C. B. Simpson, R. E. Carlson, W. G. Schrage, and F. A. Dinenno, "Endothelium-dependent vasodilatation and exercise hyperaemia in ageing humans: impact of acute ascorbic acid administration," *Journal of Physiology*, vol. 587, no. 9, pp. 1989–2003, 2009.

[39] C. Goto, K. Nishioka, T. Umemura et al., "Acute moderate-intensity exercise induces vasodilation through an increase in nitric oxide bioavailiability in humans," *American Journal of Hypertension*, vol. 20, no. 8, pp. 825–830, 2007.

[40] D. M. Gilligan, J. A. Panza, C. M. Kilcoyne, M. A. Waclawiw, P. R. Casino, and A. A. Quyyumi, "Contribution of

endothelium-derived nitric oxide to exercise-induced vasodilation," *Circulation*, vol. 90, no. 6, pp. 2853–2858, 1994.

[41] D. L. Boveris and A. Boveris, "Oxygen delivery to the tissues and mitochondrial respiration," *Frontiers in Bioscience*, vol. 12, no. 3, pp. 1014–1023, 2007.

[42] F. A. Dinenno, D. R. Seals, C. A. Desouza, and H. Tanaka, "Age-related decreases in basal limb blood flow in humans: time course, determinants and habitual exercise effects," *Journal of Physiology*, vol. 531, no. 2, pp. 573–579, 2001.

[43] S. J. Ridout, B. A. Parker, S. L. Smithmyer, J. U. Gonzales, K. C. Beck, and D. N. Proctor, "Age and sex influence the balance between maximal cardiac output and peripheral vascular reserve," *Journal of Applied Physiology*, vol. 108, no. 3, pp. 483–489, 2010.

[44] A. J. Maxwell, E. Schauble, D. Bernstein, and J. P. Cooke, "Limb blood flow during exercise is dependent on nitric oxide," *Circulation*, vol. 98, no. 4, pp. 369–374, 1998.

[45] C. A. Fahs, K. S. Heffernan, S. Ranadive, S. Y. Jae, and B. Fernhall, "Muscular strength is inversely associated with aortic stiffness in young men," *Medicine and Science in Sports and Exercise*, vol. 42, no. 9, pp. 1619–1624, 2010.

[46] M. A. Alomari, E. F. Keewan, R. A. Shammaa, K. Alawneh, S. Y. Khatib, and M. A. Welsch, "Vascular function and handgrip strength in rheumatoid arthritis patients," *The Scientific World Journal*, vol. 2012, Article ID 580863, 2012.

[47] M. Ronnback, M. Hernelahti, E. Hamalainen, P. H. Groop, and H. Tikkanen, "Effect of physical activity and muscle morphology on endothelial function and arterial stiffness," *Scandinavian Journal of Medicine and Science in Sports*, vol. 17, no. 5, pp. 573–579, 2007.

[48] E. L. Dillon, S. L. Casperson, W. J. Durham et al., "Muscle protein metabolism responds similarly to exogenous amino acids in healthy younger and older adults during NO-induced hyperemia," *American Journal of Physiology*, vol. 301, no. 5, pp. R1408–R1417, 2011.

[49] M. Ochi, K. Kohara, Y. Tabara et al., "Arterial stiffness is associated with low thigh muscle mass in middle-aged to elderly men," *Atherosclerosis*, vol. 212, no. 1, pp. 327–332, 2010.

[50] J. Deanfield, A. Donald, C. Ferri et al., "Endothelial function and dysfunction. Part I: methodological issues for assessment in the different vascular beds: a statement by the working group on endothelin and endothelial factors of the European society of hypertension," *Journal of Hypertension*, vol. 23, no. 1, pp. 7–17, 2005.

[51] M. C. Corretti, T. J. Anderson, E. J. Benjamin et al., "Guidelines for the ultrasound assessment of endothelial-dependent flow-mediated vasodilation of the brachial artery: a report of the international brachial artery reactivity task force," *Journal of the American College of Cardiology*, vol. 39, no. 2, pp. 257–265, 2002.

[52] E. A. Patvardhan, K. S. Heffernan, J. M. Ruan, M. I. Soffler, R. H. Karas, and J. T. Kuvin, "Assessment of vascular endothelial function with peripheral arterial tonometry: information at your fingertips?" *Cardiology in Review*, vol. 18, no. 1, pp. 20–28, 2010.

[53] I. B. Wilkinson, H. MacCallum, J. R. Cockcroft, and D. J. Webb, "Inhibition of basal nitric oxide synthesis increases aortic augmentation index and pulse wave velocity in vivo," *British Journal of Clinical Pharmacology*, vol. 53, no. 2, pp. 189–192, 2002.

[54] E. J. Metter, R. Conwit, J. Tobin, and J. L. Fozard, "Age-associated loss of power and strength in the upper extremities in women and men," *Journals of Gerontology*, vol. 52, no. 5, pp. B267–B276, 1997.

[55] S. V. Brooks and J. A. Faulkner, "Skeletal muscle weakness in old age: underlying mechanisms," *Medicine and Science in Sports and Exercise*, vol. 26, no. 4, pp. 432–439, 1994.

[56] K. J. Martins, I. MacLean, G. K. Murdoch, W. T. Dixon, and C. T. Putman, "Nitric oxide synthase inhibition delays low-frequency stimulation-induced satellite cell activation in rat fast-twitch muscle," *Applied Physiology, Nutrition and Metabolism*, vol. 36, no. 6, pp. 996–1000, 2011.

[57] Z. Yu, P. Li, M. Zhang, M. Hannink, J. S. Stamler, and Z. Yan, "Fiber type-specific nitric oxide protects oxidative myofibers against cachectic stimuli," *PLoS ONE*, vol. 3, no. 5, Article ID e2086, 2008.

[58] D. M. Hirai, S. W. Copp, K. S. Hageman, D. C. Poole, and T. I. Musch, "Aging alters the contribution of nitric oxide to regional muscle hemodynamic control at rest and during exercise in rats," *Journal of Applied Physiology*, vol. 111, no. 4, pp. 989–998, 2011.

[59] T. I. Musch, K. E. Eklund, K. S. Hageman, and D. C. Poole, "Altered regional blood flow responses to submaximal exercise in older rats," *Journal of Applied Physiology*, vol. 96, no. 1, pp. 81–88, 2004.

[60] R. M. McAllister, "Endothelium-dependent vasodilation in different rat hindlimb skeletal muscles," *Journal of Applied Physiology*, vol. 94, no. 5, pp. 1777–1784, 2003.

[61] K. F. Reid, G. Doros, D. J. Clark et al., "Muscle power failure in mobility-limited older adults: preserved single fiber function despite lower whole muscle size, quality and rate of neuromuscular activation," *European Journal of Applied Physiology*, vol. 112, no. 6, pp. 2289–2301, 2012.

[62] W. R. Frontera, K. F. Reid, E. M. Phillips et al., "Muscle fiber size and function in elderly humans: a longitudinal study," *Journal of Applied Physiology*, vol. 105, no. 2, pp. 637–642, 2008.

[63] M. H. Laughlin and R. B. Armstrong, "Muscle blood flow during locomotory exercise," *Exercise and Sport Sciences Reviews*, vol. 13, pp. 95–136, 1985.

[64] T. Hirai, M. D. Visneski, K. J. Kearns, R. Zelis, and T. I. Musch, "Effects of NO synthase inhibition on the muscular blood flow response to treadmill exercise in rats," *Journal of Applied Physiology*, vol. 77, no. 3, pp. 1288–1293, 1994.

[65] R. J. Morrison, C. C. Miller III, and M. B. Reid, "Nitric oxide effects on force-velocity characteristics of the rat diaphragm," *Comparative Biochemistry and Physiology Part A*, vol. 119, no. 1, pp. 203–209, 1998.

[66] R. I. Viner, D. A. Ferrington, A. F. R. Hühmer, D. J. Bigelow, and C. Schöneich, "Accumulation of nitrotyrosine on the SERCA2a isoform of SR Ca-ATPase of rat skeletal muscle during aging: a peroxynitrite-mediated process?" *FEBS Letters*, vol. 379, no. 3, pp. 286–290, 1996.

[67] B. Van Der Loo, R. Labugger, J. N. Skepper et al., "Enhanced peroxynitrite formation is associated with vascular aging," *Journal of Experimental Medicine*, vol. 192, no. 12, pp. 1731–1743, 2000.

[68] T. L. Dutka, J. P. Mollica, and G. D. Lamb, "Differential effects of peroxynitrite on contractile protein properties in fast- and slow-twitch skeletal muscle fibers of rat," *Journal of Applied Physiology*, vol. 110, no. 3, pp. 705–716, 2011.

[69] T. L. Dutka, J. P. Mollica, G. S. Posterino, and G. D. Lamb, "Modulation of contractile apparatus Ca^{2+} sensitivity and disruption of excitation-contraction coupling by S-nitrosoglutathione in rat muscle fibres," *Journal of Physiology*, vol. 589, no. 9, pp. 2181–2196, 2011.

[70] G. D. Lamb and H. Westerblad, "Acute effects of reactive oxygen and nitrogen species on the contractile function of

skeletal muscle," *Journal of Physiology*, vol. 589, no. 9, pp. 2119–2127, 2011.

[71] K. S. Heffernan, E. A. Patvardhan, N. K. Kapur, R. H. Karas, and J. T. Kuvin, "Peripheral augmentation index as a biomarker of vascular aging: an invasive hemodynamics approach," *European Journal of Applied Physiology*, vol. 112, no. 8, pp. 2871–2879, 2012.

[72] D. Green, C. Cheetham, C. Reed, L. Dembo, and G. O'Driscoll, "Assessment of brachial artery blood flow across the cardiac cycle: retrograde flows during cycle ergometry," *Journal of Applied Physiology*, vol. 93, no. 1, pp. 361–368, 2002.

[73] D. H. J. Thijssen, E. A. Dawson, T. M. Tinken, N. T. Cable, and D. J. Green, "Retrograde flow and shear rate acutely impair endothelial function in humans," *Hypertension*, vol. 53, no. 6, pp. 986–992, 2009.

[74] D. H. J. Thijssen, G. A. Rongen, P. Smits, and M. T. E. Hopman, "Physical (in)activity and endothelium-derived constricting factors: overlooked adaptations," *Journal of Physiology*, vol. 586, no. 2, pp. 319–324, 2008.

[75] D. H. Thijssen, A. J. Maiorana, G. O'Driscoll, N. T. Cable, M. T. Hopman, and D. J. Green, "Impact of inactivity and exercise on the vasculature in humans," *European Journal of Applied Physiology*, vol. 108, no. 5, pp. 845–875, 2010.

[76] J. Sugawara, K. Hayashi, F. Kaneko, H. Yamada, T. Kizuka, and H. Tanaka, "Reductions in basal limb blood flow and lumen diameter after short-term leg casting," *Medicine and Science in Sports and Exercise*, vol. 36, no. 10, pp. 1689–1694, 2004.

[77] N. M. Hamburg, C. J. McMackin, A. L. Huang et al., "Physical inactivity rapidly induces insulin resistance and microvascular dysfunction in healthy volunteers," *Arteriosclerosis, Thrombosis, and Vascular Biology*, vol. 27, no. 12, pp. 2650–2656, 2007.

[78] M. Rakobowchuk, J. Crozier, E. I. Glover et al., "Short-term unilateral leg immobilization alters peripheral but not central arterial structure and function in healthy young humans," *European Journal of Applied Physiology*, vol. 111, no. 2, pp. 203–210, 2011.

[79] M. Dhindsa, S. M. Sommerlad, A. E. DeVan et al., "Interrelationships among noninvasive measures of postischemic macro- and microvascular reactivity," *Journal of Applied Physiology*, vol. 105, no. 2, pp. 427–432, 2008.

[80] W. I. Yang, S. Park, J. C. Youn et al., "Augmentation index association with reactive hyperemia as assessed by peripheral arterial tonometry in hypertension," *American Journal of Hypertension*, vol. 24, no. 11, pp. 1234–1238, 2011.

[81] R. B. Schnabel, P. S. Wild, A. Schulz et al., "Multiple endothelial biomarkers and noninvasive vascular function in the general population: the gutenberg health study," *Hypertension*, vol. 60, no. 2, pp. 288–295, 2012.

[82] N. M. Hamburg, J. Palmisano, M. G. Larson et al., "Relation of brachial and digital measures of vascular function in the community: the framingham heart study," *Hypertension*, vol. 57, no. 3, pp. 390–396, 2011.

[83] C. R. Lee, A. Bass, K. Ellis et al., "Relation between digital peripheral arterial tonometry and brachial artery ultrasound measures of vascular function in patients with coronary artery disease and in healthy volunteers," *American Journal of Cardiology*, vol. 109, no. 5, pp. 651–657, 2012.

4

Dementia Care: Intersecting Informal Family Care and Formal Care Systems

Prabhjot Singh,[1] Rafat Hussain,[2,3] Adeel Khan,[2] Lyn Irwin,[4] and Roslyn Foskey[2]

[1] *Disability Services, Queensland Department of Communities, Child Safety and Disability Services, Brisbane, QLD 4001, Australia*
[2] *University of New England, Armidale, NSW, Australia*
[3] *School of Rural Medicine, University of New England, Armidale, NSW 2351, Australia*
[4] *Aged Care Standards and Accreditation Agency Ltd., Sydney, NSW 2124, Australia*

Correspondence should be addressed to Rafat Hussain; rhussain@une.edu.au

Academic Editor: Astrid E. Fletcher

Dementia is one of the major causes of disability and dependence amongst older people and previous research has highlighted how the well-being of people with dementia is inherently connected to the quality of their relationships with their informal carers. In turn, these carers can experience significant levels of emotional stress and physical burden from the demands of caring for a family member with dementia, yet their uptake of formal services tends to be lower than in other conditions related to ageing. This paper is based on a qualitative study undertaken in the Australian state of Queensland and explores issues of access to and use of formal services in dementia care from the perspective of the informal family carers. It identifies three critical points at which changes in policy and practice in the formal care system could improve the capability of informal carers to continue to care for their family member with dementia: when symptoms first become apparent and a diagnosis is sought; when the condition of the person with dementia changes resulting in a change to their support needs; and when the burden of informal care being experienced by the carer is so great that some form of transition appears to be immanent in the care arrangement.

1. Introduction

Dementia as one of the major causes of disability and dependence amongst older people is an important aspect of formal service provision within aged care. Dementia is an umbrella term applied to more than one hundred degenerative brain syndromes which include Alzheimer disease, vascular dementia, dementia with Lewy bodies, and frontotemporal dementia [1]. These conditions are characterised by cognitive impairment and can result in communication difficulties, loss of memory, problems in performing previous routine tasks, and personality, mood, and behavior changes [1, 2].

The well-being of people with dementia has been linked to the quality of their relationships with their informal carers [3]. In spite of research, both in Australia and elsewhere in the world, identifying the significant levels of strain and burden informal carers often experience from the emotional stress and physical burden of caring for a person with dementia the uptake of formal in-home and community care services is lower among the carers of people with dementia than for other conditions associated with ageing [4, 5]. Canadian research suggests that among the explanations for the poor uptake of services is that the informal carers of people with dementia are either unaware of the services which are available or that these services are inaccessible, inconvenient, or too expensive [6]. There are also crucial differences in power, status, and authority between the informal and formal care system that need to be considered in the intersection of the two systems [6].

The policies and practices of the formal care system are conceptualized in rational and decontextualized terms, whereas the expectations and experiences of informal family carers emerge out of a unique set of personal circumstances. This suggests a need for medical and aged care services to consider not only the impact of caring for a person with dementia on their family, but also the family's perspective on formal services [2, 7–9].

The aim of the current paper is to explore the intersection of informal family caregiving and the formal care systems from the perspective of the primary family carers of people with dementia in an Australian context. The study focuses on issues of access to and use of formal services in dementia care from the perspective of the informal family carers. Recent research has found that the decisions made by informal carers on whether to seek or reject formal service provision arise through a complex interplay of social, moral, emotional, and cultural issues [10]. Thus, negotiating the intersection between family carers and those involved in designing and delivering formal aged care services involves social actors who belong to different systems each of which has specific configurations and ideologies [11].

2. Background to the Formal Aged Care System in Australia

In Australia, each year, more than million older people (out of a total population of just under 23 million) receive some form of formal support through the aged care system [12]. Although older Australians prefer home-based care to residential care, the greatest proportion of government funding for aged care services continues to be spent on residential aged care services [13]. In June 2010 the distribution of government subsidized aged care places for people aged 70 years and over within the state of Queensland (the state where the study reported in this paper was undertaken) was 95.6 per thousand in residential care, 3.9 per thousand in high level community care, and 20.8 per thousand in low level community care [12].

The service provision responsibilities are split both at the level of funding and frontline services for people who are ageing. The Australian service system has two streams of community service provision; home and community care services are jointly funded by the national and state governments, whilst home care packages are fully funded by the national government. Within Australia, not only the national and state levels of government do provide two different forms of community and dementia care and support, but also the actual provision of services then occurs through a combination of nonprofit and for-profit providers, which, in turn, may be managed at a local, regional, and state level. As a result in the local area there can be multiple providers with whom the carer comes into contact, in some cases providing the same or similar services. This causes considerable confusion for carers due to the complicated and overlapping formal service system. At the frontline of service delivery this is often perceived to have negative impacts due to competition between providers, along with issues related to internal organizational dynamics and interorganizational relationships.

In Australia there are economic benefits to government in supporting informal carers to continue to care for people with dementia as long as possible, thus reducing admissions to residential care services. In 2010 across Australia the cost of residential aged care provision was on average $48,710 per person per year, with government bearing 69% of this cost (or $33,610); in contrast the average annual cost of providing a person with in-home formal aged care was $7,520, with government bearing 92% of the cost (or $6,918 per year); the cost of mixed informal and formal in-home care was on the average of $11,370, with government bearing 35% of the cost of care (or $3,983 per year); and in-home informal care with the person receiving no support from formal aged care services was estimated to cost $10,880 per year, with government bearing no direct cost [13].

3. Methodology

The research reported here was undertaken in the Australian state of Queensland using a qualitative research design incorporating descriptive thematic analysis. This method was chosen as was congruent with the research aims, allowed for an in-depth understanding of the informal caring experience of family carers of people with dementia, and enabled the experience of carers to be presented from their own point of view.

Seventeen family carers involved were recruited from across Queensland, the third most populous state in Australia with a population of 4.6 million people. Selection of participants included in the study was based on the person's experience of caring for a family member with dementia living at home, irrespective of the duration, frequency, or status of the care relationship. Those recruited came from throughout southeast Queensland including metropolitan Brisbane (the third most populous city in Australia), regional centres, and rural communities.

All participants were volunteers and recruited through advertisements in local papers, along with distribution of information through two key nongovernment bodies in the state: the Alzheimer's Association and Carers Queensland. Eight of the interviews were conducted face to face and nine via were conducted the telephone—including all of those with participants living in rural and remote areas of the geographically large state.

The sample included two males and fifteen females, a gender balance consistent with the distribution of primary carers of people with dementia in Australia. In the study carers were categorized into two groups based on the age of eligibility for the Australian Aged Pension—as younger carers where they were under the age of 65 years and as older carers when they were aged 65 years and over at the time of the research interview.

The sample included

(i) two sons both of whom were aged less than 65 years;
(ii) five daughters, all aged less than 65 years;
(iii) one daughter-in-law aged less than 65 years;
(iv) nine wives, of whom two were under the age of 65 years and seven aged 65 years and over.

4. Data Analysis

The individual interviews were audio-recorded, with prior consent and transcribed verbatim. The transcripts were read several times to develop a coding scheme based on thematic analysis of the data [14]. To improve audibility, other members of the research team also reviewed the transcripts and the emergent themes. The first author, who conducted all the interviews, brought to the experience both her background on dementia care as well as on policy and practice development in aged care. That is, within the research process neither the researcher nor the person being interviewed came to the interview "untouched" [15] by the experience of caring for a person with dementia, albeit from very different perspectives. Other members of the project team provided their own perspective from their work in health services management and sociology of health. Rigour was gained through incorporating three key elements—validity, reliability, and verification related to sampling, the position of the researchers, and assessment of whether the objectives of the research were met—into the analysis process [16].

The analysis included a constant comparison method with roots in grounded theory along with descriptive thematic analysis, an inductive, or data driven, method that began with the development of a coding matrix based on the questions used in the interviews. The themes were named, defined, described, and refined though a six-stage process which allowed the analysis to become richer in explanation as the process progressed [14, 15]. A subsampling technique, used as a comparative technique, was used to draw out codes by comparing each participant's experience, considered unique in its own right [17]. The clustering of thematic codes to develop higher order themes was a crucial step in the identification of patterns connected to the broader questions under investigation [18]. These higher order themes were then arranged into a conceptual clustering matrix to allow conclusions to be drawn from the data [19]. Through this rigorous process the key findings of the research were schematized to answer the question of how family carers of people with dementia living in the community were successfully managing, continuing, and sustaining informal caring in the present and how they would continue to care in the future. The coding schema was reviewed and corroborated over several face-to-face discussions by three senior academic researchers, who are also coauthors of this paper.

5. Results

The uncertain and unpredictable nature of caring for a family member with dementia was one of the key concerns of the carers, influencing their ability to manage and continue with their caring situation. The carers described the total change in their lives as a result of their caring responsibilities and expressed their desire to continue caring for their family member with dementia but noted that in order to do so they needed access to formal services capable of providing more flexible support that recognized the concerns and issues experienced by carers. From the carer's perspective recognition of the importance of their role was about ensuring timely provision of information and access to formal care early in their caring journey, rather than access to formal care only as a crisis response when their situation deteriorated.

TABLE 1: Main themes and subthemes based on carers perspectives of intersection of formal and informal dementia care services.

Main theme	Subthemes
Interaction with medical and aged care services	(i) Delays in initial diagnosis (ii) Lack of information for nonmedical support services (iii) Lack of understanding of needs of informal carers
Impediments and enablers at the level of formal community services	(i) Quality of in-home and day care services (ii) Appropriate and accessible opportunities for carer participation in formal services

The two major themes which emerged were related to the challenges they had experienced in their interaction with medical and aged care services and enablers and impediments at the level of formal community support services. The analysis revealed several distinct subthemes embedded within both the major themes. In relation to interaction with medical and aged care services the sub-themes included delays in the initial diagnosis of dementia, barriers experienced in seeking access services, and a lack of understanding of the needs of informal carers of people with dementia by service providers (see Table 1). For enablers and impediments at the level of formal community support services, the participants identified two key characteristics of formal community services which would assist in their ability to balance the effort of caring and their own capacity to continue to care: quality of in-home and day care services and appropriate and accessible opportunities for carer participation in policy formulation and training of staff employed by the aged care and community-based formal services (see Table 1).

5.1. Challenges in Carer Interaction with Medical and Aged Care Services. The family carers described the challenges they had experienced in gaining the initial diagnosis and accessing appropriate medical treatment for their family member with dementia, including timely access to appropriate specialist care. Several carers suggested that the local general practitioners familiarity with their family member interfered with the objectivity of the medical assessment impeding early diagnosis. Two of the carers explained in some detail how they felt it was their family member's past medical history, of posttraumatic stress disorder in one case and mental illness in another, which had contributed to the delay in diagnosis. In the first case it had taken seven years from the time the first symptoms of dementia became apparent and were drawn to the attention of the local general practitioner to the eventual diagnosis of dementia. As the wife/carer explained *seven years is a long time* to wait for a diagnosis. In the second case there had been a three-year delay in diagnosis, resulting in lost opportunities in medical treatment. As that man's wife/carer explained, *"You need to be on them* (referring to drug treatment) *early. So, not much use waiting for the doctor to decide that there is a problem, after three years of, of saying it's depression"* (wife carer).

Not only some of the family careers had experienced delays in diagnosis and referral to other medical services but also this had then been exacerbated, in several cases, by a poor quality response by the medical professional at the time of the disclosure of the diagnosis. Carers described doctors who failed to take the time to listen or respond to the queries which were raised in ways they felt as insensitive to the needs of both the person with dementia and their own needs as the person's primary carer.

The carers also identified the impediments they had experienced in referral to specialist medical services in dementia care. Regardless of where they lived the family carers identified timely and appropriate access to specialist services as a crucial element in their interaction with and confidence of the formal service system.

One carer described the delays she and her mother had experienced in accessing appropriate services in terms of age discrimination embedded within the health care system as follows:

> *And so now a geriatrician is taking care of her but such a long-winded process that should have been so much easier. Had it seemed to us that she mattered, but she just didn't seem to matter. So my feeling was well perhaps when you're over 65 or—and/or experiencing dementia, that you just drop to the bottom of the pile, I find that incredibly offensive.*

Several family carers described how they had been left feeling stressed and demoralized when the medical specialist failed to take the time to properly listen to and adequately respond to their questions and concerns, around the implications of changes in the person's behaviour and capabilities. The following description by a wife/carer is indicative of the absence of explanation, advice and support by some medical specialists, "*the doctor just said, just go home and live out the rest of your life as well as you can.*" "*That's it. I wasn't told anything. I wasn't given any advice, nu-nu-nothing!*"

A specialist's dismissal of the carers concerns, can also mean a misdiagnosis as in this description by a daughter/carer:

> *So she was sent to a geriatrician at the Base Hospital. He was quite good but a little bit arrogant, a little bit condescending, a little bit smug, dismissed dementia and said, no it wasn't dementia, it certainly wasn't Alzheimer's and he thought it was probably MS.*

This misdiagnosis added to the challenges being experienced by this family carer, as the care recipient continued to display symptoms associated with dementia, yet the misdiagnosis meant that the daughter was unable to access appropriate dementia-specific services and support. Fortunately not all medical practitioners consulted by those involved in the current study had acted in this dismissive way, with several of the carers describing medical practitioners who had been very helpful, ensuring both their family member with dementia, and they as the primary carer, understand the medical implications of the dementia diagnosis.

5.2. Lack of Information on How to Seek Nonmedial Support Services. Almost all the carers described challenges they had experienced in getting appropriate and timely information about the nonmedical support services available to people with dementia and their carers. Initially this was indicative of the poor intersection between medical and non-medical services in aged care. As one wifecarer explained, *my GP is very nice and very good, but he didn't mention where to go or how to access it* (non-medical information and support). *Because (medical practitioner) is the first port of call, if evenif he just had a paper with a code on it that this is Alzheimer's society or whatever name, give them a call, that was all thatwas needed.* The carers believed that information on support services was of equal importance as medical assistance in the diagnosis of dementia. Overall what emerges from the interview data was the importance of the doctor's approach in supporting the family carer's capacity to manage the caring situation, especially in planning for future care needs.

As explained by one wife/carer the compounding impact of providing informal care is invidious,

> *because you feel duty-bound to keep going, and I think because you've eased into it month by month, year by year you just eased in and you're doing more and more and more and you don't know.*

A number of carers described their frustration that even where they had been provided with information on services in their local area early in their journey as carers this had often been *out of date.* Carers had also experienced different agencies *duplicating the same information, resulting in overlap and confusion,* yet still leaving them with gaps in their understanding of the extent of the options potentially available through the formal aged care system.

Carers also described the confusion resulting from a dual stream of community service provision between national, state, and local systems which results in multiple providers with which the carer comes into contact, in some cases providing similar or the same type of services. Rather than perceiving the choice of providers as positive, the carers felt that a lot of resources were being wasted on managing an unnecessarily complicated and overlapping service system. Several carers highlighted the negative impacts of competition between providers, along with issues related to internal organizational dynamics and interorganizational relationships.

In the present study those family carers with previous experience in engaging with the health and community sectors found that being familiar with the ways support services operated advantaged them in negotiating at the intersection of formal and informal care and support. The lack of familiarity with the organizational logic and work routines that underlies such interactions served to heighten family carers sense that they have no control over the situation they have found themselves in, at a time when they are already stressed and vulnerable. To add to the confusion they found that a single term, such as respite care, was often being applied to differing forms of service provision.

For example, in relation to respite care, the same term is used for in-home care, a centre providing day respite, and a block of respite care in a residential facility.

Carers also highlighted their difficulties in accessing services soon after diagnosis, with several carers indicating that the services they had contacted appeared to give little priority to the needs of people in the early stages of dementia. In rural areas, in particular, several carers were given the choice of either accessing generic services unsuitable for the needs of their family member with dementia or dementia-specific services which were inappropriate as they were designed around the needs of those with more severe symptoms and behaviours. Other carers highlighted their frustration when they found that the generic community aged care services they had contacted effectively denied access to people with a diagnosis of dementia. Delays experienced in access to some services were also a concern for the carers with long waiting periods not only causing frustration, but also leaving the carer feeling that no one cared for them, whilst they cared for their family member with dementia.

Carers described coming into contact with a community aged care system which they felt had become a business, rather than service, a system which cared more about managing finances than meeting the complex needs of people with dementia, along with those of their informal carers. The commodification of services is paradoxical for it also raises carers expectations in relation to the availability of case management as illustrated by the following comment by a daughter/carer:

> *I also believe that if they're providing a seven-day service then there needs to be a contact number for them for all seven days because you can't actually ring them on a Saturday morning and say what's happened because there's nobody there. There's no one to answer the phones.*

5.3. Lack of Understanding of Needs of Informal Carers by Formal Care Services. A crucial factor that encouraged carers to become actively engaged with formal support services was care workers who were proactive in their contact, rather than relying on the carer to initiate all the interaction with the service provider. In these circumstances the service was more likely to be perceived by the carer as complementing, rather than undermining, their capacity to sustain their caring role. Carers expressed particular concerns about carers *effectively having to do their own case management*, with the pressure always being on them to initiate contact with services.

However, most often the assessment and monitoring processes being used by the formal services were described by the family carers as inflexible and the services as lacking in the ability to respond in a timely way to the constantly changing demands and emergent needs involved in caring for a person with dementia. A failure by assessors in the formal system to adequately consider the needs of the carer is evident in the following description by a daughter/carer:

> *We will only give you X number of minutes in service, we will only do this and we will only do that and it will cost you part of your income and it was just, I thought I honestly suspect that part of this was not meant to be easy to access.*

This is indicative of the different logics underlying formal and informal care systems. The carers in the present study believed that their active involvement in the decision-making process would allow for the best interests of the person with dementia to remain paramount in formal care provision. They explained how it was through their involvement in decisions relating to formal services that they were able to develop their confidence and trust in the system increasing the possibility that they would continue to access services. Conversely a complex assessment process, which left carers feeling excluded or peripheral, was identified as an impediment to constructing a comfortable and trusting relationship with service providers.

Whilst some carers noted that their role was nominally recognized by services, this was most often only a passive recipient of support, rather than an active participant in the support and care process. The carers emphasized that the formal community aged care system needs to be rebalanced and refocused to ensure that carers are conceived and included as equal partners at the intersection of formal and informal care systems. Carers suggested that this would assist formal care providers to be more responsive and accountable as reflected in the following comment by a daughter/carer:

> *I'd like the care providers to be more accountable to carers and have to explain why they do the things that they do and not just treat their clients like it's a bloody car service or whatever. I think they should be accountable to treat them as people and they just can't have one rule for everybody.*

Carers considered the availability of services to complement their role as informal carers as critical to the future sustainability of their informal care. With many formal services restricted to week-day provision the carers highlighted that services needed to be responsive to the continuous nature of caring by broadening their coverage to seven days a week. The impact of service rationing on the carers own sense of wellbeing and social engagement can be significant as this son/carer explained, *I get four hours a month off, which isn't much time to socialize.... "I haven't got a social life any more."* Other service-related issues experienced by carers included barriers to the transportability of care and support arrangements across the structural boundaries of local, nongovernment, state-based, and national service providers and systems.

In some situations, the carers had found that there was no appropriately flexible and responsive service available. This included those carers who still remained in the workforce and those who would have liked the option to continue working alongside their caring role, but had found it impossible as in the following description by a daughter carer:

> *I had no one to look after mum, so I couldn't go to work, and I do believe that that impacted and I do believe that that's one of the reasons that they fired me. Because I couldn't attend work because I had to look after mum.*

5.4. Quality of In-Home and Day Carer Services. A number of those receiving formal in-home services in the Queensland study described how they felt a need to monitor services when workers unknown to them came into their home. Some carers expressed particular concerns about the quality of in-home services. They described circumstances in which in-home respite care assistants were constantly changing, did not turn up when expected, did not demonstrate compassion towards the person with dementia, and did not have good communication skills or demonstrate understanding of the care needs of both the carer and their care recipient. Such issues contributed to the carer's levels of worry and stress as they believed that the vulnerability of the person with dementia and their lack of familiarity with the in-home worker were a risk that needed to be actively managed. The carers described a number of strategies they had used to handle the risks they perceived in using in-home services: staying around the home whilst care was being provided, familiarising themselves with the care system, and most importantly accessing only those services they felt to be reliable and trustworthy.

On the same vein the quality of day care services was perceived to be problematic. The poor physical and interpersonal environment within some out-of-home services encountered by carers deterred them from accessing that service for their family member, particularly when they knew that their family member would not approve the facility. For example, this carer highlights a need to improve both the physical infrastructure of day-care facilities and the education of staff, "*it is not the facility it is just a chair, and that is hard to send someone to a place for a day where they just sit in a chair.*" Central to the carers concern was the fact that this situation potentially compromised the safety and security of the person with dementia. In all types of out-of-home environments the carers sought a home-like quality and their ideal was for sufficient respite options to be available so that the most appropriate alternative could be selected, which met the particular needs of their family member with dementia.

Creating a trusting relationship with both residential and in-home respite services was factor which had helped the carers feel more confident about dealing with emergencies and sudden changes to care arrangements. Almost half of the carers described the vital role of respite care in allowing them to attend regular commitments which included, but were not limited to, paid work and carer-related support activities (e.g., attending support groups and committee meetings). Respite, in these terms, was not necessarily providing the carer with a break from engagement in instrumental tasks, just time away from the care recipient to complete necessary chores or to earn a living. The carers expressed a need for respite options to be more widely available. They also identified a need for services to be responsive to the needs of carers recovering from personal crises, including those that were health-related.

It was through consistent, good quality, service provision that the trust and confidence of the carer in formal care arrangements gradually increase. The carers considered consistency in workers providing good quality care and support to be fundamental in meeting the needs of the care recipient and through this in also supporting them to sustain their informal care.

5.5. Appropriate and Accessible Opportunities for Carer Participation in Formal Services. Almost half of the carers interviewed already played an active role in providing support for other carers, reflecting the recruitment process for interview participants through the Alzheimer's Association and carers organizations. Despite this carers also highlighted barriers in participation in consultation processes such as carer forums and carer support groups, including issues related to the timing and location of such events, as in the following comments of this daughter/carer:

> *I got an email the other day and they're actually having a forum in one of the big cities. This is the first time I've ever been asked but the thing is that I think it's at 10:30 in the morning, do you know what I mean?*

Several of the carers highlighted the vital importance of carer input into policy and planning and implementation of formal service provision. These carers felt they had inside knowledge from their caring experience that would be extremely valuable to improving formal services, as expressed by this daughter/carer, "*it doesn't matter how many university degrees and that people do, they don't know until they're a carer.*" ... *What it really involves.*

These carers indicated that a greater investment in making support and training available to ex-carers to provide peer support would bring systemic benefits, including better carer and care-recipient outcomes. They suggested that combining professional expertise and peer support would assist the carers of people with dementia to work through their specific, unique, sensitive, and complex issues. Peer support was identified as important both in helping primary carers adjust to their changing circumstances and in assisting other family members to better understand the impact of dementia on the primary carer. Several carers indicated that they would be willing to contribute to the education or training of formal dementia care workers through sharing their own experience.

These carers also expressed concern about the shortage of appropriately trained aged care workers. They also highlighted the staff retention issues within community care services, due to the poor pay and conditions of frontline workers in formal community aged care, as in the following description by a carer/daughter:

> *Well to tell you the absolute truth I think that they need to pay them more money. The actual people that come to the door and help these people are on the most terrible wage imaginable.*

These carers noted how the complex design and implementation of the service delivery system placed additional stress and strain not only on themselves as informal carers but also on frontline workers. At the interface of the two systems the frontline carer and the informal family carer come into contact within a social contract of providing care to the person with dementia in a form which exceeds the reciprocity which usually exists between adults, and therefore the continuity in workers allows for these interrelationships to develop and deepen which can be crucial to the sustainability of informal care.

6. Discussion

The present study, along with the other recent research focused on the carers experience in dementia care, indicates that the quality of interaction is key to whether the relationships established add to or reduce the burden of care on family carers. There are three key points where changes to policy and practice in the formal care system could improve the capability of informal carers to continue to care. The first occurs when the early symptoms of dementia in the care recipient become apparent and lead to initial contact of the carer with the medical system. At this point information is very much a two-way flow between the informal carer and the formal community care and support system. It needs to be recognized that family members have historical information about the person that, if shared in a timely manner, has the potential to benefit everyone involved [20].

Previous studies both in Australia and elsewhere in the western world have found that the general practitioner's role is often vital, not only in the early detection of dementia, but also in the timely referral of the person to specialist services [21–23]. The Australian Institute for Health and Welfare [1] highlighted in their recent report on dementia care in Australia that as there is not a "single or simple test that will definitively diagnose dementia" the general aim is for the medical assessment process to gather sufficient information about "changed behaviours, functional capacity, psychosocial issues, and relevant medical conditions to allow a diagnosis to be made." However, a recent survey of the dementia-related health literacy in the Australian and English general practice found that only 22 percent of general practitioners and 15 percent of practice nurses considered their dementia knowledge to be adequate [24].

It has previously been argued that when medical professionals are discussing dementia as a condition issues of concern must be considered from the perspective of both the person with dementia and the primary carer [25]. As mentioned earlier, the hierarchical organization of healthcare services and the esteemed status of health professionals particularly doctors as primary holders of knowledge leads to asymmetrical power relations in clinical encounters. Carers often feel disempowered as they have limited voice in relation to information on services and care on offer for their family member with dementia. There are also acknowledged structural constraints within the Australian medical system, with recent research finding that particularly in regional Australia general practitioners may delay referring a patient to a specialist for further testing, in part because of more limited access to specialist services [21].

The second critical point occurs when there is a change in support needs as the condition of the person with dementia changes, such as increasing concerns by the carer about the safety of their family member or the emergence of challenging behaviours. This is the point at which access to appropriate respite care may be crucial to the sustainability of informal care. Various approaches that would improve carers engagement with formal community care services, such shifting the focus of formal case management away from making referrals and providing a linking service between services, to a focus by the case manager on organizing personalised and flexible services which not only considered the present issues but also anticipated the future challenges for the carer. This includes consideration of the impact of the demands of caring the lives of people caring for a family member with dementia beyond their caring role to ensure that carers continue to have opportunities for economic and social engagement.

A recent inquiry by the Australian Human Rights and Equal Opportunity Commission highlighted the challenges faced by Australians seeking to combine work and informal caring responsibilities and identified serious implications for the emotional and economic wellbeing of carers over the long term [26, 27]. In the present study, the stress being experienced by the carers was identified by them as risking their ability to continue to fulfill their informal caring role alongside other responsibilities in their lives. It is important to note that some of the younger carers were combining their role as a primary carer with other family and work commitments, whilst several of the older carers interviewed in the present study did not have access to practical hands-on informal support on which they could readily draw in a crisis.

Health economists have conceptualized the burden of informal care in dementia as the putative cost of the time spent by the informal carer on the tasks of care. In their recent meta-review on informal dementia care Costa and colleagues [2] assessed the objective burden of informal care in two common dementia-related conditions: firstly Alzheimer disease at 55.73 hours per week and secondly Parkinsons disease at 15.8 hours per week. They then linked this objective measurement to the subjective evaluation of caregiver burden or strain noting that "the more the number of informal hours increases, the more the subjective burden is important" [2]. This is most evident where the person with dementia is exhibiting emotional difficulties and/or challenging behaviours [9, 26–28].

The assessment of the subjective burden of informal care by formal services needs to better understand the contextual, psychological, and emotional dimensions of care from the perspective of the carer [2]. The gap between apparent need and actual uptake of services points to an important mismatch between the logics operating within organizational systems and the logics within the family environments in which most of dementia care occurs [5]. For example, whilst formal systems tend to base their measurement of need around an abstract and lineal conceptualization of time, for the person with dementia and their informal carer (as well as some frontline staff) the framing of time is enmeshed with social relations and involves processes which cannot be hurried [29].

Other Australian researchers have highlighted that the gain that carers experience in receiving formal services is inherently ambiguous, for whilst formal services are providing support to family carers, they can also be undermining their sense of identity and control over their circumstances [5]. A number of those receiving formal in-home services in the present study described how they felt a need to monitor services when workers unknown to them came into their home. In their Tasmanian study Lloyd and Stirling [5] similarly noted that whilst access to formal services can offer physical, psychological, and emotional relief to informal carers it can also cause the carer to experience a threatening loss of mastery over the material and symbolic boundaries of previously private spaces.

The third critical point occurs when the burden of informal care is being experienced by the carer as so great that some form of transition is imminent in the care arrangement. As in the other research (e.g., [3, 6, 13]) the carers in the present study were committed to caring for their family member in the community as long as possible, yet also being very aware of the fact that there were limits in their capability to sustain their caring role, particularly as dementia (dependent on the condition) can be associated with progressive decline. They wished to begin to prepare in advance for the point was reached in which the person could no longer be cared for at home.

7. Conclusion

The issues which emerged through the present study, combined with other recent research in Australia, suggests that for informal dementia care to become more sustainable it is necessary to ensure that formal service provision is flexible enough to respond to the complexity of the circumstances (family, social, and economic), not only for the person with dementia but also for their informal carer/s. There is increasing recognition within Australian aged care funding and policy that the care and support of people with dementia is complex and needs to take the particular needs of carers into consideration. However, on the ground carers continue to be faced with confusing funding arrangements and a complex array of services provided by for-profit as well as non-profit organisations.

The present study has reinforced the findings of other reports [3, 26, 27] that in order to improve the sustainability of informal care of people with dementia in the community the formal community care system needs to take a more proactive approach in engaging with informal carers. In order to reduce the burden of care on the primary carers of people with dementia there is a need to ensure the carers perspective is being sought both in the development of policy and within everyday practice. Carers have noted that better services, including respite care, medical (professional and primary) services, and more responsive and appropriate information, and flexible and responsive services are the key considerations in the sustainability of informal care.

Conflict of Interests

The authors declare that there is no conflict of interests regarding the publication of this paper.

Acknowledgments

The authors would also like to thank the participants for their time and interest in the study. The authors acknowledge the contribution made by the Collaborative Research Network on Mental Health and Well-Being in Rural Communities, supported by the Department of Industry, Innovation, Science, Research and Tertiary Education, Commonwealth Government of Australia.

References

[1] Australian Institute of Health and Welfare [AIHW], *Dementia in Australia*, Australian Institute of Health and Welfare, Canberra, Australia, 2012.

[2] N. Costa, L. Ferlicoq, H. Derumeaux-Burel et al., "Comparison of informal care time and costs in different age-related dementias: a review," *BioMed Research International*, vol. 2013, Article ID 852368, 15 pages, 2013.

[3] Nuffield Council on Bioethics [NCB], *Dementia: Ethical Issues*, Nuffield Council on Bioethics, London, UK, 2009.

[4] C. Bakker, M. E. de Vugt, D. van Vliet et al., "The use of formal and informal care in early onset dementia: results from the NeedYD study," *The American Journal of Geriatric Psychiatry*, vol. 21, no. 1, pp. 37–45, 2013.

[5] B. T. Lloyd and C. Stirling, "Ambiguous gain: uncertain benefits of service use for dementia carers," *Sociology of Health and Illness*, vol. 33, no. 6, pp. 899–913, 2011.

[6] C. Ward-Griffin, J. Hall, R. DeForge et al., "Dementia home care resources: how are we managing?" *Journal of Aging Research*, vol. 2012, Article ID 590724, 11 pages, 2012.

[7] M. Algera, A. L. Francke, A. Kerkstra, and J. van der Zee, "An evaluation of the new home-care needs assessment policy in the Netherlands," *Health and Social Care in the Community*, vol. 11, no. 3, pp. 232–241, 2003.

[8] G. Mountain, "Self-management for people with early dementia: an exploration of concepts and supporting evidence," *Dementia*, vol. 5, no. 3, pp. 429–446, 2006.

[9] World Health Organization [WHO], *Dementia: A Public Health Priority*, World Health Organization, Geneva, Switzerland, 2012, http://whqlibdoc.who.int/publications/2012/9789241564458_eng.pdf.

[10] V. Edgell, "Who cares? Managing obligation and responsibility across the changing landscapes of informal dementia care," *Ageing and Society*, vol. 33, no. 5, pp. 888–907, 2013.

[11] N. Carpentier, "Caregiver identity as a useful concept for understanding the linkage between formal and informal care systems: a case study," *Sociology Mind*, vol. 2, no. 1, pp. 41–49, 2012.

[12] Australian Department of Health and Ageing, Online, 2013.

[13] C. Bridge, "Taking care: costs and benefits of providing care services in the home?" in *Proceedings of the International Federation on Ageing Conference*, Symposium Discussion Paper: Home Truths: Housing and Neighbourhood Design and Care for Ageing in Place in Australia, Melbourne, Australia, 2010, http://www.be.unsw.edu.au/sites/default/files/upload/research/centres/cf/CFpresentations/IFA_Conference.pdf.

[14] R. Boyatzis, *Transforming Qualitative Information: Thematic Analysis and Code Development*, Sage, Thousand Oaks, Calif, USA, 1998.

[15] K. Charmaz, *Constructing Grounded Theory: A Practical Guide Through Qualitative Analysis*, Sage, London, UK, 2006.

[16] J. Cresswell, Sage, Thousand Oaks, Calif, USA, 2007.

[17] M. Sandelowski, "Whatever happened to qualitative description?" *Research in Nursing and Health*, vol. 23, no. 4, pp. 334–340, 2000.

[18] A. Strauss and J. Corbin, *Basics of Qualitative Research: Techniques and Procedures for Developing Grounded Theory*, Sage, Thousand Oaks, Calif, USA, 1998.

[19] M. Miles and A. Huberman, *Qualitative Data Analysis*, Sage, Thousand Oaks, Calif, USA, 1994.

[20] A. Ryan, "Transitions in care: family carers experiences of nursing home placement," *Nursing Times Research*, vol. 7, no. 5, pp. 324–334, 2002.

[21] A. Greenway-Crombie, P. Snow, P. Disler, S. Davis, and D. Pond, "Influence of rurality on diagnosing dementia in Australian general practice," *Australian Journal of Primary Health*, vol. 18, no. 3, pp. 178–184, 2012.

[22] S. Illiffe and J. Wilcock, "The identification of barriers to the recognition of, and response to, dementia in primary care using a modified focus group approach," *Dementia*, vol. 4, no. 1, pp. 73–85, 2005.

[23] D. Scott and M. Donnelly, "The early detection of cognitive impairment: a stakeholder evaluation of a "dementia awareness service" in Belfast," *Dementia*, vol. 4, no. 2, pp. 207–232, 2005.

[24] F. B. Millard, R. L. Kennedy, and B. T. Baune, "Dementia: opportunities for risk reduction and early detection in general practice," *Australian Journal of Primary Health*, vol. 17, no. 1, pp. 89–94, 2011.

[25] M. Downs, R. Clibbens, C. Rae, A. Cook, and R. Woods, "What do general practitioners tell people with dementia and their families about the condition?" *Dementia*, vol. 1, no. 1, pp. 47–58, 2002.

[26] Australian Human Rights Commission, *Investing in Care: Recognising and Valuing Those Who Care*, vol. 1 of *Research Report*, Australian Human Rights Commission, Sydney, Australia, 2013.

[27] Australian Human Rights Commission, *Investing in Care: Recognising and Valuing Those Who Care*, vol. 2 of *Technical Papers*, Australian Human Rights Commission, Sydney, Australia, 2013.

[28] J. Gorse, J. Frost, J. Richardson, and H. Skirton, "Using meta-ethnography to understand the emotional impact of caring for people with increasing cognitive impairment," *Nursing Health Science*, vol. 15, no. 1, pp. 113–123, 2013.

[29] H. Colley, L. Henricksson, B. Niemeyer, and T. Seddon, "Competing time orders in human services work: towards a politics of time," *Time and Society*, vol. 21, no. 3, pp. 371–394, 2012.

5

Malnutrition-Sarcopenia Syndrome: Is This the Future of Nutrition Screening and Assessment for Older Adults?

Maurits F. J. Vandewoude,[1] Carolyn J. Alish,[2] Abby C. Sauer,[2] and Refaat A. Hegazi[2]

[1] *Department of Geriatrics, ZNA St. Elisabeth Leopoldstraat 26, University of Antwerp, 2000 Antwerp, Belgium*
[2] *Scientific and Medical Affairs, Abbott Nutrition, Abbott Laboratories, 3300 Stelzer Road, Columbus, OH 43219, USA*

Correspondence should be addressed to Maurits F. J. Vandewoude, maurits.vandewoude@zna.be

Academic Editor: Astrid E. Fletcher

Malnutrition is common across varying patient populations, particularly older adults, and sarcopenia prevalence increases with advancing age. Both malnutrition and sarcopenia are associated with substantial adverse outcomes affecting both the patient and the healthcare system, including increased morbidity, mortality, rehospitalization rates, and healthcare costs. Healthcare practitioners may assess patients for either malnutrition or sarcopenia; however, many patients clinically present with both conditions, resulting in the syndrome, Malnutrition-Sarcopenia Syndrome, which is the clinical presentation of both malnutrition and accelerated age-associated loss of lean body mass, strength, and/or functionality. Clinicians are urged to screen, assess, and treat these conditions currently so as to adequately address the full spectrum of patients' nutritional issues. By examining aspects of both conditions, clinicians can more fully assess their patients' clinical and nutritional status and can tailor targeted therapies to meet their needs and improve outcomes. This proposed syndrome embodies the inherent association of malnutrition and sarcopenia, highlighting their combined impact on clinical outcomes. The objective of this review paper is to characterize Malnutrition-Sarcopenia Syndrome to advance clinical practice, by providing clinicians with the necessary background information to integrate nutritional assessment along with loss of muscle mass and functionality in their everyday clinical practice.

1. Introduction

Historically, malnutrition has been defined as a condition of an imbalance of energy, protein, and other nutrients that cause measurable negative effects on body composition, physical function, and clinical outcomes [1]. Typical measures that clinicians use to screen and assess for malnutrition or the risk for malnutrition include dietary or nutrient intake, changes in body weight, and laboratory values [2]. A new definition of malnutrition has recently been proposed by an International Guideline Consensus Committee, integrating the acuity of the associated disease and inflammation [3]. The committee specified three subtypes of malnutrition using an etiology-based terminology to assist clinicians to make a nutrition diagnosis in clinical practice settings: (1) starvation-related without inflammation, (2) chronic disease or conditions that impose sustained mild-to-moderate inflammation (e.g., sarcopenic obesity, organ failure, and pancreatic cancer), and (3) acute disease or injury states, when inflammatory response is marked [3].

One critical clinical aspect often not assessed in nutrition screening or assessment is lean body mass or muscle mass loss. Lean body mass (LBM) is defined as that portion of the body mass that is everything but fat and includes water, mineral, muscle, and other protein-rich structures (e.g., enzymes, viscera, red cells, and connective tissues) [4]. Skeletal muscle mass constitutes the majority of LBM and provides strength, mobility, and balance [5]. Muscle mass also plays a critical role in whole-body protein metabolism and impacts quality of life in patients with chronic diseases [6]. The balance between muscle protein anabolism and catabolism is vitally important to maintaining skeletal muscle mass, particularly in older adults who lose muscle mass as a consequence of aging and/or illness [6, 7]. It was not until 1989, when Irwin Rosenberg introduced the term sarcopenia [8]. The European Working Group on Sarcopenia in Older People (EWGSOP) defines sarcopenia as an age-related loss of muscle mass, combined with loss of strength, functionality, or both (Figure 1) [9]. The working group also proposed a diagnostic algorithm for sarcopenia that is based on the presence of low muscle mass plus either low muscle strength (e.g., low handgrip strength) or low physical performance (e.g., 4 meter walking speed).

Sarcopenia is further classified into either primary or secondary categories. Primary sarcopenia, when no specific etiologic cause can be identified, is progressive and associated with the impact of aging: a reduction in motor neurons, alterations in skeletal muscle tissue including mitochondrial dysfunction, changes in the hormonal milieu (e.g., insulin resistance and a reduction in insulin-like growth factor-1 and an increase in proinflammatory cytokines, such as tumor necrosis factor α and interleukin 6. Next to the intrinsic, age-related processes, a multitude of extrinsic and behavioral factors can aggravate the development and/or progression of sarcopenia, leading to secondary sarcopenia, such as disuse and lack of physical activity, malnutrition, chronic inflammation, and comorbidity. As such, sarcopenia can be thought of as both a process and an outcome. Sarcopenia as a condition is a major cause of frailty and disability in older adults; as an active process, it is present in every person reaching adult life [9].

2. Malnutrition and Sarcopenia Are Prevalent among Older Adults

There are no published data demonstrating the co-occurrence of malnutrition and sarcopenia in older adults. However, research has shown that reductions in handgrip strength are common in individuals who have sarcopenia as well as in individuals who are malnourished [9, 10]. Many older adults are malnourished or at high risk for malnutrition due to many factors. Decreased appetite and food intake, poor dentition, an increased frequency and severity of acute and chronic medical conditions, multiple medications, social and economic challenges, and cognitive decline all play a role in the etiology of malnutrition among older adults. Advanced age is an independent risk factor for malnutrition and is associated with a lower body weight, body mass index (BMI), and serum albumin [11–13].

The prevalence of malnutrition is greater among older adults in health care settings than in the community (Table 1). In hospital settings, malnutrition among older patients is approximately 56% [11]. For older adults living in the community, the prevalence of malnutrition ranges from 1 to 10%, while 41–48% are at risk for malnutrition [14]. Consistently, in a large international study, malnutrition was present in 2% of those living in the community, 9% of outpatients and home care combined, 23% in the hospital, 21% in institutions, and 15% in those with cognitive impairment [15].

Age-associated loss of muscle mass is characterized by a 3–8% decline per decade after the age of 30 years with further decline in adults 60 years of age and older [7, 16]. With aging, the loss of muscle mass is accompanied by an increase in body fat [17]. On average, adults can experience annual losses of 0.23 kg of muscle and gains of 0.45 kg of fat between 30 and 60 years of age [18]. Acute illness and injury can accelerate age-related changes in body composition. Studies demonstrate that, following injury, patients can lose 5-6% of their total body weight—most of which is muscle mass — and gain between 4 and 11% in fat mass within 12 months, with the majority of LBM loss occurring within the first two to four months after the injury [19].

Using the EWGSOP diagnostic criteria, Landi et al. evaluated the baseline data of adults who were 80 years of age or older ($n = 260$) from the ilSIRENTE study. The results of the study indicated that sarcopenia is prevalent among community-dwelling older adults with no differences based on gender (25%) [20]. Using the same diagnostic algorithm, Landi et al. demonstrated that the prevalence of sarcopenia is slightly higher (32.8%) among older adults in long-term care settings and was higher among male residents (68%) than among female residents (21%) [21].

Reductions in muscle mass among older adults are common and can contribute to functional impairment, disability, increased risk for falls [20], lowered quality of life, and increased risk for mortality. For instance, using cross-sectional body composition data from the Third National Health and Nutrition Examination Survey, Janssen and colleagues determined the prevalence of class I sarcopenia (skeletal muscle mass index within one to two standard deviations below sex-specific values for young adults) and class II sarcopenia (skeletal muscle mass index two standard deviations of young adult values) in adults age 50 years of older. Among adults 50 years of age and older, the prevalence of class I sarcopenia was estimated between 37 and 47% in men and 50–61% in women, and a prevalence of class II sarcopenia between 5–7% in men and 7–11% in women. The prevalence of sarcopenia increased from the third to sixth decades and remained constant among subjects 70 years of age and older, while the prevalence of class I (59% versus 45%) and class II (10% versus 7%) was greater in women ≥50 years of age than men ($P < 0.001$). Moreover, functional impairment was 2-3-fold higher in older subjects with class II sarcopenia than those with normal muscle mass, even after adjusting for age, race, BMI, health behaviors, and comorbidities [22].

3. Malnutrition Sarcopenia Syndrome and Clinical Outcomes

In many patient populations, malnutrition and sarcopenia are present in parallel and manifest clinically through a combination of decreased nutrient intake, decreased body weight, along with a decrease in muscle mass, strength, and/or physical function. This leads us to coin the proposed clinical syndrome of Malnutrition-Sarcopenia Syndrome (MSS). MSS is the clinical presentation of both malnutrition and accelerated age-associated loss of lean body mass, strength, and/or physical performance. Malnutrition and sarcopenia are each independently associated with negative health consequences that impact older adults across health care

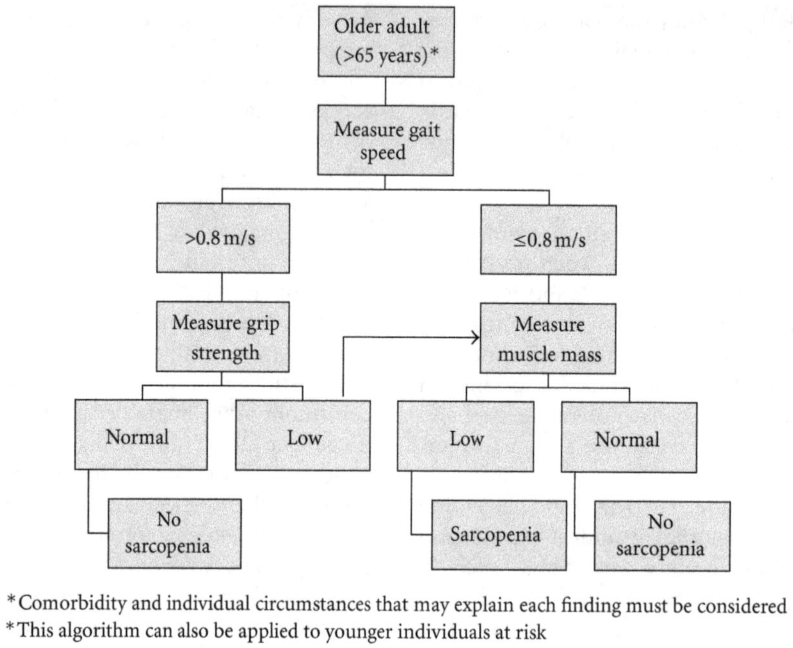

FIGURE 1: EUGMS working group-suggested algorithm for sarcopenia case finding in older individuals (used with permission) [9].

TABLE 1: Prevalence of malnutrition and sarcopenia in older adults across clinical settings.

Patient Population/Setting	Malnutrition	Sarcopenia
Hospital/Acute Care	56% [11]	
	23% [15]	
Long Term Care	21% [15]	32.8% [21]
	2–9% [15]	25% [20]
Community	1–10% [15]	37–61% (class I sarcopenia) [22]
	(41–48% at risk) [14]	5–11% (class II sarcopenia) [22]

settings. Patients with malnutrition and/or sarcopenia are at risk of increased morbidity and mortality, decreased quality of life and functioning and increased rehospitalization, length of hospital stay, and healthcare costs. Importantly, malnutrition and sarcopenia are associated with increased mortality [23–27]. Cederholm et al. found significant differences in mortality rates between malnourished patients and well-nourished patients after hospitalization (44% versus 18%, respectively) [23]. In community-dwelling older adults, unintentional weight loss and low BMI are associated with elevated 3-year mortality rates, and older adults reporting unintentional weight loss were 1.67 times more likely to experience mortality than those who reported no weight loss [28]. Newman and colleagues demonstrated that 5% weight loss over a three-year period is a significant and independent predictor of mortality in community-dwelling aging adults [17]. Similarly, Cereda et al. determined that low BMI predicted mortality in older institutionalized adults [29]. Interestingly, a prospective observational cohort of older adults demonstrated that higher lean mass and lean mass index predicted lower mortality with an 85% reduction in risk, suggesting that changes in lean mass and lean mass index, rather than BMI, are better predictors of mortality in older adults and highlighting the role of lean muscle mass loss in defining malnutrition [30]. Sarcopenia has also been linked with increased mortality in various patient populations. Recently, Landi et al. demonstrated that sarcopenia is highly prevalent in older nursing home residents and is associated with a significantly increased risk of all-cause death [31]. Additionally, Bunout et al. evaluated the relationship between the loss of fat-free mass and mortality among aging adults ($n = 1413$, 74.3 ± 5.6 years of age) and showed that low fat-free mass was significantly associated with mortality among individuals over 74 years of age [32]. Furthermore, results from a recent meta-analysis show that objective measures of physical capability, such as handgrip strength, walking speed, and chair rise, are predictors of all-cause mortality in older community-dwelling populations [33]. The loss of function associated with sarcopenia and malnutrition is a risk factor for negative outcomes.

Malnutrition and sarcopenia are associated with increased morbidity, in particular increased infection and complications rates, including falls [34] and disability [35]. In a study of hospitalized patients, malnutrition was shown to be a significant independent risk factor for nosocomial infections, with infection rates of 4.4% in the well-nourished group, 7.6% in the moderate malnutrition group as compared to 14.6% in the severely malnourished group [36]. In addition, serum albumin levels, age, weight, immunodeficiency, and nutrition risk index score were associated with increased risk of nosocomial infections [36]. Edington et al. determined that malnourished patients experience a two-fold increase in rates of infection as compared to well-nourished patients, indicating that malnutrition is associated with hospital-acquired infections [37]. Similarly, a study of hospitalized older adults demonstrated that patients identified with sarcopenia (detected by dual energy X-ray absorptiometry (DXA)) upon admission were at a greater risk of contracting a nosocomial infection during the first 3 weeks of hospitalization (relative risk of 2.1) [38].

Malnutrition and loss of muscle mass compromise the quality of life and functional capacity of aging adults. Malnutrition is associated with declines in functional capacity in hospitalized patients [39]. Moreover, reduced quality of life has been reported among malnourished patients with a total Mini-Nutritional Assessment (MNA) score <24 [40]. Malnutrition significantly impacts the clinical outcomes of community-dwelling older adults. Specifically, older patients who are malnourished are more likely to be discharged to a residential home and less likely to return home [41, 42] with an increased length of convalescence, greater disability and dependence on walking devices, and loss of muscle strength after hospitalization [43–45]. Other consequences of sarcopenia are persistent sense of fatigue, muscle weakness, increased predisposition to metabolic disorders, and increased risk of falls and fractures [46]. Studies suggest that loss of muscle mass is a predictor of functional decline in independent older adults and those with disability [22, 47] and that age-related loss of muscle mass is directly correlated with loss in strength [48]. Interestingly, Reid et al. showed that lower extremity muscle mass is a strong independent predictor of the level of functional impairment [49]. Loss of strength with aging tends to track with loss of muscle mass in physiological studies although the decline in muscle strength is steeper than the decline in muscle mass [50]. Also, interventions that increase muscle mass do not necessarily increase strength, and changes in strength that occur with resistance training precede measurable changes in muscle mass. Correlations between change in muscle mass and change in strength in older adults are therefore not consistent. Recently, the term "sarcopenia with limited mobility" was proposed as a syndrome that occurs when sarcopenia leads to loss of function and individuals become candidates for therapeutic interventions [51].

In addition to increased risk of infections and functional impairment, malnutrition and loss of muscle mass are also associated with increased hospital length of stay (LOS) [11, 37, 52–55]. Moreover, studies have shown that weight loss and malnutrition are predictors of increased rehospitalization rates in adults [56–59]. In one study, LOS is significantly shorter among well-nourished patients (5.7 days) as compared to malnourished patients (8.9 days) [60]. Leandro-Merhi et al. reported that well-nourished patients are three times more likely to be discharged sooner than patients with varying degrees of malnutrition [55]. Additionally, severely malnourished patients with a BMI < 20 kg/m^2 or weight loss of greater than 10% stayed in the hospital even longer at 18.3 and 17.5 days, respectively [37]. Hospitalization is associated with significant reductions in muscle mass and strength and functional decline in older adults [44, 61–64]. Interestingly, in a large sample of patients, Pichard et al. determined that fat-free mass (FFM) and fat-free mass index are significantly lower among elderly hospitalized patients than their nonhospitalized counterparts. Additionally, 37% of patients hospitalized for just 1-2 days had low FFM, which increased to 55.6% after 12 days of hospitalization [65]. Another study concluded that short-term hospitalization was associated with significant declines in functional capacity and muscle strength, regardless of age or baseline functional status [45]. The relationship between hospitalization—related loss of muscle mass and strength and declining functional capacity and the risk for future hospital admission needs further exploration.

Collectively, malnutrition, loss of muscle mass, strength, and functional capacity are accelerated in hospitalized older adults [55, 61, 62, 66]. Increased LOS worsens malnutrition and sarcopenia, creating a vicious cycle of disease severity, increased frequency and severity of complications, increasing LOS, and rehospitalization rates [62].

Due to their associated comorbid conditions, malnutrition and sarcopenia impose a major economic burden on healthcare systems, contributing to escalating healthcare costs. A study of hospitalized patients showed significantly increased costs in malnourished patients. The mean daily expense was $228.00 per malnourished patients versus $138.00 per well-nourished patients, a cost increase of 60.5%, after including costs for medications and tests, the cost to treat malnourished patients rose by 308.9% [53]. According to a British Association of Parenteral and Enteral Nutrition report, malnutrition in the UK costs in excess of £13 billion per year: £8 billion is for healthcare, including hospital inpatients and outpatients, and primary care (prescriptions and general medical services), and £5 billion is for nursing, residential, and home care services [67]. Additionally, sarcopenia significantly increases health care costs. A 2000 US study estimated that sarcopenia resulted in $18.5 billion dollars in direct health care expenditures, which reflected 1.5% of total healthcare expenditures. Moreover, a 10% reduction in sarcopenia prevalence would result in $1.1 billion US dollars in health care savings [68].

4. Screening and Assessing for Malnutrition Sarcopenia Syndrome

Clinicians should integrate nutrition assessment with sarcopenia screening for optimal evaluation of these two interrelated nutritional issues to help improve patients' clinical outcomes. A variety of malnutrition screening tools are available such as the Malnutrition Screening Tool (MST) [69], Malnutrition Universal Screening Tool (MUST) [70], the short form of the Mini-Nutritional Assessment (SF-MNA) [71] and Nutrition Risk Screening-2002 (NRS-2002) [72].

Table 2: The clinical signs and symptoms of Malnutrition-Sarcopenia Syndrome.

Malnutrition-Sarcopenia Syndrome	
Malnutrition	Sarcopenia
↓ Food intake	↓ Muscle mass
↓ Appetite	↓ Muscle strength and/or functionality
↓ Body weight	

A standard for nutritional assessment, the Subjective Global Assessment (SGA), is a valid and reliable method to assess nutritional status in a variety of patient populations [73]. The MNA is another reliable assessment tool validated for use with older adults in multiple settings [71, 74]. Elements of history and physical examination are commonly shared among these tools and include unintentional weight loss (e.g., 3 kg within the last 3 months), decreased food intake, gastrointestinal symptoms, and functional impairment. For sarcopenia screening, a simple clinician tool has been suggested by the European Geriatric Medical Society (EUGMS) Consensus Committee of defining sarcopenia (Figure 1), in which older adults are screened and assessed for sarcopenia using both gait speed and handgrip strength measurements [9, 75–77]. If a patient is identified to have slow gait speed or low hand grip strength, muscle mass should then be measured and evaluated. Based on the evidence presented, the combination of screening and assessing for malnutrition and sarcopenia is recommended to screen for the presence of MSS in at-risk patient populations, particularly older adults in clinical settings and in the community. The proposed clinical signs and symptoms to identify MSS are highlighted in Table 2. Specifically, to facilitate screening and assessment of MSS, we propose that patients would be at high risk for MSS if at least four of these criteria are present:

(1) recent history of reduced appetite that resulted in poor food intake,

(2) unintentional weight loss of 3 kg or more over the last 3 months,

(3) low muscle mass (as measured by DXA, CT, MRI, or BIA),

(4) decreased gait speed (less than 0.8 meter/second), and

(5) reduced hand grip strength for age and gender.

Future research is warranted to determine the reliability and validity of this assessment tool across patient populations and settings.

5. Conclusion

Malnutrition and sarcopenia are both commonly occurring conditions across patient populations, especially older adults. Both conditions result in numerous and substantial negative outcomes to both the patient and the health care system, including increased morbidity and mortality, decreased patient quality of life and functionality, and increased health care costs and rehospitalization rates. Historically, patients have been screened or assessed by healthcare practitioners for either malnutrition or sarcopenia, but rarely for both conditions concurrently. However, many patients present clinically with both conditions in parallel and this combination, or the malnutrition sarcopenia syndrome should be the focus of future nutrition screening and assessment in at-risk patient populations. Examining the entirety of the patient's nutritional and functional status through screening and assessment for both malnutrition and sarcopenia will enable healthcare practitioners to better determine the presence of MSS in their patients and target interventions to fit the patients' needs. Moreover, as the world is aging and older adults will utilize health care services at an increased rate, this could ultimately result in better patient care and outcomes in this unique and expanding patient population. Clinicians and researchers are called upon to work together to develop a practical, reliable, and valid tool for MSS that is appropriate for implementation into a variety of clinical practice settings, with the aim of identifying patients with MSS and providing the appropriately targeted interventions.

Acknowledgments

MFJV is a professor of geriatric medicine and a paid speaker and consultant to Abbott Nutrition. C. J. Alish, A. C. Sauer, and R. A. Hegazi are employees of Abbott Nutrition, Abbott Laboratories. The material presented in this paper is based on published clinical evidence and is not affected by any financial relationship.

References

[1] M. Elia and Malnutrition Advisory Group, *Guidelines for Detection and Management of Malnutrition*, BAPEN, Maidenhead, UK, 2000.

[2] R. J. Stratton, C. J. Green, and M. Elia, *Disease-Related Malnutrition: An Evidence-Based Approach to Treatment*, CABI, Wallingford, UK, 2003.

[3] G. L. Jensen, J. Mirtallo, C. Compher et al., "Adult starvation and disease-related malnutrition: a proposal for etiology-based diagnosis in the clinical practice setting from the International Consensus Guideline Committee," *Clinical Nutrition*, vol. 29, no. 2, pp. 151–153, 2010.

[4] R. H. Demling, "Nutrition, anabolism, and the wound healing process: an overview," *ePlasty*, vol. 9, pp. 65–94, 2009.

[5] R. R. Wolfe, "The underappreciated role of muscle in health and disease," *American Journal of Clinical Nutrition*, vol. 84, no. 3, pp. 475–482, 2006.

[6] J. J. McCarthy and K. A. Esser, "Anabolic and catabolic pathways regulating skeletal muscle mass," *Current Opinion in Clinical Nutrition and Metabolic Care*, vol. 13, no. 3, pp. 230–235, 2010.

[7] K. S. Nair, "Muscle protein turnover: methodological issues and the effect of aging," *Journals of Gerontology A*, vol. 50, pp. 107–112, 1995.

[8] I. H. Rosenberg, "Sarcopenia: origins and clinical relevance," *Journal of Nutrition*, vol. 127, no. 5, supplement, pp. 990S–991S, 1997.

[9] A. J. Cruz-Jentoft, J. P. Baeyens, J. M. Bauer et al., "Sarcopenia: European consensus on definition and diagnosis," *Age and Ageing*, vol. 39, no. 4, pp. 412–423, 2010.

[10] K. Norman, N. Stobäus, M. C. Gonzalez, J. D. Schulzke, and M. Pirlich, "Hand grip strength: outcome predictor and marker of nutritional status," *Clinical Nutrition*, vol. 30, no. 2, pp. 135–142, 2011.

[11] M. Pirlich, T. Schütz, K. Norman et al., "The German hospital malnutrition study," *Clinical Nutrition*, vol. 25, no. 4, pp. 563–572, 2006.

[12] M. Pirlich, T. Schütz, M. Kemps et al., "Social risk factors for hospital malnutrition," *Nutrition*, vol. 21, no. 3, pp. 295–300, 2005.

[13] S. Forster and S. Gariballa, "Age as a determinant of nutritional status: a cross sectional study," *Nutrition Journal*, vol. 4, article 28, 2005.

[14] L. C. P. G. M. de Groot, A. M. Beck, M. Schroll, and W. A. van Staveren, "Evaluating the DETERMINE your nutritional health checklist and the mini nutritional assessment as tools to identify nutritional problems in elderly Europeans," *European Journal of Clinical Nutrition*, vol. 52, no. 12, pp. 877–883, 1998.

[15] Y. Guigoz, "The Mini Nutritional Aseesment (MNA) review of the literature—what does it tell us?" *The Journal of Nutrition, Health & Aging*, vol. 10, no. 6, pp. 466–487, 2006.

[16] D. Paddon-Jones, *Lean Body Mass Loss With Age*, Abbott Nutrition, Columbus, Ohio, USA, 2009, Edited by: J. Gussler.

[17] A. B. Newman, J. S. Lee, M. Visser et al., "Weight change and the conservation of lean mass in old age: The Health, Aging and Body Composition Study," *American Journal of Clinical Nutrition*, vol. 82, no. 4, pp. 872–878, 2005.

[18] G. B. Forbes, "Longitudinal changes in adult fat-free mass: influence of body weight," *American Journal of Clinical Nutrition*, vol. 70, no. 6, pp. 1025–1031, 1999.

[19] M. Karlsson, J. Å. Nilsson, I. Sernbo, I. Redlund-Johnell, O. Johnell, and K. J. Obrant, "Changes of bone mineral mass and soft tissue composition after hip fracture," *Bone*, vol. 18, no. 1, pp. 19–22, 1996.

[20] F. Landi, R. Liperoti, A. Russo et al., "Sarcopenia as a risk factor for falls in elderly individuals: results from the ilSIRENTE study," *Clinical Nutrition*. In press.

[21] F. Landi, R. Liperoti, D. Fusco et al., "Prevalence and risk factors of sarcopenia among nursing home older residents," *Journals of Gerontology A*, vol. 67, pp. 48–55, 2012.

[22] I. Janssen, S. B. Heymsfield, and R. Ross, "Low relative skeletal muscle mass (sarcopenia) in older persons is associated with functional impairment and physical disability," *Journal of the American Geriatrics Society*, vol. 50, no. 5, pp. 889–896, 2002.

[23] T. Cederholm, C. Jagren, and K. Hellstrom, "Outcome of protein-energy malnutrition in elderly medical patients," *American Journal of Medicine*, vol. 98, no. 1, pp. 67–74, 1995.

[24] A. B. Newman, D. Yanez, T. Harris, A. Duxbury, P. L. Enright, and L. P. Fried, "Weight change in old age and its association with mortality," *Journal of the American Geriatrics Society*, vol. 49, no. 10, pp. 1309–1318, 2001.

[25] J. I. Wallace, R. S. Schwartz, A. Z. LaCroix, R. F. Uhlmann, and R. A. Pearlman, "Involuntary weight loss in older outpatients: incidence and clinical significance," *Journal of the American Geriatrics Society*, vol. 43, no. 4, pp. 329–337, 1995.

[26] D. F. Williamson and E. R. Pamuk, "The association between weight loss and increased longevity: a review of the evidence," *Annals of Internal Medicine*, vol. 119, no. 7, pp. 731–736, 1993.

[27] S. A. French, A. R. Folsom, R. W. Jeffery, and D. F. Williamson, "Prospective study of intentionality of weight loss and mortality in older women: The Iowa Women's Health Study," *American Journal of Epidemiology*, vol. 149, no. 6, pp. 504–514, 1999.

[28] J. L. Locher, D. L. Roth, C. S. Ritchie et al., "Body mass index, weight loss, and mortality in community-dwelling older adults," *Journals of Gerontology A*, vol. 62, no. 12, pp. 1389–1392, 2007.

[29] E. Cereda, C. Pedrolli, A. Zagami et al., "Body mass index and mortality in institutionalized elderly," *Journal of the American Medical Directors Association*, vol. 12, no. 3, pp. 174–178, 2011.

[30] S. S. Han, K. W. Kim, K. I. Kim et al., "Lean mass index: a better predictor of mortality than body mass index in elderly Asians," *Journal of the American Geriatrics Society*, vol. 58, no. 2, pp. 312–317, 2010.

[31] F. Landi, R. Liperoti, D. Fusco et al., "Sarcopenia and mortality among older nursing home residents," *Journal of the American Medical Directors Association*, vol. 13, no. 2, pp. 121–126, 2011.

[32] D. Bunout, M. P. de la Maza, G. Barrera, L. Leiva, and S. Hirsch, "Association between sarcopenia and mortality in healthy older people," *Australasian Journal on Ageing*, vol. 30, no. 2, pp. 89–92, 2011.

[33] R. Cooper, D. Kuh, and R. Hardy, "Objectively measured physical capability levels and mortality: systematic review and meta-analysis," *British Medical Journal*, vol. 341, Article ID c4467, 2010.

[34] E. M. Castillo, D. Goodman-Gruen, D. Kritz-Silverstein, D. J. Morton, D. L. Wingard, and E. Barrett-Connor, "Sarcopenia in elderly men and women: The Rancho Bernardo Study," *American Journal of Preventive Medicine*, vol. 25, no. 3, pp. 226–231, 2003.

[35] I. Janssen, "Influence of sarcopenia on the development of physical disability: The Cardiovascular Health Study," *Journal of the American Geriatrics Society*, vol. 54, no. 1, pp. 56–62, 2006.

[36] S. M. Schneider, P. Veyres, X. Pivot et al., "Malnutrition is an independent factor associated with nosocomial infections," *British Journal of Nutrition*, vol. 92, no. 1, pp. 105–111, 2004.

[37] J. Edington, J. Boorman, E. R. Durrant et al., "Prevalence of malnutrition on admission to four hospitals in England," *Clinical Nutrition*, vol. 19, no. 3, pp. 191–195, 2000.

[38] G. Cosquëric, A. Sebag, C. Ducolombier, C. Thomas, F. Piette, and S. Weill-Engerer, "Sarcopenia is predictive of nosocomial infection in care of the elderly," *British Journal of Nutrition*, vol. 96, no. 5, pp. 895–901, 2006.

[39] A. Vivanti, N. Ward, and T. Haines, "Nutritional status and associations with falls, balance, mobility and functionality during hospital admission," *The Journal of Nutrition, Health & Aging*, vol. 15, no. 5, pp. 388–391, 2011.

[40] S. A. Neumann, M. D. Miller, L. Daniels, and M. Crotty, "Nutritional status and clinical outcomes of older patients in rehabilitation," *Journal of Human Nutrition and Dietetics*, vol. 18, no. 2, pp. 129–136, 2005.

[41] J. Potter, K. Klipstein, J. J. Reilly, and M. Roberts, "The nutritional status and clinical course of acute admissions to a geriatric unit," *Age and Ageing*, vol. 24, no. 2, pp. 131–136, 1995.

[42] R. Muhlethaler, A. E. Stuck, C. E. Minder, and B. M. Frey, "The prognostic significance of protein-energy malnutrition in geriatric patients," *Age and Ageing*, vol. 24, no. 3, pp. 193–197, 1995.

[43] M. Lumbers, L. T. Driver, R. J. Howland, M. W. J. Older, and C. M. Williams, "Nutritional status and clinical outcome

in elderly female surgical orthopaedic patients," *Clinical Nutrition*, vol. 15, no. 3, pp. 101–107, 1996.

[44] T. M. Gill, H. G. Allore, T. R. Holford, and Z. Guo, "Hospitalization, restricted activity, and the development of disability among older persons," *Journal of the American Medical Association*, vol. 292, no. 17, pp. 2115–2124, 2004.

[45] M. M. Suesada, M. A. Martins, and C. R. Carvalho, "Effect of short-term hospitalization on functional capacity in patients not restricted to bed," *American Journal of Physical Medicine and Rehabilitation*, vol. 86, no. 6, pp. 455–462, 2007.

[46] T. Lang, T. Streeper, P. Cawthon, K. Baldwin, D. R. Taaffe, and T. B. Harris, "Sarcopenia: etiology, clinical consequences, intervention, and assessment," *Osteoporosis International*, vol. 21, no. 4, pp. 543–559, 2010.

[47] M. Visser, B. H. Goodpaster, S. B. Kritchevsky et al., "Muscle mass, muscle strength, and muscle fat infiltration as predictors of incident mobility limitations in well-functioning older persons," *Journals of Gerontology A*, vol. 60, no. 3, pp. 324–333, 2005.

[48] W. J. Evans, "Effects of exercise on body composition and functional capacity of the elderly," *Journals of Gerontology A*, vol. 50, pp. 147–150, 1995.

[49] K. F. Reid, E. N. Naumova, R. J. Carabello, E. M. Phillips, and R. A. Fielding, "Lower extremity muscle mass predicts functional performance in mobility-limited elders," *The Journal of Nutrition, Health & Aging*, vol. 12, no. 7, pp. 493–498, 2008.

[50] W. R. Frontera, D. Suh, L. S. Krivickas, V. A. Hughes, R. Goldstein, and R. Roubenoff, "Skeletal muscle fiber quality in older men and women," *American Journal of Physiology*, vol. 279, no. 3, pp. C611–C618, 2000.

[51] J. E. Morley, A. M. Abbatecola, J. M. Argiles et al., "Sarcopenia with limited mobility: an international consensus," *Journal of the American Medical Directors Association*, vol. 12, pp. 403–409, 2011.

[52] J. Dzieniszewski, M. Jarosz, B. Szczygieł et al., "Nutritional status of patients hospitalised in Poland," *European Journal of Clinical Nutrition*, vol. 59, no. 4, pp. 552–560, 2005.

[53] M. I. Correia and D. L. Waitzberg, "The impact of malnutrition on morbidity, mortality, length of hospital stay and costs evaluated through a multivariate model analysis," *Clinical Nutrition*, vol. 22, no. 3, pp. 235–239, 2003.

[54] M. Suominen, S. Muurinen, P. Routasalo et al., "Malnutrition and associated factors among aged residents in all nursing homes in Helsinki," *European Journal of Clinical Nutrition*, vol. 59, no. 4, pp. 578–583, 2005.

[55] V. A. Leandro-Merhi, J. L. de Aquino, and J. F. Sales Chagas, "Nutrition status and risk factors associated with length of hospital stay for surgical patients," *Journal of Parenteral and Enteral Nutrition*, vol. 35, no. 2, pp. 241–248, 2011.

[56] C. S. Chima, K. Barco, M. L. Dewitt, M. Maeda, J. C. Teran, and K. D. Mullen, "Relationship of nutritional status to length of stay, hospital costs, and discharge status of patients hospitalized in the medicine service," *Journal of the American Dietetic Association*, vol. 97, no. 9, pp. 975–978, 1997.

[57] D. H. Sullivan and R. C. Walls, "Protein-energy undernutrition and the risk of mortality within six years of hospital discharge," *Journal of the American College of Nutrition*, vol. 17, no. 6, pp. 571–578, 1998.

[58] N. Allaudeen, A. Vidyarthi, J. Maselli, and A. Auerbach, "Redefining readmission risk factors for general medicine patients," *Journal of Hospital Medicine*, vol. 6, no. 2, pp. 54–60, 2011.

[59] A. M. Mudge, K. Kasper, A. Clair et al., "Recurrent readmissions in medical patients: a prospective study," *Journal of Hospital Medicine*, vol. 6, no. 2, pp. 61–67, 2011.

[60] J. Edington, J. Boorman, E. R. Durrant et al., "Prevalence of malnutrition on admission to four hospitals in England," *Clinical Nutrition*, vol. 19, no. 3, pp. 191–195, 2000.

[61] P. M. Cawthon, K. M. Fox, S. R. Gandra et al., "Do muscle mass, muscle density, strength, and physical function similarly influence risk of hospitalization in older adults?" *Journal of the American Geriatrics Society*, vol. 57, no. 8, pp. 1411–1419, 2009.

[62] D. E. Alley, A. Koster, D. MacKey et al., "Hospitalization and change in body composition and strength in a population-based cohort of older persons," *Journal of the American Geriatrics Society*, vol. 58, no. 11, pp. 2085–2091, 2010.

[63] L. Ferrucci, J. M. Guralnik, M. Pahor, M. C. Corti, and R. J. Havlik, "Hospital diagnoses, medicare charges, and nursing home admissions in the year when older persons become severely disabled," *Journal of the American Medical Association*, vol. 277, no. 9, pp. 728–734, 1997.

[64] M. A. Sager, T. Franke, S. K. Inouye et al., "Functional outcomes of acute medical illness and hospitalization in older persons," *Archives of Internal Medicine*, vol. 156, no. 6, pp. 645–652, 1996.

[65] C. Pichard, U. G. Kyle, A. Morabia, A. Perrier, B. Vermeulen, and P. Unger, "Nutritional assessment: lean body mass depletion at hospital admission is associated with an increased length of stay," *American Journal of Clinical Nutrition*, vol. 79, no. 4, pp. 613–618, 2004.

[66] P. Kortebein, A. Ferrando, J. Lombeida, R. Wolfe, and W. J. Evans, "Effect of 10 days of bed rest on skeletal muscle in healthy older adults," *Journal of the American Medical Association*, vol. 297, no. 16, pp. 1772–1774, 2007.

[67] M. Elia and C. A. Russell, "Combating malnutrition: recommendations for action. Report From the Advisory Group on Malnutrition," Led By BAPEN; Output of a meeting of the Advisory Group on Malnutrition, 12 June 2008.

[68] I. Janssen, D. S. Shepard, P. T. Katzmarzyk, and R. Roubenoff, "The healthcare costs of sarcopenia in the United States," *Journal of the American Geriatrics Society*, vol. 52, no. 1, pp. 80–85, 2004.

[69] M. Ferguson, S. Capra, J. Bauer, and M. Banks, "Development of a valid and reliable malnutrition screening tool for adult acute hospital patients," *Nutrition*, vol. 15, no. 6, pp. 458–464, 1999.

[70] M. Elia, *Screening for Malnutrition: A Multidisciplinary Responsibility. Development and Use of the 'Malnutrition Universal Screening Tool' ('MUST') for Adults*, BAPEN, Worcestershire, UK, 2003.

[71] Y. Guigoz, S. Lauque, and B. J. Vellas, "Identifying the elderly at risk for malnutrition the mini nutritional assessment," *Clinics in Geriatric Medicine*, vol. 18, no. 4, pp. 737–757, 2002.

[72] J. Kondrup, H. H. Ramussen, O. Hamberg et al., "Nutritional risk screening (NRS 2002): a new method based on an analysis of controlled clinical trials," *Clinical Nutrition*, vol. 22, no. 3, pp. 321–336, 2003.

[73] H. M. Kruizenga, M. W. Van Tulder, J. C. Seidell, A. Thijs, H. J. Ader, and M. A. van Bokhorst-de van der Schueren, "Effectiveness and cost-effectiveness of early screening and treatment of malnourished patients," *American Journal of Clinical Nutrition*, vol. 82, no. 5, pp. 1082–1089, 2005.

[74] M. J. Kaiser, J. M. Bauer, C. Rämsch et al., "Frequency of malnutrition in older adults: a multinational perspective using the mini nutritional assessment," *Journal of the American Geriatrics Society*, vol. 58, no. 9, pp. 1734–1738, 2010.

[75] D. M. Buchner, E. B. Larson, E. H. Wagner, T. D. Koepsell, and B. J. de Lateur, "Evidence for a non-linear relationship between leg strength and gait speed," *Age and Ageing*, vol. 25, no. 5, pp. 386–391, 1996.

[76] H. C. Roberts, H. J. Denison, H. J. Martin et al., "A review of the measurement of grip strength in clinical and epidemiological studies: towards a standardised approach," *Age and Ageing*, vol. 40, no. 4, pp. 423–429, 2011.

[77] A. J. Cruz-Jentoft, F. Landi, E. Topinková, and J. P. Michel, "Understanding sarcopenia as a geriatric syndrome," *Current Opinion in Clinical Nutrition and Metabolic Care*, vol. 13, no. 1, pp. 1–7, 2010.

6

Efficacy of a Multimodal Cognitive Rehabilitation Including Psychomotor and Endurance Training in Parkinson's Disease

I. Reuter,[1] S. Mehnert,[1] G. Sammer,[2] M. Oechsner,[3] and M. Engelhardt[4]

[1] *Department of Neurology, Justus-Liebig University, Klinikstraße 33, 35392 Giessen, Germany*
[2] *Department of Psychiatry, Cognitive Laboratory Justus-Liebig University, Am Steg 22, 35385 Giessen, Germany*
[3] *Neurologisches Rehabilitationszentrum, HELIOS Klinik Zihlschlacht AG, Hauptstrße 2-4, 8588 Zihlschlacht, Switzerland*
[4] *Department of Orthopedic Surgery, Klinikum Osnabrück, Am Finkenhügel 1, 49076 Osnabrück, Germany*

Correspondence should be addressed to I. Reuter, iris.reuter@neuro.med.uni-giessen.de

Academic Editor: Alice Nieuwboer

Mild cognitive impairment, especially executive dysfunction might occur early in the course of Parkinson's disease. Cognitive training is thought to improve cognitive performance. However, transfer of improvements achieved in paper and pencil tests into daily life has been difficult. The aim of the current study was to investigate whether a multimodal cognitive rehabilitation programme including physical exercises might be more successful than cognitive training programmes without motor training. 240 PD-patients were included in the study and randomly allocated to three treatment arms, group A cognitive training, group B cognitive training and transfer training and group C cognitive training, transfer training and psychomotor and endurance training. The primary outcome measure was the ADAS-Cog. The secondary outcome measure was the SCOPA-Cog. Training was conducted for 4 weeks on a rehabilitation unit, followed by 6 months training at home. Caregivers received an education programme. The combination of cognitive training using paper and pencil and the computer, transfer training and physical training seems to have the greatest effect on cognitive function. Thus, patients of group C showed the greatest improvement on the ADAS-Cog and SCOPA-COG and were more likely to continue with the training programme after the study.

1. Introduction

Idiopathic Parkinson's disease (PD) is a neurodegenerative disorder characterized by loss of dopaminergic neurons and basal ganglia dysfunction. The prevalence of PD increases with age and is estimated in 100–200/100000 people [1, 2] worldwide. The clinical hallmarks of PD are akinesia, rigidity, and tremor [3, 4]. However, a spectrum of nonmotor symptoms occurs in Parkinson's disease. One of the most disabling symptoms is dementia, which is common among patients with PD with an average prevalence of 40% in cross-sectional studies and a cumulative prevalence approaching 80% [5, 6]. PD dementia is the third most common reason for dementia and is associated with rapid functional and motor decline, shortened survival [7], greater sensitivity to medication, higher risk of developing psychosis, reduced quality of life for both patients [8] and caregivers [9], increased caregivers' stress, and frequent transfer to nursing homes [10]. Clinical characteristics of PD dementia are cognitive slowing, executive deficits, visuospatial deficits, and memory impairments [11]. Pathological findings include Lewy bodies outside the substantia nigra, neurofibrillary tangles, and amyloid plaques [12]. Neurochemically, cholinergic deficits are found to be the most consistent associated with cognitive and neuropsychiatric symptoms [13].

In contrast to dementia, mild cognitive impairment (MCI) might occur early in the course of PD. Approximately, a quarter of PD-patients without dementia have mild cognitive impairment (PD-MCI). The Movement Disorder Society commissioned task force reported that MCI in PD is associated with increasing age, increasing disease duration, and disease severity [14]. However, 20% of PD-patients might have MCI at the time of diagnosis [15]. The clinical profile of PD-MCI is heterogeneous with a range of cognitive domains affected. Nonamnestic, single-domain impairment is the most common subtype of PD-MCI [14]. Criteria for the diagnosis of PD-MCI have been published recently [14]. Neuropsychological testing should include two tests within each of the five cognitive domains (attention, working memory, executive language, memory, and visuospatial). A diagnosis of PD-MCI impairment has to be found either in two neuropsychological tests in one domain or one impaired test in two different domains. Components of the executive systems are attention (focusing on relevant information), selective visual attention, inhibition (inhibition of irrelevant information) [15], overcoming of strong habitual responses or resisting temptation [16], task and time management, monitoring and coding of information for processing in the working memory, flexibility, set maintenance, and set shifting. The executive system can be viewed as a manager enabling the adaptation of the perceptive, cognitive, and motor system to new tasks [17]. Thus, patients with impaired executive functions face many difficulties in everyday life. They have a low attention span, difficulties in problem solving and decision making, in dual tasking, in set shifting, in visuospatial tasks, in adaptation to new tasks, and even in verbal learning and delayed recall. For example, PD-patients with impairment of executive functions may have difficulties in simultaneously driving a car and searching for a street or in keeping appointments. Executive dysfunctions also affect social components and the interaction with other people [15]. Patients are reported of being more irritable and having difficulties in suppressing inappropriate behaviour. PD-patients with MCI might have a higher risk to develop PD dementia. There is some evidence from previous studies that the presence of a nonamnestic single-domain MCI- subtype, executive deficits, impaired verbal fluency, visuospatial deficits, memory and language dysfunction predict PD-dementia, since patients with mild cognitive impairment have a higher risk of developing dementia. Intervention at an early stage of cognitive decline and prevention of the progress from MCI to dementia would be desirable. While treatment of motor symptoms has largely improved, treatment of cognitive dysfunction is still limited. Acetylcholine esterase inhibitors improve cognitive functioning only in some patients. Furthermore, transfer of improvements in cognitive training into activities of daily living has been extremely difficult. There is a large body of studies on animals and humans in the literature showing positive effects of exercise and sports on cognition [18–23]. Several studies suggest an enhancement of cortical plasticity by exercise [24, 25]. Executive functioning [19, 20, 26] as well as quality of daily living [27, 28] was found to be improved by aerobic endurance exercise. Patients, who complain of cognitive problems, suffer more often from cognitive deficits than patients without complaints [29]. Therefore, these patients should be offered neuropsychological testing. We have chosen a comprehensive training approach and designed a study using a multimodal cognitive training to improve cognitive functions.

The aim of the present study was to compare the effect of a multimodal cognitive training regime including paper and pencil tasks combined with transfer tasks and a psychomotor training with a cognitive training based on paper and pencil tasks only and a cognitive training consisting of various tasks requiring executive functions combined with transfer tasks.

2. Methods

2.1. Subjects. 240 patients, men and women who were between 50 and 80 years old and who had received a diagnosis of Parkinson's disease according to the UK brain bank criteria [4], were recruited for the study at the Hospital for Parkinson's Disease Bad Nauheim. Patients had been admitted at the hospital for rehabilitation. The presence of MCI was required for inclusion into the study. MCI was diagnosed when (a) patients complained of cognitive decline, preferably corroborated by a reliable source, (b) minimal effect on day-to-day functioning and the absence of dementia, and (c) presence of cognitive abnormalities which cannot be simply attributed to age. Exclusion criteria were severe concomitant diseases, which limit physical performances, a second neurodegenerative disease, and lack of motivation to improve cognitive deficits and the presence of dementia. De novo patients and those who had undergone surgery for DBS were not included into the study. All patients were assessed by a movement disorder specialist. Medical treatment was optimised prior to the study. It was aimed at keeping medication stable during the study.

2.2. Design. The study was divided into two periods. Patients were enrolled into the study during an in-patient stay on a rehabilitation ward. The first part of the study (4 weeks) took place on the rehabilitation unit with a supervised cognitive training conducted by physiotherapists, occupational therapists, and two neuropsychologists.

Patients were randomly allocated to one of the three training groups. Randomisation was conducted by using a computer-generated sequence. All groups received a cognitive training regime using paper and pencil material and a multimedial PC training. Group A received cognitive training only, while group B took part in a transfer training and a cognitive training. Group C conducted a cognitive training, and transfer and psychomotor trainings. Patients of group A and B had additional relaxation training and occupational training without transfer training to compensate for the additional training time of group C.

After randomisation medical history was taken, patients underwent medical and neurological assessments and were asked about their cognitive difficulties. They identified cognitive deficits that they want to improve. Severity of Parkinson's disease was assessed by using the Unified Parkinson's Disease Rating Scale (UPDRS) [30].

Demographic data included information about age, body mass index (BMI), duration of disease, weekly sports activity, smoking habits, medication and concomitant diseases (hypertension, chronic obstructive pulmonary disease, thyroid disease, diabetes mellitus, hypercholesterinaemia, and osteoarthritis), education, profession, family, onset and severity of disease, history of psychosis, and impairments in daily living. Patients kept an activity log one week prior to the training programme and one week prior to the third assessment. Sports activities, time spent sitting, and doing light, moderate, and heavy work were recorded. The ethical committee of the Justus-Liebig University has approved the study and all patients have given written informed consent. Figure 1 shows the study design.

2.3. Scales Used for Neurological and Neuropsychological Assessment of PD. For the assessment of the longitudinal course of the disease, the Unified Parkinson's disease rating scale (UPDRS) was applied [30].

For the assessment of the goals of the cognitive training, the Goal Attainment Scale was chosen. The Goal Attainment Scaling (GAS) was used to define individual realistic and feasible goals according to patients' needs and expectations. The cognitive difficulties of the patients were assessed and the results of the baseline test were explained to the patients. In this study, GAS was measured using a 6-point Likert scale −3 represented function that is worse than at the start of treatment, −2 no change, −1 some improvement without meeting the expected goal, 0 represented goal achievement and +1 or +2 overachievement (exceeding the defined therapeutic goal) [31].

2.3.1. Neuropsychological Tests. At the beginning of the study, all patients underwent two cognitive screening tests (PANDA and MMSE) [32, 33], followed by a detailed cognitive test battery including the ADAS-COG subscale and the SCOPA-COG as primary and secondary outcome measures, respectively. The neuropsychological assessment was repeated after the 4-week inpatient stay and after the 6-month training at home.

2.3.2. ADAS-COG (Alzheimer Assessment Scale Cognition). Although the ADAS-COG is the primary outcome measure in many clinical trials [34, 35], it is not a specific test for cognitive impairment in Parkinson's Disease. The scale was chosen as primary outcome measure in the current study, because it was the primary outcome measure in earlier trials assessing effects of medication on cognitive function in PD [6]. The study by Emre et al. [6] gave an estimate regarding the relevance of a 3-point improvement on the ADAS-COG in PD. Thus, it was possible to relate the results of the current study to previous results.

The conceptual framework underlying the ADAS-COG is to identify three reproducible factors: memory, language, and praxis [35]. The ADAS-COG score ranges in total from 0 to 70 points with higher scores indicating greater impairment.

2.3.3. SCOPA-COG (Scales for Outcome of Parkinson's Disease-Cognition). The SCOPA-COG is an instrument which was designed to assess the specific cognitive deficits found in Parkinson's disease [36]. The scale consisting of 10 items covers the following domains: memory and recall (verbal recall, digit span backward, and indicate cubes), attention (counting backward, months backward), executive function (fist-edge-palm, semantic fluency, and dice), visual-spatial functions (assembly pattern), and memory (delayed recall). The score ranges from 0 to 43 points with higher scores reflecting better performance.

2.3.4. Additional Tests. Since PD-patients show pronounced deficits in executive functions additional tests for evaluation of executive functions were conducted at baseline, second and final assessment: Information processing speed (Paced auditory serial addition test (PASAT) [37]), Executive function (Behavioural assessment of the dysexecutive syndrome (BADS) [38]), Test for premorbid performance (Mehrfach-Wortschatz-Test (MWT-B) Multiple choice word test [39]), Assessment of mood and anxiety (Hospital anxiety and depression scale was applied [40]).

2.3.5. Health-Related Quality of Life (Parkinson's Disease Questionnaire 39 (PDQ-39)). For assessment of health-related quality of life, patients filled in the PDQ-39 [41]. It consists of 8 subscales. The sum score of raw data ranges from 0 to 156 points, with high scores indicating lower health-related quality of life. For better comparison of the results, raw data were transformed and expressed in percentages of maximal possible sum score.

The assessments were performed by psychologists and movement disorders specialists who were blinded to the treatment allocation of the patients.

2.4. Training Programmes. Patients performed the training programmes in onstage and after optimisation of the medication. Dopaminergic deficits may affect the performance of patients in cognitive and physical exercises [42, 43].

2.4.1. Cognitive Training. The cognitive training programme was individually tailored to patients' requirements based on the results of the baseline tests. Four individual (one-to-one) 60 min-lessons took place each week. All patients received at least 14 cognitive training sessions.

The training included training of attention, concentration, biographical work, reasoning, memory, working memory, social rules, anticipation, cognitive information speed, prospective memory, cognitive estimation, problem solving, sequencing and planning, associations, and coping with disease.

For the training programme, a set of tasks requiring executive and memory functions was chosen from a variety of specific tests. Executive tasks of the BADS, which were not used for the baseline assessment, were included in the training. Simple patterns of the "Raven's Progressive Matrices" were used to establish problem solving strategies in the patients. Picture arrangement tasks, picture completion tasks, block design, and object assembly were adapted from the "Wechsler Intelligence test for children." For improvement of verbal fluency, patients were encouraged to tell short stories or discuss short text passages. Photos were used for training of working memory. Tasks including visual search and rule finding were practised by using a PC-based programme. The training methods were designed to improve the various cognitive deficits, diagnosed at baseline, and focused on the executive functions. Task difficulty was adapted to the individual performance level of the patients. Table 1 shows the content of the cognitive training and the percentage of time spent with different tasks.

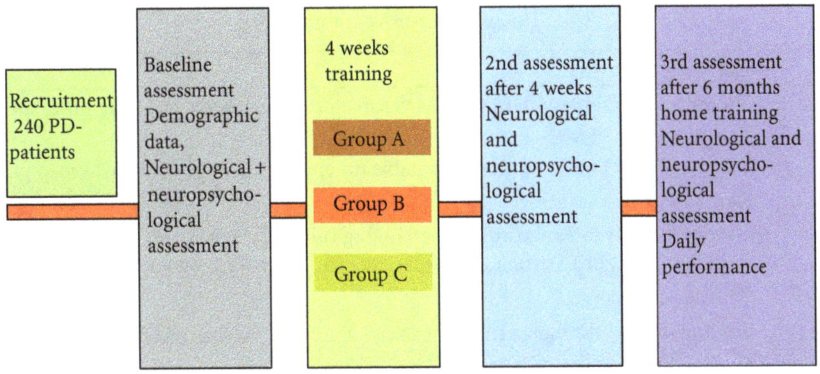

Figure 1: Study design group A: Cognitive training; group B: Cognitive + transfer training, group C: Cognitive, transfer + motor training.

2.4.2. Transfer Training. The aim of the training was to support patients to manage their daily life better and to become more self-confident. Therefore, patients were asked to practise competence in tasks of daily routines. The transfer training programme was composed according to the baseline test results. Special preferences of the patients were considered. The transfer training included training of concentration, use of mnemonics, strategy (planning), navigational skills, impulse control, decision processes, listening training and memory, behaviour, calculating, handling of money, summarising of articles read or heard, and decision making. Typical tasks were to find the way to the supermarket or to prepare a meal, to go to the bank, pay a bill, and to use mnemonics. Patients had to look after a vegetable patch and some flowers to improve prospective memory. For better evaluation of the training, tasks were allocated to different categories: concentration, strategy, orientation, planning, and the use of mnemonic devices. The training took place 3 times a week, each lasted 90 min. Patients received at least 10 sessions of transfer training (Table 2).

2.4.3. Motor Training. Group C performed a motor training resembling motor skill training or psychomotor training applied in children. The training included games and tasks designed to enhance inhibitory control, working memory, attention, visuospatial abilities, and planning and motor skills [44–47]. The training should also improve coordination, strength, speed, perception, and orientation. Patients should improve perception of their body. The therapeutic approach was based on individual capabilities and needs. Patients learned to perform motor sequences, dual tasking (walking and bouncing or throwing a ball), and spatial orientation tasks (finding items, remember hidden items). They walked through a parcours with obstacles following changing rules in order to improve anticipation and mental flexibility. For improvement of time estimation and movement performance mental imagery was used. Patients had to follow the guidance of the physiotherapist given by touch at different parts of the body. In addition, an aerobic training which should be of benefit for executive functions was performed. The training was conducted partly outdoors with inclusion of Nordic walking in summer. In winter patients walked on a treadmill. The training included at least 10, maximal 12 sessions each lasting 60 minutes.

2.5. Education of Caregivers. A long lasting training effect depends on continuing training. Thus, cognitive training and exercises need to be adapted to the home environment. Accordingly, the caregivers most often the patients' family were included into the programme. The education for the caregivers consisted of 5 modules: information about Parkinson's disease, psychological aspects and the role of a caregiver, information about help aids, information on care management, assessment of individual problems, support in cognitive (all groups) and transfer training (groups A and B), NW and movement skill training. Course instructors were a specialist nurse, a physiotherapist and a psychologist.

Phase II Continuation of Training at Home. Corresponding to the allocation to the training groups patients got written instructions for the cognitive training, transfer training, and physical exercises at home. The instructions encompassed a collection of the tasks conducted during the stay at the hospital. Caregivers were advised how to organise the training but the hospital staff did not organise the training at home. All patients were asked to perform three 45 min cognitive training sessions per week using paper, pencil, and a computer programme. Patients of groups B and C were asked to continue with two transfer trainings per week and patients of group C got instructions to conduct movement skill training and aerobic training lessons twice a week. To compensate for the additional physical training of group C, patients of group A and B were provided with prescriptions for relaxation training.

2.6. Evaluation of the Training. All patients were tested using a neuropsychological test battery at three time points: prior to the training, and prior to discharge to assess the short-term effect, and 6 months after the training to assess the long-term effect.

Caregivers were asked regarding their own well being and regarding the cognitive competence of the patients in activities of daily living. Patients and caregivers kept a diary

Table 1: Cognitive training.

Training section	Examples for tasks
Planning strategies	Shopping lists, key search of the BADS subscales, to get items out of a bottle, special wooden 3-dimensional jig saw
Mnemonics	Using memory hooks, writing of suitable mnemonics, and planning where to place them
Decision making	Computer tasks, painting
Set shifting	To solve various tasks according to changing rules, to calculate for 5 min, then to read for 10 min and to write for 5 min, or to switch tasks after every third answer, categorising items according to different rules
Calculation	Calculation tasks
Navigational skills	Finding the way through a maze on a screen, finding the way around obstacles on a paper or on a screen
Information speed processing	Connecting numbers or letters, connecting figures to an image, and finding the meaning of a fictive word
Summary	Extracting the relevant information from news or from a story or a short movie
Concentration	Finding similar or dissimilar items

Table 2: Transfer training.

Tasks	Examples
Planning and sequencing	Preparing of meals, shopping, construction of items, repairing of items, and art works
Reasoning	Finding the right solution, using deductive strategies, finding a way by incomplete instructions, to find out how things work, and use of unfamiliar tools
Concentration	Sorting and selection tasks, to fit small items, to build a model of a castle, knitting and weaving patterns, jig saw, to listen to a story and to press a button, when a previously identified word was read
Memory	Role play, music performance, singing, and learning poems
Working memory	Games, n-back tasks, dual tasks like driving on a driving simulator and listening to the news, calculating during walking, to follow complex instructions, and to extract the necessary information out of a long text
Anticipation	Walking on a crowded sidewalk, watching a movie and predict what people will do next, finish a picture story, and decipher the mood of people on pictures
Pospective memory	To look after a vegetable patch and flowers, to keep appointments, and to take over special tasks at the beginning of the week
Cognitive information speed	Follow verbal instructions given with increasing content of information and speed, card games, and complex reaction tasks
Social rules	Define the appropriate behaviour in different situations, role play,
Association	Solving tasks by association, finding common features, and categorisation
Cognitive estimation	Estimation of height, quantity of items shown, and weight

to record training lesions. The diaries were collected and analysed at the 3rd assessment.

2.7. Statistical Analysis. Statistical analysis was conducted using IBM SPSS Statistics 18.0 (IBM, Somers, USA) statistical software. Formal power analysis was performed prior to the study. The power analysis was based on an improvement of the ADAS-COG by 3 points. The results indicated that a sample size of 60 subjects per group was sufficient. Since comprehensive training programmes including several assessments imply dropouts, a drop-out rate of 20% was taken into account. Demographic data on ordinal level were analysed by using a nonparametric test (Kruskall-Wallis). The Kruskall-Wallis test was also applied for the analysis of depression and the BADS subscales. Demographic continuous data were analysed by using One-way ANOVA. Linear model for repeated measures was used for analysis of training outcomes. The repeated measure analysis provides information about "between and within subjects" effects. Within subject effects give information about training effects over the assessment period. Linear trends showed if there was a systematic change of training effects over time. The interaction between groups and the linear trend of days (assessments) provided information about the difference in the rate of improvement between groups. The between subject factor compared the overall treatment effect between the groups. Post hoc analysis was done using Bonferroni tests. Parametric data were tested for normal distribution by using the Kolmogorov-Smirnov test. Significance level was set at 0.05.

3. Results

General Results, Demographic Data and Accomplishment of the Training. In total 223 patients (97.1%) completed the programme during the in-patient stay in the hospital: 71 (90%) patients in group A, 75 (93.8%) in group B, and 76 (95%) patients in group C. The patients were on average 64 ± 4 years old and that 8 years diagnosed with PD. The patients did not differ significantly in demographic data (Table 3).

TABLE 3: Demographic data.

	Group A $N = 71$			Group B $N = 75$			Group C $N = 76$		
Gender	F = 35		M = 36	F = 36		M = 39	F = 36		M = 40
Duration of PD (months) ∅± SD		98 ± 8			95 ± 9			100 ± 6	
Stage (Hoehn and Yahr)									
II		$N = 7$			$N = 6$			$N = 10$	
III		$N = 55$			$N = 59$			$N = 58$	
IV		$N = 9$			$N = 10$			$N = 8$	
Medication									
L-Dopa		Yes: $N = 68$			Yes: $N = 64$			Yes: $N = 59$	
Dopamine agonist		Yes: $N = 53$			Yes: $N = 56$			Yes: $N = 59$	
MA0 inhibitor		$N = 43$			$N = 38$			$N = 43$	
COMT inhibitor		$N = 33$			$N = 31$			$N = 34$	
Antidepressants		$N = 7$			$N = 8$			$N = 8$	
Neuroleptic drugs		$N = 5$			$N = 8$			$N = 7$	
Formal education (years) ∅± SD		10 ± 1.2			11 ± 0.6			11 ± 1.0	
Marital status m = married, s = single, and p = partner	m = 58	s = 9	p = 5	m = 61	s = 11	p = 3	m = 63	s = 9	p = 4
Home (own home, renting)	Own: $N = 40$		Renting: $N = 32$	Own: $N = 43$		Renting; $N = 32$	Own: $N = 40$		Renting: $N = 36$
BMI ∅± SD		27.5 ± 4			26.8 ± 7			27.2 ± 3	
Smoking	Yes: $N = 7$		No: $N = 65$	Yes: $N = 10$		No: $N = 65$	Yes: $N = 9$		No: $N = 67$
Sports activities (min)/week ∅± SD		155 ± 17			163 ± 25			147 ± 17	
Physical work h/week ∅± SD									
Very hard		8.5 ± 2.6			9.2 ± 2.8			9.8 ± 2.1	
Hard		15.5 ± 4.5			14.9 ± 5			15.1 ± 5.5	
Comorbidity									
Coronary heart disease		$N = 7$			$N = 6$			$N = 8$	
Hypertension		$N = 32$			$N = 33$			$N = 36$	
Diabetes mellitus		$N = 7$			$N = 10$			$N = 8$	
COPD		$N = 5$			$N = 6$			$N = 9$	
Thyroid disease		$N = 12$			$N = 10$			$N = 11$	
Hypercholesterinaemia		$N = 36$			$N = 32$			$N = 27$	
Osteoarthritis		$N = 27$			$N = 31$			$N = 34$	

Number of patients is shown as total number, mean values are shown ∅ ± SD.

There was no difference in PD specific impairment and in the progress of PD between the groups.

Table 4 shows the percentage of time spent with different tasks. Patients of group A underwent on average 14.9 ± 0.7, patients of group B 14.7 ± 0.5, and patients of group C 14.8 ± 0.7 cognitive training sessions, respectively ($P < 0.85$). The time spent on different tasks was identical in all three groups.

Patients of group B conducted 11.2 ± 0.5 and patients of group C 11.4 ± 0.6 transfer training sessions ($P < 0.9$).

Table 5 shows the percentage of time spent on different tasks of the transfer training, which was identical in both groups.

3.1. Motor Training. Patients had many difficulties to cope with the tasks. They struggled to find strategies to solve the tasks on their own, for example, they had difficulties to find the correct path through the parcours with obstacles and to follow the changing rules (set shifting). Patients tended

Table 4: Distribution of cognitive training.

Training section	Percentage of time spent (%)
Planning strategies	17
Mnemonics	15
Decision making	15
Set shifting	15
Calculation	10
Navigational skills	10
Information speed processing	8
Summary	5
Concentration	5

Table 5: Transfer training: time spent on different tasks.

Tasks	Percentage of time spent (%)
Planning and sequencing	18
Reasoning	11
Concentration	11
Memory	10
Working memory	8
Anticipation	8
Prospective memory	7
Cognitive information speed	7
Social rules	5
Association	5
Cognitive estimation	4

to perseverate. Walking through a room with eyes closed only guided by different touches of the therapist challenged the patients as well since PD-patients have both deficits in proprioception and in perception of stimuli. The type of tasks and exercises were new to the majority of patients. PD-patients needed more time and repeated instructions to learn mental imagery. The lessons were conducted as individual lessons. It was not possible to conduct group lessons. About 40% of the training took place outdoors, 60% in the gym.

3.2. Assessment of the Caregivers. The caregivers' knowledge about Parkinson's disease was assessed with a questionnaire at the end of the training programme. They were able to answer on average 27 ± 2.1 questions out of 30 compared to 20.2 ± 4.5 questions prior to the education programme. The carers' burden scale did not reveal any significant differences compared to baseline assessment. However, the questionnaire showed low burden in 60% of carers of group A, in 58% of group B, and in 62% of group C. Moderate burden was revealed in 30% of carers in group A, in 33% in group B, and 32% in group C. However, caregivers reported in a semi structured interview at the end of the education programme that they felt more confident. There was no difference between the caregivers of group A, B, and C.

3.3. Training at Home. 60% of patients of group A continued practising cognitive tasks 3 times a week for 45 min, while 40% conducted the training only once or twice per week. All patients of group B tried to continue the transfer tasks learnt during the rehabilitation, but further assessment showed that only 60% performed transfer tasks following a regular schedule. 75% of the patients of group B practised cognitive tasks 3 times a week. 90% of patients of group C pursued the training at home with the same quantity and intensity. They conducted a motor training three times a week, most often accompanied by their partners. The partners of patients of groups B and C managed to support their patients in practising transfer tasks. They asked them to prepare meals, to write the shopping list, or to go to the bank.

3.4. Results of Neuropsychological Testing. The screening tests for cognitive functions did not reveal any differences between the groups and the results did exclude dementia. The neuropsychological baseline assessment did not reveal any differences between the groups either. Patients of all three groups had shown deficits mainly in tests addressing executive functions. Consecutively, the performance of the patients was worse on the subtests of the SCOPA-COG, semantic fluency, LURIA, dice and assembly pattern, zoo test of the BADS and PASAT. The memory tasks such as immediate and delayed recall were only mildly disturbed.

The multiple-choice word test (MWT-B) was conducted as a measure for premorbid intelligence; the groups did not differ significantly either ($P = 0.78$). Thus, the randomisation process was successful. Table 6 shows the neuropsychological test results over the course of the study.

3.5. Primary Outcome Measure

3.5.1. ADAS-COG. All groups improved on the ADAS-COG significantly shown by a significant linear trend ($F_{\text{lin}}[1, 220] = 150$; $P < 0.001$). Group C improved most indicated by a significant interaction between groups and assessments ($F_{\text{groups}\times\text{assessments}}[1, 220] = 27.26$; $P < 0.001$) and a significant group difference ($F[2, 220] = 7.7$, $P < 0.001$). Further analysis showed that 78% of the patients showed some improvement at the second assessment, 51% of patients of group A, 85% of patients of group B, and 96% of patients of group C. 50% of the patients reached a reduction of the ADAS-COG score of 3 or more points, 18% of group A, 54% of group B, and 76% of group C. Six months after discharge of the rehabilitation unit 35% of patients (50% of patients of group A, 31% of patients of group B, and 28% of group C) showed a deterioration compared to the assessment at the end of the in-patient training programme. Further improvement was observed in 21% patients of group A, 37% patients of group B, and 50% patients of group C.

3.5.2. SCOPA-COG. In accordance the SCOPA-COG test showed a significant difference between the groups (Figure 2). All groups improved, indicated by the linear trend of days ($F_{\text{lin}}[1, 220) = 46.09$; $P < 0.001$). Group C improved most resulting in a significant difference between the groups ($F[2, 220] = 31.4$, df = 2; $P < 0.001$). Since the slopes of the improvements differed between the groups,

TABLE 6: Summary of neuropsychological test results.

Test	Baseline	T1	T2	Significant differences between the groups
ADAS-Cog	∅ ± SD	∅ ± SD	∅ ± SD	
Group A	21.51 ± 2.27	20.81 ± 2.77	20.5 ± 3.6	
Group B	21.37 ± 4.11	18.33 ± 3.67	18.5 ± 4.2	$P < 0.001$
Group C	22.92 ± 4.02	17.98 ± 2.76	17.4 ± 2.5	
SCOPA-Cog				
Group A	29.07 ± 3.8	27.21 ± 3.6	26.86 ± 3.32	
Group B	29.68 ± 2.87	31.32 ± 3.24	30.71 ± 2.9	$P < 0.001$
Group C	31.83 ± 3.21	39.15 ± 2.9	39.29 ± 2.72	
BADS Zoo (profile)	∅ ± SD	∅ ± SD	∅ ± SD	
Group A	2.5 ± 0.95	3.0 ± 1.2	2.4 ± 1.2	T1: Chi-square: 49.31; $P < 0.001$
Group B	2.4 ± 0.9	2.8 ± 1.1	2.6 ± 1.1	T2: Chi-square: 14.42; $P < 0.001$
Group C	2.6 ± 0.98	3.54 ± 0.82	3.43 ± 1.0	
BADS instruction	∅ ± SD	∅ ± SD	∅ ± SD	
Group A	2.8 ± 1.3	3.3 ± 1.1	2.9 ± 0.8	T1: Chi-square: 7.1; $P < 0.03$
Group B	2.6 ± 1.3	2.9 ± 1.2	3.2 ± 1.1	T2: Chi-square: 9.1; $P < 0.01$
Group C	2.7 ± 1.1	3.5 ± 1.1	3.8 ± 0.9	
BADS 6 elements	∅ ± SD	∅ ± SD	∅ ± SD	
Group A	2.8 ± 1.2	3.14 ± 0.89	3.1 ± 0.9	T1: Chi-square: 39.4; $P < 0.001$
Group B	2.9 ± 1.2	3.0 ± 1.2	2.9 ± 1.1	T2: Chi-square: 25.3 $P < 0.01$
Group C	3.0 ± 0.7	3.55 ± 0.8	3.6 ± 0.9	
PASAT	∅ ± SD	∅ ± SD	∅ ± SD	
Group A	29.94 ± 14.32	32.8 ± 14.83	32.5 ± 13.87	
Group B	31.00 ± 13.32	37.43 ± 12.72	39.57 ± 13.65	$P < 0.001$
Group C	30.4 ± 12.98	46.5 ± 11.5	49.2 ± 13.4	

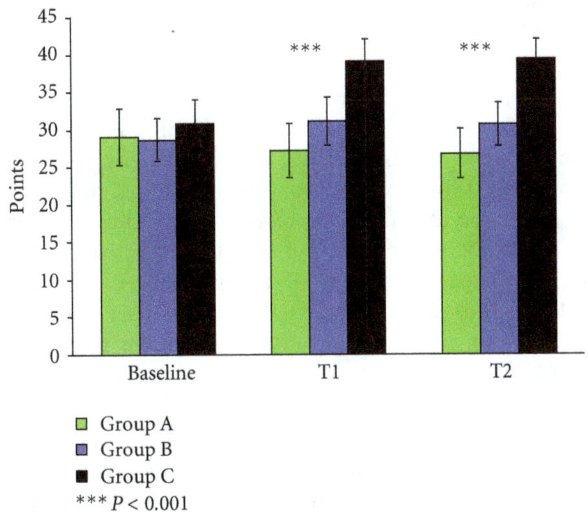

FIGURE 2: Group C improved significantly more on the SCOPA-COG test than group A and B.

a significant interaction between assessments and groups occurred ($F_{groups \times assessments}[2, 220] = 65.63$; $P < 0.001$). Post hoc tests revealed a significant difference between all groups ($P < 0.001$). Patients of group A reached 28.8 ± 3.7 points, group B 30.3 ± 2.7 points, and group C 37.6 ± 3.4 points. After completion of the in-patient training programme 31% of group A, 64% of group B, and 88% of group C had shown a significant improvement on the SCOPA-COG. Six months later at the final assessment 70% of patients of group A, 80% of patients of group B, and 94% of patients of group C had been able to keep their level of performance. Most improvement has been observed in the LURIA, dice, assembly pattern, and MOSAIC test of the SCOPA-COG. The pattern of improvement did not differ between the groups but the percentage of subjects showing an improvement and the speed of recovery.

3.5.3. Executive Function

BADS-Subscales. The BADS-subscales especially the zoo map are a very demanding task requiring excellent planning skills. The subtests of the BADS (rule shift cards, zoo map, modified 6 elements test) showed the following results.

The baseline scores of the rule shift cards did not differ between the groups. There was a mild but significant difference between the groups at the second assessment (Chi-square = 7.1; $P < 0.03$) and final assessment (Chi-square = 9.1; $P < 0.01$).

At baseline assessment group C showed a tendency to perform better on the BADS zoo test. The mean profile scores of all groups were higher at the second assessment, but significant more patients of group C improved compared to groups A and B. There was a clear group difference at the second (Chi-square = 49.31; $P < 0.03$) and third assessment (Chi-square = 14.42; 0.001). At the final assessment six months after the discharge patients of groups A and B had lost most of the previously shown improvement. Only patient of group C managed to keep their level of performance. Thus, group C has been superior to groups B and A immediately after completing the training and at the second assessment six months later.

There was no difference in the performance in the 6 elements test at baseline assessment. Group C showed a greater increase of the average profile scores leading to significant group differences at the second (Chi-square = 39.3; $P < 0.001$) and third assessments (Chi-square = 25.3; $P < 0.001$).

3.5.4. PASAT. The results of the PASAT test did not differ between the groups at baseline assessment, all groups produced on average 50% correct answers. Group A improved only marginally. Groups B and C benefitted from the training programme shown in a significant linear trend for assessments ($F_{\text{lin}}[1, 154] = 63.71$; $P < 0.001$). Since the improvement of the groups differed there was also a significant interaction between assessments and groups ($F_{\text{groups}\times\text{assessments}}[2, 154] = 18.99$; $P < 0.001$). Group C improved significantly more than groups B ($P < 0.03$) and A ($P < 0.001$) ($F[2, 154] = 15.46$; $P < 0.001$).

Only 157 patients (group A: 50, group B: 53, and group C: 54) managed the PASAT test on the first assessment and were included in the statistical model. The other patients did not succeed in finding a strategy to cope with the task. On the second and third assessment 56 patients of group A, 64 patients of group B, and 71 patients of group C scored on the test. Groups B and C showed further improvement between the second and final assessment.

3.5.5. Goal Attainment Scale. The goals were identified at the baseline assessment. On the final assessment it was reviewed whether the goals were obtained. Patients of group C reached more often the main goal than the other groups (Chi-square: 57.1; $P < 0.001$). The detailed analysis of the results is shown in Tables 7 and 8.

The patients had selected the goals based on their self-evaluation of their cognitive impairment and on the advice given by the psychologist after the baseline testing. The main cognitive impairments reported by the patients could be attributed to the following domains: dual tasking, planning of complex and sequential tasks, decision making, rule recognition, rule shifting problems, delayed recall, and difficulties in finding misplaced items.

Table 7 shows the goals patients had chosen and whether they were obtained at the final assessment.

Planning of complex tasks, rule recognition, and shifting and dual tasking were identified as goals most often. While there was no significant difference between the goals chosen

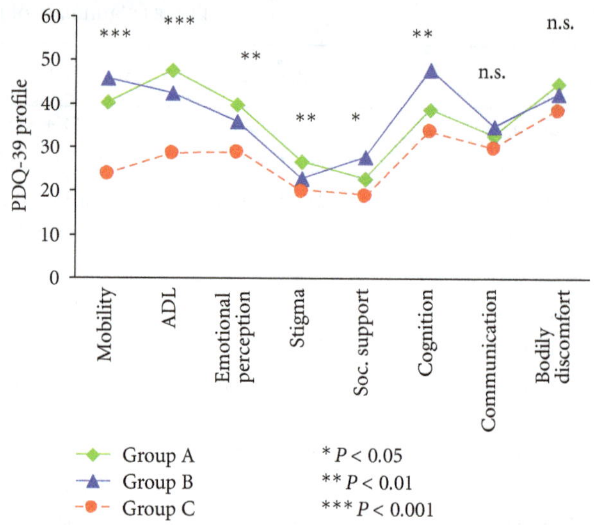

FIGURE 3: PD-patients of group C reported less PD-specific impairment at the final assessment. The y-axis shows the percentage of the maximal possible sum scores. The x-axis shows the 8 subscales of the PDQ-39. The lines represent the scores the groups have achieved in the 8 subscales.

by the three groups there was a significant difference between the percentages of patients obtaining the goals between the groups. 71% of patient obtained the goal "decision making," but only 40% of patients of group A.

Table 8 shows the improvement of the patients on the GAS scale with reference to their main goals.

More patients of group A compared to group B and C did not obtain the chosen goal or deteriorated compared to baseline, while 27.6% of patients of group C obtained the goal and 39.4% exceeded the expectations mildly and 7.6% substantially. The difference between the groups was significant (Chi-square = 48.23; $P < 0.001$).

3.6. Assessment of Mental State. 15% of the patients in group A, 20% of group B, and 18% of patients of group C reported to suffer from depression and received medication. The results on the HADS depression scale indicated in 20% of patients of group A and group C, respectively, and in 25% of patients of Group B the presence of a mild to moderate depression. The anxiety level was assessed by using the Hamilton Anxiety Scale and did not differ between the groups.

3.7. PD-Specific Impairment at the Final Assessment. The results of the PDQ-39 at the final assessment showed that patients of group C rated their health-related quality of life higher than the other groups. 13.8% of patients of group A, 38% of patients of group B, and 52% of patients of group C reported less impairment due to PD (Figure 3).

3.8. PD-Specific Functioning. The UPDRS score showed a mild improvement in all groups at the final assessment but there were no significant differences between the groups indicating that the cognitive improvement could not be

Table 7: Individual goals chosen by the patients and percentage of goal achievement.

Groups	Goal	Goals chosen		Goals obtained		Significance
		Total number	Percentage (%)	Total number	Percentage (%)	
A $N = 71$	Dual tasking	$N = 15$	21.1	$N = 3$	20	$P < 0.001$
B $N = 75$		$N = 14$	18.7	$N = 9$	64	
C $N = 76$		$N = 15$	20	$N = 10$	67	
A $N = 71$	Planning of complex tasks	$N = 15$	21.2	$N = 3$	20	$P < 0.001$
B $N = 75$		$N = 16$	21.3	$N = 9$	56.3	
C $N = 76$		$N = 17$	22.4	$N = 10$	58.9	
A $N = 71$	Decision making	$N = 10$	14.1	$N = 4$	40	$P < 0.001$
B $N = 75$		$N = 11$	14.7	$N = 6$	54.5	
C $N = 76$		$N = 14$	18.4	$N = 10$	71.4	
A $N = 71$	Rule recognition and rule shifting	$N = 13$	18.3	$N = 4$	30.8	$P < 0.01$
B $N = 75$		$N = 16$	21.3	$N = 7$	43.8	
C $N = 76$		$N = 14$	18.4	$N = 10$	71.4	
A $N = 71$	Delayed recall	$N = 12$	16.9	$N = 3$	25	$P < 0.001$
B $N = 75$		$N = 12$	16	$N = 7$	58.3	
C $N = 76$		$N = 11$	14.5	$N = 9$	82	
A $N = 71$	Search strategies	$N = 6$	8.5	$N = 4$	67	$P < 0.01$
B $N = 75$		$N = 6$	8	$N = 5$	83.3	
C $N = 76$		$N = 5$	6.6	$N = 4$	80	

Table 8: Effect of the training programme on the main goals (GAS).

GAS	Group A $N = 71$		Group B $N = 75$		Group C $N = 76$		Total	
	Total	Percent	Total	Percent	Total	Percent	Total	Percent
−3	$N = 12$	16.7	$N = 6$	8	$N = 2$	2.6	$N = 20$	8.9
−2	$N = 10$	13.8	$N = 5$	6.7	$N = 3$	3.9	$N = 18$	23.7
−1	$N = 28$	40.3	$N = 21$	28	$N = 18$	23.6	$N = 67$	30
0	$N = 13$	18.1	$N = 19$	25.3	$N = 23$	30.2	$N = 55$	24.7
1	$N = 8$	11.1	$N = 24$	32	$N = 24$	26.3	$N = 56$	25.1
2	$N = 0$	0	$N = 0$	0	$N = 6$	7.9	$N = 6$	2.7
	71		75		76		223	

−3 = worse than start of treatment, −2 = no change, −1 = some improvement, 0 = goal achievement, +1 = slight over-achievement, +2 = great over-achievement.

Table 9: UPDRS.

	Group A $N = 72$	Group B $N = 75$	Group C $N = 76$
Baseline			
UPDRS Motor scale	38.56 ± 12.44	37.53 ± 10.76	38.4 ± 11.78
UPDRS Sum Score	59.20 ± 12.4	60.3 ± 12.4	61.5 ± 12.8
Final assessment			
UPDRS Motor scale	34.1 ± 11.4	34.2 ± 11.2	35.2 ± 12.4
UPDRS Sum Score	55.4 ± 12.4	56.3 ± 11.5	57.2 ± 11.4

referred to a nonspecific effect resulting from general physical improvement (Table 9).

Performance in Activities of Daily Living at the Final Assessment and Evaluation of the Training Programme by Patients and Caregivers. The patients of group C reported that they had adapted a more active life style, felt more confident in activities of daily living, and had taken over some more chores. They perceived their partners and caregivers as being helpful. They enjoyed the participation of their partners in conjoint sports activities.

Patients of group B also regarded the training programme as helpful but reported of having still problems with activities of daily living. Patients of group A had more difficulties with transfer of skills into daily life and the carryover effect was smaller than in the other groups.

65% of the caregivers of patients in group C, 54% of caregivers of group B, and 49% of caregivers of group A found that competence and cognition of their patients had improved in activities of daily living. A deterioration of the performance in daily living was reported in 11% of group C, 17% of group B, and 25% of group A.

Caregivers felt more relaxed and competent to manage difficult situations, while patients accepted the guidance of their caregivers better than prior to the training. Caregivers felt confident to support the partners with the training at home.

Patients of group A felt that the cognitive training was arduous at times. Some patients perceived the training as stressful. Patients of groups B and C were asked to compare the training programmes. Patients of group C preferred the motor training to transfer training and cognitive pencil and paper tasks. 80% of patients judged the training as strenuous and felt sometimes exhausted. 30% of patients reported of being frustrated at times but did not ask for help or further explanations.

In summary patients who conducted a multimodal cognitive rehabilitation programme improved most on the ADAS-COG and SCOPA-COG, reported a better quality of life, were more active, and continued coping with daily tasks. Patients of group C were physically more active after the training programme and a higher percentage of patients of group C continued with the cognitive training. Physical improvement did not explain the difference in cognitive performance after the end of the study.

4. Discussion

Dementia is a part of the Parkinson's disease spectrum. Currently, there is no treatment aimed at halting or reversing disease progression [6]. Most treatment approaches are based on substituting neurotransmitter deficits. However, the effect of the drug treatment is limited and inconsistent among PD-patients. Therefore, other treatment options are needed. The current study has shown that a multimodal cognitive training programme might improve cognitive performance in PD-patients with mild cognitive impairment. The effect of the multimodal cognitive training on cognitive functioning was comparable to the effect found by Emre et al. in the rivastigmine trial [6]. The superiority of group C with respect to the cognitive assessments suggests that a diversified and challenging training is more effective. The results support our hypothesis that a special motor training might positively affect cognitive functioning. In children movement skill training is used to improve working memory, inhibition of impulses, attention, and visuospatial capacity. The expression psychomotor training is often used in Germany for physical training that combines physical and cognitive tasks. Oswald et al. [46, 47] were the first who called the physical training conducted in the SIMA project psychomotor training. They found that a combined psychomotor and memory training led to an improvement of psychomotor performance and to an improvement of cognitive performance and competence. Neither the psychomotor training nor the memory training on its own resulted in such effects. Oswald et al. [46, 47] assumed that neurophysiological changes led to a provision of reserve capacity of CNS performance. Therefore, emphasis should be placed on the reduction of cognitive load in neuropsychological training programmes. Goebel et al. [48] postulated as well to reduce instructions and working memory load during the training and to use procedures which lead to a more automated, implicit strategy application which demand less executive control [49–51].

Oswald et al. [46, 47] also suggested that the memory training affects psychomotor performance confirming the "memory-movement-hypothesis." An interaction between motor training and memory training might support remembering movement sequences. Our results confirm the hypothesis of Oswald et al. [46] that more diverse training programme enhances motivation and resulted in more regular training. Patients of group C exercised more physically and conducted more paper and pencil lesions at home than the other groups indicating that the attitude towards learning was positively influenced. In addition, the partners of patients in group C participated actively in the sport programme which helped patients to adhere to the training programme. As known from questionnaires we had sent to patients and their families inquiring about the training; social aspects are very important for PD-patients. Home-based multimodal cognitive training programme was sufficient to keep the performance of the second assessment in patients of group C. The psychomotor training combined with endurance training might have contributed to the superiority of group C. There is a huge body of literature suggesting a prevention of cognitive decline by life long exercise or even an improvement of cognitive deficits by physical activity. Executive functions may be selectively maintained or improved in people with better physical condition provided by physical training [52]. The importance of aerobic physical exercise on cognitive functions, especially on executive functions, has been shown [19–21, 26]. The studies have been mainly conducted in healthy elderly or patients with dementia but older people with PD can benefit their executive functions in the same way, as do their peers without PD. The results of some studies have shown that brain areas undergoing biological aging benefit most from endurance sports. Even structural changes have been observed [21]. Since group C conducted more training lessons at home compared to the other groups, one might argue that the superiority of group C was rather due to the quantity of the training than to the content. However, group C has already performed better at the second assessment and group A had shown poorer results than groups B and C. At this time all groups spent a similar amount of time with training and received similar attention by the therapists. Thus, the content of the training might be responsible for the different performance of the groups. The superiority of group B compared to group A suggests the efficacy of the transfer tasks. The psychomotor training helped group C to improve further, especially in the challenging executive tasks regarding rule cognition, set shifting, and decision making. The authors had also taken care during the study design that groups B and A received relaxation training and physiotherapy as compensation for the motor training of group C during the 6-month training period at home. These treatment offers were also accepted by the patients but especially patients of group A did not practise cognitive lessons at home as much as they were advised to do. Home-based cognitive training without transfer and physical training as performed by group A was less attractive for the patients.

The groups managed the executive tests very differently. The BADS zoo map is a very challenging test as mentioned above and requires various training approaches to achieve an improvement. Only patients of group C obtained a permanent improvement on this test.

Thus, the different training schedules affect the training outcome also regarding the type of tasks, which were better performed. Patients of group C managed executive tasks better than group A and B, which is shown by the better performance on the BADS test battery and the better results on the SCOPA-COG. Exercise and endurance training is thought to improve executive functions most. Furthermore, brain areas which are more vulnerable for age-related volume lose benefit most from physical exercise.

Patients with mild cognitive impairment benefit more from cognitive training than more advanced patients. Studies have shown that the effect of physical exercise on demented patients is limited. Patients have to be capable of understanding the training programme. Depression might also influence the performance in neuropsychological tests. Klepac et al. [53] have found that depression preceding PD motor signs might favour poorer cognitive abilities. However, there was no significant difference between the groups regarding the percentage of patients being depressed and the severity of depression. Thus, depression and anxiety were not confounding factors and not responsible for the different treatment outcomes of the three groups. Assessment bias in favour for one treatment can be excluded because the movement disorder specialists conducting the tests were blinded to the treatment arms.

The findings of the study confirmed as well that PD-patients benefit from a specific cognitive training. Based on the results of a previous study [54], we had chosen an individual training approach. Therefore, patients did not undergo a standardised cognitive training programme but a programme tailored to their needs. Interestingly, the results of the baseline testing and the psychologist's training suggestions were very often concordant with the requests of the patients. Therefore, the goal attainment scale was very suitable to represent both the training suggestions and the patients' requests. The fact that more patients of group C attained the selected goals might also support the strength of a multimodal training. Resembling the results of the executive tests some goals seemed to be more difficult to attain (see Tables 7 and 8). Patients struggled more to attain goals such as rule generation or rule shifting while dual tasking and memory improvement were easier to accomplish. However, group C was also more successful in achieving an improvement in planning of complex tasks, rule generation, rule shifting, and decision finding than groups B and C.

In contrast to a study by París et al. [55], the present study suggested a translation of improved cognitive performance into daily living. The patients' caregivers also reported an improved competence in real life. However, patients practised during the transfer training situations of everyday life. Hence, they did not face completely new situations in their daily life. París et al. [55] found an improvement in attention, information processing speed, memory, visuospatial and visuo-constructive abilities, semantic verbal fluency, and executive functions but no improvement of cognitive difficulties in daily living.

Sinforiani et al. [56] observed a carryover effect after completion of a 6-week cognitive rehabilitation training including cognitive and physical training. The authors suggested that the combined cognitive rehabilitation training exerts its positive effects by reinforcing cognitive strategies with improvement of frontal lobe functions.

Quality of life is closely associated with nonmotor symptoms of PD, especially cognitive function [8]. Consequentially Group C scored much higher on the PDQ-39 than the other groups. Thus, health-related quality of life was improved markedly in these patients. In contrast to our results París et al. [55] did not find any benefits of the cognitive training in self-reported quality of life. Probably, the cognitive training has to lead to improvements in daily living in order to improve quality of life.

Research over the last decade has shown that cognitive deficits affect motor performance. Patients with cognitive deficits had more difficulties in motor tests than patients without cognitive deficits. Hausdorff et al. [57] have found a close correlation between walking and executive functions. Yogev et al. [58] have shown that gait variability in dual tasking is closely associated with the performance in executive tasks. The difficulties that patients of group C experienced while solving the motor tasks have been in accordance with these results. Nevertheless, most of the patients managed to cope with the training programme, though some patients felt overstrained and quitted the programme.

4.1. Limitations of the Study. One might criticise that we compared three different treatment arms and did not include a control group without cognitive training in this study. However, patients were enrolled into the study during their stay on a rehabilitation unit and complained of a deterioration of their cognitive performance. For this reason, it was not possible to withhold treatment. Further, we had shown the superiority of a cognitive training compared to standard treatment in a previous study [54].

Another limitation is that there are no evidence-based data for the transfer training. Further research is necessary to evaluate and validate which transfer exercises are useful tools. The psychomotor training or movement skill training has been used for many years in children and has been applied in patients with dementia [53, 54]. However, it has not been validated in PD-patients so far. The selection of tasks has been based on the experience of the therapists and medical staff and published data which were based on the work with children.

One might also argue which improvement on the ADAS-COG or SCOPA-COG might be clinically relevant. However, the scales are validated and had been often applied in clinical trials. The clinical relevance of the improvements has also been shown by the observed translation into real life. Furthermore, due to the short follow-up period of 6 months we cannot report on long-term effects. However, studies assessing long-term results are very difficult to conduct since it is very difficult to keep the medication stable.

4.2. Strengths of the Study. To our knowledge, the results of the current study show for the first time, that a multimodal cognitive training in patients with Parkinson's disease can lead to improvements of cognitive function and improves quality of life. In addition, there was some translation of the cognitive improvement into real life. We also want to emphasize that it was a blinded randomised study and the drop-out rate was low.

5. Conclusion

In conclusion, we have shown that PD-patients with cognitive deficits benefit from a multimodal cognitive training. The multimodal training was superior to a paper- and pencil-based cognitive training. The combination of the cognitive training with a motor training seems to be most successful and the short-term effect of the training on cognitve functions was comparable to the effect found in the rivastigmine trial. However, we cannot predict the long-term effect of the cognitive multimodal training. The study has shown some translation of cognitive improvements into "real" life. Admittedly, the multimodal training of cognitive functions is time consuming, requires high motivation of the patients, and put demands on resources. Due to the quantity and quality of the trainings sessions it will also be costly. On the other hand dementia is a risk factor for falls, high morbidity and transfer to nursing homes, which increases the costs for the patients' care substantially and jeopardizes the patients' quality of life.

Acknowledgment

The authors would like to thank Dr. Werner Jackstädt-Stiftung for the generous support of the study.

References

[1] R. C. Chen, S. F. Chang, C. L. Su et al., "Prevalence, incidence, and mortality of PD: a door-to-door survey in Ilan County, Taiwan," *Neurology*, vol. 57, no. 9, pp. 1679–1686, 2001.

[2] A. Schrag, Y. Ben-Shlomo, and N. P. Quinn, "Cross sectional prevalence survey of idiopathic Parkinson's disease and parkinsonism in London," *British Medical Journal*, vol. 321, no. 7252, pp. 21–22, 2000.

[3] J. Douglas, D. J. Gelb, E. Oliver, and S. Gilman, "Diagnostic criteria for Parkinson disease," *Archives of Neurology*, vol. 56, no. 1, pp. 33–39, 1999.

[4] A. J. Hughes, S. E. Daniel, L. Kilford, and A. J. Lees, "Accuracy of clinical diagnosis of idiopathic Parkinson's disease: a clinico-pathological study of 100 cases," *Journal of Neurology Neurosurgery and Psychiatry*, vol. 55, no. 3, pp. 181–184, 1992.

[5] D. Aarsland, K. Andersen, J. P. Larsen, A. Lolk, and P. Kragh-Sørensen, "Prevalence and characteristics of dementia in Parkinson disease: an 8-year prospective study," *Archives of Neurology*, vol. 60, no. 3, pp. 387–392, 2003.

[6] M. Emre, D. Aarsland, A. Albanese et al., "Rivastigmine for dementia associated with Parkinson's disease," *New England Journal of Medicine*, vol. 351, no. 24, pp. 2509–2518, 2004.

[7] G. Levy, M. X. Tang, E. D. Louis et al., "The association of incident dementia with mortality in PD," *Neurology*, vol. 59, no. 11, pp. 1708–1713, 2002.

[8] A. Schrag, M. Jahanshahi, and N. Quinn, "What contributes to quality of life in patients with Parkinson's disease?" *Journal of Neurology Neurosurgery and Psychiatry*, vol. 69, no. 3, pp. 308–312, 2000.

[9] D. Aarsland, J. P. Larsen, K. Karlsen, N. G. Lim, and E. Tandberg, "Mental symptoms in Parkinson's disease are important contributors to caregiver distress," *International Journal of Geriatric Psychiatry*, vol. 14, no. 10, pp. 866–874, 1999.

[10] D. Aarsland, J. P. Larsen, E. Tandberg, and K. Laake, "Predictors of nursing home placement in Parkinson's disease: a population-based, prospective study," *Journal of the American Geriatrics Society*, vol. 48, no. 8, pp. 938–942, 2000.

[11] M. Emre, "Dementia associated with Parkinson's disease," *Lancet Neurology*, vol. 2, no. 4, pp. 229–237, 2003.

[12] H. Braak, K. Del Tredici, U. Rüb, R. A. I. De Vos, E. N. H. Jansen Steur, and E. Braak, "Staging of brain pathology related to sporadic Parkinson's disease," *Neurobiology of Aging*, vol. 24, no. 2, pp. 197–211, 2003.

[13] E. K. Perry, M. Curtis, and D. J. Dick, "Cholinergic correlates of cognitive impairment in Parkinson's disease: comparisons with Alzheimer's disease," *Journal of Neurology Neurosurgery and Psychiatry*, vol. 48, no. 5, pp. 413–421, 1985.

[14] I. Litvan, D. Aarsland, C. H. Adler et al., "MDS task force on mild cognitive impairment in Parkinson's disease: critical review of PD-MCI," *Movement Disorders*, 2011.

[15] E. E. Smith and J. Jonides, "Storage and executive processes in the frontal lobes," *Science*, vol. 283, no. 5408, pp. 1657–1661, 1999.

[16] P. W. Burgess and T. Shallice, "Response suppression, initiation and strategy use following frontal lobe lesions," *Neuropsychologia*, vol. 34, no. 4, pp. 263–272, 1996.

[17] E. K. Miller and J. D. Cohen, "An integrative theory of prefrontal cortex function," *Annual Review of Neuroscience*, vol. 24, pp. 167–202, 2001.

[18] R. D. Abbott, L. R. White, G. W. Ross, K. H. Masaki, J. D. Curb, and H. Petrovitch, "Walking and dementia in physically capable elderly men," *Journal of the American Medical Association*, vol. 292, no. 12, pp. 1447–1453, 2004.

[19] S. Colcombe and A. F. Kramer, "Fitness effects on the cognitive function of older adults: a meta-analytic study," *Psychological Science*, vol. 14, no. 2, pp. 125–130, 2003.

[20] S. J. Colcombe, K. I. Erickson, N. Raz et al., "Aerobic fitness reduces brain tissue loss in aging humans," *Journals of Gerontology A*, vol. 58, no. 2, pp. 176–180, 2003.

[21] S. J. Colcombe, K. I. Erickson, P. E. Scalf et al., "Aerobic exercise training increases brain volume in aging humans," *Journals of Gerontology A*, vol. 61, no. 11, pp. 1166–1170, 2006.

[22] D. Laurin, R. Verreault, J. Lindsay, K. MacPherson, and K. Rockwood, "Physical activity and risk of cognitive impairment and dementia in elderly persons," *Archives of Neurology*, vol. 58, no. 3, pp. 498–504, 2001.

[23] Y. Rolland, G. Abellan van Kan, and B. Vellas, "Healthy brain aging: role of exercise and physical activity," *Clinics in Geriatric Medicine*, vol. 26, no. 1, pp. 75–87, 2010.

[24] G. Nelles, "Cortical reorganization—effects of intensive therapy: results from prospective functional imaging studies," *Restorative Neurology and Neuroscience*, vol. 22, no. 3-4, pp. 239–244, 2004.

[25] R. B. Shepherd, "Exercise and training to optimize functional motor performance in stroke: driving neural reorganization?" *Neural Plasticity*, vol. 8, no. 1-2, pp. 121–129, 2001.

[26] A. F. Kramer, S. Hahn, N. J. Cohen et al., "Ageing, fitness and neurocognitive function," *Nature*, vol. 400, no. 6743, pp. 418–419, 1999.

[27] J. Baatile, W. E. Langbein, F. Weaver, C. Maloney, and M. B. Jost, "Effect of exercise on perceived quality of life of individuals with Parkinson's disease," *Journal of Rehabilitation Research and Development*, vol. 37, no. 5, pp. 529–534, 2000.

[28] I. Reuter, M. Engelhardt, K. Stecker, and H. Baas, "Therapeutic value of exercise training in Parkinson's disease," *Medicine and Science in Sports and Exercise*, vol. 31, no. 11, pp. 1544–1549, 1999.

[29] K. Dujardin, A. Duhamel, M. Delliaux, C. Thomas-Antérion, A. Destée, and L. Defebvre, "Cognitive complaints in Parkinson's disease: its relationship with objective cognitive decline," *Journal of Neurology*, vol. 257, no. 1, pp. 79–84, 2010.

[30] S. Fahn, R. L. Elton, and The Members of the UPDRS Development Committee, "Unified Parkinson's disease rating scale," in *Recent Developments in Parkinson's Disease II*, S. Fahn, C. D. Marsden, M. Goldstein et al., Eds., pp. 153–163, McMillan, New York, NY, USA, 1987.

[31] Royal College of Physicians and the Intercollegiate Stroke Working Party, *National Clinical Guideline for Stroke*, RCP, London, UK, 3rd edition, 2008.

[32] E. Kalbe, P. Calabrese, N. Kohn et al., "Screening for cognitive deficits in Parkinson's disease with the Parkinson neuropsychometric dementia assessment (PANDA) instrument," *Parkinsonism and Related Disorders*, vol. 14, no. 2, pp. 93–101, 2008.

[33] M. F. Folstein, S. E. Folstein, and P. R. McHugh, "'Mini mental state'. A practical method for grading the cognitive state of patients for the clinician," *Journal of Psychiatric Research*, vol. 12, no. 3, pp. 189–198, 1975.

[34] W. G. Rosen, R. C. Mohs, and K. L. Davis, "A new rating scale for Alzheimer's disease," *American Journal of Psychiatry*, vol. 141, no. 11, pp. 1356–1364, 1984.

[35] S. Talwalker, "Assessment of AD with the ADAS-cog," *Journal of Geriatric Psychiatry and Neurology*, vol. 9, pp. 39–46, 1996.

[36] J. Marinus, M. Visser, N. A. Verwey et al., "Assessment of cognition in Parkinson's disease," *Neurology*, vol. 61, no. 9, pp. 1222–1228, 2003.

[37] D. M. A. Gronwall, "Paced auditory serial addition task: a measure of recovery from concussion," *Perceptual and Motor Skills*, vol. 44, no. 2, pp. 367–373, 1977.

[38] B. A. Wilson, J. J. Evans, H. Emslie, N. Alderman, and P. Burgess, "The development of an ecologically valid test for assessing patients with a dysexecutive syndrome," *Neuropsychological Rehabilitation*, vol. 8, no. 3, pp. 213–228, 1998.

[39] S. Lehrl, *Mehrfach-Wortschatz-Intelligenztest: MWT-B*, Perimed Fachbuch-Verlagsgesellschaft mbH, Erlangen, Germany, 1989.

[40] A. S. Zigmond and R. P. Snaith, "The hospital anxiety and depression scale," *Acta Psychiatrica Scandinavica*, vol. 67, no. 6, pp. 361–370, 1983.

[41] C. Jenkinson, V. Peto, R. Fitzpatrick, R. Greenhall, and N. Hyman, "Self-reported functioning and well-being in patients with Parkinson's disease: comparison of the short-form wealth survey (SF-36) and the Parkinson's disease questionnaire (PDQ-39)," *Age and Ageing*, vol. 24, no. 6, pp. 505–509, 1995.

[42] S. J. G. Lewis, A. Slabosz, T. W. Robbins, R. A. Barker, and A. M. Owen, "Dopaminergic basis for deficits in working memory but not attentional set-shifting in Parkinson's disease," *Neuropsychologia*, vol. 43, no. 6, pp. 823–832, 2005.

[43] N. Fournet, O. Moreaud, J. L. Roulin, B. Naegele, and J. Pellat, "Working memory functioning in medicated Parkinson's disease patients and the effect of withdrawal of dopaminergic medication," *Neuropsychology*, vol. 14, no. 2, pp. 247–253, 2000.

[44] S. Golubović, T. Tubić, and S. Marković, "Psycho-motor re-education-movement as therapeutic method," *Medicinski Pregled*, vol. 64, no. 1-2, pp. 61–63, 2011.

[45] T. Golubović, J. Maksimović, B. Golubović, and N. Glumbić, "Effects of exercise on physical fitness in children with intellectual disability," *Research in Developmental Disabilities*, vol. 33, no. 2, pp. 608–614, 2012.

[46] W. D. Oswald, R. Rupprecht, T. Gunzelmann, and K. Tritt, "The SIMA-project: effects of 1 year cognitive and psychomotor training on cognitive abilities of the elderly," *Behavioural Brain Research*, vol. 78, no. 1, pp. 67–72, 1996.

[47] W. D. Oswald, T. Gunzelmann, R. Rupprecht, and B. Hagen, "Differential effects of single versus combined cognitive and physical training with older adults: the SimA study in a 5-year perspective," *European Journal of Ageing*, vol. 3, no. 4, pp. 179–192, 2006.

[48] S. Goebel, H. M. Mehdorn, and B. Leplow, "Strategy instruction in Parkinson's disease: influence on cognitive performance," *Neuropsychologia*, vol. 48, no. 2, pp. 574–580, 2010.

[49] A. D. Baddeley, *Working Memory*, Clarendon Press, Oxford, UK, 1986.

[50] D. A. Norman and T. Shallice, "(1980) Attention to action: willed and automatic control of behaviour," in *Cognitive Neuroscience A*, M. S. Gazzaniga, Ed., Blackwell, Oxford, UK, 2000.

[51] G. Sammer, I. Reuter, K. Hullmann, M. Kaps, and D. Vaitl, "Training of executive functions in Parkinson's disease," *Journal of the Neurological Sciences*, vol. 248, no. 1-2, pp. 115–119, 2006.

[52] J. D. Churchill, R. Galvez, S. Colcombe, R. A. Swain, A. F. Kramer, and W. T. Greenough, "Exercise, experience and the aging brain," *Neurobiology of Aging*, vol. 23, no. 5, pp. 941–955, 2002.

[53] N. Klepac, S. HajnÅek, and V. Trkulja, "Cognitive performance in nondemented nonpsychotic parkinson disease patients with or without a history of depression prior to the onset of motor symptoms," *Journal of Geriatric Psychiatry and Neurology*, vol. 23, no. 1, pp. 15–26, 2010.

[54] K. Hullmann, G. Sammer, and I. Reuter, "Training of executive functions in Parkinson's disease," in *Medimont International Proceedings*, pp. 143–148, 2004.

[55] A. P. París, H. G. Saleta, M. de la Cruz Crespo Maraver et al., "Blind randomized controlled study of the efficacy of cognitive training in Parkinson's disease," *Movement Disorders*, vol. 26, no. 7, pp. 1251–1258, 2011.

[56] E. Sinforiani, L. Banchieri, C. Zucchella, C. Pacchetti, and G. Sandrini, "Cognitive rehabilitation in Parkinson's disease.," *Archives of Gerontology and Geriatrics*, supplement 9, pp. 387–391, 2004.

[57] J. M. Hausdorff, G. Yogev, S. Springer, E. S. Simon, and N. Giladi, "Walking is more like catching than tapping: gait in the elderly as a complex cognitive task," *Experimental Brain Research*, vol. 164, no. 4, pp. 541–548, 2005.

[58] G. Yogev, N. Giladi, C. Peretz, S. Springer, E. S. Simon, and J. M. Hausdorff, "Dual tasking, gait rhythmicity, and Parkinson's disease: which aspects of gait are attention demanding?" *European Journal of Neuroscience*, vol. 22, no. 5, pp. 1248–1256, 2005.

7

Validity and Reliability of Accelerometer-Based Gait Assessment in Patients with Diabetes on Challenging Surfaces

Eling D. de Bruin,[1] Michèle Hubli,[1] Pamela Hofer,[1] Peter Wolf,[2] Kurt Murer,[1] and Wiebren Zijlstra[3,4]

[1] *Institute of Human Movement Sciences and Sport, ETH, 8093 Zurich, Switzerland*
[2] *Sensory-Motor Systems Lab, ETH, Zurich, Switzerland*
[3] *Center for Human Movement Sciences, University Medical Center Groningen, University of Groningen, Groningen, The Netherlands*
[4] *Institut für Bewegungs- und Sportgerontologie, Deutsche Sporthochschule Köln, Köln, Germany*

Correspondence should be addressed to Eling D. de Bruin, eling.debruin@hest.ethz.ch

Academic Editor: Bijan Najafi

Walking on irregular terrain influences gait of diabetic patients. We investigate the test-retest reliability and construct validity of gait measured with the DynaPort MiniMod under single and dual task conditions in diabetic patients walking on irregular terrain to identify the measurement error (precision) and minimal clinical detectable change. 29 patients with Type 2 diabetes were measured once, and 25 repeated the measurement within 7 days. Patients walked on a therapy garden walkway. Differences between three groups of diabetics with various levels of lower extremity neuropathy were analyzed with planned contrasts. ICC was excellent for intervisit measurements with ICC's > 0.824. Bland and Altman Plots, SEM, and SDD showed precise values, distributed around zero for both test conditions. A significant effect of grouping on step length performance hints at possible construct validity of the device. Good reliability of DynaPort MiniMod measurements on a therapy garden walkway and an indication for discriminatory capability suggests that DynaPort MiniMod could facilitate the study of gait in diabetic patients in conditions close to real-life situations. Good reliability, small measurement error, and values of minimal clinical detectable change recommend the further utilization of DynaPort MiniMod for the evaluation of gait parameters in diabetic patients.

1. Introduction

The World Health Organization has described type 2 diabetes as an international epidemic. Current estimates suggest that the number of persons with diabetes will reach 300 million by 2025 [1]. Fifty percent of patients who have diabetes for more than 20 years develop peripheral neuropathy (PN), which affects nerve function from the periphery to more proximal regions [2, 3]. Because the increasing prevalence of diabetes is accompanied by gait problems and a heightened risk of falling, there is an increased need for understanding the possible gait pattern changes diabetic patients are confronted with [4]. It has, furthermore, been demonstrated that patients with diabetes may also improve their gait due to specific exercise programs [5, 6].

In this context gait analysis is usually performed in specialized kinesiology laboratories. Cameras, force platforms, and magnetic and ultrasound systems are thereby often used technologies for the gait analysis [7, 8]. However, time expenditure and financial constraints limit their use in clinical practice [9]. Moreover, gait analyses are traditionally performed indoors, on a predefined, clean, and flat specific pathway. Such conditions enable precise recording but are not representative of the real-life context. Activities of daily life require us to move about in challenging environments and to walk on varied surfaces. Irregular terrain has been shown to influence gait parameters such as speed, especially in a population at risk for falling [10], for example, patients with Diabetes [11, 12]. Furthermore, the fact that falling mainly occurs in a complex environment [13] under attention demanding conditions emphasizes the need for clinicians to objectively record gait data in a real-life context [14] under dual task conditions [15].

The recent use of body-fixed sensors suggests that they could serve as a tool for analyzing the gait of patients in more challenging walking environments [16–18]. In comparison with other motion measurement devices, body-fixed sensors have the advantage of being lightweight and portable, which enables subjects to move relatively freely. They permit data collection in a challenging environment; they are easy to use, provide a good ratio in terms of cost and amount of information retrieved, and can capture data from many gait cycles. Thus they seem ideal for extending our understanding of gait changes in specific populations by performing measures in real-life conditions, for example, in diabetic patients [19]. An objective evaluation in real-life conditions might help understand the causes of diabetic gait problems and ultimately facilitate the choice or the development of appropriate physical treatment. Therefore, the potential of body-fixed sensor approaches should be investigated in the diabetic population in order to ensure the validity and the reliability of data recorded during gait analysis under single and dual task conditions on changing types of surfaces.

To be clinically useful, an assessment procedure must have a small measurement error to detect a real change and must be able to distinguish between subpopulations for example, diabetic patients with and without various stages of peripheral neuropathy. A test-retest difference in a patient with a value smaller than the standard error of the measurement (SEM) is likely to be the result of "measurement noise" and is unlikely to be detected reliably in practice; a difference greater than the smallest real difference is highly likely (with 95% confidence) to be a real difference [20]. Another example of these statistics is the smallest detectable difference (SDD) [21]. The DynaPort MiniMod body-fixed sensor has previously been shown to be reliable, valid, and valuable in elderly for the analysis of gait performed on challenging surfaces [22–25]. To date, little is known about the variability in gait measures within the diabetic population and the reliable use of accelerometers in these patients. With this in mind, we conducted this study to (a) investigate the validity and reliability of gait parameters measured with DynaPort MiniMod in diabetic patients walking under single and dual task conditions on a challenging walking course, (b) identify the measurement error (precision), and (c) identify the smallest clinical detectable difference. We hypothesized [1] that walking quality in patients with diabetes can be reliably measured with accelerometers [2], that the walking quality is different in patient subgroups (we expect diabetic neuropathy to change gait quality compared to the group with no neuropathy), and [3] we believe that severe neuropathy effects walking quality more than mild neuropathy.

2. Methods

The study was approved by the ethics committee in Canton Zurich. All participants received written and oral information and were requested to sign an informed consent statement.

2.1. Subjects. A convenience sample of 31 patients with diabetes Type 2 (with and without neuropathy) was recruited from the patients consulting the Division of Endocrinology, Diabetes and Clinical Nutrition, University Hospital of Zurich (Table 1). Patients were included if they were medically diagnosed with diabetes Type 2, were between 50 and 70 years of age, and had the ability to walk without assistive devices. Patients were excluded if they had concomitant foot ulcer, orthopaedic or surgical problems influencing gait parameters, a nondiabetic neuropathy (due to Charcot-Marie-Tooth disease, alcohol, or thyroid dysfunction), or neurological pathology influencing gait parameters.

Before gait analysis started, patients were assigned to one of three groups: "DIABETIC," "MILD NEUROPATHY," and "SEVERE NEUROPATHY" based on three tests. A Neurometer CPT electrodiagnostic device was used for sensory nerve conduction threshold (sNCT) evaluations at the great toe by determining current perception threshold (CPT) levels. CPT permits diagnosis of neuropathy due to its ability to diagnose and quantify hyperaesthesia [26]. The used Rapid Screening CPT (R-CPT) resulted in a value between 1 and 25, where the higher numbers indicate worse nerve conduction. The value was used to grade neuropathy: no neuropathy = 6–13, moderate neuropathy = 14–19, severe neuropathy = 20–25. The Rydel-Seiffer tuning fork test was used to assess the vibratory threshold perception at the base of the great toe as a good predictor for impairment of the vibratory senses and, therefore, also usable to diagnose neuropathy [27–29]. The Rydel-Seiffer tuning fork test acquires values between 0 and 8, where the higher values indicate better vibratory senses. Patients were grouped by the test in one of the three categories with application of an age-related correction [30]. The third test used was the Semmes-Weinstein monofilament test, a good test to diagnose but not to quantify neuropathy [31]. If the subjects did not notice five of seven stimuli, a neuropathy was diagnosed.

Testing and group assignment was performed by an MD unfamiliar with the study design and the patients. Based on the results of all three tests the MD categorized the patients in one of three categories. The MD principally considered the results from the Neurometer CPT/C tests where three values for every frequency were obtained for the right and the left great toe. If at least two frequencies of the worse foot had a value over 14, the subject was allocated to the "moderate neuropathy" group. If at least two frequencies of the worse foot had a value over 19, the subject was allocated to the "severe neuropathy" group. If there were any uncertainties in the group allocation according to R-CPT values, the Rydel-Seiffer tuning fork test was the next criteria considered. The loading of the group arrangement's criteria was Neurometer CPT/C > Rydel-Seiffer tuning fork > Semmes-Weinstein monofilament test.

After the analysis of nerve conduction the gait analysis started.

TABLE 1: Demographic description of the consecutively recruited subjects at baseline.

Subject (no.)	Sex (m/f)	Age (years)	Weight (kg)	Height (m)	BMI (kg/m^2)	Group*
01	m	60	82	1.76	26.5	2
02	m	70	88	1.74	29.1	2
03	f	64	92	1.73	30.7	3
04	m	63	94	1.76	30.4	3
05	m	69	84	1.76	27.1	2
06	m	57	102	1.78	32.2	2
07	f	63	67	1.55	27.9	2
08	m	70	95	1.76	30.7	3
09	m	69	73	1.79	22.8	2
10	m	57	98	1.84	29	3
11	m	61	103	1.79	32.2	1
12	m	69	66	1.72	22.3	2
13	m	53	90	1.71	30.8	3
14	m	70	102	1.85	29.8	3
15	f	67	78	1.64	29	1
16	m	65	94	1.74	31.1	1
17	m	62	81	1.75	26.5	1
18	m	62	92	1.70	31.8	1
19	m	56	108	1.82	32.6	1
20	m	59	67	1.67	24	1
21	m	60	76	1.73	25.4	1
22	m	56	93	1.70	32.2	1
23	f	64	54	1.60	21.1	2
24	m	60	92	1.78	29.0	1
25	f	50	60	1.63	22.6	2
26	m	57	85	1.80	26.2	2
27	f	60	75	1.60	29.3	1
28	m	55	85	1.78	26.8	1
29	m	65	81	1.87	23.2	2

BMI: body mass index; * 1: "diabetic," 2: "mild neuropathy," and 3: "severe neuropathy"; m/f: male/female.

2.2. Apparatus. A triaxial accelerometer (DynaPort Mini-Mod, McRoberts BV, The Hague, The Netherlands) was used to measure pelvic accelerations. The accelerometer was placed at the lower back of the subject with the center of the device at the level of the second sacral vertebrae.

2.3. Test Procedures. Each subject was assessed during usual walking at preferred velocity under two different conditions over an outdoor gait therapy walkway with different surfaces: (1) silent walking on the walkway and (2) walking on the walkway with a counting task. The walkway contained a paved trajectory, cobble stones, and gravel rocks (Figure 1(a)). The complete walkway was 31 meter long and 1.5 meter wide. To measure steady state- walking, the 16.6 meters (with the three different surfaces) of the walking course was used as the test distance. The remaining parts of the walkway were used for acceleration and deceleration. At the end of the first 31 meters the subjects had to stop for two seconds, then turn around, and walk the walkway back to the starting point. At the beginning the measurement was started (S), and, at the end, the measurement was stopped (S + M5; Figure 1(b)).

(1) Test run with subject's preferred walking speed: the subject received the most important information: no speaking, hold arms out of the pocket, and try not to stop walking during the measurement.

(2) First trial with preferred walking speed: the subject was briefed to "*walk like you would bring a letter to the mailbox*" (single task).

(3) Second trial with preferred walking speed and an additional cognitive task (count backwards aloud in steps of three): the subject had to walk and count aloud in steps of three. The subject was briefed to "*try to walk and count at the same time. Do not favour one task over the other but try to perform these concurrently*" (dual task).

The dual task was subtracting repeatedly the number three starting from 200 down and was practiced before gait

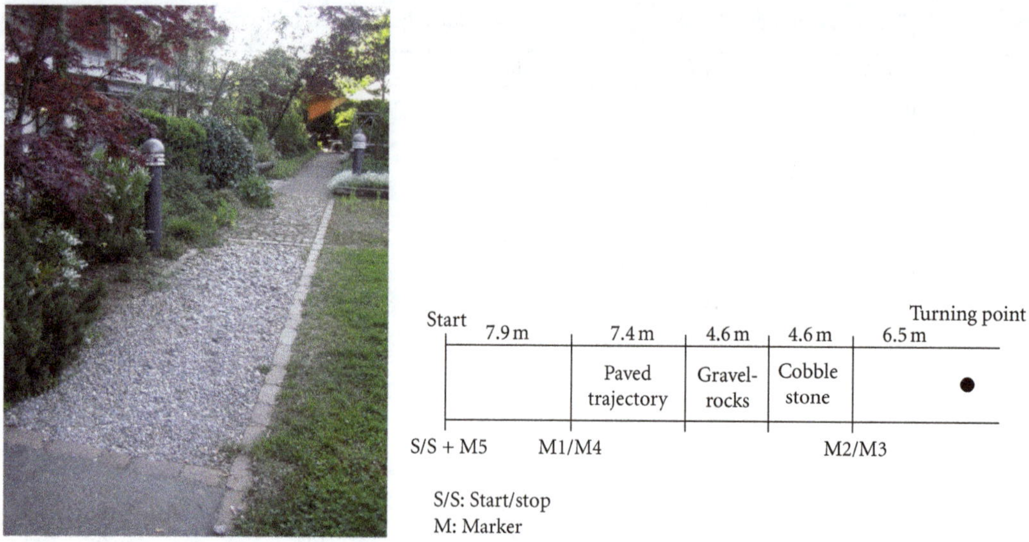

(a) (b)

FIGURE 1: (a) The gait garden walkway with paved trajectory, cobble stones, and gravel rocks. (b) Schematic representation of the walkway and test procedure used. M signifies markers that are set in the signal to recognize the gait data for analyses.

testing while sitting on a chair. Subjects were told to try and perform both tasks at the same time without prioritizing either the walking or counting. A small receiver was mounted on the accelerometer and the researcher placed a marker in the data through triggering by the use of a remote control when the subjects passed distance lines (Figure 1(b)). The researcher walked alongside the subjects to ensure their safety. At the end of the last trial the SD card was removed from the accelerometer, and the measurements were checked for completeness on a laptop. The subject was asked to come again for the retest one week later at the same time and to wear the same shoes as during the first trial.

Per trial, all measured data between the two trigger signals (M1-M2/M3-M4) were used for analysis. Walking speed (V), cadence, mean values ($\overline{X}$) of step duration (SDu) and step length (SL), and corresponding standard deviations (SD) were calculated for each subject and each trial.

3. Statistical Analyses

Normality of the data was tested with the Kolmogorov-Smirnov test. Descriptive statistics were used to define the study population and to calculate gait characteristics.

We used the intraclass correlation ($\text{ICC}_{(2,1)}$) with 95% confidence intervals to calculate intervisit reliability between visit 1 and visit 2. $\text{ICC}_{(2,1)}$ was used because individual ratings constitute the unit of analysis, and raters and subjects were conceived as being a random selection. There was one week between visit 1 and 2. To interpret $\text{ICC}_{(2,1)}$ values we used benchmarks suggested by Shrout and Fleiss [32] (>0.75 excellent reliability, 0.4–0.75 fair to good reliability, and <0.4 poor reliability). To evaluate precision the 95% limits of agreement statistics (Bland and Altman) were used. It expresses the degree of error proportional to the mean, and was calculated as $\overline{d} \pm 2\text{SD}_{\text{diff}}$ [33, 34], where $\overline{d}$ is the mean of the difference and SD_{diff} the standard deviation of the difference. The measurement error (standard error of the mean difference (SEM)) was reported, and the smallest detectable difference (SDD) for each parameter was calculated as described by de Vet et al. [35]. SEM was derived by $\sigma\sqrt{(1 - \text{ICC})}$ in which σ represents the total variance [36]. The smallest detectable change was calculated with the formula $1.96 \times \text{SEM} \times \sqrt{2}$.

To identify differences between groups we used an analysis with planned contrasts [37]. All statistical analyses were performed using SPSS 17 for Windows (SPSS Inc.).

4. Results

Of the 31 patients screened for eligibility all met the inclusion criteria. Data from two individuals were, however, not available. One person presented with hypersensibility of the feet and could not be measured. Technical problems prevented data acquisition for the second person. This resulted in complete data for 29 patients (21 male and 8 female) at baseline, mean age: 61.9 (±5.5) years; body mass index: 28.2 (±3.5)) kg/m^2; leg length 0.84 (±0.06) m (Table 1).

Twelve patients were categorized as "DIABETIC," eleven as "MILD NEUROPATHY," and six as "SEVERE NEUROPATHY." Post hoc ANOVA revealed that the groups did not differ in Age $F(2, 26) = 0.949$, $P = .40$; height $F(2, 26) = 1.26$, $P = .302$; SDu $F(2, 26) = 1.99$, $P = .157$; V $F(2, 26) = 3.01$, $P = .067$; cadence $F(2, 26) = 1.98$, $P = .159$ and showed to be different for weight $F(2, 26) = 4.729$, $P = .018$; BMI $F(2, 26) = 4.28$, $P = .025$; SL $F(2, 26) = 3.14$, $P = .048$.

Four patients were unable or refused to perform the retest due to time limitations or lack of motivation. For the reliability testing we had twenty-five patients performing retesting (17 male and 8 female); mean age: 61 (±5.7)

Table 2: Results of repeated measurements ($N = 25$).

	Test visit 1 mean ± SD	Test visit 2 mean ± SD	P value
Single task			
SDu (s)	0.54 (0.051)	0.55 (0.045)	0.771
SL (m)	0.69 (0.095)	0.69 (0.111)	0.884
V (m/s)	1.28 (0.213)	1.28 (0.243)	0.942
Cad (step/min)	111.7 (10.234)	111.0 (9.031)	0.652
Dual task			
SDu (s)	0.58 (0.079)	0.56 (0.056)	0.046
SL (m)	0.67 (0.109)	0.68 (0.107)	0.325
V (m/s)	1.17 (0.273)	1.23 (0.233)	0.154
Cad (step/min)	104.51 (12.626)	107.7 (10.170)	0.046

SD: standard deviation; SDu: step duration; SL: step length; V: velocity; Cad: cadence.

years; Body Mass Index: 28.7 (±3.5) kg/m^2, leg length 0.83 (±0.06) m. Eleven patients were "DIABETIC," eight "MILD NEUROPATHY" and six "SEVERE NEUROPATHY".

4.1. Differences between the Walking Conditions. Table 2 presents means and SDs of both tests. Significant differences between the two test conditions at baseline, single versus dual task walking, were identified for all gait parameters (walking speed: $t(28) = 3.616$, $P = .001$, cadence: $t(28) = 3.221$, $P = .003$, step duration: $t(28) = -3.112$, $P = .004$, and step length: $t(28) = 2.308$, $P = .029$. Walking speed, step length, and cadence were significantly decreased under dual tasking, and step duration was significantly increased compared to normal walking.

4.2. Reliability. All data were normally distributed and showed no heteroscedasticity. The results of the repeated measurements for the different gait parameters SDu, SL, V, and Cadence are presented in Table 2. Except for cadence under dual task condition there were no differences in walking between visit 1 and 2.

All gait parameters on the walking trajectory under single and dual task walking with regard to test retest reliability are illustrated in Figure 2 by Bland-Altman plots. The results of the test retest reliabilities are summarized in Table 3. The reliability of single task walking speed, cadence, step duration, and step length was "excellent" [32] (ICCs between 0.824–0.898 and SEMs between 0.03–5.2) and comparable to the reliability of dual task walking speed, cadence, step duration and step length (ICCs between 0.826–0.869 and SEMs between 0.1–5.38).

4.3. Validity. The mean values and standard deviations of the gait parameters of 29 evaluated patients at baseline are reported in Table 4 for their grouping. Planned contrasts showed that there was no significant effect on SDu, V, and cadence and a significant effect of grouping on step length performance. This latter parameter, however, showed a large effect [38]. The planned contrasts revealed that having mild and severe PN did not significantly alter step length compared to diabetic patients presenting without PN, $t(26) = -1.318$, $P = .101$, and having severe PN significantly influenced step length compared to mild PN, $t(26) = -2.469$, $P = .046$ (one tailed).

5. Discussion

This study has shown that the reliability of walking speed, cadence, step duration and step length on different surfaces and under dual task conditions was high with excellent ICCs, small SEMs and RLOAs in older adults with diabetes using the DynaPort MiniMod system. Results from discriminant validity were essentially non conclusive, with the exception of step length. There are, therefore, only indications that the system might also be able to distinguish between subpopulations within the population of patients with diabetes based on step length. The disease status of the elderly participants in our study varied from having diabetes without PN and having diabetes with mild or severe polyneuropathy. We thus expected our subjects to represent a heterogeneous group with regard to walking abilities. From previous studies we know that disease severity negatively influences walking velocity [4] especially in challenging environments where patients with neuropathy walk slower when compared to patients without neuropathy [12]. We think that the negative findings in our cross-sectional sample are very likely related to the limited statistical power of this analysis and might be attributed to a possible Type I error. A post hoc power analysis revealed that Power (1-β err prob) = 0.19. Our data allow for an a priori sample size calculation for a future trial with a fixed effects one-way ANOVA design and under the assumption of a moderate effect size of 0.25. To avoid a type I or II error in this future trial, we need an estimated sample size of 159 (53 individuals per group). This would result in 80% power at α-level 0.05 [39].

The gait changes that we observed in dual task walking relative to single task walking are consistent with other studies that demonstrate that cognitive tasks have a destabilizing effect on gait [40–44]. This finding seems to indicate that it is important to consider additional cognitive tasks in gait assessment of diabetic patient populations in clinical practice.

There is scarce information available about the reliability of body fixed sensor approaches to assess gait parameters in older adults with diabetes. The ICCs for walking speed and cadence that we found were, however, similar to values reported by Allet et al. [19] who were using the Physilog system in older, diabetic subjects.

The relative reliability is the degree to which individuals maintain their test results in a sample with repeated measurements and is affected by sample heterogeneity, that means the more heterogeneous a sample is, the higher the relative reliability becomes. Therefore, a high correlation may still mean unacceptable measurement error for some analytical goals, for example, for individualised assessments [36], and data about absolute reliabilities of a test are desired for clinical use. The determination of what constitutes an acceptable RLOA depends on what size difference the researcher

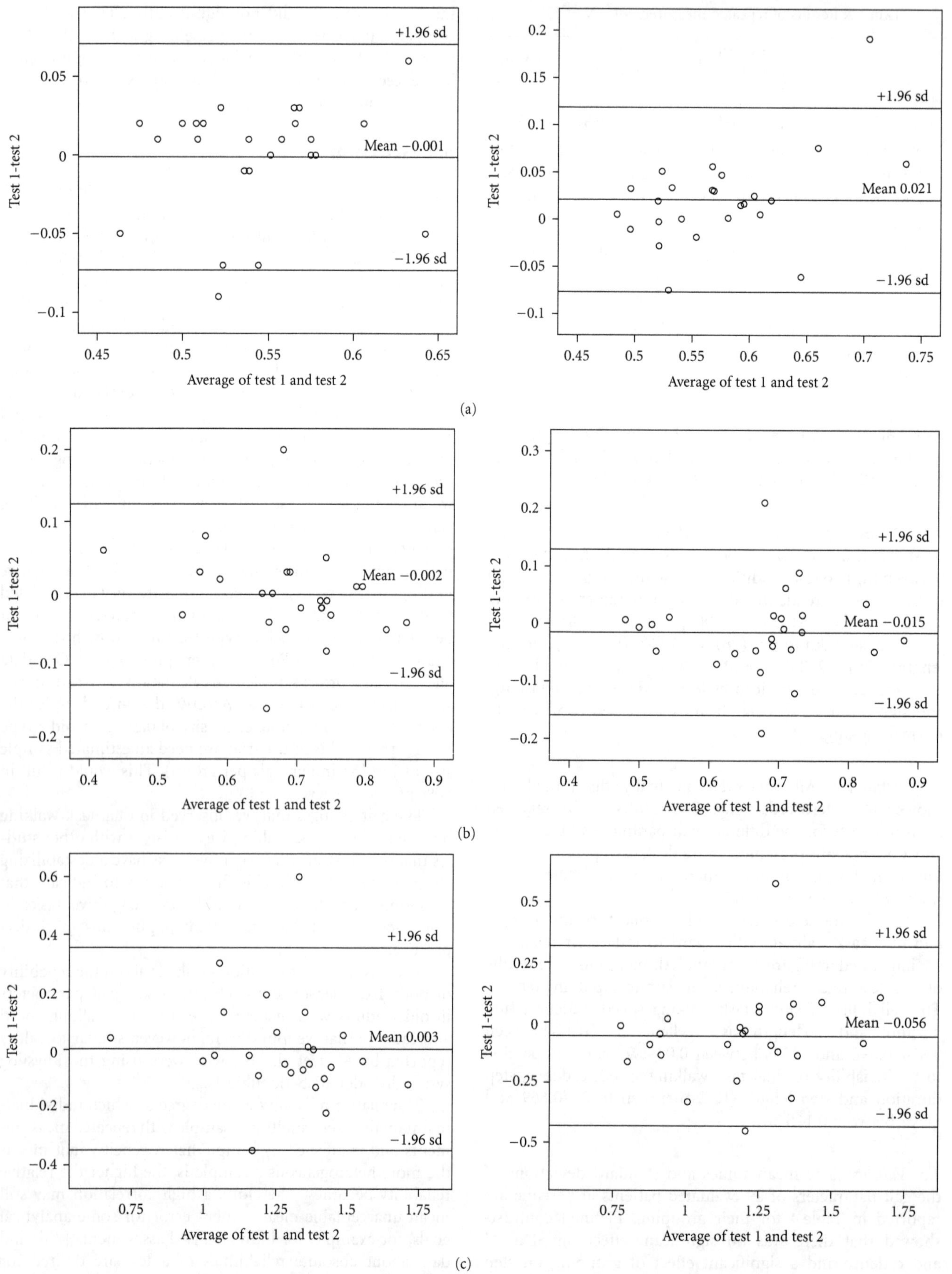

Figure 2: Continued.

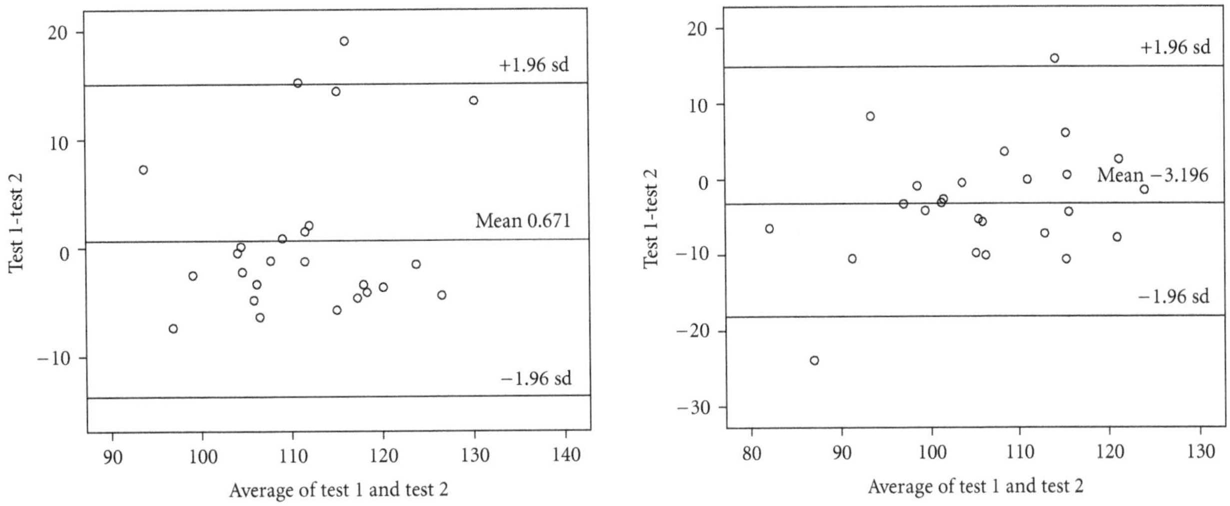

(d)

FIGURE 2: Bland-Altman plots of (a) step duration, (b) step length, (c) walking velocity, and (d) cadence (top to bottom). Left side represents the single task condition, and the right side represents the dual task walking.

TABLE 3: Reliability of different gait parameters[a] at preferred speed (ICC: intraclass correlation coefficient, CI 95% confidence interval 95%, SEM standard error of measurement, SDD smallest detectable difference, and LALB limits of agreement lower boundary, LAUB limits of agreement upper boundary).

	ICC	CI 95%	SEM	CI 95%	SDD	LALB	LAUB
Single task							
SDu (s)	0.848	0.652–0.933	0.03	±0.06	0.09	−0.072	0.071
SL (m)	0.898	0.767–0.955	0.04	±0.09	0.12	−0.128	0.124
V (m/s)	0.824	0.597–0.923	0.12	±0.25	0.35	−0.349	0.354
Cad (step/min)	0.834	0.623–0.927	5.20	±10.2	14.42	−13.754	15.096
Dual task							
SDu (s)	0.829	0.597–0.926	0.10	±0.20	0.28	−0.077	0.119
SL (m)	0.869	0.706–0.942	0.17	±0.34	0.48	−0.159	0.130
V (m/s)	0.829	0.616–0.924	0.13	±0.26	0.37	−0.431	0.318
Cad (step/min)	0.826	0.672–0.940	5.38	±10.54	14.90	−18.101	14.901

SDu: step duration; SL: step length; V: velocity; Cad: cadence.
[a]Calculations—SEM: $\sqrt{\text{Mean square error}}$; CI 95% = ±1.96 × SEM; SDD = $1.96 \times \sqrt{2} \times$ SEM.

TABLE 4: The mean and standard deviations of the gait parameters of 29 evaluated patients, grouped based on disease status, at baseline.

Performance measure	Group		
	Diabetic ($n = 12$)	Mild neuropathy ($n = 11$)	Severe neuropathy ($n = 6$)
Single task			
Step duration (SDu; s)	0.56 ± 0.03	0.53 ± 0.05	0.55 ± 0.05
Step length (SL; m)	0.72 ± 0.06	0.73 ± 0.1	0.62 ± 0.12
Velocity ($m \cdot s^{-1}$)	1.29 ± 0.14	1.39 ± 0.14	1.14 ± 0.37
Cadence (steps/min)	107 ± 5.8	115 ± 10.2	107.6 ± 15
Dual task			
Step duration (SDu; s)	0.6 ± 0.08	0.55 ± 0.05	0.6 ± 0.12
Step length (SL; m)	0.7 ± 0.07	0.7 ± 0.13	0.63 ± 0.1
Velocity ($m \cdot s^{-1}$)	1.18 ± 0.21	1.31 ± 0.28	1.09 ± 0.32
Cadence (steps/min)	101.4 ± 11	110 ± 9.3	103.4 ± 17.6

or clinician wants to detect when comparing groups or when assessing the effect of interventions [45]. Whether the absolute reliability reported here for the gait measures is sufficiently high to identify gait impairments or small effects of an intervention program to improve walking in populations suffering from diabetes should be part of future studies. In particular, the RLOAs for step length and gait velocity might be indicative for rather large needed changes to be detected with the system. A study that investigated gait recovery in a sample of patients with diabetes due to specific exercises [46], with a mean age of 63 years and that used the Physilog gait analysis system for evaluation in challenging environments, showed that changes in gait velocity of around $0.149\,\mathrm{m\cdot s^{-1}}$, and improvements of 10% for cadence are achievable with specific rehabilitation [5, 6]. Whether such changes are also clinically meaningful should be determined in future studies.

In the present study we have shown that step length measures derived from the DynaPort MiniMod are significantly different between groups of patients. There are measurable differences between individuals with mild and severe PN. Clinical detection of these differences potentially allows the division of diabetes patients into two groups with different mean step length: one with severe NP and one without severe NP. These results support the assertion that there is a relationship between quality of walking and the presence of PN. However, these are only preliminary data, and further (cross-sectional and longitudinal) research is needed with larger samples to substantiate this observation.

To obtain the diagnostic information from a walking test in a challenging environment alone, the outcomes of the gait analysis should be compared with other diagnostic tests in use. This necessitates the concurrent measurement of those tests in future research. Therefore, bigger samples of subjects should be selected in the future, and with logistic regression analysis the contribution of the DynaPort MiniMod gait assessment to existing diagnostic tests should be estimated more precisely [47].

6. Conclusions

The results of this study demonstrate that walking speed, cadence, step duration, and step length under more challenging conditions can be reliably measured in adults with diabetes using the DynaPort MiniMod system. There are first indications that the system is able to discriminate subgroups of patients with diabetes based on their step length. Further research in diabetic populations is needed to determine the value of these parameters that are derived from this measurement system in clinical settings.

Acknowledgments

The authors thank all the participants for their involvement. Furthermore, they thank Damiano Zemp, MSc for his part in the data acquisition, and they thank Prof. Roger Lehmann, MD, from the Division of Endocrinology, Diabetes and Clinical Nutrition, University Hospital of Zurich, for his support and for referring his patients to this study. The authors of this manuscript do not have a direct financial relation with the commercial identities mentioned in this paper that might lead to a conflict of interests for any of the authors.

References

[1] K. Osei, "Global epidemic of type 2 diabetes: implications for developing countries," *Ethnicity and Disease*, vol. 13, no. 2, supplement 2, pp. S102–S106, 2003.

[2] J. B. Dingwell and P. R. Cavanagh, "Increased variability of continuous overground walking in neuropathic patients is only indirectly related to sensory loss," *Gait & Posture*, vol. 14, no. 1, pp. 1–10, 2001.

[3] J. Pirart, "Diabetes mellitus and its degenerative complications: a prospective study of 4,400 patients observed between 1947 and 1973 (author's transl)," *Diabete et Metabolisme*, vol. 3, no. 2, pp. 97–107, 1977.

[4] L. Allet, S. Armand, A. Golay, D. Monnin, R. A. de Bie, and E. D. de Bruin, "Gait characteristics of diabetic patients: a systematic review," *Diabetes/Metabolism Research and Reviews*, vol. 24, no. 3, pp. 173–191, 2008.

[5] L. Allet, S. Armand, K. Aminian et al., "An exercise intervention to improve diabetic patients' gait in a real-life environment," *Gait & Posture*, vol. 32, no. 2, pp. 185–190, 2010.

[6] L. Allet, S. Armand, R. A. de Bie et al., "The gait and balance of patients with diabetes can be improved: a randomised controlled trial," *Diabetologia*, vol. 53, no. 3, pp. 458–466, 2010.

[7] H. Dejnabadi, B. M. Jolles, and K. Aminian, "A new approach to accurate measurement of uniaxial joint angles based on a combination of accelerometers and gyroscopes," *IEEE Transactions on Biomedical Engineering*, vol. 52, no. 8, pp. 1478–1484, 2005.

[8] K. Aminian, C. Trevisan, B. Najafi et al., "Evaluation of an ambulatory system for gait analysis in hip osteoarthritis and after total hip replacement," *Gait & Posture*, vol. 20, no. 1, pp. 102–107, 2004.

[9] S. R. Simon, "Quantification of human motion: gait analysis—benefits and limitations to its application to clinical problems," *Journal of Biomechanics*, vol. 37, no. 12, pp. 1869–1880, 2004.

[10] J. K. Richardson, S. B. Thies, T. K. DeMott, and J. A. Ashton-Miller, "Gait analysis in a challenging environment differentiates between fallers and nonfallers among older patients with peripheral neuropathy," *Archives of Physical Medicine and Rehabilitation*, vol. 86, no. 8, pp. 1539–1544, 2005.

[11] S. B. Thies, J. K. Richardson, T. DeMott, and J. A. Ashton-Miller, "Influence of an irregular surface and low light on the step variability of patients with peripheral neuropathy during level gait," *Gait & Posture*, vol. 22, no. 1, pp. 40–45, 2005.

[12] L. Allet, S. Armand, R. A. de Bie et al., "Gait alterations of diabetic patients while walking on different surfaces," *Gait & Posture*, vol. 29, no. 3, pp. 488–493, 2009.

[13] E. Freiberger and H. B. Menz, "Characteristics of falls in physically active community-dwelling older people: findings from the "Standfest im Alter" study," *Zeitschrift für Gerontologie und Geriatrie*, vol. 39, no. 4, pp. 261–267, 2006.

[14] K. Tong and M. H. Granat, "A practical gait analysis system using gyroscopes," *Medical Engineering & Physics*, vol. 21, no. 2, pp. 87–94, 1999.

[15] A. Zijlstra, T. Ufkes, D. A. Skelton, L. Lundin-Olsson, and W. Zijlstra, "Do dual tasks have an added value over single tasks

for balance assessment in fall prevention programs? A mini-review," *Gerontology*, vol. 54, no. 1, pp. 40–49, 2008.

[16] W. Zijlstra and K. Aminian, "Mobility assessment in older people: new possibilities and challenges," *European Journal of Ageing*, vol. 4, no. 1, pp. 3–12, 2007.

[17] E. D. de Bruin, A. Hartmann, D. Uebelhart, K. Murer, and W. Zijlstra, "Wearable systems for monitoring mobility-related activities in older people: a systematic review," *Clinical Rehabilitation*, vol. 22, no. 10-11, pp. 878–895, 2008.

[18] L. Allet, R. H. Knols, K. Shirato et al., "Wearable systems for monitoring mobility-related activities in chronic disease: a systematic review," *Sensors*, vol. 10, no. 10, pp. 9026–9052, 2010.

[19] L. Allet, S. Armand, R. A. de Bie et al., "Reliability of diabetic patients' gait parameters in a challenging environment," *Gait & Posture*, vol. 28, no. 4, pp. 680–686, 2008.

[20] A. Hartmann, R. Knols, K. Murer, and E. D. de Bruin, "Reproducibility of an isokinetic strength-testing protocol of the knee and ankle in older adults," *Gerontology*, vol. 55, no. 3, pp. 259–268, 2009.

[21] E. D. de Bruin, R. H. Rozendal, and E. Stüssi, "Reliability of phase-velocity measurements of tibial bone," *Physical Therapy*, vol. 78, no. 11, pp. 1166–1174, 1998.

[22] A. Hartmann, K. Murer, R. A. de Bie, and E. D. de Bruin, "The effect of a training program combined with augmented afferent feedback from the feet using shoe insoles on gait performance and muscle power in older adults: a randomised controlled trial," *Disability and Rehabilitation*, vol. 32, no. 9, pp. 755–764, 2010.

[23] A. Hartmann, K. Murer, R. A. de Bie, and E. D. de Bruin, "The effect of a foot gymnastic exercise programme on gait performance in older adults: a randomised controlled trial," *Disability and Rehabilitation*, vol. 31, no. 25, pp. 2101–2110, 2009.

[24] A. Hartmann, K. Murer, R. A. de Bie, and E. D. de Bruin, "Reproducibility of spatio-temporal gait parameters under different conditions in older adults using a trunk tri-axial accelerometer system," *Gait & Posture*, vol. 30, no. 3, pp. 351–355, 2009.

[25] A. Hartmann, S. Luzi, K. Murer, R. A. de Bie, and E. D. de Bruin, "Concurrent validity of a trunk tri-axial accelerometer system for gait analysis in older adults," *Gait & Posture*, vol. 29, no. 3, pp. 444–448, 2009.

[26] R. Matsutomo, K. Takebayashi, and Y. Aso, "Assessment of peripheral neuropathy using measurement of the current perception threshold with the neurometer in patients with type 2 diabetes mellitus," *The Journal of International Medical Research*, vol. 33, no. 4, pp. 442–453, 2005.

[27] T. Kästenbauer, S. Sauseng, H. Brath, H. Abrahamian, and K. Irsigler, "The value of the Rydel-Seiffer tuning fork as a predictor of diabetic polyneuropathy compared with a neurothesiometer," *Diabetic Medicine*, vol. 21, no. 6, pp. 563–567, 2004.

[28] I. S. J. Martina, R. van Koningsveld, P. I. M. Schmitz, F. G. A. van der Meché, and P. A. van Doorn, "Measuring vibration threshold with a graduated tuning fork in normal aging and in patients with polyneuropathy," *Journal of Neurology, Neurosurgery, and Psychiatry*, vol. 65, no. 5, pp. 743–747, 1998.

[29] I. S. J. Merkies, P. I. M. Schmitz, F. G. A. van der Meché, and P. A. van Doorn, "Reliability and responsiveness of a graduated tuning fork in immune mediated polyneuropathies," *Journal of Neurology, Neurosurgery, and Psychiatry*, vol. 68, no. 5, pp. 669–671, 2000.

[30] C. Liniger, A. Albeanu, D. Bloise, and J. P. Assal, "The tuning fork revisited," *Diabetic Medicine*, vol. 7, no. 10, pp. 859–864, 1990.

[31] Y. Feng, F. J. Schlösser, and B. E. Sumpio, "The Semmes Weinstein monofilament examination as a screening tool for diabetic peripheral neuropathy," *Journal of Vascular Surgery*, vol. 50, no. 3, pp. 675.e1–682.e1, 2009.

[32] P. E. Shrout and J. L. Fleiss, "Intraclass correlations: uses in assessing rater reliability," *Psychological Bulletin*, vol. 86, no. 2, pp. 420–428, 1979.

[33] G. Rankin and M. Stokes, "Reliability of assessment tools in rehabilitation: an illustration of appropriate statistical analyses," *Clinical Rehabilitation*, vol. 12, no. 3, pp. 187–199, 1998.

[34] J. M. Bland and D. G. Altman, "Statistical methods for assessing agreement between two methods of clinical measurement," *The Lancet*, vol. 1, no. 8476, pp. 307–310, 1986.

[35] H. C. W. de Vet, C. B. Terwee, D. L. Knol, and L. M. Bouter, "When to use agreement versus reliability measures," *Journal of Clinical Epidemiology*, vol. 59, no. 10, pp. 1033–1039, 2006.

[36] G. Atkinson and A. M. Nevill, "Statistical methods for assessing measurement error (reliability) in variables relevant to sports medicine," *Sports Medicine*, vol. 26, no. 4, pp. 217–238, 1998.

[37] A. Field, *Discovering Statistics Using SPSS*, Sage, Los Angeles, Calif, USA, 3rd edition, 2009.

[38] R. E. Kirk, "Practical significance: a concept whose time has come," *Educational and Psychological Measurement*, vol. 56, no. 5, pp. 746–759, 1996.

[39] F. Faul, E. Erdfelder, A. G. Lang, and A. Buchner, "G*Power 3: a flexible statistical power analysis program for the social, behavioral, and biomedical sciences," *Behavior Research Methods*, vol. 39, no. 2, pp. 175–191, 2007.

[40] H. B. Menz, S. R. Lord, and R. C. Fitzpatrick, "Age-related differences in walking stability," *Age and Ageing*, vol. 32, no. 2, pp. 137–142, 2003.

[41] P. C. Grabiner, S. T. Biswas, and M. D. Grabiner, "Age-related changes in spatial and temporal gait variables," *Archives of Physical Medicine and Rehabilitation*, vol. 82, no. 1, pp. 31–35, 2001.

[42] M. Woollacott and A. Shumway-Cook, "Attention and the control of posture and gait: a review of an emerging area of research," *Gait & Posture*, vol. 16, no. 1, pp. 1–14, 2002.

[43] J. H. Hollman, F. M. Kovash, J. J. Kubik, and R. A. Linbo, "Age-related differences in spatiotemporal markers of gait stability during dual task walking," *Gait & Posture*, vol. 26, no. 1, pp. 113–119, 2007.

[44] M. B. van Iersel, H. Ribbers, M. Munneke, G. F. Borm, and M. G. O. Rikkert, "The effect of cognitive dual tasks on balance during walking in physically fit elderly people," *Archives of Physical Medicine and Rehabilitation*, vol. 88, no. 2, pp. 187–191, 2007.

[45] L. G. Portney and M. P. Watkins, *Foundations of Clinical Research: Applications to Practice*, Prentice Hall, Upper Saddle River, NJ, USA, 2000.

[46] E. D. de Bruin and K. Murer, "Effect of additional functional exercises on balance in elderly people," *Clinical Rehabilitation*, vol. 21, no. 2, pp. 112–121, 2007.

[47] Y. T. van der Schouw, A. L. M. Verbeek, and S. H. J. Ruijs, "Guidelines for the assessment of new diagnostic tests," *Investigative Radiology*, vol. 30, no. 6, pp. 334–340, 1995.

8

Letrozole Potentiates Mitochondrial and Dendritic Spine Impairments Induced by β Amyloid

P. K.-Y. Chang, S. Boridy, R. A. McKinney, and D. Maysinger

Department of Pharmacology and Therapeutics, Faculty of Medicine, McGill University, 3655 Promenade Sir William Osler, Montreal, QC, Canada H3G 1Y6

Correspondence should be addressed to R. A. McKinney; anne.mckinney@mcgill.ca and D. Maysinger; dusica.maysinger@mcgill.ca

Academic Editor: Holly M. Brown-Borg

Reduced estrogens, either through aging or postsurgery breast cancer treatment with the oral nonsteroidal aromatase inhibitor letrozole, are linked with declined cognitive abilities. However, a direct link between letrozole and neuronal deficits induced by pathogenic insults associated with aging such as beta amyloid ($A\beta_{1-42}$) has not been established. The objective of this study was to determine if letrozole aggravates synaptic deficits concurrent with $A\beta_{1-42}$ insult. We examined the effects of letrozole and oligomeric $A\beta_{1-42}$ treatment in dissociated and organotypic hippocampal slice cultures. Changes in glial cell morphology, neuronal mitochondria, and synaptic structures upon letrozole treatment were monitored by confocal microscopy, as they were shown to be affected by $A\beta_{1-42}$ oligomers. Oligomeric $A\beta_{1-42}$ or letrozole alone caused decreases in mitochondrial volume, dendritic spine density, synaptophysin (synaptic marker), and the postsynaptic protein, synaptopodin. Here, we demonstrated that mitochondrial and synaptic structural deficits were exacerbated when letrozole therapy was combined with $A\beta_{1-42}$ treatment. Our novel findings suggest that letrozole may increase neuronal susceptibility to pathological insults, such as oligomeric $A\beta_{1-42}$ in Alzheimer's disease (AD). These changes in dendritic spine number, synaptic protein expression, and mitochondrial morphology may, in part, explain the increased prevalence of cognitive decline associated with aromatase inhibitor use.

1. Introduction

Currently, aromatase inhibitors, leading to reduction of estradiol synthesis from testosterone, have been favoured in the treatment of breast cancer of postmenopausal women [1]. Letrozole is one such oral nonsteroidal aromatase inhibitor which prevents the aromatase from producing estrogens by competitive, reversible binding to the heme of its cytochrome P450 unit [2, 3]. Patients receiving letrozole have shown deficits in learning and memory [4]. However, it is still unclear if these functional impairments occur because of neurosteroid deficits and if they become exacerbated in the presence of an additional insult associated with aging, such as an excess of soluble, conformationally altered $A\beta_{1-42}$. Such forms of $A\beta_{1-42}$ can interact with synapses and cause pronounced degenerative changes, an observation made in brain tissue from postmortem Alzheimer's disease (AD) patients and animal models [5]. It has been well documented in AD that there are changes in neuronal and glial morphologies such as dendritic spine atrophy and increased glial growth [5, 6]. In contrast to these negative effects caused by $A\beta_{1-42}$, it is well established that the neurosteroid estradiol can increase the number of dendritic spines and proteins in humans, as well as promoting synaptogenesis and cellular models of learning such as long-term potentiation (LTP) in hippocampal cultures [7, 8]. Despite these well-established positive effects of neuroestrogens in the CNS, 17-β-estradiol hormone therapy in postmenopausal women did not exhibit clear cognitive benefits [9–13]. These clinical studies did not provide conclusive evidence whether exogenous estrogen exposure in early menopause affects AD or cognitive aging [14] and to what extent (if any) peripheral estrogen in blood could play a role in patients or animal models of AD [15–17].

To investigate whether aromatase suppression in the CNS affects synaptic responses to pathological insults, we used confocal microscopy to examine the effect of letrozole and $A\beta_{1-42}$ on two model systems, dissociated hippocampal neurons, and organotypic slice cultures. The slice cultures have a preserved neural circuitry, exhibit similar synaptic transmission as *in vivo*, and permit long-term studies allowing for the assessment of synapse morphology and function following pharmacological aromatase inhibition. The objective of the present study was to investigate the response of hippocampal neurons and glia to soluble $A\beta_{1-42}$ species upon inhibition of CNS aromatase by letrozole. We have found significant decrease in neuronal mitochondrial volume, dendritic spine density, synapse number, and the synaptic protein, synaptopodin, in cultures that were either treated with letrozole or $A\beta_{1-42}$ alone. With letrozole and $A\beta_{1-42}$ co-treatment, the synaptic and mitochondrial deficits were further enhanced in the hippocampal neurons. These findings could explain why women on letrozole have a higher incidence of cognitive decline and may be more vulnerable to the detrimental effect of $A\beta_{1-42}$.

2. Materials and Methods

2.1. Preparation of β-Amyloid ($A\beta_{1-42}$). $A\beta_{1-42}$ (Sigma-Aldrich, St. Louis, MO, USA) was dissolved in 5% NH4OH in Tris Buffered Saline and vortexed until fully dissolved (several minutes) at a concentration of 1 mM. Aliquots were stored at −80°C. Upon reconstitution, aliquots are dissolved directly in media prior to treatment at a final concentration of 1 μM [18].

2.2. Preparation of Dissociated Neural Cell Cultures. All procedures for animal handling were carried out according to the guidelines of the Canadian Council on Animal Care (CCAC) and approved by the Animal Resource Committee of the School of Medicine, McGill University. Hippocampal tissues from mouse pups of 3–5 days old were dissected, trypsinized, dissociated, and incubated as described previously [19]. Briefly, hippocampi of P3–5mice were isolated, mechanically and enzymatically (0.25% trypsin; Gibco, Life Technologies Inc, Burlington, ON, Canada) dissociated, and plated onto coated (poly-l-ornithine, 100 μg/mL (Sigma-Aldrich) and laminin, 0.587 μg/mL (Invitrogen, Life Technologies Inc, Burlington, ON, Canada) glass coverslips and maintained at 37°C and 5% CO_2 in a 24-well plate (Corning; Lowell, MA, USA). Culture medium consisted of neurobasal A (Invitrogen) supplemented with 2% (v/v) B-27 supplement (Invitrogen), 1% (v/v) PSN (Invitrogen), and 1 mM L-glutamine (Sigma-Aldrich).

2.3. Pharmacological Treatments of Dissociated Neural Cell Cultures. Dissociated cells were treated on day *in vitro* (DIV) 8 with 1 μM letrozole (Novartis, Dorval, QC, Canada) and/or 1 μM $A\beta_{1-42}$ (American Peptide Company, Sunnyvale, CA, USA) [20] according to the respective design outlined in the results section and corresponding figure legends.

2.4. Preparation of Slice Cultures. Hippocampal slices (400 μm) from P6–8 transgenic mice expressing membrane-targeted MARCKS-eGFP under the Thy-1 promoter in a subpopulation of CA1 cells [21] were prepared as previously described using the roller-tube method [22]. Slice cultures were maintained in the incubator with a roller-drum for three weeks before experimentation to allow for spine maturation [23].

2.5. Pharmacological Treatments of Slice Cultures. Slice cultures were maintained for at least 3 weeks *in vitro* to allow for maturation prior to treatment. In addition, all treatments were done on sister cultures (slice cultures that were prepared from the same mice litter and handled the same way at the same time). To prevent the effects of estradiol known to be present in serum, which is normally included in the culture media, we placed our preparations in serum free media prior to testing the effects of $A\beta_{1-42}$ or letrozole [24]. Following preincubation, cultures were then treated with media containing either, vehicle, $A\beta_{1-42}$ (1 μM), letrozole (1 μM), or $A\beta_{1-42}$ + letrozole for 24 or 72 hours. No media change was performed during the time course.

2.6. Immunocytochemistry for Dissociated Cells. Following treatments, the hippocampal cells were fixed in 4% formaldehyde for 10 min at room temperature (RT), and routine immunocytochemical protocol was followed using mouse monoclonal anti-GFAP (1 : 250; Molecular Probes, Life Technologies Inc, Burlington, ON, Canada), β-III tubulin (1 : 100; Molecular Probes), and Alexa488-conjugated goat anti-mouse IgG (1 : 800; Invitrogen). The samples were counterstained with Hoechst 33258 (Molecular Probes), mounted onto glass slides (Vectashield H-1000, Vector, Burlingame, CA, USA), and sealed with clear nail polish.

2.7. Mitochondrial Labeling and Morphological Status. Morphological status of mitochondria was determined by labelling live cells (treated or untreated) with 500 nM Mitotracker Deep Red FM (Molecular Probes) for 3 minutes and imaged with a confocal microscope at 63× (Zeiss LSM510, Carl Zeiss MicroImaging GmbH, Jena, Germany); 633 nm HeNe laser at 20% max excitation intensity. Z-stacks (10 slices, 0.33 μm steps) were acquired of dendritic segments from 4–6 different neurons per coverslip, and 2-3 coverslips per condition were analyzed. 3D deconvolution of the raw stack was performed using Huygen's Deconvolution Software (Scientific Volume Imaging, Hilversum, The Netherlands) with maximum likelihood extrapolation, and images were further analyzed for volumetric measurements using Imaris (Bitplane, Zurich, Switzerland).

2.8. Image Acquisition and Quantification of Dendritic Spines. Following treatments, slice cultures were transferred to a temperature-controlled chamber (30°C) mounted on an upright confocal microscope equipped with W Plan-APOCHROMAT 63×/1.0 objective (Zeiss LSM710, Carl Zeiss MicroImaging GmbH) and continuously perfused with Tyrode solution containing (in mM): NaCl, 137; KCl, 2.7; $CaCl_2$, 2.5; $MgCl_2$, 2; $NaHCO_3$, 11.6; NaH_2PO_4, 0.4; and glucose, 5.6 (pH 7.4). Secondary and tertiary dendritic branches from either apical or basal dendrites of CA1 pyramidal neurons were imaged using 488 nm argon-ion laser line. Spine

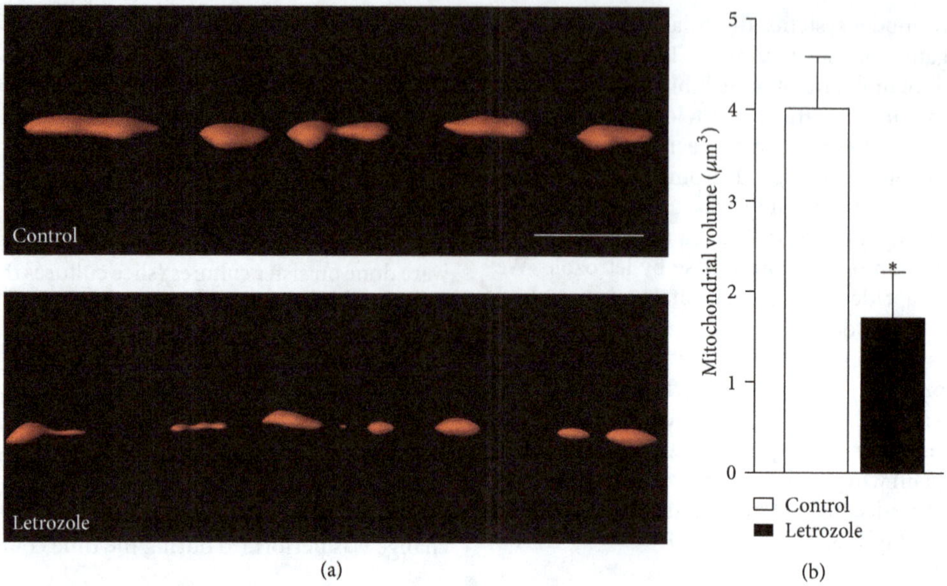

FIGURE 1: Mitochondrial impairments following $A\beta_{1-42}$ and letrozole treatment. (a) Representative 3D reconstructions of MitoTracker Deep Red-positive mitochondria from hippocampal dendritic segments treated with letrozole (1 μM) for 72 hours. Scale bar 5 μm. (b) Quantifications of mitochondrial volumes. Significant differences in mitochondrial volume relative to control ($4.03 \pm 0.56\,\mu m^3$) were observed for letrozole ($1.72 \pm 0.49\,\mu m^3$, $P = 0.015$) and indicated by an asterix (*).

classification was based on previously established criteria and separated into three main morphological subtypes, stubby, mushroom, and thin-type spines based on the ratio between the diameter and length of spine heads and necks [23].

2.9. Immunohistochemical Staining of Synaptic Proteins. Following treatment, hippocampal slice cultures were removed from the cover glass and fixed in 4% paraformaldehyde dissolved in 0.1 M phosphate buffer (PB) overnight at 4°C. Primary antibodies were incubated for five days at 4°C in the permeabilizing solution containing 0.4% Triton X 100. Rabbit monoclonal anti-synaptophysin primary antibody was used at 1 : 400 dilution (Zymed, CA, USA) and mouse monoclonal anti-synaptopodin primary antibody was used at 1 : 400 dilution (Abcam, MA, USA), as well. Secondary antibodies (Texas Red (Invitrogen); Cy-5 (Jackson ImmunoResearch Laboratories Inc., West Grove, PA, USA)) were prepared at 1 : 250 dilutions in 0.1 M PB containing 1.5% horse serum and incubated overnight at 4°C. Slices were then mounted with DAKO fluorescent mounting medium (Dako Canada, ON, Canada) onto microscope slides and imaged. Secondary and tertiary dendrites of CA1 pyramidal neurons were imaged using a Leica TCS SP2 scanhead (Leica Microsystems, Concord, ON Canada) on a Leica DM6000 B upright microscope (Leica Microsystems).

2.10. Statistical Analysis. Two-tailed, one-way ANOVA followed by Tukey's or Dunnet's multiple comparison tests or Student's t-tests is performed, and Bonferroni's correction is applied when appropriate. Results are expressed as mean ± SEM. All data analyses were performed blind.

3. Results

It has been previously shown that abnormalities in spine structure and composition are observed in response to aromatase inhibition; the present study considers the effects of soluble oligomeric $A\beta_{1-42}$ on characterized dendritic spine subtypes and mitochondrial structures in hippocampal neurons exposed to letrozole. Estrogens mediate neuroprotective effects in part through maintenance of mitochondrial structure and metabolic function [25, 26], and, thus far, letrozole's effect on mitochondrial network plasticity has not been considered. Live dissociated mixed neural cultures treated for 24 hrs with 1 μM letrozole were labelled with the mitochondrial-specific probe, MitoTracker Deep Red FM (see methods and materials). Sectioning of isolated hippocampal neuronal dendrites followed by 3D reconstruction of the resultant image stacks using Imaris software allowed for mitochondrial volume measurement acquisition and thus a readout of mitochondrial integrity, following aromatase inhibition (Figure 1(a)). We found that letrozole treatment resulted in mitochondrial fragmentation, measured as a significant reduction in volume (Figure 1(b), control, $4.03 \pm 0.56\,\mu m^3$; letrozole, $1.72 \pm 0.49\,\mu m^3$; $P = 0.015$), implying mitochondrial dysfunction. Next, we thought to address the question of how does blockade of estrogen synthesis affect neuronal circuitry.

To this end, we examined the effects of estrogen synthesis inhibition on the morphological characteristics of neurons and glial cells using letrozole (Figure 2). Immunohistochemical analyses of colabelled neurons and glia from these mice using β-III tubulin as a neuronal marker and anti-glial fibrillary acidic protein (GFAP) as an astrocytic marker revealed profound changes in those cultures that

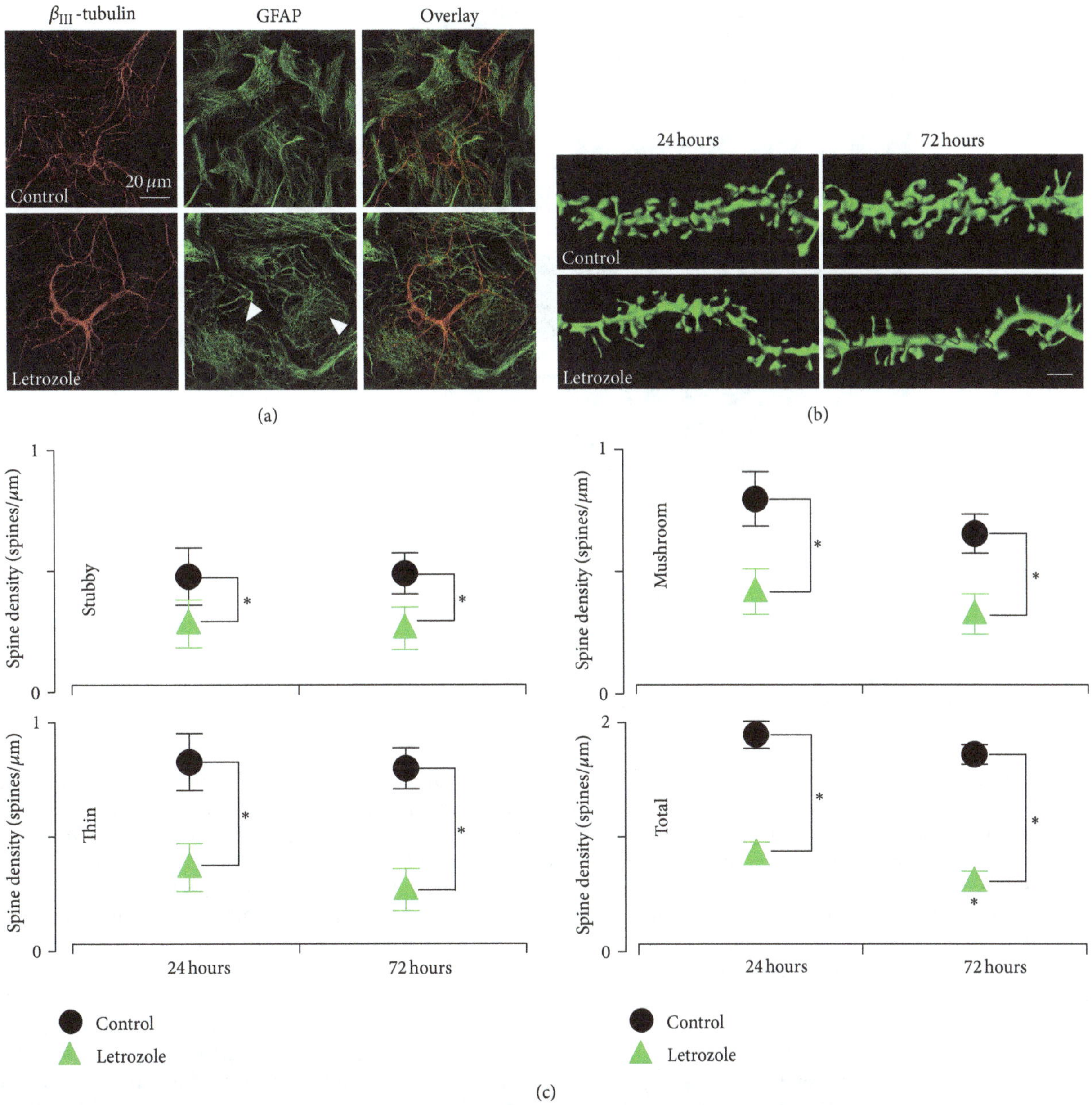

FIGURE 2: Hypertrophy of astroglia and a loss of dendritic spines following 3-day letrozole treatment. (a) Gender mixed hippocampal neural cells were isolated from 3-day old C57/BL6 mouse pups and fixed in 10% Formalin on DIV7. Shown is confocal images of immunocytochemically labelled hippocampal cell cultures with GFAP (astroglia, green) and β-III tubulin (neurons, red). Arrowheads outline astrocytic hypertrophy in letrozole-treated cultures after 72 hours. Scale bar, 20 μm. (b) Representative 3D reconstructions of dendritic segments from organotypic hippocampal sister slice cultures that were treated with either control or letrozole (1 μm)-containing media for either 24 or 72 hours. Scale bar, 2 μm. (c) Quantification of the spine subtype densities following treatments. There is a significant decrease in the densities for all spine subtypes following letrozole treatment compared to control. 24-hour treatment, control, n = total dendritic segment lengths of 441 μm from 10 cells in 4 cultures; letrozole, n = 433 μm of dendrite from 9 cells in 4 cultures. 72-hour treatment, control, n = 500 μm of dendrite from 12 cells in 4 cultures; letrozole, n = 489 μm of dendrite from 11 cells in 4 cultures.

were treated with letrozole (1 μM) for 72 hours: primary cultures that were treated with control media have extensive neuronal arbors and normal astrocytic morphology while striking changes were revealed in the letrozole-treated cultures where hippocampal neurons were sparse, with thin dendritic extensions, coupled with massive astrocytic hypertrophy (Figure 2(a)). When the letrozole treatments were repeated using organotypic hippocampal slice cultures, a culture system with more intact neuronal circuitry, we observed a significant loss of dendritic spines following 24 and 72 hours of letrozole treatment. These findings suggest that the aromatase-mediated blockade of estradiol synthesis with letrozole adversely affects neuronal circuitry in the hippocampus.

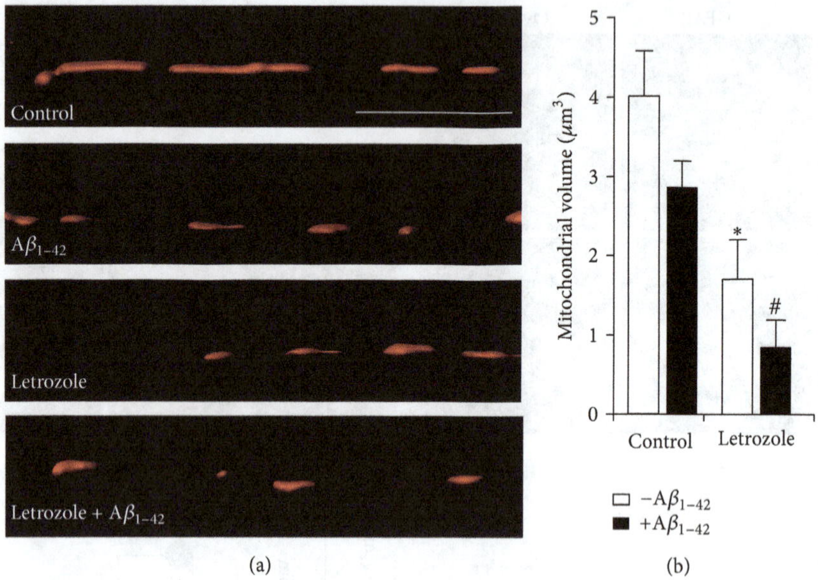

FIGURE 3: Letrozole and $A\beta_{1-42}$ cause significant changes in mitochondrial morphology. (a) Representative 3D reconstructions of MitoTracker Deep Red FM-positive mitochondria from hippocampal dendritic segments treated with $A\beta_{1-42}$ (1 μM) for 24 hours in the presence and absence of 3-day letrozole (1 μM) treatment. Scale bar, 5 μm. (b) Quantifications of mitochondrial volumes. Significant differences in mitochondrial volume, compared to control cultures ($4.03 \pm 0.56\,\mu m^3$), were observed for letrozole- ($1.72 \pm 0.49\,\mu m^3$, $P = 0.015$) treated cultures, as indicated by (∗). Although there is no significant difference in mitochondrial volume between control and $A\beta_{1-42}$ ($P = 0.25$), it is noteworthy that further reduction in mitochondrial volume relative to $A\beta_{1-42}$ ($2.88 \pm 0.32\,\mu m^3$) was observed in letrozole + $A\beta_{1-42}$ treated cultures ($0.86 \pm 0.33\,\mu m^3$, $P = 3.37 \times 10^{-4}$) and is signified by (#).

As the densities of dendritic spines are known to be modulated by estrogens [8], we investigated the effect of letrozole on spine density and shape (Figure 2(b) and Supplementary Table 1). See Supplementary material available online at http://dx.doi.org/10.1155/2013/538979. Treatments for 24 hours with letrozole led to a significant reduction in the number of CA1 dendritic spines compared to control slices (Figure 2(c) and Supplementary Table 1, stubby, $P = 2.1 \times 10^{-4}$; mushroom, $P = 1.0 \times 10^{-7}$; thin, $P = 2.1 \times 10^{-4}$; total, $P = 1.1 \times 10^{-6}$). Given the observed decrease in spine density, we subsequently investigated whether the significant decrease in spine density was subtype dependent (thin, stubby, and mushroom), which could serve as a correlate of the number of glutamatergic α-amino-3-hydroxy-5-methyl-4-isoxazolepropionic (AMPA)-type receptors and synapse strength [27]. All subtypes of the spines were affected with the different treatments after 24 hours. Next, we determined if the dendritic spine loss following the treatment is time dependent, and we examined spine densities after 72 hours of letrozole treatment (Figure 2(c) and Supplementary Table 1, stubby, $P = 7.6 \times 10^{-8}$; mushroom, $P = 3.3 \times 10^{-8}$; thin, $P = 1.8 \times 10^{-10}$; total, $P = 1.8 \times 10^{-10}$). We found, at 72 hours, a continued loss of dendritic spines compared to treatments after 24 hours. These findings show that reduction of estradiol concentrations due to the aromatase inhibition affects all spine subclasses with the most marked reduction in mushroom and thin spines.

Given that letrozole alone caused mitochondrial impairments and synaptic deficits, we next determined whether it could exacerbate changes in response to soluble oligomeric $A\beta_{1-42}$, an established mediator of neuronal deficits associated with AD pathology. First, we examined the effect of oligomeric $A\beta_{1-42}$ in conjunction with letrozole treatment on neuronal mitochondrial integrity (Figure 3). Mixed dissociated neural cultures were treated with 1 μM letrozole every 24 hours from DIV 6 to 8. On DIV 8, letrozole treatment was combined with oligomeric $A\beta_{1-42}$ species (1 μM) for a subsequent 24 hours, following which mitochondria were labelled and imaged as described above. As shown in Figure 3(b), we observed a trend towards a decrease ($P = 0.26$) in mitochondrial volume when the neuronal cultures were treated with $A\beta_{1-42}$ alone. We found a further reduction of mitochondrial volume when the cultures were pretreated with letrozole prior to oligomeric $A\beta_{1-42}$ species exposure compared to either letrozole ($P = 0.17$) or $A\beta_{1-42}$ alone ($P = 3.37 \times 10^{-4}$). Our data suggest that letrozole treatment sensitizes neuronal mitochondria to alterations induced by $A\beta_{1-42}$ oligomers. Next, we examined whether these treatments can also lead to changes in synaptic structures.

Previously, it was shown that the addition of soluble oligomeric $A\beta_{1-42}$ can cause a decrease in dendritic spine density [20]. Hence, we determined if the combined treatment with $A\beta_{1-42}$ and letrozole exerts even greater impairments of mitochondrial integrity and synaptic structures. Treatments for 24 and 72 hours with either letrozole or $A\beta_{1-42}$ alone lead to a significant reduction in the number of CA1 dendritic spines compared to control slices (Figure 4 and Supplemantary Table 2, $P = 4.7 \times 10^{-5}$, $P = 1.1 \times 10^{-6}$, resp.). The decrease in spines can be attributed to a drop in mushroom and thin-type spines (Figure 4 and Supplemantary

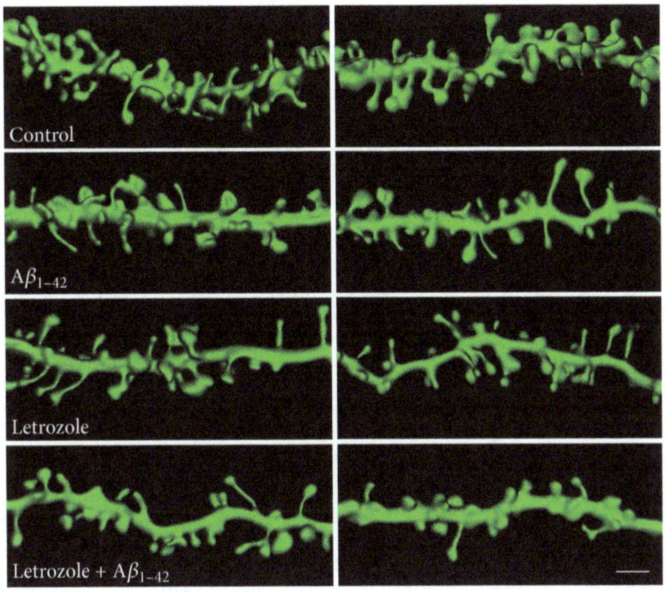

(a)

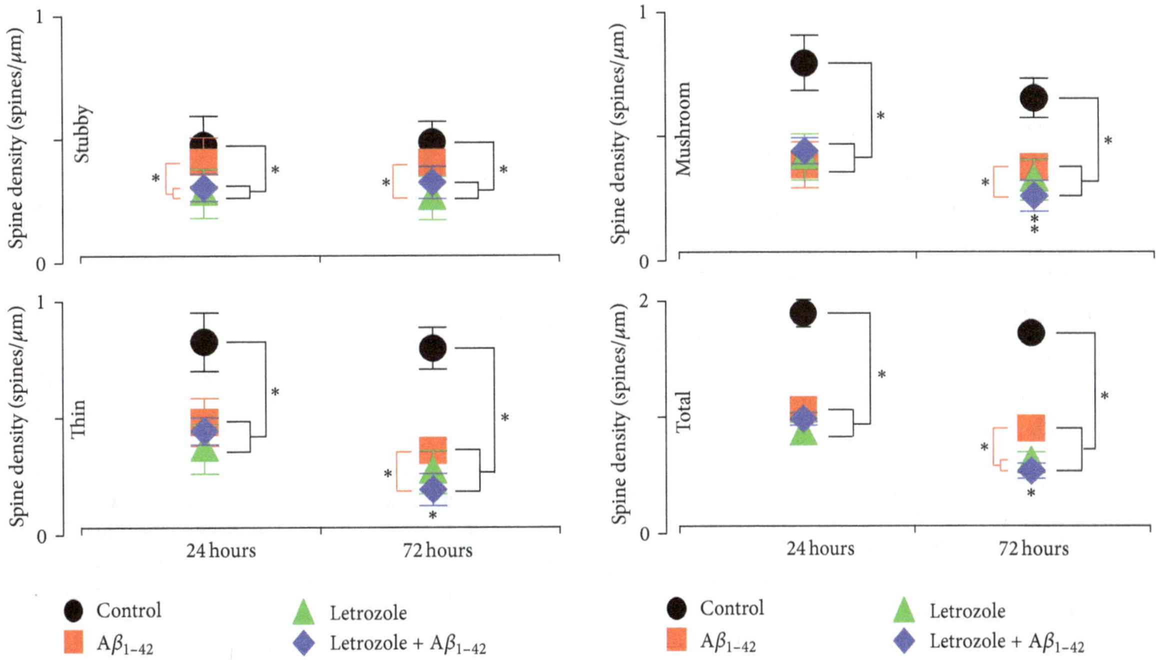

(b)

FIGURE 4: Letrozole and $A\beta_{1-42}$ reduce the number of dendritic spines. (a) Representative 3D reconstructions of dendritic segments from sister cultures that were treated with either control, $A\beta_{1-42}$ (1 μM), and letrozole (1 μM) or $A\beta_{1-42}$ + letrozole (1 μM) for 24 or 72 hours. Scale bar, 2 μm. (b) Quantification of the spine subtype densities following treatments. There is a significant decrease in the total dendritic spine densities for $A\beta_{1-42}$, letrozole, and $A\beta_{1-42}$ + letrozole-treated cultures compared to control after 24 hours. When spine subtypes are examined, there are significant differences between control and treated cultures in mushroom and thin-type spines while spine density for stubby spines is only significantly different between letrozole and $A\beta_{1-42}$ + letrozole compared to control and between $A\beta_{1-42}$ and letrozole. Control, n = total dendritic segment lengths of 441 μm from 10 cells in 4 cultures; $A\beta_{1-42}$, n = 428 μm of dendrite from 11 cells in 4 cultures; letrozole, n = 433 μm of dendrite from 9 cells in 4 cultures; $A\beta_{1-42}$ + letrozole, n = 431 μm of dendrite from 10 cells in 4 cultures. There is a significant decrease in the total dendritic spine densities compared to control cultures after 72 hours as well. In total spine density, cultures treated with either letrozole or $A\beta_{1-42}$ + letrozole had lower spine counts compared to cultures treated with $A\beta_{1-42}$ alone. For mushroom and thin-type spines, cultures treated with both $A\beta_{1-42}$ and letrozole had significantly lower spine densities compared to $A\beta_{1-42}$ alone while stubby spine density was lower for letrozole-treated compared to $A\beta_{1-42}$ alone. Control, n = 500 μm of dendrite from 12 cells in 4 cultures; $A\beta_{1-42}$, n = 465 μm of dendrite from 10 cells in 4 cultures; letrozole, n = 489 μm of dendrite from 11 cells in 4 cultures; $A\beta_{1-42}$ + letrozole, n = 441 μm of dendrite from 9 cells in 4 cultures. Only cultures treated with $A\beta_{1-42}$ + letrozole had significant decrease in total spine densities between 24 and 72 hours of treatment. This difference is contributed by significant decrease in spine density in both mushroom and thin type spines.

Table 2, mushroom: $A\beta_{1-42}$, $P = 1.7 \times 10^{-8}$; letrozole, $P = 1.0 \times 10^{-7}$, thin: $A\beta_{1-42}$, $P = 2.1 \times 10^{-3}$; letrozole, $P = 2.1 \times 10^{-4}$); while spine density for stubby spines is only significantly different between letrozole and $A\beta_{1-42}$ + letrozole compared to control (letrozole, $P = 2.1 \times 10^{-4}$; $A\beta_{1-42}$ + letrozole, $P = 2.1 \times 10^{-4}$) and between $A\beta_{1-42}$ and letrozole ($P = 0.014$). In addition, treatments at 72 hours revealed a further reduction in dendritic spine densities in the slice cultures that were treated with both $A\beta_{1-42}$ and letrozole compared to $A\beta_{1-42}$ alone (Figure 4 and Supplemantary Table 2, $P = 1.9 \times 10^{-11}$). In total spine density, cultures treated with either letrozole or $A\beta_{1-42}$ + letrozole had lower spine count compared to cultures treated with $A\beta_{1-42}$ alone ($P = 0.036$ and 3.3×10^{-4} resp.). For mushroom and thin-type spines, cultures treated with both $A\beta_{1-42}$ and letrozole had significantly lower spine densities compared to $A\beta_{1-42}$ alone (mushroom, $P = 0.024$; thin, $P = 0.013$) while stubby spine density was lower for letrozole-treated cultures compared to $A\beta_{1-42}$ alone ($P = 7.0 \times 10^{-3}$). Furthermore, to examine whether the observed dendritic spine loss was indeed caused by estradiol depletion using letrozole, we treated the slice cultures with letrozole, $A\beta_{1-42}$, and letrozole + $A\beta_{1-42}$ in the presence of estradiol (Supplemantary Figure 1, Supplemantary Tables 1 and 4, estradiol). We have found that cotreatment with estradiol successfully prevented the decrease in dendritic spine density caused by letrozole and/or $A\beta_{1-42}$, as no change in spine densities was observed compared to control at 24 or 72 hours (24 hours: estradiol, $P = 0.13$; estradiol + letrozole, $P = 0.38$; estradiol + $A\beta_{1-42}$, $P = 0.22$; estradiol + letrozole + $A\beta_{1-42}$, $P = 0.37$; 72 hour, estradiol, $P = 0.57$; estradiol + letrozole, $P = 0.18$; estradiol + $A\beta_{1-42}$, $P = 0.69$; estradiol + letrozole + $A\beta_{1-42}$, $P = 0.61$). These data provide substantial evidence that letrozole can worsen neuronal deficits caused by oligomeric $A\beta_{1-42}$.

Although dendritic spines density was decreased after letrozole and $A\beta_{1-42}$ treatment, it has been shown that the loss of spine does not necessary mean the loss of synapses [28]. In some instances, presynaptic terminals may be pulled back onto the dendrite to form asymmetric shaft synapses [28]. To answer the question if the observed loss of postsynaptic dendritic spines is accompanied by a loss of presynaptic terminals, we performed immunohistochemistry labelling of synaptophysin (presynaptic terminal marker). This presynaptic marker allows the determination of a loss or gain of presynaptic terminals when there is a loss (or gain) of dendritic spines induced by therapeutic treatments or insults to the CNS (Figure 5 and Supplemantary Table 3). There was a significant decrease in synaptophysin puncta after 24 hours which became more pronounced at 72 hours of letrozole or $A\beta_{1-42}$ + letrozole treatments compared to control conditions (24 hours: $A\beta_{1-42}$, $P = 6.1 \times 10^{-2}$; letrozole, $P = 7.3 \times 10^{-6}$; $A\beta_{1-42}$ + letrozole, $P = 1.2 \times 10^{-5}$; 72 hour, $A\beta_{1-42}$, $P = 4.0 \times 10^{-6}$; letrozole, $P = 4.0 \times 10^{-6}$; $A\beta_{1-42}$ + letrozole, $P = 4.0 \times 10^{-6}$). After 72 hours, the number of synaptophysin puncta was significantly lower in letrozole and $A\beta_{1-42}$ + letrozole-treated cultures compared to $A\beta_{1-42}$ or letrozole alone (letrozole, $P = 0.043$; $A\beta_{1-42}$ + letrozole, $P = 2.0 \times 10^{-3}$). When synaptophysin puncta densities were compared between 24- and 72-hour treated cultures there was a significant decrease in $A\beta_{1-42}$, letrozole, and $A\beta_{1-42}$ + letrozole-treated cultures after 72 hours ($A\beta_{1-42}$, $P = 1.1 \times 10^{-4}$; letrozole, $P = 1.0 \times 10^{-7}$; and $A\beta_{1-42}$ + letrozole, $P = 1.4 \times 10^{-8}$).

We next investigated if there was also a loss of synaptopodin, an actin-binding protein mainly found in a subgroup of mature spines. Synaptopodin is known to be downregulated upon exposure to estradiol [29]. It also plays a role in learning and memory; synaptopodin knockout animals have reduced LTP and have deficits in spatial learning [30]. We found that there is a change in synaptopodin staining after treatment with $A\beta_{1-42}$, letrozole, and $A\beta_{1-42}$ + letrozole (Figure 5 and Supplemantary Table 3). There was a significant decrease in synaptopodin puncta after 24 and 72 hours of treatments compared to control (Figure 5 and Supplemantary Table 3; 24 hours, $A\beta_{1-42}$, $P = 4.1 \times 10^{-6}$; letrozole, $P = 4.0 \times 10^{-6}$; $A\beta_{1-42}$ + letrozole, $P = 4.0 \times 10^{-6}$; 72 hours, $A\beta_{1-42}$, $P = 2.2 \times 10^{-4}$; letrozole, $P = 3.9 \times 10^{-6}$; $A\beta_{1-42}$ + letrozole, $P = 3.9 \times 10^{-6}$). After 72 hours, the number of synaptopodin puncta was significantly lower in letrozole and $A\beta_{1-42}$ + letrozole-treated cultures compared to $A\beta_{1-42}$ alone (letrozole, $P = 1.2 \times 10^{-5}$; $A\beta_{1-42}$ + letrozole, $P = 3.9 \times 10^{-6}$). When synaptopodin puncta densities were compared between 24- and 72-hour treated cultures, there was a significant decrease in $A\beta_{1-42}$ ($P = 4.1 \times 10^{-6}$), letrozole ($P = 4.0 \times 10^{-6}$), and $A\beta_{1-42}$ + letrozole ($P = 4.0 \times 10^{-6}$)-treated cultures after 72 hours. Difference between controls was not significant ($P = 0.09$). Decreases in estrogen levels reduced the number of synaptic connections, and this was more pronounced in the presence of $A\beta_{1-42}$.

4. Discussion

Chronic estrogen deficit, similar to that experienced by menopausal women, is a recognized risk factor for AD [31]. The neurological deficits known to result from estrogen deficiency are accompanied by morphological deterioration of postsynaptic spines and functional impairments of mitochondria. We have now shown similar pathological features in an animal model with estrogen deficiency [32] and in neural cells of normal animals with estrogen deficiency induced by letrozole, a therapeutic agent for breast cancer. However, in both instances, the more marked dendritic spine degeneration was produced only when letrozole treatment was together with oligomeric $A\beta_{1-42}$.

Dendritic atrophy and astrocytic hypertrophy are common observations in many neurological disorders [6], including AD [33]. Although it was very clear that both circulating and brain estrogens were reduced in animal models and can lead to learning deficits, the contribution of neuroestrogens versus circulating estradiol could not be determined [15, 34]. To circumvent this, we used hippocampal organotypic cultures treated with the aromatase inhibitor, letrozole. This experimental paradigm allowed us to control the concentration and duration of aromatase inhibition and estrogen deficit. Moreover, this model is optimal for studying neuronal connections and glial input in a spatiotemporal (longitudinal)

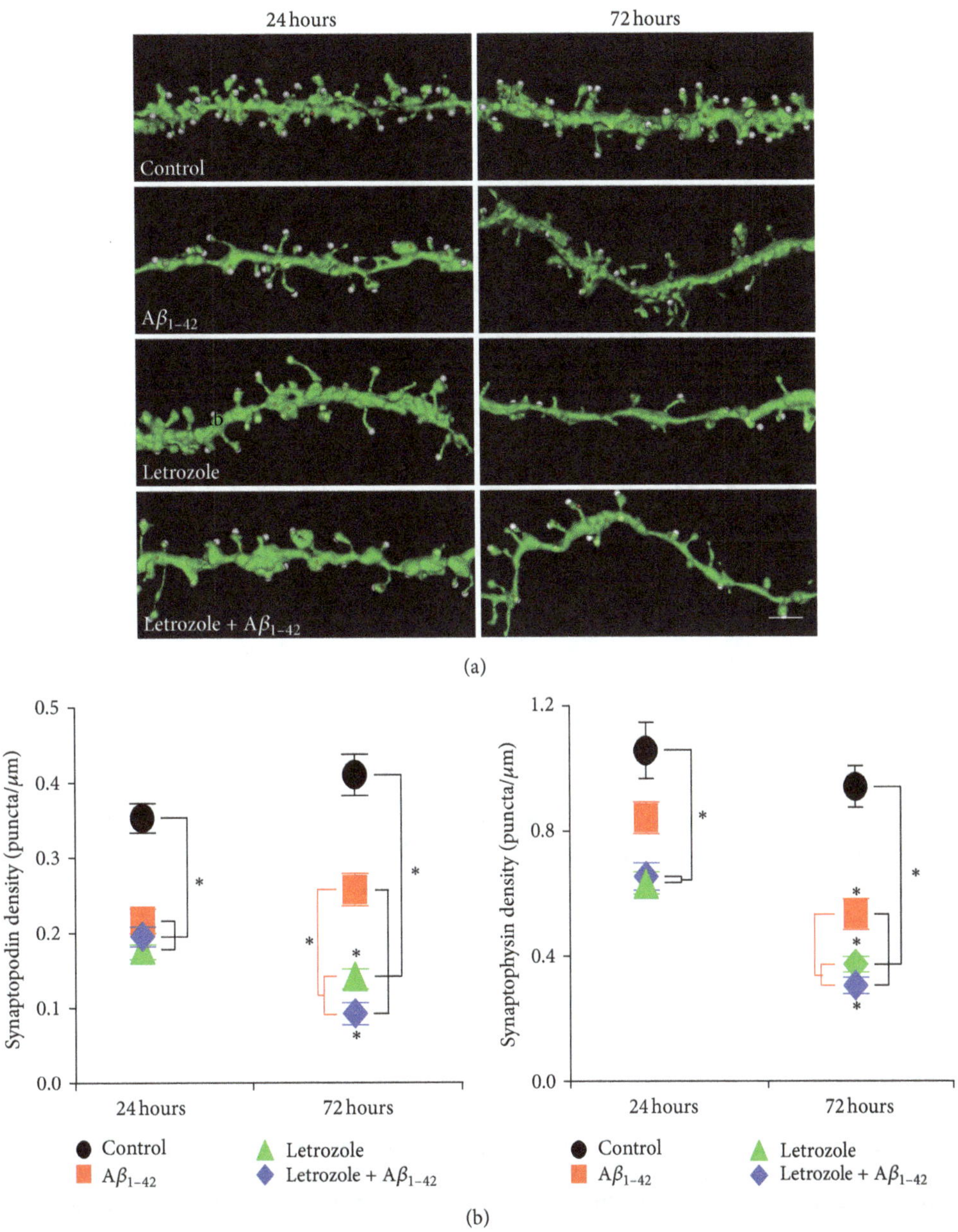

FIGURE 5: Letrozole and $A\beta_{1-42}$ reduce synaptic proteins. (a) Representative 3D reconstructions of dendritic segments from sister cultures that were treated with either control, $A\beta_{1-42}$ (1 μM), and letrozole (1 μm) or $A\beta_{1-42}$ + letrozole (1 μm) for 24 or 72 hours and immunostained for synaptophysin (white) and synaptopodin (red). Scale bar, 2 μm. (b) Quantification of the densities of synaptopodin-positive puncta following treatments. There is a significant decrease in synaptopodin puncta after 24 and 72 hours of $A\beta_{1-42}$, letrozole or $A\beta_{1-42}$ + letrozole treatments compared to control conditions. After 72 hours, the number of synaptopodin puncta was significantly lower in letrozole and $A\beta_{1-42}$ + letrozole-treated cultures compared to $A\beta_{1-42}$ alone. When synaptopodin puncta densities were compared between 24- and 72-hour treated cultures there was a significant decrease only in letrozole and $A\beta_{1-42}$ + letrozole-treated cultures after 72 hours. 24 hours: control, n = total dendritic segment lengths of 1041 μm from 12 cells in 4 cultures; $A\beta_{1-42}$, n = 633 μm of dendrite from 8 cells in 4 cultures; letrozole, n = 952 μm of dendrite from 10 cells in 4 cultures; $A\beta_{1-42}$ + letrozole, n = 1007 μm of dendrite from 10 cells in 4 cultures. 72 hours: control, n = total dendritic segment lengths of 559 μm from 10 cells in 3 cultures; $A\beta_{1-42}$, n = 472 μm of dendrite from 9 cells in 4 cultures; letrozole, n = 838 μm of dendrite from 9 cells in 4 cultures; $A\beta_{1-42}$ + letrozole, n = 750 μm of dendrite from 8 cells in 4 cultures. There is a significant decrease in synaptophysin puncta after 24 and 72 hours of $A\beta_{1-42}$, letrozole, or $A\beta_{1-42}$ + letrozole treatments compared to control conditions. After 72 hours, the number of synaptophysin puncta was significantly lower in letrozole and $A\beta_{1-42}$ + letrozole-treated cultures compared to $A\beta_{1-42}$ alone When synaptophysin puncta densities were compared between 24- and 72-hour treated cultures there was a significant decrease in $A\beta_{1-42}$, letrozole, and $A\beta_{1-42}$ + letrozole-treated cultures after 72 hours. 24 hours: control, n = total dendritic segment lengths of 1041 μm from 12 cells in 4 cultures; $A\beta_{1-42}$, n = 633 μm of dendrite from 8 cells in 4 cultures; letrozole, n = 952 μm of dendrite from 10 cells in 4 cultures; $A\beta_{1-42}$ + letrozole, n = 1007 μm of dendrite from 10 cells in 4 cultures. 72 hours: control, n = total dendritic segment lengths of 559 μm from 10 cells in 3 cultures; $A\beta_{1-42}$, n = 472 μm of dendrite from 9 cells in 4 cultures; letrozole, n = 838 μm of dendrite from 9 cells in 4 cultures; $A\beta_{1-42}$ + letrozole, n = 750 μm of dendrite from 8 cells in 4 cultures.

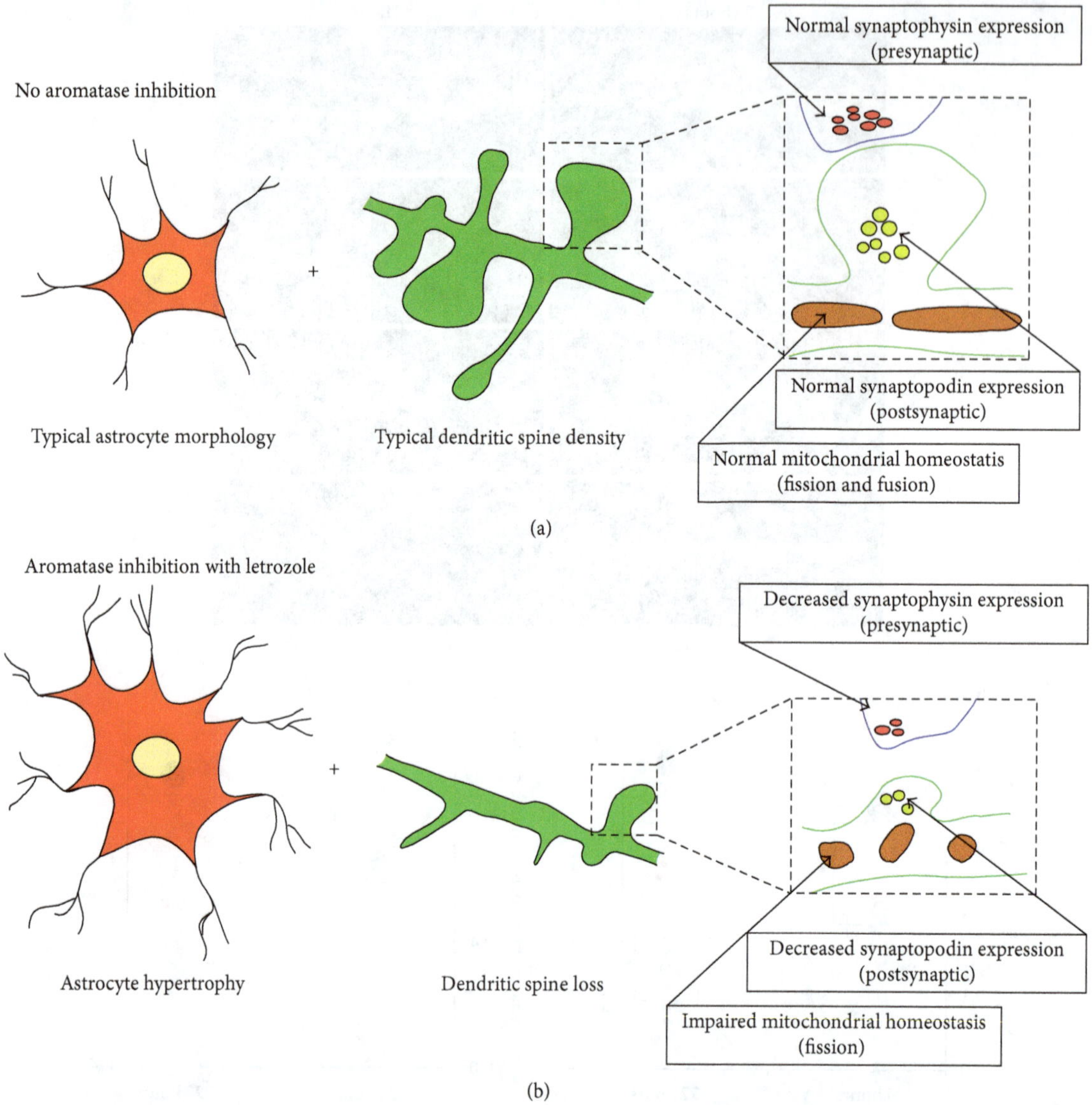

FIGURE 6: Summarising schematic: aromatase inhibition leads to synaptic and mitochondrial deficits. (a) Aromatase-mediated conversion of testosterone to estrogen in astrocytes serves as a local reservoir of neuroestrogens to promote maintenance of dendritic spines and synaptic mitochondrial integrity. (b) Aromatase inhibition by letrozole leads to spine loss, pre- and postsynaptic protein deficits, and compromised mitochondrial integrity.

manner, in parallel with studies of mitochondrial responses to local estrogen deficits.

Functional and morphological impairment of synaptic mitochondria was associated with accumulation of $A\beta_{1-42}$ in AD animal models [35, 36]. How does this relate to synaptic functions? Neuronal activity was shown to increase mitochondrial fission and entry of mitochondria into dendritic spines [37]; however fission is also initiated to sequester dysfunctional mitochondrial components and to facilitate apoptosis associated with neurodegenerative changes [38]. Recently, it has been suggested that mitochondria associated with dendritic spines may play an important role in regulating AMPA receptor trafficking, which is altered in the presence of $A\beta_{1-42}$ oligomers [5, 39]. We were interested in whether changes in mitochondrial morphology under conditions of reduced estrogen synthesis in the presence of $A\beta_{1-42}$ oligomers, were associated with synaptic deficits. We noted a significant decrease in mitochondrial volume, suggesting fission after $A\beta_{1-42}$, letrozole, or combined treatments with both. These observations are therefore in line with our present understanding of how synaptic degeneration relates to mitochondrial impairment.

Our results also suggest that estradiol may play a role in regulating the balance between the two opposing processes of mitochondrial fission and fusion. Dynamics between these two processes maintains mitochondrial homeostasis in healthy cells but is disrupted in AD [40, 41]. Findings reported in this study are in accordance with recent findings indicating a role for $A\beta_{1-42}$ in the regulation of mitochondrial fission in AD [40, 42]. Further emphasizing the importance of mitochondria in spine maintenance, impairment of mitochondrial transport to synapses by $A\beta_{1-42}$ has been reported to contribute to AMPAR removal and trafficking defects leading to synaptic inhibition [39].

In order to further understand how these disturbances in mitochondrial dynamics affect neuronal plasticity and function, we next investigated dendritic spine morphology, density, and synaptic proteins, following similar treatments. We examined changes in synaptophysin, a presynaptic marker, and synaptopodin, an actin binding protein, mainly found in a subgroup of mature spines and is regulated by estradiol [29]. The precise role of synaptopodin in hippocampal neurons is still unclear but has been shown to be important in learning and memory and in glutamate functions [30]. Our data show a significant reduction of pre- and postsynaptic components and synaptopodin with $A\beta_{1-42}$ and letrozole treatment.

Taken together, present results suggest that the neurological deficits seen in women on letrozole therapy for breast cancer could result, at least in part, from the therapy-induced hippocampal estrogen deficiency (Figure 6). Herein, we demonstrate that dendritic spine and mitochondrial deteriorations are particularly prominent in states of central hypoestrogenicity (Figure 6, lower half) and can further increase hippocampal susceptibility to spine/synaptic loss or mitochondrial functional impairment induced by a pathological insult. An important outcome of the current studies is the recognition that caution must be exercised in the use of letrozole as a therapy for breast cancer, and that account must be taken especially of the age of the female patient and/or presence of other recognised risk factors for AD. Given that letrozole is highly lipophilic and can cross the blood brain barrier, its incorporation into a nanodelivery system to prevent its access to the brain and at the same time enhance accumulation in the tumor warrants consideration.

Conflict of Interests

The authors declare they have no competing financial interests.

Author's Contribution

D. Maysinger and R. A. McKinney designed the experiments and consulted the students. P. K.-Y. Chang, S. Boridy, D. Maysinger, and R. A. McKinney wrote the draft and edited the final version of the paper. P. K.-Y. Chang performed all the experiments with hippocampal organotypic cultures, analyzed the data, and prepared Figures 2, 4, and 5. S. Boridy performed experiments with primary cultures and data analyses and prepared Figures 1 and 3. P. K.-Y. Chang and S. Boridy contributed equally to this paper.

Acknowledgments

The authors would like to thank François Charron for all his technical expertise in preparing the organotypic slice cultures. The work was supported by Grants from the Canadian Institute of Health Research and the Alzheimer's Society of Canada.

References

[1] V. F. Semiglazov, V. V. Semiglazov, G. A. Dashyan et al., "Phase 2 randomized trial of primary endocrine therapy versus chemotherapy in postmenopausal patients with estrogen receptor-positive breast cancer," *Cancer*, vol. 110, no. 2, pp. 244–254, 2007.

[2] J. V. A. Choate and J. A. Resko, "Paradoxical effect of an aromatase inhibitor, CGS 20267, on aromatase activity in guinea pig brain," *Journal of Steroid Biochemistry and Molecular Biology*, vol. 58, no. 4, pp. 411–415, 1996.

[3] B. P. Haynes, M. Dowsett, W. R. Miller, J. M. Dixon, and A. S. Bhatnagar, "The pharmacology of letrozole," *Journal of Steroid Biochemistry and Molecular Biology*, vol. 87, no. 1, pp. 35–45, 2003.

[4] V. Shilling, V. Jenkins, L. Fallowfield, and T. Howell, "The effects of hormone therapy on cognition in breast cancer," *Journal of Steroid Biochemistry and Molecular Biology*, vol. 86, no. 3-5, pp. 405–412, 2003.

[5] P. Penzes, M. E. Cahill, K. A. Jones, J.-E. Vanleeuwen, and K. M. Woolfrey, "Dendritic spine pathology in neuropsychiatric disorders," *Nature Neuroscience*, vol. 14, no. 3, pp. 285–293, 2011.

[6] M. V. Sofroniew and H. V. Vinters, "Astrocytes: biology and pathology," *Acta Neuropathologica*, vol. 119, no. 1, pp. 7–35, 2010.

[7] J. Prange-Kiel, L. Fester, L. Zhou, H. Jarry, and G. M. Rune, "Estrus cyclicity of spinogenesis: underlying mechanisms," *Journal of Neural Transmission*, vol. 116, no. 11, pp. 1417–1425, 2009.

[8] R. Vierk, G. Glassmeier, L. Zhou et al., "Aromatase inhibition abolishes LTP generation in female but not in male mice," *The Journal of Neuroscience*, vol. 32, no. 24, pp. 8116–8126, 2012.

[9] P. Polo-Kantola, R. Portin, O. Polo, H. Helenius, K. Irjala, and R. Erkkola, "The effect of short-term estrogen replacement therapy on cognition: a randomized, double-blind, cross-over trial in postmenopausal women," *Obstetrics and Gynecology*, vol. 91, no. 3, pp. 459–466, 1998.

[10] E. Hogervorst, J. Williams, M. Budge, W. Riedel, and J. Jolles, "The nature of the effect of female gonadal hormone replacement therapy on cognitive function in post-menopausal women: a meta-analysis," *Neuroscience*, vol. 101, no. 3, pp. 485–512, 2000.

[11] O. T. Wolf, B. M. Kudielka, D. H. Hellhammer, S. Törber, B. S. McEwen, and C. Kirschbaum, "Two weeks of transdermal estradiol treatment in postmenopausal elderly women and its effect on memory and mood: verbal memory changes are associated with the treatment induced estradiol levels," *Psychoneuroendocrinology*, vol. 24, no. 7, pp. 727–741, 1999.

[12] T. Duka, R. Tasker, and J. F. McGowan, "The effects of 3-week estrogen hormone replacement on cognition in elderly healthy females," *Psychopharmacology*, vol. 149, no. 2, pp. 129–139, 2000.

[13] A. Kugaya, C. N. Epperson, S. Zoghbi et al., "Increase in prefrontal cortex serotonin2A receptors following estrogen treatment in postmenopausal women," *American Journal of Psychiatry*, vol. 160, no. 8, pp. 1522–1524, 2003.

[14] V. W. Henderson, "Action of estrogens in the aging brain: dementia and cognitive aging," *Biochimica et Biophysica Acta*, vol. 1800, no. 10, pp. 1077–1083, 2010.

[15] D. Caruso, A. M. Barron, M. A. Brown et al., "Age-related changes in neuroactive steroid levels in 3xTg-AD mice," *Neurobiol Aging*, vol. 34, pp. 1080–1089, 2013.

[16] C. R. Overk, P.-Y. Lu, Y.-T. Wang et al., "Effects of aromatase inhibition versus gonadectomy on hippocampal complex amyloid pathology in triple transgenic mice," *Neurobiology of Disease*, vol. 45, no. 1, pp. 479–487, 2012.

[17] J. C. Carroll, E. R. Rosario, L. Chang et al., "Progesterone and estrogen regulate Alzheimer-like neuropathology in female 3xTg-AD mice," *Journal of Neuroscience*, vol. 27, no. 48, pp. 13357–13365, 2007.

[18] W. Wei, L. N. Nguyen, H. W. Kessels, H. Hagiwara, S. Sisodia, and R. Malinow, "Amyloid beta from axons and dendrites reduces local spine number and plasticity," *Nature Neuroscience*, vol. 13, no. 2, pp. 190–196, 2010.

[19] S. Boridy, H. Takahashi, K. Akiyoshi, and D. Maysinger, "The binding of pullulan modified cholesteryl nanogels to Aβ oligomers and their suppression of cytotoxicity," *Biomaterials*, vol. 30, no. 29, pp. 5583–5591, 2009.

[20] H. Hsieh, J. Boehm, C. Sato et al., "AMPAR removal underlies Aβ-induced synaptic depression and dendritic spine loss," *Neuron*, vol. 52, no. 5, pp. 831–843, 2006.

[21] V. De Paola, S. Arber, and P. Caroni, "AMPA receptors regulate dynamic equilibrium of presynaptic terminals in mature hippocampal networks," *Nature Neuroscience*, vol. 6, no. 5, pp. 491–500, 2003.

[22] B. H. Gähwiler, M. Capogna, D. Debanne, R. A. McKinney, and S. M. Thompson, "Organotypic slice cultures: a technique has come of age," *Trends in Neurosciences*, vol. 20, no. 10, pp. 471–477, 1997.

[23] R. A. McKinney, M. Capogna, R. Dürr, B. H. Gähwiler, and S. M. Thompson, "Miniature synaptic events maintain dendritic spines via AMPA receptor activation," *Nature Neuroscience*, vol. 2, no. 1, pp. 44–49, 1999.

[24] P. Mendez, L. M. Garcia-Segura, and D. Muller, "Estradiol promotes spine growth and synapse formation without affecting pre-established networks," *Hippocampus*, vol. 21, no. 12, pp. 1263–1267, 2011.

[25] A. Grimm, Y. A. Lim, A. G. Mensah-Nyagan, J. Gotz, and A. Eckert, "Alzheimer's disease, oestrogen and mitochondria: an ambiguous relationship," *Molecular Neurobiology*, vol. 46, pp. 151–160, 2012.

[26] J. W. Simpkins, K. D. Yi, S.-H. Yang, and J. A. Dykens, "Mitochondrial mechanisms of estrogen neuroprotection," *Biochimica et Biophysica Acta*, vol. 1800, no. 10, pp. 1113–1120, 2010.

[27] M. Matsuzaki, G. C. R. Ellis-Davies, T. Nemoto, Y. Miyashita, M. Iino, and H. Kasai, "Dendritic spine geometry is critical for AMPA receptor expression in hippocampal CA1 pyramidal neurons," *Nature Neuroscience*, vol. 4, no. 11, pp. 1086–1092, 2001.

[28] J. M. Mateos, A. Lüthi, N. Savic et al., "Synaptic modifications at the CA3-CA1 synapse after chronic AMPA receptor blockade in rat hippocampal slices," *Journal of Physiology*, vol. 581, no. 1, pp. 129–138, 2007.

[29] L. Fester, L. Zhou, C. Voets et al., "The opposing roles of estradiol on synaptic protein expression in hippocampal cultures," *Psychoneuroendocrinology*, vol. 34, supplement 1, pp. S123–S129, 2009.

[30] A. Vlachos, E. Korkotian, E. Schonfeld, E. Copanaki, T. Deller, and M. Segal, "Synaptopodin regulates plasticity of dendritic spines in hippocampal neurons," *Journal of Neuroscience*, vol. 29, no. 4, pp. 1017–1033, 2009.

[31] S. C. Janicki and N. Schupf, "Hormonal influences on cognition and risk for Alzheimer's disease," *Current Neurology and Neuroscience Reports*, vol. 10, no. 5, pp. 359–366, 2010.

[32] A. Prat, M. Behrendt, E. Marcinkiewicz et al., "A novel mouse model of Alzheimer's disease with chronic estrogen deficiency leads to glial cell activation and hypertrophy," *Journal of Aging Research*, vol. 2011, Article ID 251517, 12 pages, 2011.

[33] J. L. Furman, D. M. Sama, J. C. Gant et al., "Targeting astrocytes ameliorates neurologic changes in a mouse model of Alzheimer's disease," *The Journal of Neuroscience*, vol. 32, pp. 16129–16140, 2012.

[34] F. Liu, M. Day, L. C. Muñiz et al., "Activation of estrogen receptor-β regulates hippocampal synaptic plasticity and improves memory," *Nature Neuroscience*, vol. 11, no. 3, pp. 334–343, 2008.

[35] H. Du, L. Guo, S. Yan, A. A. Sosunov, G. M. McKhann, and S. S. Yan, "Early deficits in synaptic mitochondria in an Alzheimer's disease mouse model," *Proceedings of the National Academy of Sciences of the United States of America*, vol. 107, no. 43, pp. 18670–18675, 2010.

[36] S. J. Baloyannis, "Mitochondria are related to synaptic pathology in Alzheimer's disease," *International Journal of Alzheimer's Disease*, Article ID 305395, 2011.

[37] J. Y. Sung, O. Engmann, M. A. Teylan, A. C. Nairn, P. Greengard, and Y. Kim, "WAVE1 controls neuronal activity-induced mitochondrial distribution in dendritic spines," *Proceedings of the National Academy of Sciences of the United States of America*, vol. 105, no. 8, pp. 3112–3116, 2008.

[38] R. J. Youle and A. M. van der Bliek, "Mitochondrial fission, fusion, and stress," *Science*, vol. 337, pp. 1062–1065, 2012.

[39] Y. Rui, J. Gu, K. Yu, H. C. Hartzell, and J. Q. Zheng, "Inhibition of AMPA receptor trafficking at hippocampal synapses by -amyloid oligomers: the mitochondrial contribution," *Molecular Brain*, vol. 3, no. 1, article 10, 2010.

[40] X. Zhu, G. Perry, M. A. Smith, and X. Wang, "Abnormal mitochondrial dynamics in the pathogenesis of Alzheimer's disease," *Journal of Alzheimer's Disease*, vol. 33, pp. S253–S262, 2013.

[41] E. Trushina, E. Nemutlu, S. Zhang et al., "Defects in mitochondrial dynamics and metabolomic signatures of evolving energetic stress in mouse models of familial alzheimer's disease," *PLoS ONE*, vol. 7, no. 2, Article ID e32737, 2012.

[42] B. Westermann, "Nitric oxide links mitochondrial fission to alzheimer's disease," *Science Signaling*, vol. 2, no. 69, p. pe29, 2009.

9

Effects of Medicare Coverage of a "Welcome-to-Medicare" Visit on Use of Preventive Services among New Medicare Enrollees

Boon Peng Ng,[1] Gail A. Jensen,[2] and Heather Fritz[3]

[1]*Department of Economics, Wayne State University, 656 W Kirby St., 2074 FAB, Detroit, MI 48202, USA*
[2]*Department of Economics and Institute of Gerontology, Wayne State University, 87 East Ferry St., Detroit, MI 48202, USA*
[3]*Eugene Applebaum College of Pharmacy and Health Sciences and Institute of Gerontology, Wayne State University, 259 Mack Ave., Detroit, MI 48201, USA*

Correspondence should be addressed to Boon Peng Ng; bng@wayne.edu

Academic Editor: F. R. Ferraro

In January 2005, Medicare began covering a one-time initial preventive physical examination (IPPE), also called a "Welcome-to-Medicare" visit, during a beneficiary's first 6 months under Part B. This paper examines the effects of offering Medicare IPPE coverage on the use of mammograms, breast self-exams, Pap smears, prostate cancer screenings, cholesterol screenings, and flu vaccines among beneficiaries new to Part B. We adopt a difference-in-difference estimator and estimate a set of multivariate logit models to quantify the effects of introducing Medicare IPPE coverage on the use of preventive services. Models are estimated separately for men and women. Data for the analysis come from the 1996–2008 Health and Retirement Study. Among both men and women, having coverage for a one-time IPPE under Medicare had no effects on the utilization of any of the preventive services listed above. In this study, we find that offering coverage for a one-time IPPE under Medicare was insufficient to spur greater use of preventive services among new Medicare beneficiaries. These findings are important and suggest that policy-makers may need to consider other approaches to increase the use of recommended preventive services.

1. Introduction

Expanding Medicare benefits in ways to increase older adults' utilization of preventive healthcare has been a hallmark of changes to Medicare over the last 15 years. The 2003 Medicare Modernization Act (MMA), the 2008 Medicare Improvements for Patients and Providers Act (MIPPA), and most recently, the 2010 Affordable Care Act (ACA) all contained provisions intended to enhance older adults' access to affordable preventive services. The argument to encourage greater use of preventive services is that they can or will prevent more serious illnesses that are costly to treat or potentially deadly. There is broad consensus that preventive measures and quality healthcare improve overall health [1].

One key provision of the MMA involved the introduction in 2005 of Medicare coverage for a one-time initial preventive physical examination (IPPE) during a beneficiary's first six months under Medicare Part B. An IPPE, also known as a "Welcome-to-Medicare" visit, is a visit with a physician (or a physician's designee) for the purpose of introducing the beneficiary to Medicare and what it covers, talking with the beneficiary about health promotion, early disease detection, and preventive services that can help him/her stay well, and providing actual referrals for recommended preventive services [2].

In this paper, we use data from the ongoing Health and Retirement Study (HRS) to evaluate whether the introduction of Medicare IPPE coverage in 2005 improved rates of preventive services use among beneficiaries new to Part B. We examine the use of flu vaccines and cholesterol screenings among men and women, prostate cancer screenings among men, and mammograms, breast self-exams, and Pap smears among women. Because past studies have shown gender differences in health-related behaviors and medical care utilization, we examine the use of flu vaccines and cholesterol screenings separately for men and women.

We are aware of one previous study of the effects of covering an IPPE on the use of mammography and Pap smears among women aged 65 and 66 and new to Medicare Part B. Salloum and colleagues found that the use of mammograms and Pap smears among new female beneficiaries did not change following the introduction of IPPE coverage [3]. Our study examines the effects of IPPE coverage on the use of six different preventive services, including flu immunizations and five disease screening procedures, and examines these effects separately for men and women. Given that fewer than half of seniors are up-to-date on recommended preventive services [4], and expanding the use of recommended preventive services continues to be a national priority [5], the effectiveness of covering an IPPE under Medicare remains an interesting issue.

Since an IPPE is an opportunity for patients and physicians to discuss the need to use preventive services and to develop a preventive care plan, Medicare's introduction of coverage for it in 2005 may have increased the use of preventive care services among those eligible for the benefit. In this paper, we examine whether the introduction of IPPE coverage influenced the use of flu shots, cholesterol checks, and five types of cancer screening among men and women newly insured under Part B.

2. Methods

We analyze data from the Health and Retirement Study (HRS) and the RAND HRS. These data were chosen because the longitudinal nature of the HRS allows us to account for the effects of an individual's past utilization patterns on their current use of services, separate from the effects of Medicare IPPE coverage. (Cross-sectional data sources, such as the Medicare Current Beneficiary Survey, the Medical Expenditure Panel Survey, and the Behavioral Risk Factor Surveillance System, all lack information on individuals' past behavior regarding preventive services.) In addition, HRS data have not been used before to evaluate the effects of introducing IPPE coverage, so they may shed new light on this topic.

The HRS is a nationally representative sample survey of older adults in the US that has been conducted every two years since 1992. The survey contains copious self-reported information on health, healthcare use, insurance coverage, and sociodemographic information. The HRS first surveyed a sample of adults aged 51–61 in 1992, and this sample is called the "original HRS cohort." A second survey, conducted in 1993 and called the Study of Assets and Health Dynamics among the Oldest Old (AHEAD), was a survey of individuals aged 70 and older. As with the HRS, spouses were also surveyed in AHEAD [7, 8]. Participants in both surveys were reinterviewed every two years, and in 1998 these two surveys were combined and have since been referred to simply as the HRS. (More information is available on the HRS website, http://hrsonline.isr.umich.edu/.)

The RAND HRS is derived from the HRS and contains many (but not all) key variables from the HRS. RAND HRS files are constructed for ease of use, and variables in the file are named and formatted to be consistent across HRS waves [6, 9].

2.1. Sampling Criteria. Data are drawn from the 1996, 2000, 2004, and 2008 waves (or odd number waves) of the HRS. Information on the use of preventive services is available for all HRS participants only in these waves [10]. As noted earlier, as of January 1, 2005, Medicare began covering an IPPE for beneficiaries but only during their first six months under Part B. Since most people enter Medicare when they turn 65, their eligibility for a covered IPPE would have occurred during six months when they were 65 years old. We restrict our focus to Medicare beneficiaries, aged 66–69 at the time of an HRS interview, who were insured under Part B, who were not also enrolled in Medicaid, and who were not enrolled in an HMO. We exclude beneficiaries with Medicaid because, during the period we examine (1996–2008), Medicaid already offered an ongoing preventive screening benefit, and we exclude beneficiaries with HMO coverage (Medicare Part C) because coverage of an IPPE did not apply to them; rather it was a benefit under Medicare Part B.

We divide this sample into two groups: a "treatment group" of Medicare beneficiaries aged 66 or 67 at the time of an HRS interview and a "comparison group" of Medicare beneficiaries aged 68 or 69 at the time of an HRS interview. The treatment group consists of beneficiaries aged 66 or 67 because for these individuals, at least from 2005 onward, HRS questions regarding preventive service use would have captured their six-month eligibility window for IPPE coverage. The comparison group consists of beneficiaries aged 68 or 69 because, for these individuals, HRS questions covered a two-year period well past their eligibility window for IPPE coverage.

Given our sampling criteria, each observation in our analytic sample is a distinct HRS participant and no individual contributes multiple observations across waves. Our final sample sizes by type of services are as follows:

(i) Mammograms: treatment group of 325 women, comparison group of 1,036 women

(ii) Breast self-exams: treatment group of 326 women, comparison group of 1,037 women

(iii) Pap smears: treatment group of 327 women, comparison group of 1,030 women

(iv) Prostate cancer screenings: treatment group of 249 men, comparison group of 783 men

For cholesterol tests and flu vaccines, models are estimated separately for men and women, with sample sizes as follows:

(i) Cholesterol testing women: treatment group of 326, comparison group of 1,029

(ii) Cholesterol testing men: treatment group of 254, comparison group of 784

(iii) Flu vaccine women: treatment group of 323, comparison group of 1,031

(iv) Flu vaccine men: treatment group of 254, comparison group of 786

2.2. Data Analysis. Since all of the preventive services here are binary variables, we estimate a multivariate logit model for each one and use a different-in-differences (DID) methodology to estimate the effects of introducing Medicare coverage for an IPPE [11]. The general form of the model to be estimated is

$$\begin{aligned}\text{logit}\{\text{pr}(Y_i = 1 \mid X)\} = \beta_0 &+ \beta_1 \text{Post 2005} \\ &+ \beta_2 \text{Treatment} \\ &+ \beta_3 \text{Post 2005} \cdot \text{Treatment} \\ &+ \beta_4 X_i + \varepsilon_i,\end{aligned} \tag{1}$$

where Y_i is a binary indicator for the occurrence of screening (1 if yes, 0 if no), Post 2005 indicates whether the individual's interview occurred when Medicare covered an IPPE (1 if yes, 0 if no), Treatment is a binary variable indicating membership in the treatment group (1 if yes, 0 if no), Post 2005 · Treatment is the interaction term between Post 2005 and Treatment, X_i is a vector of other covariates in the model, and ε_i is a random error term. The coefficient on the interaction term, Post 2005 · Treatment, (β_3) quantifies the effect of eligibility for IPPE coverage on use of the preventive service. This estimation strategy essentially computes a difference-in-differences estimate of the effect of a beneficiary having IPPE coverage [12]. All statistical analyses were conducted in 2015 using Stata, Version 11.2 from StataCrop in College Station, Texas.

Variables in X_i include predisposing, enabling, and need-related variables suggested by Andersen's behavioral model of factors affecting the use of preventive healthcare [13, 14]. Predisposing factors include demographic characteristics, social structure, and health beliefs. Enabling factors encompass the economic accessibility of services (e.g., insurance and income), as well as the availability of services nearby [15, 16]. Finally, need factors account for an individual's current state of health, as well as their attitudes about their needs for healthcare based on how they perceive their own health [17]. Although past experience with preventive services is not explicit in Andersen's model, we think it may reflect an individual's attitudes regarding the value of such services and may also reflect their past health habits. As such, it belongs to behavioral models of the use of preventive services.

Andersen's model was adapted by Walsh and McPhee (1992) to account for the potential effects of patient-physician interactions on the use of services. In their "Systems Model of Clinical Preventive Care" Walsh and McPhee posit that seven categories of factors affect the use of preventive healthcare services: predisposing factors, enabling factors, reinforcing factors, healthcare delivery system factors, situational factors (cues to action), and preventive activity factors [18]. Situational factors are particular circumstances or cues that may trigger the use of preventive services. An example is a patient receiving a physician's recommendation or a reminder to use preventive services [19]. Past studies have shown that recommendations from physicians are a strong predictor of use of preventive services among older adults, and patients who have discussions about preventive services with their physician are much more likely to use such services [20–22].

Our predisposing variables include marital status, race, education, and whether the individual previously used that particular preventive service. Enabling-related variables include access to additional insurance beyond Medicare, such as an employer-sponsored policy or a Medigap plan, income, region of residence, urban/rural location, employment status, and whether the individual is able to drive. Need-related variables in each model include whether the individual smokes, drinking habits, whether the individual is overweight, the presence of chronic diseases, self-rated health, eyesight, exercise habits, performance on activities of daily living (ADL), and mental health, as measured by the Center for Epidemiologic Studies Depression Scale (CES-D).

3. Results

Table 1 reports definitions and descriptive statistics for variables used in this analysis. During the preperiod, that is, before Medicare covered an IPPE, 76% of women in the treatment group and 80% in the comparison group reported receiving a mammogram during the past two years. Sixty-five percent of women in the treatment group and 61% in the comparison group reported they were checking their breasts for lumps monthly. Sixty-four percent of women in the treatment group and 63% in the comparison group reported receiving a Pap smear during the past two years. Seventy-eight percent of men in the treatment group and 81% in the comparison group reported receiving a prostate exam during the past two years. Sixty-eight percent of men in the treatment group and 67% in the comparison group reported receiving a flu vaccine during the past two years. Sixty-seven percent of women in the treatment group and 70% in the comparison group reported receiving a flu vaccine during the past two years. Eighty-seven percent of men in the treatment group and 84% in the comparison group reported receiving a cholesterol test. Finally, 82 percent of women in the treatment group and 84% in the comparison group reported receiving a cholesterol test during the past two years.

Tables 2 and 3 report the odds ratios from the estimated logit regressions for the use of various preventive services. For each model the odds ratio of key interest is the one corresponding to the row labeled "Post 2005 $*$ Treatment." For all six preventive services, the estimated coefficient of policy effect indicator is statistically insignificant. This implies that having a six-month window of Medicare coverage for a one-time IPPE had no effects on the use of mammograms, breast self-exams, Pap smears, prostate cancer screenings, cholesterol tests, or flu vaccines among new Medicare enrollees.

Several other factors, however, were highly predictive of preventive services utilization, and we briefly discuss them here. Among women, those who previously received a mammogram were 10.81 times more likely to have one again (Table 2). Having employer-provided insurance (in addition to Medicare) increased a woman's likelihood of having a mammogram by 1.56. Full-time employment, nondrinkers, and the absence of any chronic diseases reduced the likelihood of having a mammogram by 0.48, 0.68, and 0.55 times,

TABLE 1: Variable definitions and descriptive statistics for the treatment and comparison groups before Medicare introduced IPPE coverage, Health and Retirement Study, 1996–2004.

Variable	Definition	Treatment Group Mean (SE)		Comparison Group Mean (SE)	
Dependent variables					
Mammogram[a]	1 if having a mammogram; 0 otherwise	0.76 (0.42)		0.80 (0.39)	
Check for breast lumps[a]	1 if conducting a monthly self-exam for breast lumps; 0 otherwise	0.65 (0.47)		0.61 (0.48)	
Pap smear[a]	1 if having a Pap smear; 0 otherwise	0.64 (0.47)		0.63 (0.48)	
Prostate exam[a]	1 if having a prostate examination; 0 otherwise	0.78 (0.41)		0.81 (0.38)	
		Men	Women	Men	Women
Cholesterol test[a]	1 if having a cholesterol blood test; 0 otherwise	0.87 (0.33)	0.82 (0.38)	0.84 (0.36)	0.84 (0.36)
Flu vaccine[a]	1 if having a flu shot; 0 otherwise	0.68 (0.46)	0.67 (0.47)	0.67 (0.46)	0.70 (0.45)
Control variables					
Previous use of mammogram[a]	1 if previously having a mammogram; 0 otherwise	0.74 (0.43)		0.77 (0.41)	
Previous breast self-exam[a]	1 if previously conducting a monthly self-exam for breast lumps; 0 otherwise	0.62 (0.48)		0.63 (0.48)	
Previous use of Pap smear[a]	1 if previously having a Pap smear; 0 otherwise	0.67 (0.47)		0.70 (0.45)	
Previous use of prostate exam[a]	1 if previously having a prostate examination; 0 otherwise	0.76 (0.42)		0.75 (0.43)	
		Men	Women	Men	Women
Previous use of cholesterol test[a]	1 if previously having a cholesterol blood test; 0 otherwise	0.74 (0.43)	0.74 (0.43)	0.77 (0.41)	0.79 (0.40)
Previous use of flu vaccine shot[a]	1 if previously having a flu shot; 0 otherwise	0.51 (0.50)	0.53 (0.49)	0.49 (0.50)	0.54 (0.49)
Race					
White	1 if White/Caucasian; 0 otherwise	0.76 (0.42)		0.83 (0.37)	
Black	1 if Black/African American; 0 otherwise	0.14 (0.35)		0.11 (0.32)	
Hispanic	1 if Hispanic/Latino; 0 otherwise	0.06 (0.25)		0.03 (0.18)	
Other	1 if a race/ethnicity other than White, Black, or Hispanic; 0 otherwise	0.08 (0.28)		0.05 (0.22)	
Education					
Less than high school	1 if less than 12 years of education; 0 otherwise	0.22 (0.41)		0.17 (0.37)	
High school/GED	1 if 12 years of education; 0 otherwise	0.41 (0.49)		0.41 (0.49)	
Some college and beyond	1 if more than 12 years of education; otherwise	0.36 (0.48)		0.41 (0.49)	
Employment	1 if employed full time; 0 otherwise	0.09 (0.28)		0.08 (0.28)	
CES-D score[b]	1 if scored 0 in CESD; 0 otherwise	0.42 (0.49)		0.51 (0.50)	
Chronic diseases	1 if reporting 0 chronic diseases; 0 otherwise	0.13 (0.34)		0.13 (0.34)	
Married	I if married; 0 otherwise	0.71 (0.45)		0.73 (0.44)	

TABLE 1: Continued.

Variable	Definition	Treatment Group Mean (SE)	Comparison Group Mean (SE)
Census region			
Northeast	1 if census region is northeast; 0 otherwise	0.13 (0.34)	0.11 (0.32)
Midwest	1 if census region is midwest; 0 otherwise	0.28 (0.45)	0.32 (0.46)
South	1 if census region is south; 0 otherwise	0.44 (0.49)	0.44 (0.49)
West	1 if census region is west; 0 otherwise	0.13 (0.34)	0.11 (0.32)
Rural	1 if population is less than 250,000; 0 otherwise	0.39 (0.48)	0.38 (0.48)
Exercise	1 if performing physical activity; 0 otherwise	0.74 (0.43)	0.75 (0.42)
Not drinking	1 if not drinking; 0 otherwise	0.71 (0.45)	0.67 (0.46)
Not smoking	1 if not smoking; 0 otherwise	0.82 (0.37)	0.87 (0.32)
Driving	1 if being able to drive; 0 otherwise	0.90 (0.29)	0.94 (0.23)
Total household real income (in year 2007 dollars)			
Income 1	1 if total household income is less than $25000; 0 otherwise	0.28 (0.45)	0.23 (0.42)
Income 2	1 if total household income is between $25,000 and $50,000; 0 otherwise	0.32 (0.46)	0.34 (0.47)
Income 3	1 if total household income is more than $50,000, 0 otherwise	0.39 (0.48)	0.42 (0.49)
Employer provided insurance	1 if covered by employer insurance; 0 otherwise	0.43 (0.490	0.44 (0.49)
ADL[c]	1 if reporting 0 ADL limitations; 0 otherwise	0.86 (0.34)	0.90 (0.29)
Overweight	1 if BMI is equal to and greater than 25; 0 otherwise	0.70 (0.45)	0.68 (0.46)
Self-reported health			
Better than good	1 if reporting better than good health; 0 otherwise	0.36 (0.48)	0.48 (0.50)
Good	1 if reporting good health; 0 otherwise	0.30 (0.46)	0.31 (0.46)
Less than good	1 if reporting worse than good health; 0 otherwise	0.32 (0.46)	0.20 (0.40)
Rate eyesight			
Better than good	1 if reporting better than good eyesight; 0 otherwise	0.32 (0.47)	0.39 (0.48)
Good	1 if reporting good eyesight; 0 otherwise	0.45 (0.49)	0.44 (0.49)
Less than Good	1 if reporting worse than good eyesight; 0 otherwise	0.22 (0.41)	0.15 (0.36)

Note. SE = standard error.

[a]Among a specific preventive care group only.

[b]Center for Epidemiologic Studies Depression Scale (CES-D) is the sum of indicators: feeling depressed, everything being an effort, sleep being restless, feeling unhappy, feeling lonely, feeling sad, could not get going, and not enjoying life [6].

[c]The activities of daily living (ADL) index covers walking across a room, dressing, bathing, eating, getting in and out of bed, and using the toilet [6].

TABLE 2: Odds ratios derived from multivariate logit models for having a mammogram, breast self-exam, Pap smear, or prostate cancer screening (Health and Retirement Study data, 1996–2008).

	Mammogram Odds ratio (95% CI)	Breast self-exam Odds ratio (95% CI)	Pap smear Odds ratio (95% CI)	Prostate Odds ratio (95% CI)
Post 2005	0.94 (0.62–1.41)	0.97 (0.69–1.36)	0.75[a] (0.55–1.03)	0.64[b] (0.42–0.97)
Treatment	0.87 (0.55–1.37)	1.33 (0.89–1.99)	1.23 (0.84–1.80)	0.85 (0.51–1.40)
Post 2005 * Treatment	0.89 (0.42–1.88)	0.85 (0.43–1.65)	1.19 (0.64–2.21)	1.70 (0.74–3.89)
Previous use of the service	10.81[c] (7.80–14.99)	13.88[c] (10.52–18.32)	7.50[c] (5.70–9.88)	4.75[c] (3.29–6.86)
Married	1.13 (0.78–1.65)	1.50[b] (1.08–2.09)	1.19 (0.88–1.62)	1.13 (0.71–1.81)
White	0.36 (0.09–1.40)	0.88 (0.29–2.64)	0.55 (0.20–1.46)	0.64 (0.15–2.67)
Black	0.65 (0.15–2.75)	0.75 (0.24–2.39)	0.87 (0.30–2.44)	0.92 (0.20–4.12)
Hispanic	0.34 (0.07–1.50)	0.45 (0.13–1.53)	0.62 (0.20–1.90)	0.67 (0.13–3.31)
High school/GED	0.99 (0.64–1.53)	0.64[b] (0.43–0.96)	1.10 (0.77–1.59)	1.58[a] (0.98–2.55)
Some college and beyond	1.12 (0.69–1.80)	0.81 (0.53–1.24)	1.16 (0.79–1.70)	1.65[a] (0.98–2.76)
Employer provided insurance	1.56[b] (1.10–2.22)	0.89 (0.67–1.18)	1.34[b] (1.02–1.76)	1.12 (0.77–1.62)
Employment	0.48[b] (0.27–0.86)	1.82[b] (1.03–3.23)	0.94 (0.57–1.54)	1.30 (0.76–2.24)
Driving	1.53 (0.91–2.57)	0.95 (0.58–1.58)	0.71 (0.45–1.12)	2.27 (0.72–7.09)
Income 2	1.30 (0.85–1.99)	1.08 (0.73–1.57)	1.24 (0.87–1.76)	1.00 (0.61–1.63)
Income 3	1.25 (0.77–2.02)	0.95 (0.62–1.44)	1.34 (0.90–1.98)	1.27 (0.74–2.19)
Northeast	1.02 (0.54–1.92)	1.21 (0.70–2.10)	1.65[a] (0.99–2.76)	0.61 (0.30–1.25)
Midwest	0.79 (0.46–1.35)	0.71 (0.45–1.12)	1.06 (0.69–1.62)	0.74 (0.40–1.36)
South	1.20 (0.72–2.02)	0.86 (0.56–1.34)	1.12 (0.74–1.68)	0.83 (0.46–1.47)
Rural	1.18 (0.84–1.67)	1.33[a] (0.99–1.78)	0.97 (0.74–1.28)	1.07 (0.74–1.55)
Not smoking	2.15[c] (1.40–3.30)	1.24 (0.82–1.86)	1.11 (0.76–1.63)	2.17[c] (1.37–3.43)
Not drinking	0.68[a] (0.45–1.03)	1.05 (0.75–1.46)	0.79 (0.57–1.09)	1.09 (0.76–1.56)
Overweight	0.84 (0.59–1.21)	1.03 (0.76–1.39)	0.97 (0.72–1.29)	1.03 (0.69–1.53)
Exercise	1.19 (0.79–1.79)	0.86 (0.60–1.25)	1.17 (0.83–1.66)	1.25 (0.76–2.04)
No chronic diseases	0.55[b] (0.34–0.89)	1.17 (0.75–1.81)	0.88 (0.58–1.33)	0.46[c] (0.28–0.76)
No ADL	1.38 (0.85–2.24)	0.79 (0.50–1.26)	1.25 (0.82–1.89)	0.55[a] (0.30–1.02)
Zero CES-D	1.30 (0.91–1.84)	0.88 (0.65–1.18)	1.11 (0.84–1.47)	1.64[c] (1.13–2.39)
Better than good health	0.73 (0.48–1.10)	0.85 (0.60–1.19)	1.03 (0.75–1.42)	0.93 (0.61–1.43)
Less than good health	0.84 (0.54–1.32)	0.90 (0.60–1.34)	0.91 (0.63–1.31)	1.49 (0.91–2.44)
Better than good eyesight	1.47[b] (1.01–2.14)	0.80 (0.59–1.10)	1.29[a] (0.96–1.73)	1.42[a] (0.94–2.15)
Less than good eyesight	1.12 (0.71–1.76)	0.97 (0.65–1.46)	1.02 (0.70–1.48)	0.90 (0.55–1.45)
Pseudo R-squared	0.25	0.26	0.17	0.16
Sample size	$N = 1365$	$N = 1363$	$N = 1357$	$N = 1032$

Notes. CI = confidence interval. Sample sizes vary across models because some individuals are missing data on some items and because there are different numbers of women and men in the sample.

[a]Significant at 10%, [b]significant at 5%, and [c]significant at 1%.

respectively. Women who were nonsmokers were 2.15 times more likely to receive a mammogram.

For breast self-exams (Table 2), women who had previously checked their breasts for lumps were 13.88 times more likely to check them again. Women living in a rural area, who were employed, or who were married were more likely to check for breast lumps; and those with only a high school education or GED were less likely to perform a breast self-exam.

Women who previously received a Pap smear (Table 2) were 7.50 times more likely to receive another one. Having employer-provided insurance also improved the odds of receiving a Pap smear.

Men who previously received a prostate exam (Table 2) were 4.75 times more likely to receive another one. Men who were more highly educated were also more likely to be screened. Nonsmokers and men who scored zero on the CES-D were also more likely to be screened. Having no chronic diseases and having no ADL limitations had negative effects on receiving a prostate exam.

For cholesterol tests (Table 3), women who previously had a cholesterol test were 5.11 times more likely to have another one, whereas men who previously had the test were 7.73 times more likely to have another one. Both women and men who do not smoke and who exercised regularly were more likely to have their cholesterol checked. In contrast, women and

TABLE 3: Odds ratios derived from multivariate logit models for the receipt of cholesterol testing and flu vaccine (Health and Retirement Study data, 1996–2008).

	Cholesterol testing		Flu vaccine	
	Women	Men	Women	Men
	Odds ratio (95% CI)	Odds ratio (95% CI)	Odds ratio (95% CI)	Odds ratio (95% CI)
Post 2005	1.40 (0.88–2.25)	1.06 (0.62–1.80)	0.76 (0.52–1.12)	0.63^b (0.42–0.96)
Treatment	0.97 (0.60–1.55)	2.11^b (1.09–4.08)	0.87 (0.56–1.35)	1.08 (0.67–1.73)
Post 2005 * Treatment	1.19 (0.48–2.91)	0.83 (0.26–2.60)	0.85 (0.41–1.77)	0.79 (0.36–1.73)
Previous use of the service	5.11^c (3.57–7.32)	7.73^c (4.94–12.10)	17.57^c (12.55–24.59)	16.55^c (11.41–23.99)
Married	1.29 (0.84–1.95)	1.63^a (0.94–2.83)	1.39^a (0.96–2.01)	1.38 (0.87–2.20)
White	0.27 (0.05–1.55)	0.96 (0.19–4.92)	1.51 (0.50–4.55)	0.56 (0.14–2.24)
Black	0.24 (0.04–1.42)	0.84 (0.15–4.67)	0.65 (0.20–2.07)	0.39 (0.09–1.69)
Hispanic	0.26 (0.04–1.72)	0.85 (0.13–5.44)	0.32^a (0.09–1.16)	0.54 (0.11–2.53)
High school/GED	0.99 (0.61–1.60)	1.63 (0.90–2.94)	1.27 (0.83–1.94)	1.63^b (1.01–2.64)
Some college and beyond	1.40 (0.83–2.39)	2.12^b (1.11–4.03)	1.55^a (0.98–2.45)	1.79^b (1.07–2.98)
Employer provided insurance	1.20 (0.82–1.76)	0.88 (0.55–1.40)	1.09 (0.79–1.50)	1.05 (0.75–1.49)
Employment	0.78 (0.41–1.47)	1.14 (0.60–2.17)	0.76 (0.42–1.35)	0.88 (0.54–1.43)
Driving	0.83 (0.45–1.54)	9.28^c (2.57–33.43)	0.87 (0.49–1.52)	1.28 (0.32–5.09)
Income 2	1.56^a (0.97–2.51)	0.68 (0.36–1.28)	0.81 (0.53–1.24)	1.14 (0.70–1.87)
Income 3	1.32 (0.78–2.25)	0.65 (0.32–1.30)	0.72 (0.45–1.15)	0.84 (0.50–1.41)
Northeast	1.42 (0.66–3.04)	0.51 (0.18–1.43)	1.28 (0.67–2.41)	0.85 (0.42–1.69)
Midwest	0.91 (0.49–1.69)	0.42^a (0.17–1.02)	0.62^a (0.36–1.04)	0.70 (0.39–1.25)
South	0.79 (0.44–1.41)	0.45^a (0.19–1.04)	0.67 (0.40–1.11)	0.68 (0.40–1.17)
Rural	0.88 (0.61–1.27)	0.66^a (0.42–1.04)	1.11 (0.80–1.54)	1.06 (0.75–1.51)
Not smoking	1.44 (0.90–2.28)	1.98^b (1.12–3.50)	1.90^c (1.22–2.96)	1.62^a (0.99–2.64)
Not drinking	0.88 (0.57–1.36)	1.64^b (1.05–2.56)	0.94 (0.65–1.36)	0.92 (0.65–1.29)
Overweight	1.02 (0.69–1.49)	1.43 (0.90–2.29)	1.31 (0.93–1.83)	1.22 (0.82–1.80)
Exercise	1.76^c (1.14–2.69)	1.69^a (0.96–2.96)	1.20 (0.80–1.81)	0.98 (0.61–1.58)
No chronic diseases	0.36^c (0.23–0.57)	0.30^c (0.17–0.53)	0.63^b (0.40–0.99)	0.64^a (0.39–1.03)
No ADL	1.22 (0.68–2.20)	0.45^a (0.18–1.09)	0.93 (0.55–1.54)	1.01 (0.55–1.88)
Zero CES-D	0.86 (0.58–1.25)	2.01^c (1.25–3.22)	1.07 (0.77–1.48)	1.00 (0.70–1.43)
Better than good health	0.69 (0.44–1.07)	0.94 (0.55–1.60)	1.17 (0.80–1.70)	0.81 (0.54–1.21)
Less than good health	0.97 (0.57–1.64)	2.46^c (1.28–4.70)	1.99^c (1.26–3.14)	1.42 (0.87–2.29)
Better than good eyesight	0.95 (0.64–1.42)	1.22 (0.73–2.03)	1.06 (0.75–1.50)	1.43^a (0.98–2.10)
Less than good eyesight	0.98 (0.58–1.64)	0.59^a (0.32–1.07)	1.01 (0.66–1.57)	1.00 (0.62–1.60)
Pseudo R-squared	0.16	0.26	0.32	0.28
Sample size	$N = 1355$	$N = 1038$	$N = 1354$	$N = 1040$

Notes. CI = confidence interval. Sample sizes vary across models because some individuals are missing data on some items and because there are different numbers of women and men in the sample.

[a]Significant at 10%, [b]significant at 5%, and [c]significant at 1%.

men without chronic diseases were less likely to be tested for cholesterol levels. Men with less-than-good health, with some college education and beyond, who were currently married, who were able to drive, who do not drink, and who scored zero on the CES-D were more likely to take a cholesterol test. Men having no ADL limitations were less likely to have had a cholesterol test. Finally, higher income had a positive effect on the use of cholesterol tests, but only among women.

Women and men who previously received a flu vaccine (Table 3) were 17.57 and 16.55 times more likely to receive another one, respectively. Women and men who were nonsmokers, and who had at least some college education were more also likely to receive a flu vaccine. However, among both women and men, those with no chronic diseases were less likely to receive one. Hispanic women were less likely to be vaccinated against flu, compared to both (non-Hispanic) White or Black women. Finally, women who were married and with less-than-good health were more likely to be vaccinated.

4. Discussion

This analysis of data from the 1996–2008 HRS reveals that covering a one-time IPPE had no effects on the use of mammograms, breast self-exams, Pap smears, prostate cancer screenings, cholesterol tests, or flu vaccines among new Medicare enrollees. Neither men nor women changed their use of preventive services in response to the availability of IPPE coverage.

For all six preventive care services, the single strongest predictor of use was previous utilization of that service. It has not been widely used by many empirical studies and should be taken into consideration as a key factor that can affect the use of preventive services. Other factors such as having no chronic diseases, having no ADL limitations, not smoking, having supplemental health insurance, being married, being more educated, and being able to drive also affected the use of preventive services.

In our analysis of cholesterol screenings and flu vaccines, models were estimated separately for men and women. We found that the estimated coefficients of explanatory variables in these models differ for men and women. This finding, which is consistent with past studies cited, reveals that the demand for these services indeed differs by gender.

In general, the equations we estimated accord with an Andersen-type model of healthcare utilization. Our finding that an individual's prior screening habits were the strongest predictor of their current utilization, for example, suggests that reinforcing factors and overall health beliefs play a critical role when it comes to preventive care. Education, which is a predisposing factor, and having additional health insurance beyond Medicare, which is an enabling factor, were also found to be important. Our measures of need-related factors, likewise, were often predictive of actual use of services.

To ensure the robustness of our key result, namely, that covering an IPPE had no effects on the use of preventive services, several sensitivity analyses were also conducted. Yet with every robustness check the same finding of no effects emerged. Specifically, we first reestimated the models using different specifications, excluding and including key variables [11]. We also reestimated all of them without the "previous use of preventive care" as an independent variable. We then reestimated them excluding those variables that were not statistically significant. In each case, the results remained the same: the policy indicator was still statistically insignificant. We also reestimated the model only using data from waves 7 (year 2004) and 9 (year 2008), to provide evenly balanced sample counts across the pre- and postperiods. Yet, in this case too, the policy indicator remained insignificant, except for prostate cancer screenings, where it showed a positive effect on receiving a prostate cancer screening. The models were also reestimated using an alternative comparison group of individuals aged 72 and 73 (not affected by the policy change), and in these models the coefficient on the policy indicator remained insignificant. The results therefore suggest that the use of preventive services by new Medicare enrollees was not affected by coverage of an IPPE.

There are likely multiple reasons for why beneficiaries have not fully utilized the IPPE benefit. Some beneficiaries may have been simply unaware of Medicare's coverage of an IPPE, or they may have first learned about it too late to take advantage of it. Recall when the IPPE benefit was first introduced in 2005 it was only available during a beneficiary's first six months under Medicare. For example, if someone learned about it four or five months after enrollment, they may not have been able to schedule an IPPE inside their six-month window. Another explanation is that some people simply do not assign high value to this sort of visit. It is unrealistic, for example, to think that all individuals would suddenly prioritize preventive services if they had not been doing so in the past, simply because a cost barrier had been removed. Moreover, although the IPPE benefit is "free," beneficiaries still must often coordinate transportation and expend the time and energy to attend the appointment.

Time, motivation, and awareness aside, there are also logistic issues that may have prevented some providers from fully embracing the IPPE. On the provider side one concern is that an IPPE visit is supposed to be separate from other routine primary care procedures. In essence, Medicare intends for the IPPE to focus on discussing health promotion and disease prevention. If, in the middle of an IPPE, a patient asks the physician to look at a rash or examine a sore throat, addressing this violates the intent of an IPPE. Yet, patients are not accustomed to going to the doctor to *not* discuss problems, and, understandably, physicians may be reticent to tell a patient who is already in front of them that they should make another appointment to discuss their sore throat. While it is possible for a physician to add a second service code to an IPPE visit claim with a modifier that enables payment for both services, the modifier pays less than a separate evaluation and management visit would pay. This creates a reimbursement dilemma for the physician: should they accept lower payment and address the patient's ailment then-and-there or suggest the patient make another appointment? Complicating the issue is that many physicians simply do not have extra time available to squeeze in an additional same-day visit for an IPPE patient, and even if they could, that patient might be unable or unwilling to stay and wait. In short, after spending the time and energy to attend a primary care appointment many, if not all, patients expect to be able to discuss any issue with their physician that is relevant at the time and not to have to make second appointments.

Another complication arises from patients' likely confusion over what can and cannot be done during the IPPE. Many patients liken their annual physical to a health promotion and prevention visit and, therefore, may not understand why a second visit, namely, the IPPE, is necessary. This may be especially confusing for a patient because the physician does not have them undress, check their vitals, or conduct a physical exam during the IPPE. Furthermore, some physicians may have already been combining the principles of the IPPE in their patients' routine physicals and since Medicare does not cover physicals, they do not submit a claim for the IPPE.

The various explanations discussed above for why the IPPE has not been embraced under Medicare are largely speculative on our part. As far as we know, empirical studies have not yet been conducted to pin down the reasons for the low utilization of IPPEs.

This study has two limitations which should be noted. The HRS asked participants about their use of preventive services over the past two years. We would have preferred it to have asked "over the last year," as this would have allowed us to capture the effects of IPPE coverage more accurately. Some might question the validity of using self-reported healthcare utilization data, especially in a sample of older adults.

5. Conclusions

Efforts to improve the use of preventive services are important as the aging population increases in the US, and as quality healthcare, including preventive care, becomes imperative. In addition, fewer than half of seniors are up-to-date on recommended preventive services [4]. Despite this need, the findings presented here strongly suggest that, at least as it was initially designed, covering an IPPE under Medicare had no significant effects on the use of preventive services, suggesting that time-limiting benefits or health policies may not provide desired public health outcomes. Policy-makers should be aware of this limitation and consider other approaches to increase the use of preventive services under Medicare.

Conflicts of Interest

The authors declare that there are no conflicts of interest regarding the publication of this paper.

References

[1] D. C. Colby, B. C. Quinn, and S. Goodell, *Cost Savings and Cost-Effectiveness of Clinical Preventive Care*, The Robert Wood Johnson Foundation, 2009.

[2] Government Accountability Office, *Medicare Preventive Services: Most Beneficiaries Receive Some but Not All Recommended Services*, 2004, http://www.gao.gov/new.items/d041004t.pdf.

[3] R. G. Salloum, G. A. Jensen, and A. K. Biddle, "The 'welcome to medicare' visit: a missed opportunity for cancer screening among women?" *Journal of Women's Health*, vol. 22, no. 1, pp. 19–25, 2013.

[4] Centers for Disease Control and Prevention, *Clinical Preventive Services*, 2013, http://www.cdc.gov/aging/services/index.htm.

[5] Department of Health and Human Services, Centers for Medicare, and Medicaid Services, *Prevention-General Information*, 2011, http://www.cms.gov/PrevntionGenInfo/20_prevserv.asp.

[6] P. S. Clair, D. Blake, D. Bugliari et al., *RAND HRS Data Documentation*, Version K. HRS, 2011.

[7] Health and Retirement Study, *About the Health and Retirement Study*, 2012, http://hrsonline.isr.umich.edu/.

[8] F. T. Juster, R. J. Willis, and D. R. Weir, *Growing Older in America: The Health and Retirement Study*, Institute for Social Research at the University of Michigan, Mich, USA, 2012.

[9] Research And Development, *RAND Contributions to HRS*, 2004, http://hrsonline.isr.umich.edu/modules/meta/rand/index.html.

[10] K. R. Jenkins, M. B. Ofstedal, and D. Weir, *Documentation of Health Behaviors and Risk Factors Measured in the Health and Retirement Study (HRS/AHEAD)*, HRS, 2008.

[11] P. J. Gertler, S. Martinez, P. Premand, L. B. Rawlings, and M. J. V. Christel, *Impact Evaluation in Practice: Ancillary Material*, The World Bank, Wash, USA, 2010.

[12] J. M. Wooldridge, *Introductory Econometrics A Modern Approach*, Thomson Higher Education, 3rd edition, 2006.

[13] R. M. Andersen, "Revisiting the behavioral model and access to medical care: does it matter?" *Journal of Health and Social Behavior*, vol. 36, no. 1, pp. 1–10, 1995.

[14] K.-M. Lo and K. G. Fulda, "Impact of predisposing, enabling, and need factors in accessing preventive medical care among U.S. children: results of the national survey of children's health," *Osteopathic Medicine and Primary Care*, vol. 2, no. 12, Article ID PMC2615756, 2008.

[15] S. M. Yu, H. A. Bellamy, M. D. Kogan, J. L. Dunbar, R. H. Schwalberg, and M. A. Schuster, "Factors that influence receipt of recommended preventive pediatric health and dental care," *Pediatrics*, vol. 110, no. 6, article e73, 2002.

[16] M. Inkelas, P. W. Newacheck, L. M. Olson, B. Zuckerman, and M. A. Schuster, "Does having a regular primary care clinician improve quality of preventive care for young children?" *Medical Care*, vol. 46, no. 3, pp. 323–330, 2008.

[17] E. H. Bradley, S. A. McGraw, L. Curry et al., "Expanding the andersen model: the role of psychosocial factors in long-term care use," *Health Services Research*, vol. 37, no. 5, pp. 1221–1242, 2002.

[18] J. M. E. Walsh and S. J. McPhee, "A systems model of clinical prevenitve care: an analysis of factors influencing patient and physician," *Health Education & Behavior*, vol. 19, pp. 157–175, 1992.

[19] D. S. Lane, J. Zapka, N. Breen, C. R. Messina, and D. J. Fotheringham, "A systems model of clinical preventive care: The case of breast cancer screening among older women," *Preventive Medicine*, vol. 31, no. 5, pp. 481–493, 2000.

[20] C. Lerman, B. Rimer, B. Trock, A. Balshem, and P. F. Engstrom, "Factors associated with repeat adherence to breast cancer screening," *Preventive Medicine*, vol. 19, no. 3, pp. 279–290, 1990.

[21] B. K. Rimer, "Improving the use of cancer screening for older women," *Cancer*, vol. 72, no. 3, pp. 1084–1087, 1993.

[22] R. M. Weinick and K. M. Beauregard, "Women's use of preventive screening services: a comparison of hmo versus fee-for-service enrollees," *Medical Care Research and Review*, vol. 54, no. 2, pp. 176–199, 1997.

10

Association of Leukocyte Telomere Length with Fatigue in Nondisabled Older Adults

Laila Bendix,[1,2] Mikael Thinggaard,[1,3] Masayuki Kimura,[4] Abraham Aviv,[4] Kaare Christensen,[1,3,5,6,7] Merete Osler,[1,2,7,8] and Kirsten Avlund[1,2,7]

[1] *Danish Aging Research Center, Universities of Southern Denmark, Aarhus, and Copenhagen, Denmark*
[2] *Section of Social Medicine, Department of Public Health, University of Copenhagen, P.O. Box 2099, 1014 Copenhagen K, Denmark*
[3] *Epidemiology, Institute of Public Health, University of Southern Denmark, JB Winslowsvej 9B, 5000 Odense C, Denmark*
[4] *The Center of Human Development and Aging, University of Medicine and Dentistry of New Jersey, New Jersey Medical School, Newark, NJ 07103, USA*
[5] *The Danish Twin Registry, Institute of Public Health, University of Southern Denmark, JB Winslowsvej 9B, 5000 Odense C, Denmark*
[6] *Department of Clinical Genetics and Department of Biochemistry and Pharmacology, Odense University Hospital, 5000 Odense C, Denmark*
[7] *Center for Healthy Aging, University of Copenhagen, 2200 Copenhagen N, Denmark*
[8] *Research Center for Prevention and Health, The Capital Region of Denmark, 2600 Glostrup, Denmark*

Correspondence should be addressed to Merete Osler; merete.osler@regionh.dk

Academic Editor: Gustavo Duque

Introduction. Fatigue is often present in older adults with no identified underlying cause. The accruing burden of oxidative stress and inflammation might be underlying factors of fatigue. We therefore hypothesized that leukocyte telomere length (LTL) is relatively short in older adults who experience fatigue. *Materials and Methods.* We assessed 439 older nondisabled Danish twins. LTL was measured using Southern blots of terminal restriction fragments. Fatigue was measured by the Mob-T Scale based on questions on whether the respondents felt fatigued after performing six mobility items. *Results.* LTL was significantly associated with fatigue ($P = 0.023$), showing an increase of 0.038 kb/fatigue score unit. Aging-related diseases and mental health did not explain the association, while lifestyle factors slightly attenuated the estimates. *Conclusion.* Our results support an association between LTL and fatigue. Further studies are required to confirm this finding and the link of LTL with oxidative stress/inflammation over the life course.

1. Introduction

Fatigue is a common complaint among older adults. While it is often a symptom of psychiatric or medical illness, for many older persons, it is not possible to identify the underlying cause. Studies during the last 15 years have consistently shown that fatigue in older adults is a strong predictor of functional limitations [1], disability [2], and mortality [3]. Thus, fatigue might represent an early stage of frailty, defined as a physiologic state of increased vulnerability to stressors that results from decreased reserves in multiple physiologic and biologic systems [4].

Cellular and organismal damages caused by an accruing burden of oxidative stress could be an underlying factor to fatigue. Increased oxidative stress can be caused by defective mitochondria as well as by chronic low-grade inflammation. Both these conditions are known to be associated with increasing age, and evidence suggests that oxidative stress and inflammation are associated with frailty [5].

It is generally accepted that oxidative stress and inflammation are important contributors to the pathology of aging-related diseases such as cardiovascular disease [6], dementia [7], and cancer [8]. Such conditions often predispose to frailty [4]. Leukocyte telomere length (LTL) ostensibly undergoes an accelerated shortening due to inflammation and increased oxidative stress [6, 9]. This might explain the association of shortened LTL with aging-related diseases and some of their risk factors, including coronary heart disease, dementia, and insulin resistance [10, 11].

Potentially, shortened LTL and the consequent cellular aging could thus be an underlying mechanism to fatigue.

Woo et al. [12] found no apparent association between LTL and frailty in a study that applied a composite frailty index score but had not examined directly the potential connection between LTL and fatigue. To examine whether a link in fact exists between LTL and fatigue, we have exploited the same-sex twin design that has previously made it possible to show relationsships of LTL with mortality [13], and physical ability [14]. In the present study we show results supporting the association between LTL and fatigue.

2. Material and Methods

2.1. Description of Twin Sample. The Longitudinal Study of Aging Danish Twins (LSADT) began in 1995 with an assessment of same-sex twin pairs born in Denmark before 1920 [15]. Since 1995 twins from the LSADT have participated in a comprehensive face-to-face interview including detailed questions about health, lifestyle, and physical functioning [16]. This interview has been repeated every second year for a total of six examinations. At the second examination, blood samples were collected from 283 twin pairs. Of these, a total of 274 pairs (548 individuals) had their LTL measured [13].

For this study, the population was restricted to the 439 individuals who were nondisabled, that is, who were able to rise from a chair or bed, walk indoors, get outdoors, walk outdoors in nice weather, walk outdoors in bad weather, and climb stairs without help. Further, we excluded persons who had answered the questionnaire by a proxy. These restrictions were applied as previous studies have shown fatigue to be related to onset of disability [2], functional limitations [1], and even cardiovascular disease [17] among nondisabled and nondiseased. We also repeat the analyses in a restricted sample of persons below 80 years, as these persons are more likely to be without conditions, which we have not been able to adjust for.

For further information on the participants, see Table 1.

The study has been approved by the local scientific-ethical Committee. All participants provided written informed consent.

2.2. LTL Measurement. Leukocyte DNA was extracted using standard techniques. DNA quality was assessed by electrophoresis. LTL was measured using Southern blots of the terminal restriction fragments after digestion with HphI and MnlI restriction enzymes; for 377 of the nondisabled twins the terminal restriction fragments were also generated by HinfI and RsaI digestion [18]. The HphI/MnlI products include predominantly true telomeric repeats, whereas the HinfI/RsaI product includes a proximal telomere segment that is not strictly TTAGGG. The HphI/MnlI products were on average 1.1 kb shorter than the HinfI/RsaI products, and the two LTL measures correlated strongly ($r = 0.88$, $P < 0.001$).

Samples from the cotwins in each twin pair were resolved in adjacent lanes of the same gel. Running DNA digests from the two cotwins in adjacent lanes on the same gel diminished the methodological variation within twin-pairs. In between-pair analysis the "gel effect" was included as covariate.

Each sample was measured in duplicate (performed on different gels) and the mean of the two samples was used. The interassay coefficient of variation was 2.5% for the HinfI/RsaI digest and 3.4% for the HphI/MnlI digest.

We present data from the HphI/MnlI digest, while results obtained with HinfI/RsaI digest can be found in the corresponding Supplementary (S) Material (see tables in the Supplementary Material).

2.3. Fatigue. Fatigue was measured by the Mob-T Scale based on questions about six mobility items ((a) rising from a chair or bed, (b) walking indoors, (c) getting outdoors, (d) walking outdoors in nice weather, (e) walking outdoors in bad weather, and (f) climbing stairs). Every activity was described relative to whether the respondents did or did not feel fatigued afterwards. The mobility-tiredness Scale (Mob-T) counts the number of activities managed without fatigue. The highest scale value thus describes no fatigue. The construct validity of the scale was tested by the Rasch model for item analysis, which showed that the scale had satisfactory homogeneity [19, 20]. The data have recently been reanalyzed using a new test based on the Rasch model on the assumption of equal item discrimination—with satisfactory results [21]. Reliability tests showed agreement from 94.3% to 98.3% and kappa values from 0.72 to 0.88 for the included items on intrarater and interrater tests [22]. As this measure of fatigue focuses on fatigue in performing certain activities it is likely that it reflects the physiologic and biologic consequences of doing these activities.

2.4. Covariates. Covariates of lifestyle, mental health, and aging-related somatic diseases were included as potential confounding factors since previous studies have shown that they might be associated with fatigue and LTL [10, 23–29].

2.4.1. Lifestyle. Smoking status was divided in never, former, and current smokers. BMI was deduced from self-reported height and weight. Physical activity was scored on a five-point scale deducted from self-reported level and frequency of physical activity. The answers were scored as follows: 0: "no physical activity," 1: "seldom low intensity physical activity," 2: "frequent low intensity physical activity," 3: "seldom high and frequent low intensity physical activity," and 4: "frequent high intensity physical activity."

2.4.2. Mental Health Status. Cognitive performance was scored by a cognitive composite score. This was evaluated by a battery of five brief cognitive tests, which were selected to be sensitive to age-related changes. The tasks included

TABLE 1: Descriptive statistics of the study population, including data on mean LTL, fatigue and lifestyle, mental health and somatic disease covariates.

Characteristics		Total (N = 439)	Female (N = 294)	Male (N = 145)	P value (sex diff.)
LTL (in kb)	Mean (SD)	4.59	4.67	4.47	0.005*
Fatigue score	Mean (SD)	5.35	5.29	5.46	0.170
0	N (%)	4 (0.9%)	4 (1.4%)	0 (0.0%)	
1	N (%)	3 (0.7%)	3 (1.0%)	0 (0.0%)	
2	N (%)	17 (3.9%)	11 (3.7%)	6 (4.1%)	
3	N (%)	21 (4.8%)	15 (5.1%)	6 (4.1%)	
4	N (%)	29 (6.6%)	19 (6.5%)	10 (6.9%)	
5	N (%)	58 (13.2%)	42 (14.3%)	16 (11.0%)	
6	N (%)	307 (69.9%)	200 (68.0%)	107 (73.8%)	
Age	Mean(SD)	78.4	78.5	78.1	0.334
Zygosity	MZ N (%)	204 (46.5%)	138 (46.9%)	66 (45.5%)	
	DZ N (%)	235 (53.5%)	156 (53.1%)	79 (54.5%)	
Smoking	Never N (%)	154 (35.1%)	129 (43.9%)	25 (17.2%)	
	Former N (%)	155 (35.3%)	86 (29.3%)	69 (47.6%)	
	Current N (%)	139 (29.6%)	79 (26.9%)	51 (35.2%)	
BMI	Mean (SD)	24.13	23.65	25.09	<0.001*
<18.5	N (%)	25 (5.7%)	23 (7.8%)	2 (1.4%)	
18.5–24.9	N (%)	236 (53.8%)	174 (59.2%)	62 (42.8%)	
25–29.9	N (%)	157 (35.8%)	80 (27.2%)	77 (53.1%)	
>30	N (%)	17(3.9%)	13 (4.4%)	4 (2.8%)	
Physical activity	Mean (SD)	2.52	2.52	2.52	0.979
0	N (%)	62 (14.1%)	43 (14.6%)	19 (13.1%)	
1	N (%)	14 (3.2%)	9 (3.1%)	5 (3.4%)	
2	N (%)	152 (34.6%)	98 (33.3%)	54 (37.2%)	
3	N (%)	55 (12.9%)	40 (13.6%)	15 (10.3%)	
4	N (%)	156 (35.5%)	104 (35.4%)	52 (35.8%)	
Cognitive comp.	Mean (SD)	1.46	1.63	1.11	0.113
Depression sympt.	Mean (SD)	20.76	20.87	20.54	0.434
Rheumatic disease	No N	283	172	115	
	Yes N (%)	156 (35.5%)	122 (41.5%)	34 (23.4%)	
CVD	No N	280	182	98	
	Yes N (%)	159 (36.2%)	112 (38.1%)	47 (32.4%)	
Cancer	No N	389	258	131	
	Yes N (%)	50 (11.4%)	36 (12.2%)	14 (9.7%)	
Diabetes	No N	419	280	139	
	Yes N (%)	20 (4.6%)	14 (4.8%)	6 (4.1%)	

*Significant difference between sexes. †The P value for sex-differences has been adjusted for age.
LTL: leukocyte telomere length; CVD: cardiovascular disease; MZ: monozygotic twins; DZ: dizygotic twins.

a verbal fluency test, forward and backward digit span, and immediate and delayed recall of a 12-item list. The standard scores for each task were summed to give an overall score. Higher cognitive composite scores indicated better cognitive function [30].

Depression symptomatology was assessed using an adaptation of the depression section of the Cambridge Mental Disorders of the Elderly Examination (CAMDEX) [31]. McGue and Christensen [15] factor analyzed the LSADT depression items identifying two factor scales (9-item affective and 8-item somatic scales). Because these scales were highly correlated ($r > 0.50$), a 17-item total scale score has been defined [15]. Analyses reported here are based on the total scale score.

2.4.3. Somatic Disease. Cardiovascular disease included angina pectoris, heart failure, hypertension, irregular heart rhythm, and myocardial infarction. For diabetes and cancer any positive history is regarded as being a positive outcome and no distinction is done between type and duration. Rheumatologic disease covers the presence of either of the following conditions: rheumatic arthritis, osteoarthritis, and/or gout.

2.4.4. Statistical Methods. We applied a multiple regression modeling to test if fatigue was associated with LTL. A random intercept regression model was considered to account for nonindependence within pairs [32].

Possible association was further studied using an intrapair twin design in which difference in LTL was regressed on the difference in fatigue. This design enables us to control for age, sex, zygosity, and gel effect, as well as for early common environment and genetic factors. MZ twins share 100% of their genes while DZ twins only share 50%. If an association is attenuated among MZ twins it suggests genetic confounding. If an association is attenuated among MZ and DZ twins it suggests early environmental confounding.

A P value of 0.05 was chosen as significance level for all tests and the statistical analyses were done using STATA 11.1 (STATA Corp, College Station, TX, USA).

3. Results

3.1. General Characteristics. A total of 439 twins representing 257 twin pairs were studied. 145 (33%) were men, and 294 (67%) were women; 235 (53.5%) came from a dizygotic twin pair (DZ) and 204 (46.5%) from a monozygotic twin pair (MZ). Descriptive statistics of participants are presented in Table 1. The mean ages of the participants were 78.1 years for men (range 73–88) and 78.5 years for women (range 73–94).

Women were found to have longer LTL than men (age adjusted: 4.65 kb and 4.46 kb, resp.). The age-related attrition in this population was 0.020 kb per year. There was no significant difference in fatigue score between men and women. Fatigue was inversely correlated with age ($R = -0.25$, $P < 0.001$), that is, the higher the age the more fatigued (lower score).

The association between the examined covariates and, respectively, LTL and fatigue is presented in Table 2. Only smoking and depression symptomatology were significantly associated with LTL, while BMI, physical activity, cognitive function, depression symptomatology, and rheumatic disease were significantly associated with fatigue.

3.2. Multivariate Analysis. The regression model revealed a positive association between LTL and fatigue when adjusting for effects of sex and age. For every unit increase in fatigue score, LTL increased by 0.038 kb after adjustment for sex and age ($P = 0.023$; Table 2), which is equivalent to two years of age-related LTL attrition. There was no effect of zygosity nor was there an interaction effect of sex and age (data not shown) on the association. Hence, the association between fatigue and LTL was similar for each gender and zygosity.

The examined lifestyle factors had a minimal effect on the association between LTL and fatigue (Table 3, model 3), diminishing the association coefficient from 0.038 to 0.032. Including mental health in the model (Table 3, model 4) only slightly attenuated the association. However, inclusion of these covariates was not found to give a significantly better fit by a likelihood ratio test. Adjusting for somatic diseases separately or jointly did not influence the association between LTL and fatigue (Table 3, model 5).

Including all covariates, that is, sex, age, gel effect, zygosity, somatic diseases, mental health, and lifestyle resulted in slight attenuation of the association between LTL and fatigue (Table 3, model 6) ($P = 0.166$). However, likelihood ratio test indicated that the optimal model of the LTL-fatigue association includes only sex and age (model 2).

The analyses were repeated in a subsample of the study population restricted to individuals below 80 years. The LTL-fatigue association was found to be stronger in this younger subpopulation.

3.3. Intrapair Analysis. 87 pairs were intact and discordant for the fatigue score. The intrapair analysis confirmed that for every one unit change in fatigue score, LTL differed by 0.039 kb ($P = 0.054$) within the pair (Table 4). This effect was not significantly different between MZ and DZ twin pairs; however, the effect only reached significance in MZ twin pairs.

The association was attenuated when including lifestyle factors from Coef = 0.039 to Coef = 0.030 due to a small confounding effect of smoking and physical activity not seen in the regression analysis. Likelihood ratio test suggested the inclusion of smoking in the model. Also inclusion of depression symptoms provided a better fit of the data but hardly influenced the association (Coef = 0.036, $P = 0.097$) (data not shown).

3.4. Results from HinfI/RsaI Digest. This subpopulation consisted of 377 individuals representing 219 twin pairs. There was no noteworthy difference on the demographics of two populations (Table S1). There were similar associations between the examined covariates and, respectively, LTL and fatigue (Table S2).

The association with fatigue was of lesser magnitude and no longer reached significance (Table S3, model 2), neither for the younger subpopulation. Likelihood ratio test showed that the inclusion of lifestyle factors (especially smoking) as well as depression symptomatology had a better fit of data. Including these factors completely attenuated the association (Coef = 0.005, $P = 0.846$).

The intrapair analyses were in agreement with findings from the HphI/MnlI digest, however not significant, and could mostly be attributed to physical activity and smoking, as well as depression symptomatology.

4. Discussion

In this study we observed an association between fatigue and LTL in nondisabled older twins. Previous studies have found fatigue to be related to onset of several adverse health outcomes [33], also when adjusted for multiple covariates. The predictive value of fatigue has been especially strong in nondisabled older persons and in persons without cardiovascular disease, indicating that fatigue may be an early marker of the aging process, before the onset of diseases and

TABLE 2: The association between covariates and, respectively, LTL, and fatigue.

Covariates	Association with LTL						Association fatigue					
	Raw			Adjusted (sex, age)			Raw			Adjusted (sex, age)		
	Coef†	CI (95%)	*P*	Coef†	CI (95%)	*P*	Coef†	CI (95%)	*P*	Coef†	CI (95%)	*P*
Fatigue (Score 0–6)	0.039	0.006–0.071	0.019	**0.038**††	**0.005–0.070**	**0.023**						
Age	−0.019	−0.035–−0.003	0.018	**−0.20**	**−0.036–−0.004**	**0.012**	−0.041	−0.073–−0.009	0.012	**−0.040**	**−0.072–−0.008**	**0.014**
Sex												
Male	Ref			Ref			Ref			Ref		
Female	0.161	0.032–0.290	0.014	**0.169**	**0.041–0.297**	**0.009**	−0.169	−0.426–0.088	0.197	−0.154	−0.408–0.099	0.233
Zygosity												
MZ	Ref			Ref			Ref			Ref		
DZ	−0.027	−0.150–0.097	0.672	−0.039	−0.159–0.081	0.530	−0.020	−0.263–0.223	0.871	−0.047	−0.286–0.192	0.700
Geleffect	0.007	0.000–0.014	0.040	0.002	−0.008–0.011	0.688						
Smoking												
Never	Ref			Ref			Ref			Ref		
Former	−0.076	−0.172–0.021	0.124	−0.063	−0.160–0.035	0.206	−0.132	−0.408–0.144	0.349	−0.208	−0.490–0.074	0.148
Current	−0.127	−0.234–−0.020	0.020	**−0.122**	**−0.230–−0.014**	**0.027**	−0.156	−0.448–0.135	0.293	−0.252	−0.547–0.043	0.095
Physical activity (Score 0–4)	0.024	−0.006–0.054	0.122	0.020	−0.011–0.049	0.213	0.344	0.266–0.423	<0.001	**0.336**	**0.257–0.415**	**<0.001**
BMI	−0.010	−0.022–0.003	0.137	−0.010	−0.023–0.003	0.127	−0.039	−0.072–−0.006	0.019	**−0.052**	**−0.085–−0.018**	**0.002**
Cognitive function	0.014	−0.000–0.027	0.053	0.011	−0.009–0.025	0.111	0.041	0.005–0.077	0.025	**0.038**	**0.002–0.074**	**0.037**
Depression symptomatology	−0.012	−0.022–−0.002	0.022	**−0.012**	**−0.022–−0.002**	**0.024**	−0.120	−0.145–−0.094	<0.001	**−0.118**	**−0.143–−0.093**	**<0.001**
Cancer												
No	Ref			Ref			Ref			Ref		
Yes	−0.005	−0.122–0.113	0.940	−0.010	−0.127–0.107	0.868	−0.230	−0.588–0.129	0.209	−0.236	−0.592–0.120	0.194
CVD												
No	Ref			Ref			Ref			Ref		
Yes	−0.009	0.095–0.076	0.829	−0.013	−0.098–0.072	0.763	−0.173	−0.414–0.068	0.160	−0.167	−0.406–0.072	0.171
Diabetes												
No	Ref			Ref			Ref			Ref		
Yes	0.001	−0.191–0.192	0.997	0.006	−0.184–0.196	0.952	−0.297	−0.852–0.257	0.293	−0.266	−0.817–0.284	0.343
Rheumatic												
No	Ref			Ref			Ref			Ref		
Yes	0.004	−0.080–0.087	0.933	−0.011	−0.095–0.072	0.788	−0.414	−0.656–−0.179	0.001	**−0.419**	**−0.659–−0.179**	**<0.001**

Bold values mark the significant adjusted coeffients.

†The coefficients shows the magnitude of the linear association between covariates and LTL respectively fatigue. First columns are raw data, while second columns are adjusted for sex and age.

††There is a significant association between LTL and fatigue when adjusting for age and sex. The coefficient of 0.038 tells that for every increase on the fatigue score (i.e. the less fatigued) the LTL is 0.038 kb longer.

TABLE 3: The association between LTL and fatigue.

Population		Model 1 Raw	Model 2 Age, sex	Model 3 Lifestyle	Model 4 Mental	Model 5 Somatic	Model 6 Full
All $N = 439$	Coef	0.039	0.038	0.032	0.032	0.038	0.026
	CI 95%	0.006–0.071	0.005–0.070	−0.003–0.070	−0.002–0.067	0.005–0.071	−0.011–0.064
	P-value	0.019	0.023	0.074	0.066	0.025	0.166
<80 y $N = 315$	Coef	0.050	0.051	0.044	0.051	0.050	0.044
	CI 95%	0.007–0.093	0.008–0.094	−0.002–0.090	0.003–0.099	0.006–0.094	−0.007–0.095
	P-value	0.024	0.019	0.058	0.037	0.025	0.093

Model 1: raw model.
Model 2: adjusted for sex and age.
Model 3: as Model 2 including adjustment for lifestyle factors.
Model 4: as Model 2 including adjustment for mental health.
Model 5: as Model 2 including adjustment for somatic disease.
Model 6: full model that is as Model 2 including adjustment for lifestyle factors, mental health, somatic disease as well as zygosity and gel-effect.

TABLE 4: Intrapair analysis.

		All	MZ	DZ
All $N = 174$	Coef	0.039	0.057	0.026
	CI 95%	−0.001–0.079	0.007–0.107	−0.035–0.086
	P-value	0.054	0.027	0.398
<80 y $N = 110$	Coef	0.058	0.069	0.049
	CI 95%	0.003–0.112	0.002–0.138	−0.035–0.132
	P-value	0.040	0.049	0.247

The intrapair analysis is shown for the whole sample as well as for the younger subpopulation. Further the analysis has been run for only MZ and DZ twins respectively.
The simple model is intrinsically adjusted for sex, age, geleffect and zygosity due to the intrapair twin design.
LTL: leukocyte telomere length; MZ: monozygotic twins; DZ: dizygotic twins.

disability. We have earlier shown that LTL was related to physical ability, measured by a self-reported strength scale, in a study population of 70–93-year-old participants in the LSADT study [14]. The present study shows that LTL is associated with fatigue before the onset of disablement, thus suggesting that shortening of LTL is an early detectable event in this process.

Fatigue is a central symptom in many organic and psychiatric diseases. We have chosen to include four major aging-related diseases (CVD, diabetes, rheumatic disease, and cancer) as well as cognitive function as potential confounders since these have previously been suggested to be associated with LTL dynamics. However, we found no influence of either diseases or cognitive function on the LTL-fatigue association. Depression is a condition closely correlated with fatigue and is evidently associated with short LTL [34]. Thus, we considered depression a possible confounder. The inclusion of the available depression symptomatology score [15] slightly attenuated the association. It is likely that this finding is merely an over adjustment since the depression symptomatology score contains questions on feeling of lack of energy, which was highly correlated with fatigue ($R = 0.323$, $P < 0.001$). The coexistence of fatigue and depression has previously been reported [35] and found to be associated with an increased risk of death in older adults [36], as has the coexistence of depression and other diseases predisposing to fatigue. A common inflammatory and oxidative stress pathway has been suggested [37], necessitating a clarification of this coexistence in future studies.

Of the included lifestyle factors, we found that only smoking had a slight effect on the association between LTL and fatigue. We have previously found that physical activity level was associated with LTL [14]. In this subpopulation the association was of the same magnitude but not significant. We suggest that this is simply due to lack of power and therefore chose to include physical activity as a possible confounder. However, physical activity seemed only to have an effect on the association when LTL was measured with the HInfI/RsaI digest. Smoking is therefore the only of the analyzed covariates that we suggest as a confounder to be included in the model besides sex and age.

A study by Woo et al. [12] found no association between frailty and LTL. The discrepancy is likely due to the focus on fatigue in the present study, while Woo and colleagues used a composite frailty index. Methodological variation could also have an impact, as Woo et al. reported a CV of 11.1% in their qPCR based method, while the CV of the TRF assay for this cohort was only 3.4%. Moreover, although our cohort was of limited size, we gained statistical power by exploiting the twin design.

Some limitations and strengths should be considered when interpreting the results. The low coefficient of variation is a strength to our study, as well as the twin design. We have included lifestyle factors and major aging-related diseases as covariates; in future studies inclusion of medications could be of value since these could contribute to fatigue. Various tools to evaluate fatigue exist [38]. Many scales have been suggested, some focusing on the severity of fatigue. Further different performance based measures are often used (e.g., an oxygen uptake measure or accelerometers) [39]. The used fatigue measure is reliable [1, 22] and has the advantage that it is a self-reported measure of fatigue in performing certain activities and is therefore likely to reflect the physiologic and biologic consequences of doing these activities [33]. Our study suggests a possible common physiological pathway between LTL attrition and fatigue; however, to establish a better insight into the dynamics in fatigue and cellular aging, future studies should examine changes over time of LTL and fatigue score in the same individuals.

5. Conclusion

Overall, our findings indicate that LTL is associated with fatigue and that this cannot be explained by common lifestyle factors, aging-related diseases, or cognitive function. These findings largely agree with previous studies showing that fatigue is a strong indicator of adverse health outcomes in nondisabled older adults [33] and in middle-aged healthy men [17]. The findings are suggestive of oxidative stress and inflammation being underlying factors of fatigue and should spur the search for more biomarkers leading to a better understanding of the physiology behind fatigue.

Conflict of Interests

The authors declare that there is no conflict of interests regarding the publication of this paper.

Acknowledgments

This study was supported by Grants from the US National Institutes of Health (Grant no. NIA P01 AG008761 and NIH Grant AG0306778). The Danish Aging Research Center is supported by a grant from the VELUX Foundation. We remember professor Kirsten Avlund who passed away too early September 2013 for her great contribution to our work.

References

[1] M. Mänty, C. F. Mendes De Leon, T. Rantanen et al., "Mobility-related fatigue, walking speed, and muscle strength in older people," *Journals of Gerontology A*, vol. 67, no. 5, pp. 523–529, 2012.

[2] K. Avlund, T. Rantanen, and M. Schroll, "Tiredness and subsequent disability in older adults: the role of walking limitations," *Journals of Gerontology A*, vol. 61, no. 11, pp. 1201–1205, 2006.

[3] S. E. Hardy and S. A. Studenski, "Fatigue predicts mortality in older adults," *Journal of the American Geriatrics Society*, vol. 56, no. 10, pp. 1910–1914, 2008.

[4] L. P. Fried, L. Ferrucci, J. Darer, J. D. Williamson, and G. Anderson, "Untangling the concepts of disability, frailty, and comorbidity: implications for improved targeting and care," *Journals of Gerontology A*, vol. 59, no. 3, pp. 255–263, 2004.

[5] R. E. Hubbard and K. W. Woodhouse, "Frailty, inflammation and the elderly," *Biogerontology*, vol. 11, no. 5, pp. 635–641, 2010.

[6] A. Aviv, "Leukocyte telomere length, hypertension, and atherosclerosis are there potential mechanistic explanations?" *Hypertension*, vol. 53, no. 4, pp. 590–591, 2009.

[7] K. Chopra, S. Misra, and A. Kuhad, "Neurobiological aspects of Alzheimer's disease," *Expert Opinion on Therapeutic Targets*, vol. 15, no. 5, pp. 535–555, 2011.

[8] S. Reuter, S. C. Gupta, M. M. Chaturvedi, and B. B. Aggarwal, "Oxidative stress, inflammation, and cancer: how are they linked?" *Free Radical Biology and Medicine*, vol. 49, no. 11, pp. 1603–1616, 2010.

[9] T. Von Zglinicki, "Role of oxidative stress in telomere length regulation and replicative senescence," *Annals of the New York Academy of Sciences*, vol. 908, pp. 99–110, 2000.

[10] A. Benetos, J. P. Gardner, M. Zureik et al., "Short telomeres are associated with increased carotid atherosclerosis in hypertensive subjects," *Hypertension*, vol. 43, no. 2, pp. 182–185, 2004.

[11] R. M. Cawthon, K. R. Smith, E. O'Brien, A. Sivatchenko, and R. A. Kerber, "Association between telomere length in blood and mortality in people aged 60 years or older," *The Lancet*, vol. 361, no. 9355, pp. 393–395, 2003.

[12] J. Woo, N. L. S. Tang, E. Suen, J. C. S. Leung, and P. C. Leung, "Telomeres and frailty," *Mechanisms of Ageing and Development*, vol. 129, no. 11, pp. 642–648, 2008.

[13] M. Kimura, J. V. B. Hjelmborg, J. P. Gardner et al., "Telomere length and mortality: a study of leukocytes in elderly danish twins," *American Journal of Epidemiology*, vol. 167, no. 7, pp. 799–806, 2008.

[14] L. Bendix, M. M. Gade, P. W. Staun et al., "Leukocyte telomere length and physical ability among Danish Twins age 70+," *Mechanisms of Ageing and Development*, vol. 132, no. 11-12, pp. 568–572, 2011.

[15] M. McGue and K. Christensen, "Genetic and environmental contributions to depression symptomatology: evidence from Danish twins 75 years of age and older," *Journal of Abnormal Psychology*, vol. 106, no. 3, pp. 439–448, 1997.

[16] K. Andersen, H. Nybo, D. Gaist et al., "Cognitive impairment and mortality among nonagenarians: the Danish 1905 cohort survey," *Dementia and Geriatric Cognitive Disorders*, vol. 13, no. 3, pp. 156–163, 2002.

[17] A. Ekmann, M. Osler, and K. Avlund, "The predictive value of fatigue for nonfatal ischemic heart disease and all-cause mortality," *Psychosomatic Medicine*, vol. 74, no. 5, pp. 464–470, 2012.

[18] M. Kimura, R. C. Stone, S. C. Hunt et al., "Measurement of telomere length by the Southern blot analysis of terminal restriction fragment lengths," *Nature Protocols*, vol. 5, no. 9, pp. 1596–1607, 2010.

[19] K. Avlund, K. Schultz-Larsen, and S. Kreiner, "The measurement of Instrumental ADL: content validity and construct validity," *Aging*, vol. 5, no. 5, pp. 371–383, 1993.

[20] K. Avlund and B. E. Holstein, "Functional ability among elderly people in three service settings: the discriminatory power of a new functional ability scale," *European Journal of Epidemiology*, vol. 14, no. 8, pp. 783–790, 1998.

[21] K. B. Christensen and S. Kreiner, "Monte carlo tests of the rasch model based on scalability coefficients," *British Journal of Mathematical and Statistical Psychology*, vol. 63, no. 1, pp. 101–111, 2010.

[22] K. Avlund, D. Thudium, M. Davidsen, and B. Fuglsang Sorensen, "Are selfratings of functional ability reliable?" *Scandinavian Journal of Occupational Therapy*, vol. 2, no. 1, pp. 10–16, 1995.

[23] K. Avlund, T. Rantanen, and M. Schroll, "Factors underlying tiredness in older adults," *Aging*, vol. 19, no. 1, pp. 16–25, 2007.

[24] L. F. Cherkas, J. L. Hunkin, B. S. Kato et al., "The association between physical activity in leisure time and leukocyte telomere length," *Archives of Internal Medicine*, vol. 168, no. 2, pp. 154–158, 2008.

[25] E. S. Epel, E. H. Blackburn, J. Lin et al., "Accelerated telomere shortening in response to life stress," *Proceedings of the National Academy of Sciences of the United States of America*, vol. 101, no. 49, pp. 17312–17315, 2004.

[26] J. A. Martin, T. D. Brown, A. D. Heiner, and J. A. Buckwalter, "Chondrocyte senescence, joint loading and osteoarthritis," *Clinical Orthopaedics and Related Research*, supplement 427, pp. S96–S103, 2004.

[27] U. Svenson and G. Roos, "Telomere length as a biological marker in malignancy," *Biochimica et Biophysica Acta*, vol. 1792, no. 4, pp. 317–323, 2009.

[28] O. Uziel, J. A. Singer, V. Danicek et al., "Telomere dynamics in arteries and mononuclear cells of diabetic patients: effect of diabetes and of glycemic control," *Experimental Gerontology*, vol. 42, no. 10, pp. 971–978, 2007.

[29] O. M. Wolkowitz, S. H. Mellon, E. S. Epel et al., "Leukocyte telomere length in major depression: correlations with chronicity, inflammation and oxidative stress—preliminary findings," *PLoS ONE*, vol. 6, no. 3, Article ID e17837, 2011.

[30] M. McGue and K. Christensen, "The heritability of cognitive functioning in very old adults: evidence from Danish twins aged 75 years and older," *Psychology and Aging*, vol. 16, no. 2, pp. 272–280, 2001.

[31] M. Roth, E. Tym, and C. Q. Mountjoy, "CAMDEX. A standardised instrument for the diagnosis of mental disorder in the elderly with special reference to the early detection of dementia," *British Journal of Psychiatry*, vol. 149, pp. 698–709, 1986.

[32] L. Wu, *Mixed Effects Models for Complex Data*, Chapman & Hall, Boca Raton, Fla, USA, 2010.

[33] K. Avlund, "Fatigue in older adults: an early indicator of the aging process?" *Aging*, vol. 22, no. 2, pp. 100–115, 2010.

[34] M. Wikgren, M. Maripuu, T. Karlsson et al., "Short telomeres in depression and the general population are associated with a hypocortisolemic state," *Biological Psychiatry*, vol. 71, no. 4, pp. 294–300, 2012.

[35] R. Fuhrer and S. Wessely, "The epidemiology of fatigue and depression: a French primary-care study," *Psychological Medicine*, vol. 25, no. 5, pp. 895–905, 1995.

[36] P. J. Brown, S. P. Roose, R. Fieo et al., "Frailty and depression in older adults: a high-risk clinical population," *The American Journal of Geriatric Psychiatry*, 2013.

[37] M. Maes, P. Ruckoanich, Y. S. Chang, N. Mahanonda, and M. Berk, "Multiple aberrations in shared inflammatory and oxidative & nitrosative stress (IO&NS) pathways explain the co-association of depression and cardiovascular disorder (CVD), and the increased risk for CVD and due mortality in depressed patients," *Progress in Neuro-Psychopharmacology and Biological Psychiatry*, vol. 35, no. 3, pp. 769–783, 2011.

[38] A. Poluri, J. Mores, D. B. Cook, T. W. Findley, and A. Cristian, "Fatigue in the elderly population," *Physical Medicine and Rehabilitation Clinics of North America*, vol. 16, no. 1, pp. 91–108, 2005.

[39] N. B. Alexander, G. E. Taffet, F. M. Horne et al., "Bedside-to-bench conference: research agenda for idiopathic fatigue and aging," *Journal of the American Geriatrics Society*, vol. 58, no. 5, pp. 967–975, 2010.

11

Physical Activity among Veterans and Nonveterans with Diabetes

Erin D. Bouldin[1,2] **and Gayle E. Reiber**[1,2,3]

[1] *Health Services Research and Development Service, Department of Veterans Affairs, VA Puget Sound Health Care System, Seattle, WA 98101, USA*
[2] *Department of Epidemiology, University of Washington, Seattle, WA 98195, USA*
[3] *Department of Health Services, University of Washington, Seattle, WA 98195, USA*

Correspondence should be addressed to Erin D. Bouldin, erin.bouldin@va.gov

Academic Editor: Iris Reuter

Engaging in regular physical activity (PA), with or without a corresponding decrease in weight, is associated with improved health outcomes. The purpose of this study was to quantify the extent to which PA differed between veterans and nonveterans and to determine how diabetes and age influenced this association. Data from the 2009 Behavioral Risk Factor Surveillance System were used in this study. Respondents were classified as having diabetes if they reported ever being diagnosed with diabetes except during pregnancy. Respondents who reported ever serving on active military duty were classified as veterans. Based on self-report, we calculated the average minutes per week of moderate, vigorous, and total activity. After adjusting for sex, race and ethnicity, household income, education level, body mass index (BMI), and recent health checkup, veteran status was associated with a small but significantly larger amount of average weekly moderate PA (2.2 minutes, $P = 0.0058$) but not average weekly vigorous PA (-0.02 minutes, $P = 0.98$). Diabetes and prediabetes were associated with significantly lower mean levels of both moderate and vigorous intensity PA, as was increasing age. Consistent with prior research, veterans engaged in more PA than nonveterans. The association between diabetes, age, and physical activity did not differ by veteran status.

1. Introduction

Engaging in regular physical activity, with or without a corresponding decrease in weight, is associated with improved health outcomes among people with diabetes [1–4] and older adults [4–6]. Healthy People 2020 objectives include increasing glycemic, lipid, and blood pressure control among people with diabetes [7], all of which may be facilitated by increased physical activity [1]. Healthy People 2020 also includes an objective to increase the proportion of older adults with functional impairments who engage in leisure-time physical activity [7]. Guidelines from the National Institutes of Health [8] and the American College of Sports Medicine [9, 10] recommend that all adults, including those with diabetes, engage in regular moderate to vigorous physical activity. The 2008 Physical Activity Guidelines for Americans recognizes that any level of physical activity is beneficial, though the evidence is strongest for physical activity at or above the level of the recommended 150 minutes per week of moderate or 75 minutes per week of vigorous activity [4, 8]. They also recognize that older adults may have functional impairments that limit their ability to engage in physical activity, but recommend being as active as possible within safe limits [8]. Although physical activity is increasing among adults in the United States, only half of US adults meet these recommendations [11, 12]. Among older adults, the trend in physical activity is less clear [12], and roughly 40% of adults age 65 and older meet the physical activity guidelines [13].

Veterans in the United States are older, on average, than nonveterans [14] and are more likely than their nonveteran peers to meet physical activity guidelines [15]. Adults with diabetes are less likely to participate in regular exercise and less likely to meet recommendations than their peers without diabetes [16, 17]. Disability status, age, and concurrent health conditions are known to influence physical activity levels among adults [17–19], including among adults with diabetes [2, 18], but it is not clear whether veteran status influences these associations or whether veterans with diabetes and nonveterans with diabetes engage in different levels of physical activity. Therefore, the purpose of this study was to quantify the extent to which physical activity (PA) differed between veterans and nonveterans and to determine how diabetes and age influenced this association.

2. Methods

We used data from the Behavioral Risk Factor Surveillance System (BRFSS), a nationally representative cross-sectional telephone survey of noninstitutionalized adults in the United States and its territories coordinated by the Centers for Disease Control and Prevention (CDC), in this study. The BRFSS has demonstrated validity and reliability [20–22]. BRFSS respondents self-report their age. We categorized age into 18–34, 35–44, 45–54, 55–64, 65–74, and 75 and older in order to describe the sample, to calculate mean physical activity by age groups and veteran status, and to assess for effect modification. We used age as a continuous variable in the linear regression models. Respondents were classified as having diabetes if they reported ever being diagnosed with diabetes. Respondents who reported ever being told by their doctor that they have prediabetes or borderline diabetes were classified as having prediabetes. Women with gestational diabetes only and respondents who said they had never been told they have diabetes or pre-diabetes were classified as not having diabetes.

BRFSS respondents were asked about the amount and frequency of their weekly, nonwork moderate and vigorous intensity physical activity (PA). Moderate activities were defined as causing small increases in breathing or heart rate, while vigorous activities were defined as causing large increases in breathing or heart rate. We calculated the mean minutes of moderate, vigorous, and total (moderate plus vigorous) physical activity per week among respondents and also classified respondents as meeting or not meeting physical activity recommendations according to the 2008 Physical Activity Guidelines for Americans [8].

Respondents who reported ever serving on active duty in the military, National Guard, or reserve but who were not currently on active duty at the time of the survey were classified as veterans. Age, gender, educational attainment, race, ethnicity, and annual household income were used as categorical variables. Respondents were classified as having a disability if they reported an activity limitation or reported that they had a health problem requiring the use of special equipment (e.g., cane or wheelchair). We used the question "Would you say that in general your health is excellent, very good, good, fair, or poor?" to assess health-related quality of life and categorized responses into excellent/very good/good and fair/poor.

All measures used in this study were based on respondent self-report. In 2009, the BRFSS included 432,607 respondents; we excluded 70,469 respondents (16.3%) who were missing data on diabetes status, veteran status, age, sex, race/ethnicity, education, disability, time of most recent health checkup, body mass index (BMI), or average amount of moderate or vigorous physical activity per week. We retained respondents with missing income information but created a separate category for these respondents. Among our final study sample of 362,138, there were 43,048 (8.9%) who reported ever being diagnosed with diabetes, 5,678 who reported ever being diagnosed with pre-diabetes (1.2%), and 48,582 respondents (11.0%) who were veterans.

To describe the sample by veteran and diabetes status, we calculated proportions and Wald confidence intervals based on the binomial random variables. We used linear regression to model the mean frequency of moderate, vigorous, and total physical activity in an average week in three separate models. We report the β coefficients from these regression models, which represent the change in minutes of average physical activity per week associated with a one-unit change in the predictor. Because we assessed three physical activity outcomes, we used the Bonferroni correction for multiple comparisons and used an alpha value of 0.0167. We considered sex, race/ethnicity, household income, highest level of education, and body mass index (BMI) to be potential confounders based on previous studies [15–17]. The variables for recent health check-up, health insurance coverage, and having at least one personal health care provider were highly collinear, so we chose the single variable—recent health check-up—that best captured health service utilization since respondents who visited a health care professional may have been advised to engage in regular physical activity. Additionally, we were interested in whether veteran status modified the relationship between diabetes and physical activity or between age and physical activity and used an *a priori* P value of 0.05 to indicate statistical significance of the interaction. Although disability is associated with both diabetes and physical activity [18, 19], we considered disability to be in the causal pathway between diabetes and physical activity and therefore did not adjust for it. With the exception of the physical activity outcomes and age, all variables were categorical.

All analyses were conducted using SAS 9.2 with survey procedures and CDC-assigned weights to account for the complex sampling design of the BRFSS and to represent the US population by age, sex, and race/ethnicity. This study was reviewed as exempt by the VA Puget Sound Health Care System Institutional Review Board.

3. Results

Among veterans, the prevalence of diabetes was 15.4% (95% confidence interval [CI]: 14.9, 16.0), and the prevalence of pre-diabetes was 1.8% (95% CI: 1.5, 2.0; Table 1). Among nonveterans, the prevalence of diabetes and pre-diabetes was 8.0% (95% CI: 7.9, 8.2) and 1.2% (95% CI: 1.1, 1.2), respectively. Veterans were older than nonveterans (mean age 59.1 years [SE = 0.2] compared to 44.7 years [SE = 0.1]), and respondents with diabetes were older than respondents without diabetes (mean age with diabetes: 59.3 years [SE = 0.2], mean age with pre-diabetes: 55.6 [SE = 0.5], and mean age with no diabetes: 44.9 years [SE = 0.1]). More than 90% of veterans were male, while 44% of nonveterans were male. The majority of both Veterans and nonveterans

Table 1: Demographic and health characteristics of veterans and nonveterans in the United States, 2009 Behavioral Risk Factor Surveillance System.

Variable	Categories	Veterans weighted % (95% CI)	Nonveterans weighted % (95% CI)
Diabetes diagnosis	Diabetes	15.4 (14.9, 16.0)	8.0 (7.9, 8.2)
	Pre-diabetes	1.8 (1.5, 2.0)	1.2 (1.1, 1.2)
	No diabetes	82.8 (82.1, 83.4)	90.8 (90.6, 91.0)
Age	18–34	9.5 (8.7, 10.3)	32.5 (32.1, 32.9)
	35–44	12.4 (11.7, 13.1)	20.1 (19.8, 20.4)
	45–54	15.2 (14.6, 15.8)	19.9 (19.7, 20.2)
	55–64	23.2 (22.5, 23.8)	13.7 (13.5, 13.9)
	65–74	19.0 (18.5, 19.6)	7.7 (7.6, 7.9)
	75+	20.7 (20.1, 21.2)	5.9 (5.8, 6.0)
Sex	Male	91.8 (91.3, 92.3)	44.4 (44.0, 44.8)
Race, ethnicity	White, non-Hispanic	78.3 (77.4, 79.2)	61.7 (68.5, 69.3)
	Black, non-Hispanic	9.7 (9.0, 10.3)	9.7 (9.5, 9.9)
	Other race, non-Hispanic	5.2 (4.7, 5.6)	6.7 (6.5, 6.9)
	Any race, Hispanic	6.8 (6.1, 7.5)	14.7 (14.3, 15.0)
Highest level of education	Less than high school	5.0 (4.6, 5.3)	10.2 (10.0, 10.5)
	High school degree or equivalent	28.3 (27.5, 29.1)	27.4 (27.1, 27.7)
	Some college	31.2 (30.3, 32.0)	26.5 (26.2, 26.8)
	College or beyond	35.5 (34.7, 36.3)	35.8 (35.5, 36.2)
Annual household income	< $15,000	4.9 (4.5, 5.2)	9.2 (9.0, 9.5)
	$15,000–$24,999	13.2 (12.6, 13.8)	13.7 (13.5, 14.0)
	$25,000–$49,999	26.9 (26.1, 27.6)	21.7 (21.4, 22.0)
	$50,000–$74,999	17.7 (17.1, 18.4)	14.4 (14.1, 14.7)
	≥ $75,000	28.6 (27.8, 29.4)	30.2 (29.8, 30.5)
	Missing	8.9 (8.2, 9.2)	10.8 (10.5, 11.0)
Disability status	Disability	29.9 (29.1, 30.7)	19.4 (19.2, 19.7)
General health rating	Fair or poor	19.2 (18.5, 19.8)	14.9 (14.6, 15.1)
Body mass index (BMI)	Ideal (<25.0)	25.4 (24.6, 26.2)	37.4 (37.1, 37.8)
	Overweight (25.0–29.9)	44.7 (43.8, 45.5)	35.2 (34.8, 35.5)
	Obese (≥30.0)	29.9 (29.1, 30.7)	27.4 (27.0, 27.7)
Health insurance coverage	Any (including government/VA)	91.7 (91.0, 92.3)	84.7 (84.3, 85.0)
Health care cost	Time in past 12 months when could not see doctor because of cost	8.3 (7.7, 8.9)	15.2 (14.9, 15.5)
Health provider	No personal doctor	13.3 (12.5, 14.0)	18.9 (18.6, 19.3)
Last health check-up	Within past year	77.4 (76.6, 78.2)	67.1 (66.8, 67.5)
	1–5 years ago	16.4 (15.7, 17.1)	23.6 (23.2, 23.9)
	Never	6.2 (5.8, 6.6)	9.3 (9.0, 9.5)

CI: confidence interval.

reported their race and ethnicity as white, non-Hispanic, though veterans were more likely to be so than nonveterans (78.3% of veterans and 61.7% of nonveterans reported white, non-Hispanic race/ethnicity). Veterans and nonveterans had similar levels of education and annual household income. Disability was significantly more common among veterans: 29.9% of veterans were classified as having a disability compared to 19.4% of nonveterans. Veterans tended to have higher BMI than nonveterans and were more frequently classified as overweight (25.4% of Veterans and 37.4% of nonveterans were classified as ideal weight based on their BMI, and 44.7% of veterans compared to 35.2% of nonveterans were overweight). Veterans were more likely than nonveterans to have any form of health insurance (91.7% versus 84.7%) and less likely to report that cost had been a barrier to accessing health care when needed within the past year (8.3% compared to 15.2%). Veterans also were less likely to report that they did not have a personal doctor (13.3%

TABLE 2: Mean minutes of moderate, vigorous, and total physical activity in an average week reported by veterans and nonveterans with and without diabetes in the United States, 2009 Behavioral Risk Factor Surveillance System.

Demographic group	Moderate mean (SE)	Vigorous mean (SE)	Total mean (SE)
Veterans (n = 48,582)	57.2 (0.6)	35.3 (0.5)	92.5 (0.9)
With diabetes (n = 8,515)	48.7 (1.3)	24.4 (1.3)	73.1 (2.0)
With pre-diabetes (n = 947)	48.5 (3.1)	29.7 (2.8)	78.1 (4.9)
Without diabetes (n = 39,120)	59.0 (0.7)	37.4 (0.6)	96.5 (1.1)
Age 18–54 (n = 10,471)	60.4 (1.3)	42.7 (1.1)	103.2 (2.0)
Age 55–64 (n = 12,664)	57.5 (1.0)	36.1 (1.1)	93.6 (1.7)
Age 65–74 (n = 12,507)	58.3 (1.0)	31.5 (0.8)	89.9 (1.5)
Age ≥ 75 (n = 12,940)	50.2 (1.1)	24.5 (0.8)	74.6 (1.5)
Nonveterans (n = 313,556)	53.3 (0.3)	33.2 (0.2)	86.5 (0.4)
With diabetes (n = 34,533)	42.8 (0.7)	19.0 (0.5)	61.8 (1.0)
With pre-diabetes (n = 4,731)	51.3 (3.0)	26.4 (1.7)	77.7 (4.2)
Without diabetes (n = 274,292)	54.3 (0.3)	34.5 (0.3)	88.8 (0.5)
Age 18–54 (n = 158,990)	55.1 (0.4)	37.3 (0.3)	92.4 (0.6)
Age 55–64 (n = 68,919)	50.6 (0.5)	26.4 (0.4)	76.9 (0.7)
Age 65–74 (n = 49,040)	50.8 (0.5)	21.9 (0.4)	72.7 (0.7)
Age ≥ 75 (n = 36,607)	40.8 (0.6)	13.6 (0.4)	54.5 (0.8)

SE: standard error.

versus 18.9%) and were more likely to have had a health check-up within the past year (77.4% compared to 67.1%).

The mean amount of moderate physical activity (PA) among veterans was 57.2 minutes per week (standard error [SE] = 0.6), and the mean amount of vigorous physical activity was 35.3 minutes per week (SE = 0.5) for a total mean of 92.5 minutes of physical activity weekly (SE = 0.9; Table 2). The mean minutes of moderate, vigorous, and total PA were 53.3 (SE = 0.3), 33.2 (SE = 0.2), and 86.5 (SE = 0.4) per week, respectively, among nonveterans. Regardless of veteran status, people with diabetes engaged in less moderate PA and vigorous PA per week than people without diabetes. Among veterans with diabetes, the mean moderate, vigorous, and total PA amounts per week were 48.7 (SE = 1.3) minutes, 24.4 (SE = 1.3) minutes, and 73.1 (SE = 2.0) minutes, respectively, while among veterans without diabetes, the means were 59.0 (SE = 0.7) minutes of moderate PA, 37.4 (SE = 0.6) minutes of vigorous PA, and 96.5 (SE = 1.1) minutes of total PA weekly. Veterans with pre-diabetes averaged 48.5 (SE = 3.1) minutes of moderate PA, 29.7 (SE = 2.8) minutes of vigorous PA, and 78.1 (SE = 4.9) minutes of total PA weekly. Among nonveterans with diabetes, mean moderate PA was 42.8 (SE = 0.7) minutes per week, mean vigorous PA was 19.0 (SE = 0.5) minutes per week, and mean total PA was 61.8 (SE = 1.0) minutes per week compared to 54.3 (SE = 0.3) minutes, 34.5 (SE = 0.3) minutes, and 88.8 (SE = 0.5) minutes, respectively, among nonveterans without diabetes. Nonveterans with pre-diabetes averaged 51.3 (SE = 3.0) minutes of moderate PA, 26.4 (SE = 1.7) minutes of vigorous PA, and 77.7 (SE = 4.2) minutes of total PA weekly. Among both veterans and nonveterans, respondents with diabetes had a larger proportion of their total physical activity from moderate physical activity (66.6% of PA among veterans with diabetes, 62.1% of PA among veterans with prediabetes, 69.3% among nonveterans with diabetes, 66.0% among nonveterans with prediabetes, and 61.1% of PA among veterans and nonveterans without diabetes was moderate intensity). Among both veterans and nonveterans, total physical activity decreased with age, with much of the decrease related to a decrease in vigorous activity. Veterans age 18–54 averaged 60.4 (SE = 1.3) minutes of moderate, 42.7 (SE = 1.1) minutes of vigorous, and 103.2 (SE = 2.0) minutes of total PA weekly. Among veterans age 75 and older, the averages were 50.2 (SE = 1.1) minutes of moderate, 24.5 (SE = 0.8) minutes of vigorous, and 74.6 (SE = 1.5) minutes of total PA per week. Nonveterans age 18–54 averaged 55.1 (SE = 0.4) minutes of moderate, 37.3 (SE = 0.3) minutes of vigorous, and 92.4 (SE = 0.6) minutes of total PA weekly. Among nonveterans age 75 and older, the averages were 40.8 (SE = 0.6) minutes of moderate, 13.6 (SE = 0.4) minutes of vigorous, and 54.5 (SE = 0.8) minutes of total PA per week.

When physical activity was categorized based on the Physical Activity Guidelines for Americans recommendations, nearly half of veterans and nonveterans met PA recommendations (48.7% and 49.3%, resp.). Additionally, 37.1% of veterans and 38.3% of nonveterans engaged in some physical activity in an average week but did not meet recommendations, and 14.1% of veterans and 12.3% of nonveterans engaged in no physical activity.

We adjusted each linear regression model for sex, race and ethnicity, household income, education level, BMI category, and recent health check-up. In the fully adjusted models (Table 3), we found no evidence of effect modification by veteran status (P = 0.07 for diabetes and P = 0.89 for age in categories) so report results adjusted by veteran status rather than stratified.

Table 3: Adjusted* estimated differences in mean minutes of moderate, vigorous, and total physical activity (PA) per week among veterans and nonveterans in the United States, 2009 Behavioral Risk Factor Surveillance System.

Variable	Category	Moderate PA minutes (β) (95% CI)	Vigorous PA minutes (β) (95% CI)	Total[†] PA minutes (β) (95% CI)
Veteran status	Veteran	2.2 (0.6, 3.8)	−0.02 (−1.3, 1.3)	2.2 (−0.1, 4.5)
	Nonveteran	Reference	Reference	Reference
Diagnosed diabetes status	Diabetes	−8.0 (−9.4, −6.5)	−7.2 (−8.3, −6.1)	−15.2 (−17.3, −13.1)
	Pre-diabetes	−1.3 (−6.3, 3.7)	−1.5 (−4.4, 1.3)	−2.8 (−9.8, 4.2)
	Neither diabetes nor pre-diabetes	Reference	Reference	Reference
Age	One-year increase	−0.1 (−0.2, −0.1)	−0.3 (−0.4, −0.3)	−0.5 (−0.5, −0.4)

*Adjusted for sex, race/ethnicity, education, household income, body mass index, and last health check-up.
[†]Total physical activity is the sum of moderate and vigorous physical activity.
β: linear regression coefficient, indicating the minutes per week associated with a one-unit change in the exposure variable.
CI: confidence interval.

In the adjusted moderate PA model, veterans engaged in a small but statistically significantly higher amount of PA on average (2.2 minutes; 95% CI: 0.6, 3.8; $P = 0.0058$). Respondents with diabetes averaged 8.0 (95% CI: -9.4, −6.5; $P < 0.0001$) fewer minutes, and respondents with pre-diabetes averaged 1.3 fewer minutes, (95% CI: −6.3, 3.7; $P =$ 0.62) of moderate PA weekly than respondents without diabetes after adjusting for covariates. For each one year increase in age, respondents averaged 0.1 fewer minutes (95% CI: −0.2, −0.1; $P < 0.001$) of moderate PA weekly, adjusted for covariates.

In the adjusted vigorous PA model, there was no statistically significant difference in average weekly PA by veteran status (−0.02 minutes; 95% CI: −1.3, 1.3; $P = 0.98$). Respondents with diabetes averaged 7.2 (95% CI: −8.3, −6.1; $P < 0.0001$) fewer minutes and respondents with pre-diabetes averaged 1.5 fewer minutes (95% CI: −4.4, 1.3; $P =$ 0.30) of vigorous PA weekly than respondents without diabetes after adjusting for covariates. For each one year increase in age, respondents averaged 0.3 fewer minutes (95% CI: −0.4, −0.3; $P < 0.001$) of vigorous PA weekly, adjusted for covariates.

In both models, women averaged significantly less weekly PA than men (data not shown; available upon request). Respondents who reported Hispanic ethnicity had a small but statistically significantly lower mean amount of moderate PA weekly compared to white, non-Hispanic respondents. For other categories of race and ethnicity, the trend was not statistically significant in either model. People with lower levels of education had significantly higher weekly PA than people with a college degree or higher, on average. The relationship between income and PA differed by the type of PA: for moderate PA, people with lower income tended to have higher mean PA, while for vigorous PA, people with lower income had a higher mean PA. Across both moderate PA and vigorous PA models, overweight and obesity were associated with a significantly lower amount of PA per week, on average.

4. Discussion

We identified a strong and statistically significant association between diabetes and physical activity and between age and physical activity among both veterans and nonveterans. The association between pre-diabetes and physical activity was much weaker. The demographic profile of veterans in this study was similar to a previous analysis of BRFSS data and VA records [23]. Consistent with the limited prior research on the topic [15], veterans engaged in more physical activity than their nonveteran peers. As suggested by Littman et al. [15], this may be a result of their fitness for military service or a result of the tendency to continue physical activity after the high level of activity associated with military training and service. Factors associated with lower physical activity were consistent across veterans and nonveterans.

We classified respondents who had been told by a doctor that they had pre-diabetes or borderline diabetes as a separate category in this study. These individuals likely had impaired fasting glucose or glucose tolerance or high hemoglobin A1c [24] and are therefore at higher risk for developing diabetes and for poor cardiovascular health [24, 25]. In this study, respondents with pre-diabetes had, on average, higher levels of physical activity and lower levels of disability than respondents with full-blown diabetes; including these respondents in the group with diabetes would have attenuated differences between respondents with and without diabetes. Diabetes and pre-diabetes are known to be underdiagnosed: according to an analysis of National Health and Nutrition Examination Survey (NHANES) data by Cowie et al. [26], 19.0% of adults had undiagnosed diabetes, and an additional 3.5% were at high risk for diabetes based on their hemoglobin A1c. In a BRFSS reliability study, Martin and colleagues found that the sensitivity of BRFSS diabetes question had moderate sensitivity and high specificity compared to medical record review [22]. The underdiagnosis of diabetes and pre-diabetes and the moderate sensitivity of the diabetes question used in this study likely led to misclassification in this study which may have resulted in underestimating the association between diabetes or pre-diabetes and physical activity.

Data from the BRFSS are designed to represent the non-institutionalized adult population; therefore, these results are generalizable to the community-dwelling residents of the United States and its territories who age 18 and older. These data are cross-sectional, so the temporal sequence of the associations reported is unclear. It may not be true that veteran status or diabetes causes people to be more or less physically active. Nonetheless, there is a public health benefit to quantifying the amount of PA among people with diabetes, and the relationship between diabetes, pre-diabetes, and physical activity identified in this study may be useful to health care providers advising patients. Likewise, because of the cross-sectional nature of the data, we cannot be sure from this study that aging causes a decline in physical activity since individuals were not followed over time. However, given the body of existing research on the topic, we feel the decline in activity and the capacity for exercise associated with aging has been well established [4, 27, 28].

All data in this study were self-reported and therefore are subject to recall and social desirability biases. Based on data from the 2003-2004 NHANES, in which height and weight were measured directly and accelerometers were used to capture physical activity information, the proportion of US adults who meet physical activity guidelines was below 5% [29], much lower than the 50% estimate in this study and others (e.g., [15, 17]) obtained from self-reported data. This overreporting may result in nondifferential misclassification (if all respondents overreported their physical activity). It is possible that a differential social desirability bias exists since respondents with diabetes may have received physician advice to exercise more often than adults without diabetes. For these reasons, the difference in estimates between groups in this study may be more appropriate than treating the means or proportions themselves as accurate reflections of physical activity among veterans and people with diabetes in the general population.

Although the estimated differences in physical activity minutes per week were small, they are meaningful in terms of health outcomes. For example, Buman et al. [30] found that replacing 30 minutes of sedentary behavior each day with light intensity physical activity was associated with improved physical health among older adults; this benefit increased as the intensity of activity increased. Likewise, Healy et al. [31] found that light intensity physical activity was associated with improved glucose control, as measured by the two-hour postchallenge plasma glucose but not fasting glucose. Additional research is needed to understand whether self-reported moderate physical activity includes light intensity physical activity, particularly among older adults [32], including veterans and individuals with diabetes [33]. Such research may include an assessment of whether additional categories of physical activity should be routinely added to health surveys like the BRFSS.

Acknowledgments

This paper is based upon work in part by the U.S. Department of Veterans Affairs, Office of Research and Development, Health Services Research and Development, and Dr. Reiber's Research Career Scientist Award RCS no. 98-353.

References

[1] American Diabetes Association, "Standards of medical care in diabetes-2011," *Diabetes Care*, vol. 34, supplement 1, pp. S11–S61, 2011.

[2] S. R. Colberg, R. J. Sigal, B. Fernhall et al., "Exercise and type 2 diabetes: the American College Of Sports Medicine and The American Diabetes Association: joint position statement executive summary," *Diabetes Care*, vol. 33, no. 12, pp. 2692–2696, 2010.

[3] S. Mora, I. M. Lee, J. E. Buring, and P. M. Ridker, "Association of physical activity and body mass index with novel and traditional cardiovascular biomarkers in women," *Journal of the American Medical Association*, vol. 295, no. 12, pp. 1412–1419, 2006.

[4] Physical Activity Guidelines Advisory Committee, *Physical Activity Guidelines Advisory Committee Report, 2008*, US Department of Health and Human Services, Washington, DC, USA, 2008.

[5] I. A. Lang, J. M. Guralnik, and D. Melzer, "Physical activity in middle-aged adults reduces risks of functional impairment independent of its effect on weight," *Journal of the American Geriatrics Society*, vol. 55, no. 11, pp. 1836–1841, 2007.

[6] D. R. Berk, H. B. Hubert, and J. F. Fries, "Associations of changes in exercise level with subsequent disability among seniors: a 16-year longitudinal study," *Journals of Gerontology A*, vol. 61, no. 1, pp. 97–102, 2006.

[7] Healthy People, Office of Disease Prevention and Health Promotion, and United States Department of Health and Human Services, DC. Healthy People 2020, http://www.healthypeople.gov/.

[8] United States Department of Health and Human Services, Physical Activity Guidelines for Americans, 2008, http://www.health.gov/paguidelines/.

[9] W. L. Haskell, I. M. Lee, R. R. Pate et al., "Physical activity and public health: updated recommendation for adults from the American College of Sports Medicine and the American Heart Association," *Circulation*, vol. 116, no. 9, pp. 1081–1093, 2007.

[10] M. E. Nelson, W. J. Rejeski, S. N. Blair et al., "Physical activity and public health in older adults: recommendation from the American College of Sports Medicine and the American Heart Association," *Circulation*, vol. 116, no. 9, pp. 1094–1105, 2007.

[11] J. Kruger, H. W. Kohl, and I. J. Miles, "Prevalence of regular physical activity among adults-United States, 2001 and 2005," *Morbidity and Mortality Weekly Report*, vol. 56, no. 46, pp. 1209–1212, 2007.

[12] A. G. Knuth and P. C. Hallal, "Temporal trends in physical activity: a systematic review," *Journal of Physical Activity and Health*, vol. 6, no. 5, pp. 548–559, 2009.

[13] "CDC Web-Enabled Analysis Tool: cross-tabulation of age (18–64, 65+) and physical activity (Meets recommendation for moderate or vigorous physical activity) using 2009 national BRFSS data," 2012, http://apps.nccd.cdc.gov/s_broker/WEAT-SQL.exe/weat/freq_year.hsql.

[14] US Census Bureau, "Sex by age by Veteran status for the civilian population 18 years and over," American Community Survey 1-year estimates, 2010, http://factfinder2.census.gov/faces/tableservices/jsf/pages/productview.xhtml?pid=ACS_10_1YR_B21001&prodType=table.

[15] A. J. Littman, C. W. Forsberg, and T. D. Koepsell, "Physical activity in a national sample of veterans," *Medicine and Science in Sports and Exercise*, vol. 41, no. 5, pp. 1006–1013, 2009.

[16] E. H. Morrato, J. O. Hill, H. R. Wyatt, V. Ghushchyan, and P. W. Sullivan, "Physical activity in U.S. adults with diabetes and at risk for developing diabetes, 2003," *Diabetes Care*, vol. 30, no. 2, pp. 203–209, 2007.

[17] G. Zhao, E. S. Ford, C. Li, and L. S. Balluz, "Physical activity in U.S. older adults with diabetes mellitus: prevalence and correlates of meeting physical activity recommendations," *Journal of the American Geriatrics Society*, vol. 59, no. 1, pp. 132–137, 2011.

[18] S. E. Boslaugh and E. M. Andresen, "Correlates of physical activity for adults with disability," *Preventing Chronic Disease*, vol. 3, no. 3, p. A78, 2006.

[19] J. H. Rimmer, L. A. Wolf, B. S. Armour, and L. B. Sinclair, "Physical activity among adults with a disability-United States, 2005," *Morbidity and Mortality Weekly Report*, vol. 56, no. 39, pp. 1021–1024, 2007.

[20] E. M. Gentry, W. D. Kalsbeek, and G. C. Hogelin, "The behavioral risk factor surveys: II. Design, methods, and estimates from combined state data," *American Journal of Preventive Medicine*, vol. 1, no. 6, pp. 9–14, 1985.

[21] P. L. Remington, M. Y. Smith, D. F. Williamson, R. F. Anda, E. M. Gentry, and G. C. Hogelin, "Design, characteristics, and usefulness of state-based behavioral risk factor surveillance: 1981–87," *Public Health Reports*, vol. 103, no. 4, pp. 366–375, 1988.

[22] L. M. Martin, M. Leff, N. Calonge, C. Garrett, and D. E. Nelson, "Validation of self-reported chronic conditions and health services in a managed care population," *American Journal of Preventive Medicine*, vol. 18, no. 3, pp. 215–218, 2000.

[23] G. E. Reiber, T. D. Koepsell, C. Maynard, L. B. Haas, and E. J. Boyko, "Diabetes in Nonveterans, Veterans, and Veterans Receiving Department of Veterans Affairs Health Care," *Diabetes Care*, vol. 27, supplement 2, pp. B3–B9, 2004.

[24] American Diabetes Association, "Diagnosis and classification of diabetes mellitus," *Diabetes Care*, vol. 33, supplement 1, pp. S62–S69, 2010.

[25] S. Y. Rhee and J. T. Woo, "The prediabetic period: review of clinical aspects," *Diabetes and Metabolism Journal*, vol. 35, no. 2, pp. 107–116, 2011.

[26] C. C. Cowie, K. F. Rust, D. D. Byrd-Holt et al., "Prevalence of diabetes and high risk for diabetes using A1C criteria in the U.S. population in 1988-2006," *Diabetes Care*, vol. 33, no. 3, pp. 562–568, 2010.

[27] American College of Sports Medicine, "American college of sports medicine position stand: exercise and physical activity for older adults," *Medicine and Science in Sports and Exercise*, vol. 41, no. 7, pp. 1510–1530, 2009.

[28] S. A. Hawkins and R. A. Wiswell, "Rate and mechanism of maximal oxygen consumption decline with aging: implications for exercise training," *Sports Medicine*, vol. 33, no. 12, pp. 877–888, 2003.

[29] R. P. Troiano, D. Berrigan, K. W. Dodd, L. C. Mâsse, T. Tilert, and M. Mcdowell, "Physical activity in the United States measured by accelerometer," *Medicine and Science in Sports and Exercise*, vol. 40, no. 1, pp. 181–188, 2008.

[30] M. P. Buman, E. B. Hekler, W. L. Haskell et al., "Objective light-intensity physical activity associations with rated health in older adults," *American Journal of Epidemiology*, vol. 172, no. 10, pp. 1155–1165, 2010.

[31] G. N. Healy, D. W. Dunstan, J. Salmon et al., "Objectively measured light-intensity physical activity is independently associated with 2-h plasma glucose," *Diabetes Care*, vol. 30, no. 6, pp. 1384–1389, 2007.

[32] T. Prohaska, E. Belansky, B. Belza et al., "Physical activity, public health, and aging: critical issues and research priorities," *Journals of Gerontology B*, vol. 61, no. 5, pp. S267–S273, 2006.

[33] D. E. Rosenberg, C. H. Bombardier, J. M. Hoffman, and B. Belza, "Physical activity among persons aging with mobility disabilities: shaping a research agenda," *Journal of Aging Research*, vol. 2011, Article ID 708510, 16 pages, 2011.

12

Understanding Muscle Dysfunction in Chronic Fatigue Syndrome

Gina Rutherford,[1] Philip Manning,[1] and Julia L. Newton[1,2]

[1] *Institute of Cellular Medicine, Newcastle University, Newcastle NE2 4HH, UK*
[2] *Newcastle Hospitals NHS Foundation Trust, UK NIHR Biomedical Research Centre in Ageing and Age Related Disease, Newcastle University, Newcastle NE2 4HH, UK*

Correspondence should be addressed to Gina Rutherford; ginarutherford20@gmail.com

Academic Editor: Arshad Jahangir

Introduction. Chronic fatigue syndrome/myalgic encephalomyelitis (CFS/ME) is a debilitating disorder of unknown aetiology, characterised by severe disabling fatigue in the absence of alternative diagnosis. Historically, there has been a tendency to draw psychological explanations for the origin of fatigue; however, this model is at odds with findings that fatigue and accompanying symptoms may be explained by central and peripheral pathophysiological mechanisms, including effects of the immune, oxidative, mitochondrial, and neuronal pathways. For example, patient descriptions of their fatigue regularly cite difficulty in maintaining muscle activity due to perceived lack of energy. This narrative review examined the literature for evidence of biochemical dysfunction in CFS/ME at the skeletal muscle level. *Methods.* Literature was examined following searches of PUB MED, MEDLINE, and Google Scholar, using key words such as CFS/ME, immune, autoimmune, mitochondria, muscle, and acidosis. *Results.* Studies show evidence for skeletal muscle biochemical abnormality in CFS/ME patients, particularly in relation to bioenergetic dysfunction. *Discussion.* Bioenergetic muscle dysfunction is evident in CFS/ME, with a tendency towards an overutilisation of the lactate dehydrogenase pathway following low-level exercise, in addition to slowed acid clearance after exercise. Potentially, these abnormalities may lead to the perception of severe fatigue in CFS/ME.

1. Introduction

Chronic fatigue syndrome (CFS) also known as Myalgic Encephalomyelitis (ME) is a heterogeneous disorder of unknown aetiology [1]. The condition is characterised by severe disabling fatigue in the absence of alternative diagnosis and is associated with a myriad of other symptoms, including but not limited to postexertional malaise, sleep disturbance, and cognitive dysfunction [1–6]. The prevalence of CFS/ME in the adult population is estimated at around 0.2%–2.6% worldwide [5, 7–9]. For example, the Centre for Disease Control 1994 criteria (CDC4) [10] and the Canadian criteria [11] provide a strict definition and estimate prevalence to be lower (0.2%) than previously reported in a primary care setting whereby a less stringent criteria was applied [5]. In the UK, the condition affects approximately 600,000 individuals, with a peak incidence in the 20–40 age group and a preponderance in females, at a ratio of 6 : 1 [8, 12].

It is important to note that recently there has been intense interest surrounding the naming of the condition. Early in 2015 the Institute of Medicine (IOM) [13] issued a report that proposed a new case definition for CFS/ME, recommending the renaming the illness as Systemic Exertion Intolerance Disease (SEID). This new case definition requires a substantial reduction in ability to complete preillness activities, unrefreshing sleep, postexertional malaise, and either cognitive or orthostatic intolerance. In a recent study conducted by Jason et al. [14], the new SEID criteria were reported to identify a group of patients comparable in size to the Fukuda criteria but a larger group than the Canadian criteria. Additionally, the name was reported to select more patients who had less impairment and fewer symptoms than four-item empiric criteria. Presently, there is considerable debate among scientists as regards which case definition to use for clinical and research purposes. As indicated in the IOM report [13] funding was limited so an inadequate number of studies have focused on the validity and reliability of the case definition [14]. Thus, further research utilising empirical methods is required to fully evaluate the criteria and develop a consensus among researchers, clinicians, and the patient community [14].

One of the primary symptoms of CFS/ME is generalised abnormal muscle fatigue that occurs after relatively mild activity [3, 10, 15]. Fatigue can be defined as a progressive impairment in maximal force generating capacity that develops during muscular activity [16].

Historically, there has been a tendency to draw psychological explanations for the origin of fatigue in CFS/ME; however this model is at odds with patient perceptions of the nature of their condition, with many suggesting a "peripheral" as opposed to "central" origin [15]. For example, patient descriptions of their fatigue regularly cite difficulty in maintaining muscle activity due to perceived lack of energy or through muscle pain, which can be serious enough to lead to the avoidance of exercise [17].

In terms of the pathophysiological basis of peripheral muscle fatigue in CFS/ME, a wide range of potential mechanisms have been suggested. Recent studies [2, 15] using novel magnetic resonance spectroscopy (MRS) techniques have reported distinctive and reproducible muscle bioenergetic abnormality in patients following repeat exercise, contrasting previous work that has reported an absence in increased glycolytic metabolism and lactic acid production in the majority of CFS/ME study participants [18–20]. Additionally, the role of enhanced oxidative stress in CFS/ME has also been reported as a potential mechanism in muscle fatigue, with CFS/ME exhibiting elevated blood oxidative status at rest [21, 22] which is accentuated during exercise [22]. Furthermore, there is evidence to suggest a role of mitochondrial dysfunction in CFS/ME, illustrated by lowered ATP production, impaired oxidative phosphorylation, and mitochondrial damage [23, 24]. Moreover, a key symptom associated with CFS/ME is postexertional malaise (PEM), following physical or emotional stress [25]. Studies have reported exercise in CFS/ME patients to exhibit the potential to amplify preexisting immune dysfunction. Finally, a recent study [26] reported abnormality in AMP-activated protein kinase (AMPK) activation and glucose uptake, when CFS/ME patient skeletal muscle function was assessed via a novel in vitro technique.

Evidence exists to suggest that a wide range of biochemical abnormalities exist at the skeletal muscle level in CFS/ME. This narrative review will explore current evidence regarding the various proposed mechanisms underlying peripheral muscle dysfunction in CFS/ME, which are outlined in Table 1. Ultimately, to gain an improved understanding of muscle dysfunction and the end point of severe disabling fatigue associated with this debilitating condition, improved understanding of the aetiology underlying CFS/ME is pivotal within the field of ageing research, with CFS/ME recognised as an ageing related condition, with symptoms perpetuated amongst older patients.

In terms of methodology, this narrative review examines literature following searches of the electronic databases: PUB MED, MEDLINE, and Google scholar. All papers published up until August 2015 were eligible for inclusion in this review. The search included the following terms: CFS, ME, Immune, autoimmune, mitochondria, muscle, oxidative and nitrosative stress, acidosis, bioenergetics, and AMPK. A total of 435 papers were defined by search, with a total of 67 papers included in this review.

2. Central Sensitisation

Central sensitisation is defined as an alteration in the responsiveness of central neurons to input from unimodal and polymodal receptors [44]. Central sensitisation involves a number of top-down and bottom-up mechanisms, which contribute to the hyperresponsiveness of the central nervous system to a variety of stimuli [28]. It is important to note that an alteration in central pathways may impact upon peripheral muscle fatigue.

In terms of central impairment, the perception of fatigue during exercise is not always abnormal and serves an important function during significant physical exertion [2]. For example, in a study conducted by Amann and Dempsey [45] peripheral muscle fatigue was induced in patients and consequently fatiguing muscle was reported to play a pivotal role in the determination of central motor drive and force output. Therefore, suggesting the presence of a feedback signal from peripheral muscle to the central nervous system, to ensure fatigue, is confined to a certain level, preventing damage to the individual. However, it is plausible that peripheral fatigue experienced in CFS/ME is the direct result of excessive signal feedback, leading to a disproportionate perception of fatigue early in the fatiguing process associated with physical activity [15].

Interestingly, evidence exists to suggest the role of central impairment in CFS/ME patients. For example, Whiteside and colleagues [25] reported CFS/ME patients to exhibit a dysfunction of nociceptive inhibition during exercise. This was demonstrated by a decrease in pain threshold following exercise, which is abnormal as pain threshold normally increases during exercise due to a greater release of endogenous opioids and additional inhibitory mechanisms (descending inhibition). This exercise-induced abnormality was also reported in two additional studies [17, 27]. For example, Meeus and colleagues [27] compared CFS/ME patients with chronic pain ($n = 26$), healthy control participants ($n = 31$), and chronic back pain patients ($n = 21$). Participants all completed a submaximal aerobic exercise protocol, which was followed by venous blood sampling (nitric oxide) and algometry (hand, arm, calf, and lower back). Results demonstrated patients with CFS/ME to exhibit lower pain threshold compared to both the healthy control participants and chronic lower back pain participants. Taken together the results demonstrate CFS/ME patients to have a lack of descending inhibition during exercise. The implication of a lack of endogenous inhibition has been suggested to account in part for the PEM experienced by CFS/ME patients.

Evidence also exists to suggest a role of generalised hyperalgesia in CFS/ME as outlined by Nijs and colleagues [28]. It has been suggested that lower pain thresholds in symptomatic locations represents primary hyperalgesia due

TABLE 1: Summary of various proposed mechanisms underlying muscle dysfunction in CFS/ME.

Proposed mechanism underlying muscle dysfunction in CFS/ME	Study
Central sensitisation	
Decreased pain threshold in patients.	Whiteside et al. (2004) [25], Meeus et al. (2010) [27]
Generalised hyperalgesia.	Nijs et al. (2012) [28], Vecchiet et al. (2003) [29]
Oxidative and nitrosative stress	
Elevated TBARS prior to exercise in patients with history of severe infection.	Jammes et al. (2013) [22]
Elevated TBARS in patients with history of stress factors.	Jammes et al. (2012) [30]
Oxidative damage to endogenous epitopes, autoimmunity, and links with muscle fatigue.	Maes et al. (2006) [31]
Mitochondrial dysfunction	
Mitochondrial function influenced by increased immune-inflammatory stress pathways in patients.	Broderick et al. (2010) [32]
Reduction in Th1 and Th17 function and movement toward Th2 dominant immunity.	Brenu et al. (2011) [33]
Reduction in mitochondrial enzyme level citrate synthase in patient muscle samples.	Skowera et al. (2004) [34]
Reduction in mitochondrial enzymes succinate reductase and cytochrome-C oxidase in skeletal muscle of patients.	McArdle et al. (1996) [35]
No difference in cytochrome-C oxidase levels in muscle biopsies.	Edwards et al. (1993) [36]
Patients reported to exhibit reduced levels of coenzyme Q10, with a significant inverse relationship between plasma coenzyme Q10 and fatigue severity measured via fibro fatigue scale.	Maes et al. (2009) [37]
Postexertional malaise (PEM) and immune function	
Moderate intensity exercise and symptom flare (PEM) in patients, directly linked to IL-β, IL-12, IL-8, IL-10, and IL-13. Increased TNF-α postexercise in patient cohort postexercise.	White et al. (2004) [38]
Moderate intensity exercise also reported to induce a larger 48-hour postexercise area under the curve for IL-10 in patients.	Light et al. (2012) [39]
In comparison of 23 case control studies no evidence of a significant change in circulating pro/anti-inflammatory cytokines was reported. However, exaggerated complement system response, indicated by C4C split product level, enhanced oxidative stress and combined delayed and reduced antioxidant response.	Nijs et al. (2014) [40]
Muscle bioenergetic dysfunction	
Evidence of significant ($P < 0.05$) suppression in proton efflux immediately after exercise and significantly prolonged time to reach maximum proton efflux following low-level exercise (plantar flexion, 35% MVC).	Jones et al. (2010) [15]
Prolonged postexercise recovery from exercise in patients, indicated by marked increase in intramuscular acidosis compared to controls at a similar work rate. After each 3-minute bout of exercise (plantar flexion, 35% MVC), a 4-fold increase in the time taken to recover to baseline.	Jones et al. (2012) [2, 41]
No difference in intramuscular pH at rest, exhaustion, and early or late recovery following graded exercise to exhaustion. However, evidence of accelerated glycolysis at onset of exercise was illustrated by more rapid PCr depletion.	Wong et al. (1992) [42]
No consistent abnormalities in pH regulation following exercise when patient cohort is taken as a whole. However, 6 patients exhibited increased intramuscular acidification in relation to PCr depletion.	Barnes et al. (1993) [18]
In subanaerobic threshold exercise protocol only small subgroup of patients reported to have increased blood lactate responses to exercise.	Lane et al. (1998) [20, 43]
Abnormal AMPK activation and glucose uptake	
No increase in AMPK phosphorylation or glucose uptake 16 hours following electrical pulse stimulation in CFS/ME patients. Compared to significant increases in both parameters in control participants.	Brown et al. (2015) [26]

to sensitised nociceptors within injured peripheral muscle tissue. However, the authors also commented that when pain thresholds are detected in asymptomatic areas, then central sensitisation is at play. Two studies conducted by Vecchiet and colleagues [29] investigated the effect of electrical stimulation of muscle tissue, skin, and subcutis in relation to pain threshold in CFS/ME patients and healthy control participants. Interestingly, in both studies CFS/ME participants reported there to be no significant difference between groups for electrical pain threshold of skin and subcutis. Nevertheless, a much lower electrical pain threshold was observed in all sites of muscle tissue (trapezius, quadriceps, and deltoid) for the CFS/ME group only, illustrative of hyperalgesia in CFS/ME.

3. Oxidative and Nitrosative Stress

Enhanced oxidative and nitrosative stress has been reported in CFS/ME patients. For example, studies have demonstrated patients to exhibit excessive production of reactive oxygen species (ROS) following physical exertion, as well as altered resting blood oxidant to antioxidant status [21, 22].

Biochemical markers associated with oxidative stress have also been reported to play a pivotal role in skeletal muscle fatigue [46], which is often cited as a debilitating symptom experienced by CFS/ME patients [22]. Effectively, oxidative and nitrosative stress involve the enhanced production of ROS and reactive nitrogen species (RNS), in addition to other free radicals; these reactive species have the potential to disrupt cell membrane function through lipid peroxidation, as well as damage to functional proteins and DNA. This can ultimately lead to alterations in cell structure and disease initiating mutations [47].

Elevated ROS/RNS exhibit the capacity to profoundly impair mitochondrial function, which has been suggested to be due to the accumulation of oxidative modified mitochondrial proteins, lipids, and DNA [48]. Moreover, these factors exhibit the potential to induce electron transport chain dysfunction, impairment in cellular bioenergetics, and ultimately skeletal muscle fatigue. Furthermore, skeletal muscle is a postmitotic tissue so it is extremely susceptible to mitochondrial oxidative damage; this is due to being terminally differentiated and because of a slow cellular turnover and high metabolic rate [48].

Mitochondria are a major source of ROS and RNS generation in cells and are therefore highly susceptible to oxidative damage. For example, they exhibit reduced levels of antioxidants such as glutathione in comparison to levels found in the cytosol [49]. This relative lack of protection enables mitochondrial DNA (mtDNA) to be damaged, leading to major changes in polypeptide synthesis. Finally, mtDNA repair enzyme activity is considerably lower than found in the nucleus [50]. The combined effects lead to a reduced electron transfer rate with subsequent reduction in the rate of ATP synthesis [51].

In relation to the impact of elevated oxidative stress on muscle dysfunction, muscle specific symptoms of fatigue have been reported to be proportional to the blood levels of a marker of ROS induced lipid peroxidation, thiobarbituric acid reactive substances (TBARS) [21]. TBARS occurs in the serum due to the peroxidation of low-density lipoproteins and oxygen mediated injury of myocyte membranes [29, 52]. Lipid peroxidation of skeletal muscle fibres induces a loss of membrane excitability because of altered activation of K^+ channels [27, 53]. Additionally, muscle biopsies from healthy adults indicated that the intensity of membrane excitation was proportional to K^+ efflux measured in plasma [54], with an increase in ROS generation acting to inhibit Na^+-K^+ pump activity, thus reducing the K^+ outflow and muscle membrane excitability [55, 56]. Furthermore, in another study [57] CFS/ME patients were reported to exhibit a reported a loss of Na^+/K^+ and Ca^{2+}-ATPase pump regulation, as well as alterations in the ryanodine channels within the sarcoplasmic reticulum membrane. This was related to increased fluidity of the sarcoplasmic membrane due to ROS induced formation of lipid hydroperoxides, which the authors suggested to support the hypothesis that sarcolemma conduction system with some aspects of Ca^{2+} transport was negatively influenced in CFS/ME.

Furthermore, in an additional study [22] blood oxidant status and muscle membrane excitability were measured before and after exercise. The case control study compared CFS/ME patients ($n = 55$) and healthy matched controls ($n = 40$). However, within the CFS/ME cohort two subgroups emerged, firstly, those who had reported severe infection (e.g., pneumonia, sepsis, encephalomyelitis, and H1N1 influenza) within 3–7 months preceding onset of CFS/ME symptoms (infected CFS/ME group (I-CFS/ME)); secondly, those who had practiced sport to a high level (>6 hrs per week) for 6 years prior to the onset of CFS/ME symptoms and with no history of severe infection (i.e., noninfected CFS/ME [NI-CFS/ME]). Participants were required to complete a maximal incremental cycle based protocol to reach the point of maximal oxygen uptake. In relation to markers of oxidative stress, blood samples were obtained before, during, and after exercise time points, enabling plasma concentration of TBARS and endogenous antioxidant (reduced ascorbic acid) to be measured. Additionally, action potentials (M-wave) were evoked in the vastus lateralis to explore muscle excitability.

Results demonstrated all CFS/ME patients to exhibit abnormal biochemical and electrophysiological measures indicated by elevated TBARS levels prior to exercise and altered M-wave configuration during and after exercise. These findings are in agreement with other studies [19, 22, 58] which have also reported an elevated blood oxidant status at rest, which was accentuated by exercise, in addition to reduced muscle excitability. For example, one study described enhanced exercise-induced oxidative stress in CFS/ME patients, which was indicated by early changes in TBARS and reduced ascorbic acid in response to incremental exercise. Furthermore, CFS/ME patients also exhibited marked alterations in muscle membrane excitability, indicated by lengthened M-wave duration during the recovery period [58].

However, a pivotal finding of the more recent study [22] was that I-CFS/ME patients exhibited significant accentuation of blood oxidant status at rest, in addition to muscle hypoexcitability at work, as well as significantly reduced K^+ outflow in response to maximal exercise. Therefore, CFS/ME patients with a history of previous severe infection exhibited greater biological and EMG disorders compared to those who reported completing a high level of physical activity before the onset of fatigue related symptoms. The authors concluded severe infection to act as a stressor responsible for the alteration in blood oxidant status, which may help to explain impaired exercise-induced K^+ outflow and altered membrane excitability. However, it is important to acknowledge that the NI-CFS patients self-reported their physical activity level for the 6 yrs prior to the onset of CFS/ME symptoms. Therefore, it is possible that CFS/ME patients overestimated their physical activity habits prior to developing CFS/ME symptoms.

Jammes et al. [30] also measured TBARS at rest and following exercise in a CFS/ME patient cohort. Effectively, CFS/ME patients were separated into 4 distinct groups. These were as follows: group I (no relevant previous history), group II (previous high-level sport), group III (previous severe acute infection), and group IV (high-level sport and severe acute infection). Patients were required to complete a maximal cycle protocol before blood samples were collected and plasma was analysed for TBARS and heat shock proteins HSP27 and HSP70. Interestingly, in agreement with other studies [22] the authors reported elevated TBARS at rest in CFS/ME patients compared to controls; however this was only demonstrated in CFS/ME groups II, III, and IV. In contrast to the previously described studies, the authors also measured HSP levels at rest and reported significantly lower levels in all CFS/ME patient groups compared to controls. Following exercise, the peak level of TBARS was increased in CFS/ME groups II, III, and IV. HSP27 and HSP70 were suppressed with the greatest effect in groups III and IV. Therefore, the authors concluded a history of previous stress factors in a CFS/ME patient cohort to be associated with severe and the suppression of protective HSP response to exercise. Similarly, Thambirajah et al. [59] investigated HSP expression at rest and following exercise in a CFS/ME patient cohort. The authors reported basal HSP27 to be elevated in CFS/ME patients compared to controls. Additionally, HSP27 levels decreased immediately after exercise and remained below basal level at day 1 after exercise. In contrast, HSP27 levels were constant at basal and following exercise in the control group. There was also an observed decline in HSP60 and HSP90 in the CFS/ME patient group at 7 days after exercise. The findings were postulated to be evidence of an abnormal or defective adaptive response to oxidative stress in CFS/ME.

Moving on, excessive oxidative and nitrosative stress has also been suggested to be associated with secondary autoimmune responses. Prolonged oxidative and nitrosative stress may cause damage to protein and lipid structures to such an extent that they lose immunogenic tolerance and autoantibodies begin to be formed against them [60]. For example, secondary IgM and IgG mediated autoimmune reactions have been reported to occur in patients with CFS/ME. For example, Maes et al. [31] examined whether CFS/ME was accompanied by a response to neoepitopes and a variety of modified lipids and proteins indicative of damage caused by excessive oxidative and nitrosative stress. Specifically, the authors examined serum antibodies to fatty acids (oleic, palmitic, and myristic acid), by-products of lipid peroxidation (azelaic acid, malondialdehyde, acetylcholine, and S-farnesyl-L-cysteine), and N-oxide modified amino acid in 14 CFS/ME patients and 11 controls. Results indicated mean IgM serum levels directed against oleic, palmitic, and myristic acid, azelaic acid, S-farnesyl-L-cysteine, and the N-oxide derivatives to be significantly greater in CFS/ME patients when compared to controls. In addition, significant and positive correlations were exhibited in the CFS/ME group for serum IgM levels directed against fatty acid malondialdehyde and azelaic acid, N-oxide derivatives, and the severity of illness as measured by the fibro fatigue scale. Furthermore, positive correlations were also reported for the aforementioned products and measures of muscle tension and fatigue. Therefore, it would appear that autoimmune responses as a consequence of oxidative damage to endogenous lipid epitopes could play a pivotal role in CFS/ME associated muscle fatigue.

4. Mitochondrial Dysfunction

There is evidence to suggest that mitochondrial dysfunction plays a key role in CFS/ME aetiology. Lowered ATP production, impaired oxidative phosphorylation, and mitochondrial damage have been reported in patients with CFS/ME [23, 24]. Moreover, CFS/ME patients share common skeletal muscle symptoms associated with diseases linked to mitochondrial dysfunction, for example, muscle pain, fatigue, and cramping [61, 62].

There is accumulating evidence to suggest that abnormally high lactate levels and intracellular acidosis exhibited in patients with CFS/ME are the result of impaired mitochondrial function [61, 63]. For example, CFS/ME patients exhibit profound and sustained intracellular acidosis of the peripheral musculature following relatively low-level exercise. This results in a decreased anaerobic threshold (AT) due to an overutilisation of the lactate dehydrogenase pathway [15, 41]. Upon the point of exhaustion CFS/ME patients have been reported to exhibit intracellular ATP concentrations that are lower than those found in nondiseased control participants, which could be indicative of dysfunction in oxidative metabolism. Moreover, in a recent review [61] the authors concluded the response to exercise exhibited by CFS/ME patients to be typical of that reported in individuals with mitochondrial disease. Additionally, there were also a number of similarities between symptoms of mitochondrial disease and the physiosomatic symptoms of CFS/ME. For example, muscle pain, cramps, weakness, and myalgia's [54, 62, 64].

Mitochondrial dysfunction in CFS/ME may be explained by not only elevated oxidative and nitrosative stress but also increased immune-inflammatory stress pathways [65]. Interestingly, chronic low-grade inflammation in CFS/ME has been demonstrated through increased levels of proinflammatory cytokines (IL-1, TNF-α) and a movement towards a Th2 dependant immune response, in addition to inflammatory mediators including NF-κB and elastase [64]. Further evidence of elevated oxidative and nitrosative stress has also been demonstrated by increased isoprostane levels, peroxides, and protein carbonyl levels, indicating damage to lipids, protein, and mT as previously discussed [22].

In relation to immune dysfunction, one study examined cytokine networks in 40 female CFS/ME patients and 40 case matched controls [32]. The authors examined a total of 16 cytokines and results revealed a diminution of Th1 and Th17 function and a movement towards Th2 type immunity. Similarly, several other groups have reported a shift for a

Th1 to Th2 cytokine profile in CFS/ME patients [33, 34, 66]. For example, Skowera and colleagues [34] examined the frequency of type 1 and type 2 regulator CD4 and CD8 T cells in 35 patients with CFS. Results illustrated a bias towards a Th2 immune response.

Elevated levels of the inflammatory mediator NF-κB [67, 68] have also been reported in CFS/ME. NF-κB is a major upstream intracellular mechanism, which regulates inflammatory and oxidative stress mediators [68]. For example, it functions to trigger inducible nitric oxide synthetase (iNOS) expression, which promotes the production of nitric oxide (NO) by monocytes and macrophages [68].

Juel and colleagues [55, 56] examined the production of NF-κB P50 in unstimulated 10 ng/mL TNF-α and 50 ng/mL PMA (phorbol 12-myristate 13-acetate, PMA) stimulated peripheral blood lymphocytes in 18 CFS/ME patients and 18 age-matched controls. Results demonstrated both unstimulated (10 ng/mL) TNF-α ($P = 0.0009$) and PMA (0.008) stimulated production of NF-κB to be significantly higher in CFS/ME patients compared to controls. Additionally, positive correlations were reported between the production of NF-κB and severity of illness in CFS/ME patients (as measured by fibro fatigue scale) and with symptoms, including muscular fatigue and tension. The function of p53 is pivotal in the regulation of glycolysis and mitochondrial respiration as it reduces the activity of the glycolytic pathway and stimulates mitochondrial O_2 consumption and aerobic respiration. However, when inhibited there is a shift to anaerobic glycolysis and reduced O_2 consumption [65].

Aside from immune dysfunction, several studies have reported mitochondrial dysfunction to be caused by abnormal levels of key mitochondrial enzymes. For example, in a paper by Smits and colleagues [69] a significant reduction in citrate synthase in biopsies (quadriceps region) from patients with CFS/ME was reported when compared to healthy control samples. Citrate synthase is an enzyme located in the mitochondrial matrix, which plays a critical role in the tricarboxylic cycle [70]. Similarly, the McArdle group [35] reported a decrease in citrate synthase as well as succinate reductase and cytochrome- C oxidase (Complex IV), which are two of the four mitochondrial transmembrane enzyme complexes of the electron transport chain. Nevertheless, in contrast to the McArdle group [35], Smits and colleagues [69] attributed the decrease in transmembrane enzymes to be the result of reduced physical activity levels, frequently present in CFS/ME patients as opposed to underlying mitochondrial dysfunction. Nonetheless, a paper by Edwards and colleagues [36] reported there to be no significant difference in partial cytochrome-C oxidase in skeletal muscle biopsies between CFS/ME patients and healthy matched controls.

Evidence also exists to suggest that CFS/ME patients exhibit significantly reduced levels of coenzyme Q10, an important mitochondrial nutrient that functions as a cofactor for the production of ATP in the mitochondria and displays significant antioxidant activity [71]. In a study conducted by Maes and colleagues [37], CFS/ME patients ($n = 58$) displayed significantly lowered plasma coenzyme Q10 concentration compared to healthy controls ($n = 22$). Moreover, in CFS/ME patients there was a significant inverse relationship exhibited between plasma coenzyme Q10 concentration and fatigue severity measured by means of the fibro fatigue scale.

Furthermore, CFS/ME patients may also exhibit alterations in L-carnitine and acylcarnitine homeostasis [72]. L-carnitine is a ubiquitously occurring trimethylated amino acid that plays an important role in the transport of long chain fatty acids across the inner mitochondrial membrane, which is essential for energy production via fatty acid metabolism [72]. Previous studies have reported a reduction in endogenous plasma L-carnitine and total carnitine levels in patients with CFS/ME [73, 74]. Nevertheless, other studies have not always replicated these findings [75, 76]. Reuter and Evans [72] postulated this to be related to the use of varying methodological approaches, with some studies solely focused on free carnitine and total carnitine rather than the level of each individual acylcarnitine, which may be "cancelled out" by normal levels of other acylcarnitines in CFS/ME patients. To overcome this weakness Reuter and Evans [72] utilised tandem mass spectrometry to quantify individual acylcarnitine levels in plasma samples to provide a more detailed carnitine profile. Results demonstrated significant alterations in C8:1, C12DC, C14, C16:1, C18, C18:1, C18:2, and C18:1-Oh acylcarnitines. What is more, significant correlations between acylcarnitine and clinical symptomology were observed.

5. Postexertional Malaise and Immune Function

CFS/ME patients report a changeable pattern to their symptoms and physical and cognitive capabilities, often with severe symptom exacerbation following physical exercise [10, 25]. This is termed PEM, with approximately 95% of CFS/ME patients experiencing PEM [77]. As regards the cause of PEM, it has been suggested that exercise may exhibit the ability to amplify preexisting immune abnormalities, in addition to oxidative and nitrosative stress [78]. Immunological abnormalities have been reported following exercise in CFS/ME. For example, observations in CFS/ME symptom flare after moderate intensity exercise have been reported to be directly linked to the levels of interleukin-1β (IL-1β), IL-12, IL-8, IL-10, and IL-13, 8 hours after exercise [38]. Additionally, sustained increase in plasma TNF-α in CFS/ME patients and not in healthy controls has been observed after exercise [38]. Moderate intensity exercise has also been reported to induce a larger 48-hour postexercise area under the curve for IL-10 [39].

However, a recent systematic review [40] compared 23 case control studies regarding exercise-induced immunological changes in CFS/ME patients versus healthy control participants. The authors reported in comparison to healthy participants that CFS/ME patients exhibited a more exaggerated response in the complement system, indicated by C4a split product level and enhanced oxidative stress, combined with a delayed and reduced antioxidant response. Finally, the authors also reported there to be an apparent alteration in immune cell gene expression profile, which was evidenced by an increase in postexercise IL-10 and toll-like receptor 4 gene expression. Nonetheless, in contrast to previous work there was no reported change in circulating pro- and/or anti-inflammatory cytokines. Effectively, the review confirmed CFS/ME patients to respond differently to an exercise-based stimulus, resulting in a more pronounced immune response.

6. Muscle Bioenergetic Dysfunction

Even a minimal decrease in muscle pH interferes with cross bridge binding and ATPase activity due to competitive binding and reduced enzyme function [71]. Decreased intracellular pH impairs oxidative enzyme activity and may adversely affect ryanodine receptor function [79]. Recent studies have also confirmed the presence of a peripheral bioenergetic abnormality in CFS/ME patients [15, 41, 63].

In a cross-sectional study conducted by Jones et al. [15] novel MRS techniques were utilised to investigate muscle acid handling following exercise in CFS/ME patients and the relationship with autonomic dysfunction. CFS/ME patients ($n = 16$) and age- and sex-matched normal controls ($n = 8$) performed an exercise protocol, which consisted of 3 minutes of plantar flexion at 35% load maximum voluntary contraction (MVC) at a rate of 0.5 Hz, followed by 3-minute recovery. After the period of exercise, phosphorus magnetic resonance spectroscopy (PMRS) was utilised to investigate intramuscular acid handling. Results demonstrated a significant suppression of proton efflux immediately after exercise ($P < 0.05$) in CFS/ME patients and significantly ($P < 0.05$) prolonged time taken to reach maximum proton efflux. In controls, a strong inverse correlation between maximum proton efflux and nadir pH following exercise ($r^2 = 0.6$, $P < 0.01$) was reported. However, in CFS/ME the significance of this relationship was lost ($r^2 = 0.003$; $P =$ ns). Collectively, these findings demonstrated CFS/ME patients to exhibit abnormalities in the recovery of intramuscular pH following standardised exercise. Effectively, proton efflux is crucial for acidosis resolution, with the immediate postexercise period associated with maximum proton efflux in healthy individuals; however this initial fast phase does not appear to occur in all CFS/ME patients [15]. Furthermore, the authors also acknowledged there to be a close relationship between the degree of intramuscular acidosis and proton efflux, demonstrating a closely regulated process, which has been observed in healthy individuals [80] in addition to the study control group. Nevertheless, they concluded this relationship to be lost in CFS/ME patients. However, the relatively small sample size of this study made it difficult to draw firm conclusions. Therefore, further adequately powered studies are required to investigate the relationship further.

In contrast, Wong et al. [42] reported no difference in intramuscular pH at rest and exhaustion and during early and late recovery, following a graded exercise test to exhaustion. Measurement of intramuscular pH of the gastrocnemius muscle was performed via 31P nuclear magnetic resonance (NMR) spectroscopy. However, the authors did report changes in PCr and pH to occur more rapidly at the onset of exercise in CFS/ME patients compared to controls, which was suggested to be indicative of accelerated glycolysis. Nevertheless, the authors postulated this finding to reflect a lower level of physical endurance due to inactivity in the CFS/ME patient cohort. Nonetheless, it is important to interpret this study with caution, as the CFS/ME patients were able to complete a maximal exercise test to exhaustion. Therefore, it suggests that the patients in this study were not severely incapacitated by the condition and therefore may not be representative of the wider CFS/ME population.

Alternatively, Jones et al. [41] reported prolonged postexercise recovery from acidosis. In this investigation CFS/ME patients and age/sex-matched healthy controls performed a similar exercise protocol (35% MVC plantar flexion for 180 s and 390 s recovery, repeated 3 times). In addition, participants were also required to perform a MVC assessment and a cycle based cardiorespiratory fitness test. Results revealed the ability to divide patients into two distinct groups; 8 (45%) demonstrated normal phosphocreatine (PCr) depletion in response to exercise at 35% MVC, with MVC strength values comparable to controls. In the second grouping, 10 CFS/ME patients exhibited low PCr depletion (generating abnormally low MVC values). Results demonstrated anaerobic threshold (AT), VO_2, and VO_2 peak to be significantly reduced in all CFS/ME patients compared to controls. Essentially, one implication of a reduced AT would be a reliance upon anaerobic as opposed to aerobic metabolism, with the predicted consequence of greater short-term acid generation within the muscle as a result of an overutilisation of the lactate dehydrogenase pathway [15]. This was further confirmed by MRS demonstrating CFS/ME patients to exhibit markedly increased intramuscular acidosis compared to controls at a similar work rate following each 3-minute bout, with prolongation (almost 4-fold) in the time taken for pH to recover to baseline, replicating previous findings [15].

Based on the findings the authors suggested that the profound intramuscular acidosis exhibited with repeat exercise to be at least in part related to poor aerobic capacity. This in relation to the physiology of fatigue closely mirrors that observed in patients with the autoimmune disease primary biliary cirrhosis (PBC). PBC exhibits a comparable peripheral pattern and a similar level to fatigue to CFS/ME [81]. In a study by Hollingsworth and colleagues [81] PBC patients exhibited profound and comparable intramuscular acidosis to the CFS/ME patients in the Luin et al. study [53] following the same repeat exercise protocol. However, one pivotal difference between the conditions, which may contribute to the severity of fatigue in CFS/ME, relates to acid homeostasis. In contrast to CFS/ME patients, when PBC patients undergo repeat exercise the extent of acidosis within the muscle decreases with each repeated exercise bout. This may suggest a compensatory mechanism, which operates to resolve excess acidosis. One potential mechanism that may account for this is increased proton flux and the speed of onset of maximum proton excretion with repeat exercise [41, 81]. This mechanism also plays a role in mitochondrial disease whereby increased proton efflux postexercise helps to compensate for decreased aerobic capacity [82]. Nevertheless, it would appear that in comparison to other conditions that exhibit reduced aerobic capacity and acidosis, CFS/ME patients are unable to compensate for an increased reliance upon anaerobic energy pathways during exercise [41].

While the production of protons as a by-product of anaerobic metabolism is a feature of normal metabolism, the body requires mechanisms to effectively manage protons as even small changes in pH dramatically alter enzyme kinetics, decrease muscle function, and cause fatigue [83]. Thus, slow recovery from acidosis in CFS/ME may relate to the ineffective exporting of protons from the recovering muscle. Protons are actively transported out of the muscle by 3 main groups of proton transporters [55, 56]: Na^+/H^+ antiporters, namely, NHE1 [84], sodium/bicarbonate cotransporters (NBCs) [85], and most predominantly monocarboxylate transporters (MCT), whereby in the latter group MCT-1 and MCT-4 isoforms seem to be of particular importance in human skeletal muscle [86]. During rest, intramuscular pH is primarily influenced by NHEs, with MCTs and NBCs playing a greater role during the recovery from muscular contraction. These transporter systems are under autonomic regulation [87]. It is possible that the impaired function of acid transporters occurs in CFS/ME, which may be a consequence of autonomic dysfunction [88–90]. Additionally, it is also possible that reduced vascular runs off (related to autonomic dysfunction), resulting in decreased vascular flow into and out of the muscle following exercise which may have an effect on O_2 delivery, potentially limiting the function of the three-enzyme complex pyruvate dehydrogenase complex (PDC) [91].

A subgroup of patients (low PCr depletion) exhibited no excess acidosis, which appeared to be entirely the consequence of lower MVC values compared to normal PCr depletion controls. Interestingly, despite markedly lower MVC values the patients perceived themselves to be working maximally immediately following the MVC assessment. However, despite this perception the authors postulated that these findings related to a type of exercise avoidance behaviour. Kinesiophobia is defined as an excessive, irrational, and debilitating fear of movement and activity resulting from a fear of vulnerability to painful injury or reinjury [64, 71] and has been reported to play a role in a variety of musculoskeletal disorders including CFS/ME patients who experience widespread pain [92, 93]. Therefore, the fear of the consequence of an action such as exercise may lead to avoidance behaviour in patients with CFS/ME patients [41]. However, the study was limited, as it did not include a repeat assessment.

Interestingly, previous studies have also reported the existence of subgroups within CFS/ME patient cohorts in relation to glycolytic metabolism and intramuscular pH regulation [18, 20, 42, 43]. However, unlike the studies conducted by Jones et al. [15, 41], the earlier studies have reported an absence in abnormal glycolytic metabolism in the majority of the CFS/ME patients. Barnes et al. [18] explored intramuscular pH regulation in 46 CFS/ME patients via 31P MRS. Results demonstrated no consistent abnormalities in glycolysis or pH regulation at rest or following exercise when the group was taken as a whole. Nonetheless, 12 patients did exhibit abnormal PCr depletion following exercise, with 6 patients within this group displaying increased intramuscular acidification in relation to PCr depletion and the other 6 demonstrating reduced acidification. This study illustrates the heterogeneity within the CFS/ME patient population and suggests that subgroups do exist in CFS/ME that display abnormal glycolytic metabolism and intramuscular pH. Similarly, in Lane et al.'s studies [20, 43] CFS/ME patients completed a subanerobic threshold exercise protocol. Results revealed only a small subgroup (8%) of CFS/ME patients to have an increased blood lactate response to exercise and muscle biopsies revealed a relative increase in type 2 glycolytic fibres for this subgroup.

7. Acidosis because of Impaired PDC Function

It is possible that the previously demonstrated muscle cell acidosis in CFS/ME is the consequence of downregulated PDC function and a concomitant increase in the metabolism of pyruvate to lactic acid (overutilisation of lactate dehydrogenase (LDH) pathway). PDC is a 3-protein complex responsible for a series of reactions that convert pyruvate to acetyl coA during aerobic respiration. Principally, when the function of this complex is reduced, pyruvate that has been generated by glycolysis accumulates within the cells and is metabolised anaerobically to lactic acid. This accumulation causes a drop in pH and concurrent deterioration in muscle function [94].

The phenotype of fatigue exhibited by CFS/ME patients closely mirrors that seen in fatigue associated primary biliary cirrhosis patients (PBC). For example, Hollingsworth et al. [81] reported PBC patients to exhibit significant acidosis due to an overutilisation of the lactate dehydrogenase pathway, following a low-level repeat exercise protocol [81]. Furthermore, the authors postulated that the increased dependence on anaerobic pathways of energy production resulted in the fatigue associated with PDC. The idea that impaired PDC function leads to an overutilisation of the lactate dehydrogenase pathway is in agreement with other studies. For example, Murrough et al. [95] reported significantly higher levels of lactate in ventricular cerebrospinal fluid in CFS/ME patients when compared to healthy controls. Similarly, Constantin-Teodosiu and colleagues [96] in an experimental exercise model using rats demonstrated that when PDC function was decreased via the use of PPAR modulating drugs which upregulated PDK function, lactate accumulated intramuscularly which led to decreased muscle function.

Therefore, impaired energy generation in muscle, an increase in the lactate/pyruvate ratio in CFS/ME patients, and a propensity towards excess intramuscular acidosis following limited exercise suggest PDC dysfunction in the muscle of CFS/ME patients, which has implications in relation to the expression of fatigue. Furthermore, as previously discussed CFS/ME patients display significant intramuscular abnormalities relating to both acid generation and clearance from tissue, which has been postulated to relate to a centrally perceived "stop signal," leading to a disproportionate perception of fatigue [71].

8. Abnormal AMPK Activation and Glucose Uptake

A recent study [26] reported striking biochemical differences in skeletal muscle cultures established from 10 CFS/ME patients and 7 age-matched controls. Samples were subjected to electrical pulse stimulation (EPS), for 24 hours, and examined for exercise-associated changes. Key differences emerged, in the basal state; there was increased myogenin expression in CFS/ME samples but a decrease in IL-6 secretion during differentiation when compared to control samples. Following 16 hours of EPS there was a significant increase ($P < 0.006$) in AMP-activated protein kinase (AMPK) phosphorylation and glucose uptake ($P < 0.0001$) in control samples when compared to unstimulated control cultures. Alternatively, CFS/ME samples demonstrated no increase in AMPK phosphorylation or glucose uptake. Nevertheless, glucose uptake remained responsive to insulin, suggesting exercise related dysfunction. Furthermore, IL-6 secretion in response to EPS was significantly reduced ($P < 0.05$ versus corresponding control) across all time points measured.

As regards the function of AMPK, it is a phylogenetically conserved fuel-sensing enzyme, consisting of a heterotrimeric complex composed of a catalytic α subunit and regulatory β and γ subunits [97]. During exercise under normal physiological conditions, AMPK is activated in the skeletal muscle of healthy humans, with exercise suggested to be the most powerful physiological activator of AMPK [98, 99]. Upon activation AMPK sets into motion processes that increase ATP production, such as glucose transport and fatty acid oxidation [97], while decreasing others that consume ATP, for example, lipid and protein synthesis and cell growth and proliferation [97, 99, 100]. Evidence also suggests AMPK to have a broader range of actions including mitochondrial biogenesis [99, 101] and skeletal muscle angiogenesis [102], suggesting AMPK activation to play a key role in peripheral muscle function during exercise.

However, it is important to consider the role of physical activity on AMPK activation. For example, trained subjects have been reported to express higher levels of $\alpha 1$ AMPK in comparison to untrained individuals [103]. Furthermore, a 3-week endurance training intervention with young male participants resulted in increases in $\alpha 1$ and $\alpha 2$ AMPK protein expression in addition to ACC-β phosphorylation, which suggested basal activity of AMPK to be increased [104].

Therefore, it should be considered that the decreased AMPK activation reported in CFS/ME muscle samples after EPS might be the result of lowered physical activity levels of the CFS/ME sample donors, when compared to control donors. As regards study recruitment criteria, although participants were age-matched, it was not specified whether any measures had been taken to ensure donors were matched in terms of physical activity habits. Future work is required with patients and controls that are matched in terms of physical activity.

In addition to impaired activation of AMPK, the study also reported reduced IL-6 secretion in response to EPS. Interestingly, previous studies have reported IL-6 to activate AMPK in skeletal muscle by increasing the concentration of cAMP and secondly by increasing the AMP : ATP ratio [105].

The inability of CFS/ME muscle cells to activate AMPK and glucose uptake in addition to reduced IL-6 secretion in response to EPS is suggestive of underlying peripheral muscle dysfunction in CFS/ME. However, further work is required to investigate the mechanisms that lead to impaired activation of AMPK in those with CFS/ME.

9. Conclusion

CFS/ME patient perceptions of the nature of their condition frequently cite "peripheral" as opposed to a central origin, with many descriptions of their fatigue regularly referring to difficulty in maintaining muscle activity due to perceived lack of energy, or through muscle fatigue [15, 17]. There is increasing evidence to suggest that muscular biochemical abnormality may play a major role in CFS/ME associated fatigue. The literature suggests patients to exhibit profound intramuscular dysfunction regarding acid generation and clearance, with a tendency towards an overutilisation of the lactate dehydrogenase pathway following relatively low-level activity. However, the precise mechanisms underlying the dysfunction are yet to be fully elucidated. There is a real need for adequately powered studies to examine PDC function in vitro, to determine the mechanisms responsible for bioenergetic dysfunction and peripheral fatigue.

Conflict of Interests

None of the authors have any conflict of interests.

Acknowledgments

This paper is funded by Action for ME and NIHR Newcastle Biomedical Research.

References

[1] A. S. Bradley, B. Ford, and A. S. Bansal, "Altered functional B-cell subset populations in patients with chronic fatigue syndrome compared to healthy controls," *Clinical and Experimental Immunology*, vol. 172, no. 1, pp. 73–80, 2013.

[2] D. E. J. Jones, K. G. Hollingsworth, D. G. Jakovljevic et al., "Loss of capacity to recover from acidosis on repeat exercise in chronic fatigue syndrome: a case-control study," *European Journal of Clinical Investigation*, vol. 42, no. 2, pp. 186–194, 2012.

[3] A. Macintyre, *CFS, Post-Viral Fatigue Syndrome. How to Live with It*, Thorsons, London, UK, 1992.

[4] R. N. Perrin, J. D. Richards, V. Pentreath, and D. F. Percy, "Muscle fatigue in chronic fatigue syndrome/myalgic encephalomyelitis (CFS/ME) and its response to a manual therapeutic approach: a pilot study," *International Journal of Osteopathic Medicine*, vol. 14, no. 3, pp. 96–105, 2011.

[5] S. Wessely, T. Chalder, S. Hirsch, P. Wallace, and D. Wright, "The prevalence and morbidity of chronic fatigue and chronic fatigue syndrome: a prospective primary care study," *American Journal of Public Health*, vol. 87, no. 9, pp. 1449–1455, 1997.

[6] H. Knoop, J. B. Prins, M. Stulemeijer, J. W. van der Meer, and G. Bleijenberg, "The effect of cognitive behaviour therapy for chronic fatigue syndrome on self-reported cognitive impairments and neuropsychological test performance," *Journal of Neurology and Neurosurgery Psychiatry*, vol. 78, no. 4, pp. 434–436, 2007.

[7] L. C. Nacul, E. M. Lacerda, D. Pheby et al., "Prevalence of myalgic encephalomyelitis/chronic fatigue syndrome (ME/CFS) in three regions of England: a repeated cross-sectional study in primary care," *BMC Medicine*, vol. 9, article 91, pp. 1–12, 2011.

[8] NICE-National Institute for Health and Clinical Excellence, *Chronic Fatigue/Myalgic Encephalomyelitis (or Encephalopathy): Diagnosis and Management of CFS/ME in Adults and Children*, vol. 53 of *NICE Clinical Guideline*, 2007.

[9] J. B. Prins, J. W. M. Van Der Meer, and G. Bleijenberg, "Chronic fatigue syndrome," *The Lancet*, vol. 367, no. 9507, pp. 346–355, 2006.

[10] K. Fukuda, S. E. Straus, I. Hickie, M. C. Sharpe, J. G. Dobbins, and A. Komaroff, "The chronic fatigue syndrome: a comprehensive approach to its definition and study," *Annals of Internal Medicine*, vol. 121, no. 12, pp. 953–959, 1994.

[11] B. M. Carruthers, A. K. Jain, K. L. De Meirleir et al., "Myalgic encephalomyelitis/chronic fatigue syndrome: clinical working case definition, diagnostic and treatment protocols," *Journal of Chronic Fatigue Syndrome*, vol. 11, no. 1, pp. 7–115, 2003.

[12] Action for ME, An investigation into NHS specific service provision for people with ME/CFS. 1-34, 2012.

[13] IOM Institute of Medicine, *Beyond Myalgic Encephalomyelitis/Chronic Fatigue Syndrome: Redefining the Illness*, National Academies, Washington, DC, USA, 2015.

[14] L. A. Jason, M. Sunnquist, A. Brown, J. L. Newton, E. B. Strand, and S. D. Vernon, "Chronic fatigue syndrome versus systemic exertion intolerance disease," *Fatigue: Biomedicine, Health & Behavior*, vol. 3, no. 3, pp. 127–141, 2015.

[15] D. E. J. Jones, K. G. Hollingsworth, A. M. Blamire, R. Taylor, and J. L. Newton, "Abnormalities in pH handling by peripheral muscle and potential regulation by the autonomic nervous system in chronic fatigue syndrome," *Journal of Internal Medicine*, vol. 267, no. 4, pp. 394–401, 2010.

[16] "Fatigue," *The Lancet*, vol. 332, no. 8610, pp. 546–548, 1998.

[17] J. Van Oosterwijck, J. Nijs, M. Meeus et al., "Pain inhibition and postexertional malaise in myalgic encephalomyelitis/chronic fatigue syndrome: an experimental study," *Journal of Internal Medicine*, vol. 268, no. 3, pp. 265–278, 2010.

[18] P. R. J. Barnes, D. J. Taylor, G. I. Kemp, and G. K. Radda, "Skeletal muscle bioenergetics in the chronic fatigue syndrome," *Journal of Neurology, Neurosurgery and Psychiatry*, vol. 56, no. 6, pp. 679–683, 1993.

[19] Y. Jammes, J. G. Steinberg, O. Mambrini, F. Brégeon, and S. Delliaux, "Chronic fatigue syndrome: assessment of increased oxidative stress and altered muscle excitability in response to incremental exercise," *Journal of Internal Medicine*, vol. 257, no. 3, pp. 299–310, 2005.

[20] R. J. M. Lane, M. C. Barrett, D. Woodrow, J. Moss, R. Fletcher, and L. C. Archard, "Muscle fibre characteristics and lactate responses to exercise in chronic fatigue syndrome," *Journal of Neurology, Neurosurgery & Psychiatry*, vol. 64, no. 3, pp. 362–367, 1998.

[21] S. Brkic, S. Tomic, D. Maric, M. A. Novakov, and V. Turkulov, "Lipid peroxidation is elevated in female patients with chronic fatigue syndrome," *Medical Science Monitor*, vol. 16, no. 12, pp. CR628–CR632, 2010.

[22] Y. Jammes, J. G. Steinberg, R. Guieu, and S. Delliaux, "Chronic fatigue syndrome with history of severe infection combined altered blood oxidant status, and reduced potassium efflux and muscle excitability at exercise," *Open Journal of Internal Medicine*, vol. 3, no. 3, pp. 98–105, 2013.

[23] K. Filler, D. Lyon, J. Bennett et al., "Association of mitochondrial dysfunction and fatigue: a review of the literature," *BBA Clinical*, vol. 1, pp. 12–23, 2014.

[24] S. Myhill, N. E. Booth, and J. McLaren-Howard, "Chronic fatigue syndrome and mitochondrial dysfunction," *International Journal of Clinical and Experimental Medicine*, vol. 2, no. 1, pp. 1–16, 2009.

[25] A. Whiteside, S. Hansen, and A. Chaudhuri, "Exercise lowers pain threshold in chronic fatigue syndrome," *Pain*, vol. 109, no. 3, pp. 497–499, 2004.

[26] A. E. Brown, D. E. Jones, M. Walker, and J. L. Newton, "Abnormalities of AMPK activation and glucose uptake in Chronic Fatigue Syndrome," *PLoS ONE*, vol. 10, no. 4, Article ID e0122982, 2015.

[27] M. Meeus, N. A. Roussel, S. Truijen, and J. Nijs, "Reduced pressure pain thresholds in response to exercise in chronic fatigue syndrome but not in chronic low back pain: an experimental study," *Journal of Rehabilitation Medicine*, vol. 42, no. 9, pp. 884–890, 2010.

[28] J. Nijs, M. Meeus, J. Van Oosterwijck et al., "In the mind or in the brain? Scientific evidence for central sensitisation in chronic fatigue syndrome," *European Journal of Clinical Investigation*, vol. 42, no. 2, pp. 203–212, 2012.

[29] J. Vecchiet, F. Cipollone, K. Falasca et al., "Relationship between musculoskeletal symptoms and blood markers of oxidative stress in patients with chronic fatigue syndrome," *Neuroscience Letters*, vol. 335, no. 3, pp. 151–154, 2003.

[30] Y. Jammes, J. G. Steinberg, and S. Delliaux, "Chronic fatigue syndrome: acute infection and history of physical activity affect resting levels and response to exercise of plasma oxidant/antioxidant status and heat shock proteins," *Journal of Internal Medicine*, vol. 272, no. 1, pp. 74–84, 2012.

[31] M. Maes, I. Mihaylova, and C. Leunis, "Chronic fatigue syndrome is accompanied by an IgM-related immune response directed against neopitopes formed by oxidative or nitrosative damage to lipids and proteins," *Neuro Endocrinology Letters*, vol. 27, no. 5, pp. 615–621, 2006.

[32] G. Broderick, J. Fruite, A. Kreitz et al., "A formal analysis of cytokine networks in chronic fatigue syndrome," *Brain Behaviour and Immunity*, vol. 24, no. 7, pp. 1209–1217, 2010.

[33] E. W. Brenu, M. L. van Driel, D. R. Staines et al., "Immunological abnormalities as potential biomarkers in Chronic Fatigue Syndrome/Myalgic Encephalomyelitis," *Journal of Translational Medicine*, vol. 9, article 81, 2011.

[34] A. Skowera, A. Cleare, D. Blair, L. Bevis, S. C. Wessely, and M. Peakman, "High levels of type 2 cytokine-producing cells in chronic fatigue syndrome," *Clinical and Experimental Immunology*, vol. 135, no. 2, pp. 294–302, 2004.

[35] A. McArdle, F. McArdle, M. J. Jackson, S. F. Page, I. Fahal, and R. H. T. Edwards, "Investigation by polymerase chain reaction of enteroviral infection in patients with chronic fatigue syndrome," *Clinical Science*, vol. 90, no. 4, pp. 295–300, 1996.

[36] R. H. Edwards, H. Gibson, J. E. Clague, and T. Helliwell, "Muscle histopathology and physiology in chronic fatigue syndrome," *Ciba Foundation Symposia*, vol. 173, pp. 102–117, 1993.

[37] M. Maes, I. Mihaylova, M. Kubera, M. Uytterhoeven, N. Vrydags, and E. Bosmans, "Coenzyme Q10 deficiency in myalgic encephalomyelitis/chronic fatigue syndrome (ME/CFS) is related to fatigue, autonomic and neurocognitive symptoms and is another risk factor explaining the early mortality in ME/CFS due to cardiovascular disorder," *Neuro Endocrinology Letters*, vol. 30, no. 4, pp. 470–476, 2009.

[38] P. D. White, K. E. Nye, A. J. Pinching et al., "Immunological changes after both exercise and activity in chronic fatigue syndrome: a pilot study," *Journal of Chronic Fatigue Syndrome*, vol. 12, no. 2, pp. 51–66, 2004.

[39] A. R. Light, L. Bateman, D. Jo et al., "Gene expression alterations at baseline and following moderate exercise in patients with chronic fatigue syndrome and fibromyalgia syndrome," *Journal of Internal Medicine*, vol. 271, no. 1, pp. 64–81, 2012.

[40] J. Nijs, A. Nees, M. De Kooning, K. Ickmans, M. Meeus, and J. Van Oosterwijck, "Altered immune response to exercise in patients with chronic fatigue syndrome/ myalgic encephalomyelitis: a systematic review," *Exercise Immunology Review*, vol. 20, pp. 94–116, 2014.

[41] D. E. J. Jones, K. G. Hollingsworth, D. G. Jakovljevic et al., "Loss of capacity to recover from acidosis on repeat exercise in chronic fatigue syndrome: a case–control study," *European Journal of Clinical Investigation*, vol. 42, no. 2, pp. 186–194, 2012.

[42] R. Wong, G. Lopaschuk, G. Zhu et al., "Skeletal muscle metabolism in the chronic fatigue syndrome; in vivo assessment by 31P nuclear magnetic resonance spectroscopy," *Chest*, vol. 102, no. 6, pp. 1716–1722, 1992.

[43] R. J. M. Lane, M. C. Barrett, D. J. Taylor, G. J. Kemp, and R. Lodi, "Heterogeneity in chronic fatigue syndrome: evidence from magnetic resonance spectroscopy of muscle," *Neuromuscular Disorders*, vol. 8, no. 3-4, pp. 204–209, 1998.

[44] R. A. Meyer, J. N. Campbell, and S. N. Raja, "Peripheral neural mechanisms of nociceptors," in *Textbook of Pain*, R. Meizack, Ed., pp. 13–144, Churchill Livingstone, Edinburgh, UK, 3rd edition, 1995.

[45] M. Amann and J. A. Dempsey, "Locomotor muscle fatigue modifies central motor drive in healthy humans and imposes a limitation to exercise performance," *Journal of Physiology*, vol. 586, part 1, pp. 161–175, 2008.

[46] J. Finsterer, "Biomarkers of peripheral muscle fatigue during exercise," *BMC Musculoskeletal Disorders*, vol. 13, article 218, pp. 1-13, 2012.

[47] R. J. Bloomer, A. H. Goldfarb, L. Wideman, M. J. McKenzie, and L. A. Consitt, "Effects of acute aerobic and anaerobic exercise on blood markers of oxidative stress," *Journal of Strength and Conditioning Research*, vol. 19, no. 2, pp. 276–285, 2005.

[48] J. D. Crane, A. Abadi, B. P. Hettinga et al., "Elevated mitochondrial oxidative stress impairs metabolic adaptations to exercise in skeletal muscle," *PLoS ONE*, vol. 8, no. 12, Article ID e81879, 2013.

[49] J. C. Fernández-Checa, C. García-Ruiz, A. Colell et al., "Oxidative stress: role of mitochondria and protection by glutathione," *BioFactors*, vol. 8, no. 1-2, pp. 7–11, 1998.

[50] M. Yu, Y. Wan, Q. Zou, and Y. Xi, "High frequency of mitochondrial DNA D-loop mutations in Ewing's sarcoma," *Biochemical and Biophysical Research Communications*, vol. 390, no. 3, pp. 447–450, 2009.

[51] M. L. Genova, M. M. Pich, A. Bernacchia et al., "The mitochondrial production of reactive oxygen species in relation to aging and pathology," *Annals of the New York Academy of Sciences*, vol. 1011, pp. 86–100, 2004.

[52] A. J. Hulbert, "On the importance of fatty acid composition of membranes for aging," *Journal of Theoretical Biology*, vol. 234, no. 2, pp. 277–288, 2005.

[53] E. Luin, R. Giniatullin, and M. Sciancalepore, "Effects of H_2O_2 on electrical membrane properties of skeletal myotubes," *Free Radical Biology and Medicine*, vol. 50, no. 2, pp. 337–344, 2011.

[54] E. Marcos and J. Ribas, "Kinetics of plasma potassium concentrations during exhausting exercise in trained and untrained men," *European Journal of Applied*, vol. 71, no. 2-3, pp. 207–214, 1995.

[55] C. Juel, "Muscle fatigue and reactive oxygen species," *The Journal of Physiology*, vol. 576, pp. 279–288, 2006.

[56] E. Marcos and J. Ribas, "Kinetics of plasma potassium concentrations during exhausting exercise in trained and untrained men," *European Journal of Applied Physiology*, vol. 71, pp. 207–214, 1995.

[57] S. Fulle, S. Belia, J. Vecchiet, C. Morabito, L. Vecchiet, and G. Fanò, "Modification of the functional capacity of sarcoplasmic reticulum membranes in patients suffering from chronic fatigue syndrome," *Neuromuscular Disorders*, vol. 13, no. 6, pp. 479–484, 2003.

[58] Y. Jammes, J. G. Steinberg, S. Delliaux, and F. Brégeon, "Chronic fatigue syndrome combines increased exercise-induced oxidative stress and reduced cytokine and Hsp responses," *Journal of Internal Medicine*, vol. 266, no. 2, pp. 196–206, 2009.

[59] A. A. Thambirajah, K. Sleigh, H. G. Stiver, and A. W. Chow, "Differential heat shock protein responses to strenuous standardized exercise in chronic fatigue syndrome patients and matched healthy controls," *Clinical and Investigative Medicine*, vol. 31, no. 6, pp. E319–E327, 2008.

[60] G. Morris and M. Maes, "Oxidative and nitrosative stress and immune-inflammatory pathways in patients with Myalgic Encephalomyelitis (ME)/Chronic Fatigue Syndrome (CFS)," *Current Neuropharmacology*, vol. 12, no. 2, pp. 168–185, 2014.

[61] G. Morris and M. Maes, "Mitochondrial dysfunctions in Myalgic Encephalomyelitis/chronic fatigue syndrome explained by activated immuno-inflammatory, oxidative and nitrosative stress pathways," *Metabolic Brain Disease*, vol. 29, no. 1, pp. 19–36, 2014.

[62] S. Fulle, T. Pietrangelo, R. Mancinelli, R. Saggini, and G. Fanò, "Specific correlations between muscle oxidative stress and chronic fatigue syndrome: a working hypothesis," *Journal of Muscle Research and Cell Motility*, vol. 28, no. 6, pp. 355–362, 2007.

[63] J. M. VanNess, S. R. Stevens, L. Bateman, T. L. Stiles, and C. R. Snell, "Postexertional malaise in women with chronic fatigue syndrome," *Journal Womens Health*, vol. 19, no. 2, pp. 239–244, 2010.

[64] J. Nijs, K. De Meirleir, M. Meeus, N. R. McGregor, and P. Englebienne, "Chronic fatigue syndrome: intracellular immune deregulations as a possible etiology for abnormal exercise response," *Medical Hypotheses*, vol. 62, no. 5, pp. 759–765, 2004.

[65] G. Morris and M. Maes, "Increased nuclear factor-κB and loss of p53 are key mechanisms in Myalgic Encephalomyelitis/chronic fatigue syndrome (ME/CFS)," *Medical Hypotheses*, vol. 79, no. 5, pp. 607–613, 2012.

[66] M. A. Fletcher, X. R. Zeng, K. Maher et al., "Biomarkers in chronic fatigue syndrome: evaluation of natural killer cell function and dipeptidyl peptidase IV/CD26," *PLoS ONE*, vol. 5, no. 5, Article ID e10817, 7 pages, 2010.

[67] M. Maes, F. N. M. Twisk, M. Kubera, and K. Ringel, "Evidence for inflammation and activation of cell-mediated immunity in Myalgic Encephalomyelitis/Chronic Fatigue Syndrome (ME/CFS): increased interleukin-1, tumor necrosis factor-α, PMN-elastase, lysozyme and neopterin," *Journal of Affective Disorders*, vol. 136, no. 3, pp. 933–939, 2012.

[68] M. Maes, I. Mihaylova, M. Kubera, and E. Bosmans, "Not in the mind but in the cell: increased production of cyclo-oxygenase-2 and inducible NO synthase in chronic fatigue syndrome," *Neuro Endocrinology Letters*, vol. 28, no. 4, pp. 463–469, 2007.

[69] B. Smits, L. van den Heuvel, H. Knoop et al., "Mitochondrial enzymes discriminate between mitochondrial disorders and chronic fatigue syndrome," *Mitochondrion*, vol. 11, no. 5, pp. 735–738, 2011.

[70] J. Tymoczko, J. Berg, and L. Stryer, *Biochemistry: A Short Course*, W. H. Freeman and Company, New York, NY, USA, 2010.

[71] D. A. Jones, D. L. Turner, D. B. McIntyre, and D. J. Newham, "Energy turnover in relation to slowing of contractile properties during fatiguing contractions of the human anterior tibialis muscle," *The Journal of Physiology*, vol. 587, no. 17, pp. 4329–4338, 2009.

[72] S. E. Reuter and A. M. Evans, "Long-chain acylcarnitine deficiency in patients with chronic fatigue syndrome. Potential involvement of altered carnitine palmitoyltransferase-I activity," *Journal of Internal Medicine*, vol. 270, no. 1, pp. 76–84, 2011.

[73] H. Kuratsune, K. Yamaguti, M. Takahashi, H. Misaki, S. Tagawa, and T. Kitani, "Acylcarnitine deficiency in chronic fatigue syndrome," *Clinical Infectious Diseases*, vol. 18, supplement 1, pp. S62–S67, 1994.

[74] H. Karatsune, K. Yamaguti, and G. Lindh, "Low-levels of serum acyl-carnitine in chronic fatigue syndrome and chronic hepatitis type C but not other disease," *International Journal of Molecular Medicine*, vol. 2, no. 1, pp. 51–56, 1998.

[75] M. G. Jones, C. S. Goodwin, S. Amjad, and R. A. Chalmers, "Plasma and urinary carnitine and acylcarnitines in chronic fatigue syndrome," *Clinica Chimica Acta*, vol. 360, no. 1-2, pp. 173–177, 2005.

[76] T. Majeed, C. De Simone, G. Famularo, S. Marcellini, and P. O. Behan, "Abnormalities of carnitine metabolism in chronic fatigue syndrome," *European Journal of Neurology*, vol. 2, no. 5, pp. 425–428, 1995.

[77] H. Knoop, G. Bleijenberg, M. F. M. Gielissen, J. W. M. Van Der Meer, and P. D. White, "Is a full recovery possible after cognitive behavioural therapy for chronic fatigue syndrome?" *Psychotherapy and Psychosomatics*, vol. 76, no. 3, pp. 171–176, 2007.

[78] F. N. M. Twisk, "The 4I hypothesis: a neuro-immunological explanation for characteristic symptoms of myalgic encephalomyelitis/chronic fatigue syndrome," *International Journal of Neurology Research*, vol. 8, no. 2, pp. 20–38, 2015.

[79] A. M. Bellinger, M. Mongillo, and A. R. Marks, "Stressed out: the skeletal muscle ryanodine receptor as a target of stress," *Journal of Clinical Investigation*, vol. 118, no. 2, pp. 445–453, 2008.

[80] G. J. Kemp, C. H. Thompson, D. J. Taylor, and G. K. Radda, "Proton efflux in human skeletal muscle during recovery from exercise," *European Journal of Applied Physiology and Occupational Physiology*, vol. 76, no. 5, pp. 462–471, 1997.

[81] K. G. Hollingsworth, J. L. Newton, L. Robinson, R. Taylor, A. M. Blamire, and D. E. J. Jones, "Loss of capacity to recover from acidosis in repeat exercise is strongly associated with fatigue in primary biliary cirrhosis," *Journal of Hepatology*, vol. 53, no. 1, pp. 155–161, 2010.

[82] M. I. Trenell, C. M. Sue, G. J. Kemp, T. Sachinwalla, and C. H. Thompson, "Aerobic exercise and muscle metabolism in patients with mitochondrial myopathy," *Muscle and Nerve*, vol. 33, no. 4, pp. 524–531, 2006.

[83] D. G. Allen, J. Lannergren, and H. Westerblad, "Muscle cell function during prolonged activity: cellular mechanisms of fatigue," *Experimental Physiology*, vol. 80, no. 4, pp. 497–527, 1995.

[84] D. Street, J. Bangsbo, and C. Juel, "Interstitial pH in human skeletal muscle during and after dynamic graded exercise," *Journal of Physiology*, vol. 537, no. 3, pp. 993–998, 2001.

[85] J. M. Kristensen, M. Kristensen, and C. Juel, "Expression of Na^+/HCO_3^- co-transporter proteins (NBCs) in rat and human skeletal muscle," *Acta Physiologica Scandinavica*, vol. 182, no. 1, pp. 69–76, 2004.

[86] M. C. Wilson, V. N. Jackson, C. Heddle et al., "Lactic acid efflux from white skeletal muscle is catalyzed by the monocarboxylate transporter isoform MCT3," *The Journal of Biological Chemistry*, vol. 273, no. 26, pp. 15920–15926, 1998.

[87] A. P. Halestrap and N. T. Price, "The proton-linked monocarboxylate transporter (MCT) family: structure, function and regulation," *Biochemical Journal*, vol. 343, no. 2, pp. 281–299, 1999.

[88] P. De Becker, J. Roeykens, M. Reynders, N. McGregor, and K. De Meirleir, "Exercise capacity in chronic fatigue syndrome," *Archives of Internal Medicine*, vol. 160, no. 21, pp. 3270–3277, 2000.

[89] J. L. Newton, O. Okonkwo, K. Sutcliffe, A. Seth, J. Shin, and D. E. J. Jones, "Symptoms of autonomic dysfunction in chronic fatigue syndrome," *QJM*, vol. 100, no. 8, pp. 519–526, 2007.

[90] A. S. Winkler, D. Blair, J. T. Marsden, T. J. Peters, S. Wessely, and A. J. Cleare, "Autonomic function and serum erythropoietin levels in chronic fatigue syndrome," *Journal of Psychosomatic Research*, vol. 56, no. 2, pp. 179–183, 2004.

[91] E. B. Andersen, F. Boesen, and O. Henriksen, "Local and central sympathetic reflex control of blood flow in skeletal muscle and subcutaneous tissue in normal man," *Clinical Physiology*, vol. 11, no. 5, pp. 451–458, 1991.

[92] S. H. Kori, R. P. Miller, and D. D. Todd, "Kinisophobia: a new view of chronic pain behavior," *Pain Management*, vol. 3, no. 1, pp. 35–43, 1990.

[93] A. Silver, M. Haeney, P. Vijayadurai, D. Wilks, M. Pattrick, and C. J. Main, "The role of fear of physical movement and activity in chronic fatigue syndrome," *Journal of Psychosomatic Research*, vol. 52, no. 6, pp. 485–493, 2002.

[94] F. O. Forque, M. Brivet, A. Boutron et al., "Differential effect of DCA treatment on the pyruvate dehydrogenase complex in patients with severe PCHC deficiency," *Paediatric Research*, vol. 53, no. 5, pp. 793–799, 2003.

[95] J. W. Murrough, X. Mao, K. A. Collins et al., "Increased ventricular lactate in chronic fatigue syndrome measured by ^1H MRS imaging at 3.0 T. II: comparison with major depressive disorder," *NMR in Biomedicine*, vol. 23, no. 6, pp. 643–650, 2010.

[96] D. Constantin-Teodosiu, D. J. Baker, D. Constantin, and P. L. Greenhaff, "PPAR-δ agonism inhibits skeletal muscle PDC activity, mitochondrial ATP production and force generation during prolonged contraction," *Journal of Physiology*, vol. 587, no. 1, pp. 231–239, 2009.

[97] E. A. Richter and N. B. Ruderman, "AMPK and the biochemistry of exercise: implications for human health and disease," *Biochemical Journal*, vol. 418, no. 2, pp. 261–275, 2009.

[98] Z.-P. Chen, T. J. Stephens, S. Murthy et al., "Effect of exercise intensity on skeletal muscle AMPK signaling in humans," *Diabetes*, vol. 52, no. 9, pp. 2205–2212, 2003.

[99] W. W. Winder, B. F. Holmes, D. S. Rubink, E. B. Jensen, M. Chen, and J. O. Holloszy, "Activation of AMP-activated protein kinase increases mitochondrial enzymes in skeletal muscle," *Journal of Applied Physiology*, vol. 88, no. 6, pp. 2219–2226, 2000.

[100] B. B. Kahn, T. Alquier, D. Carling, and D. G. Hardie, "AMP-activated protein kinase: ancient energy gauge provides clues to modern understanding of metabolism," *Cell Metabolism*, vol. 1, no. 1, pp. 15–25, 2005.

[101] S. B. Jørgensen, J. F. P. Wojtaszewski, B. Viollet et al., "Effects of α-AMPK knockout on exercise-induced gene activation in mouse skeletal muscle," *The FASEB Journal*, vol. 19, no. 9, pp. 1146–1148, 2005.

[102] N. Ouchi, R. Shibata, and K. Walsh, "AMP-activated protein kinase signaling stimulates VEGF expression and angiogenesis in skeletal muscle," *Circulation Research*, vol. 96, no. 8, pp. 838–846, 2005.

[103] J. N. Nielsen, K. J. W. Mustard, D. A. Graham et al., "5′-AMP-activated protein kinase activity and subunit expression in exercise-trained human skeletal muscle," *Journal of Applied Physiology*, vol. 94, no. 2, pp. 631–641, 2003.

[104] C. Frøsig, S. B. Jørgensen, D. G. Hardie, E. A. Richter, and J. F. P. Wojtaszewski, "5′-AMP-activated protein kinase activity and protein expression are regulated by endurance training in human skeletal muscle," *American Journal of Physiology—Endocrinology and Metabolism*, vol. 286, no. 3, pp. 411–417, 2004.

[105] M. Kelly, M.-S. Gauthier, A. K. Saha, and N. B. Ruderman, "Activation of AMP-activated protein kinase by interleukin-6 in rat skeletal muscle: association with changes in cAMP, energy state, and endogenous fuel mobilization," *Diabetes*, vol. 58, no. 9, pp. 1953–1960, 2009.

13

Physical Activity across Frailty Phenotypes in Females with Parkinson's Disease

Kaitlyn P. Roland,[1] Kayla M. D. Cornett,[1] Olga Theou,[2] Jennifer M. Jakobi,[3] and Gareth R. Jones[3]

[1] *Interdisciplinary Graduate Studies, Health and Exercise Sciences, University of British Columbia Okanagan, Kelowna, BC, Canada V1V 1V7*
[2] *Faculty of Geriatrics Medicine, Dalhousie University, Halifax, NS, Canada B3H 2E1*
[3] *School of Health and Exercise Sciences, Faculty of Health and Social Development, University of British Columbia Okanagan, 3333 University Way, Kelowna, BC, Canada V1V 1V7*

Correspondence should be addressed to Gareth R. Jones, gareth.jones@ubc.ca

Academic Editor: Barbara Tettenborn

Females with Parkinson's disease (PD) are vulnerable to frailty. PD eventually leads to decreased physical activity, an indicator of frailty. We speculate PD results in frailty through reduced physical activity. *Objective.* Determine the contribution of physical activity on frailty in PD ($n = 15$, 65 ± 9 years) and non-PD ($n = 15$, 73 ± 14 years) females. *Methods.* Frailty phenotype (nonfrail/prefrail/frail) was categorized and 8 hours of physical activity was measured using accelerometer, global positioning system, and self-report. Two-way ANCOVA (age as covariate) was used to compare physical activity between disease and frailty phenotypes. Spearman correlation assessed relationships, and linear regression determined associations with frailty. *Results.* Nonfrail recorded more physical activity (intensity, counts, self-report) compared with frail. Self-reported physical activity was greater in PD than non-PD. In non-PD, step counts, light physical activity time, sedentary time, and self-reported physical activity were related to frailty ($R = 0.91$). In PD, only carbidopa-levodopa dose was related to frailty ($r = 0.61$). *Conclusion.* Physical activity influences frailty in females without PD. In PD females, disease management may be a better indicator of frailty than physical activity. Further investigation into how PD associated factors contribute to frailty is warranted.

1. Introduction

Frailty is a geriatric syndrome that results in an increased vulnerability to acute and chronic illness, falls and related injuries, and a general loss of functional independence [1–4]. The cardiovascular health study frailty index (CHS*fi*), proposes that frailty develops across a spectrum of phenotypes ranging from nonfrail to prefrail to frail [5]. All stages of frailty are evident within community-dwelling populations, with over 70% of older adults expressing some frailty characteristics [6]. Frailty is twice as prevalent in females as males and females typically display more frailty characteristics than males [5, 7]. Females experience increased frailty severity than males since they live longer and spend a greater proportion of life managing disability and disease [7–9].

Females with Parkinson's disease (PD) are at an increased risk of frailty [10], yet the presence of frailty in persons with PD may be misinterpreted as disease-related functional decline [11]. Females with PD are typically older [12], cite greater disability [13] and experience more difficulty performing activities of daily living (ADL) than males with PD [14, 15]. Recent evidence suggests that of the five CHS*fi* criteria, self-reported exhaustion best determines frailty phenotype in females with PD [10]. Exhaustion is a common complaint among older females, especially those with PD, and is strongly associated with inhibiting physical activity and ADL participation [16–18]. The established relationship between reduced physical activity and frailty severity [19] leads us to speculate that PD influences frailty through decreased participation in physical activity. Understanding how physical activity contributes to frailty in females with PD is important in directing management strategies aimed at maintaining functional independence. The objective of this study was to determine the contribution of daily physical activity on frailty phenotype in community-dwelling females with PD, compared to non-PD females.

2. Methods

Females greater than 50 years of age, living independently in the community, with mild to moderate PD severity (Hoehn & Yahr stage 1–3) were recruited through advertisements and support group presentations. Non-PD females were similarly recruited from the same local region. All participants were able to ambulate independently (with or without walk-aid). Females with PD were in a steady clinical state (controlled by medication) and cognitively intact. Females with PD were instructed to continue daily dopamine medication as prescribed and no incidence of freezing of gait or severe dyskinesia episodes were reported during the testing day. All participants provided written informed consent. The Clinical Research Ethics Board of the University of British Columbia granted ethical approval for this investigation.

Health history questionnaires, physical frailty criteria (CHS*fi*), self-reported physical activity, and setup of daily physical activity monitors (accelerometer, GPS) were completed at the participant's home in the morning (8~10 am). All PD participants were assessed between 1 and 2 hours post anti-Parkinson's medication, and controls were assessed 1 hour after breakfast. In older adults, reduction in daily physical activity, and associated physiological change, can be quantified using continuous objective physical activity monitors (i.e., accelerometers and global positioning systems, GPS) [20]. In this study, a waist-borne accelerometer and wrist-born GPS recorded physical activity; and the participant wore these devices continuously for the entire testing day. The participant was then instructed to go about their typical daily activities, which they recorded in a written hourly log. The accelerometer, GPS, and physical activity logbook were collected approximately 7 hours later (between 4–7 pm) at the participant's home.

2.1. Frailty Phenotype. Frailty was categorized according to CHS*fi* [5] that includes five select criteria to determine a frailty phenotype (nonfrail, prefrail, and frail). These criteria include: (1) Unintended weight loss (>10 lbs in past 12 months); (2) Weakness (maximal handgrip strength classified by body mass index, BMI); (3) Walk speed (15 ft at usual pace classified by height); (4) Self-reported energy expenditure (Minnesota Leisure Time Activities Questionnaire, MLTA); (5) Self-reported exhaustion (Center for Epidemiological Studies depression scale, CES-D). Participants were considered nonfrail if they satisfied none of the phenotypic criteria, prefrail if they satisfied 1 or 2 criteria, and frail if they satisfied 3 or more criteria [5].

2.2. Accelerometer. Daily physical activity was measured using an ActiTrainer accelerometer (Actigraph, LLC, Fort Walton Beach, FL) secured in a holster worn at the waist on the dominant side. The ActiTrainer ($8.6 \times 3.3 \times 1.5$ cm; 51 grams) is a triaxial solid-state accelerometer that was programmed to record 60-second epochs of data. Data was uploaded to ActiLife5 v.5.8.3 software (ActiGraph, LLC, Fort Walton Beach, FL). Physical activity intensity levels were categorized according to the cut-points described by Copeland and Eslinger for older adults [21]. Sedentary activity was defined as 0 to 50 counts per minute, light physical activity as 51 to 1,040 counts per minute, and moderate-to-vigorous physical activity as greater than 1,041 counts per minute. Percentage of time spent at each level of activity was reported. Measurement outputs included total counts (i.e., daily step and activity counts, total minutes of activity) and intensity (i.e., percentage of time spent at sedentary, light, and moderate-vigorous activity intensity levels).

2.3. Global Positioning System (GPS). Global Positioning System (GPS) examines gross mobility outside the individuals' home. GPS used in combination with the accelerometer can accurately assess physical activity within real-life environments [22], and this can be applied to categorize stages of frailty [23]. Participants wore a Garmin Forerunner 405 GPS watch (Garmin International Inc., Olathe, KS). GPS data were uploaded to the Garmin training center software (http://connect.garmin.com/). Both the GPS and accelerometer units were synchronized to record minute-by-minute data. The GPS and accelerometer data were time-matched using the ActiGraph GPS Correlation Wizard v.1.0.0 (Actigraph, LLC, Fort Walton Beach, FL) and exported in a Microsoft Excel compatible format for analysis. Only physical activity completed outside the home, defined using Garmin Training Software and an accompanying Google Earth Map, was included in the analysis. Participants' hourly physical activity log was also compared to GPS outputs to confirm physical activity participation. Vehicle-generated activity was considered any recording that measured greater than 3 m/sec for >1 min. All activity at speeds less than 3 m/sec >1 min were included as participant physical activity. GPS measurement outputs included; total GPS distance (km, vehicle- and participant-generated) and total amount of physical activity time (min).

2.4. Self-Reported Physical Activities. Self perceived energy expenditure was assessed using the self-reported MLTA [24], which was also used to determine energy expenditure as part of the CHS*fi* frailty assessment [5]. Twenty activities were specified, including walking for exercise, moderately strenuous household chores, mowing the lawn, raking the lawn, gardening, hiking, jogging, biking, exercise cycling, dancing, aerobics, bowling, golfing, calisthenics/general exercise, swimming, doubles tennis, singles tennis, and racquetball. Participants who engaged in any physical activity during the previous 2-weeks recorded the number of sessions and their duration. Energy (kcal/week) expenditure was determined using metabolic equivalent (MET) score: (activity-specific MET) × ((activity duration in minutes)/60) × ((number of sessions in past two weeks)/2). Total energy expenditure was calculated by summing expenditures over all activities.

2.5. Statistical Analysis. All analysis was performed using Statistical Package for Social Science 18.0 (PASW Statistics 18.0, SPSS Inc. IBM Somers, NY). Subject characteristics were compared between groups (non-PD, PD) and between frailty phenotype (nonfrail, prefrail, and frail) with a one-way ANOVA. The non-PD females were older than PD (P = 0.005), nonfrail females were younger than prefrail and frail (P = 0.007), and prefrail were younger than frail (P = 0.03). Thus, age was used as a covariate in a two-way ANCOVA to assess differences in physical activity between disease states (PD; non-PD) and frailty phenotype (nonfrail; prefrail; frail). To evaluate the main effects a univariate analysis was performed for each dependent variable to identify contributions to the main effects of disease states and frailty phenotypes. Probability level was set at $P < 0.05$ and Tukey post hoc tests were used to probe statistical interactions. Spearman's rank correlation was used to evaluate physical activity measures relative to frailty phenotype in each group. The physical activity measures that were significantly correlated with frailty phenotype were entered into a multiple regression analysis model with frailty phenotype as the dependent variable and physical activity measures as the independent variables.

3. Results

Fifteen persons with PD (65 ± 9 years) and 15 non-PD controls (73 ± 14 years) participated. Both groups were categorized into frailty phenotypes according to the CHS*fi* (Table 1). In females with PD, tremor in the upper limb was controlled with medication and participants self-reported no freezing of gait or periods of dyskinesia over the course of the day. Further, any reports of rigidity and/or slowness of movement (bradykinesia) were mild and did not restrict ADL. Comparison of physical activity between disease states and frailty phenotypes with age as a covariate determined nonfrail recorded less sedentary time, participated in more light-intensity physical activity and accumulated more steps compared with frail (Table 2). Also, self-reported physical activity was lower in frail compared with the nonfrail and prefrail phenotypes (Table 2). However, higher self-reported physical activity was reported in PD compared with non-PD, although the other physical activity variables did not differ between disease groups (Table 2).

3.1. Physical Activity and Frailty. In PD, no physical activity variables were significantly related to frailty ($P > 0.29$); however, daily dose of carbidopa-levodopa, including both controlled-release and active-release forms, was correlated with frailty (r = 0.61; P = 0.01) (Figure 1). Other medication regimes for the management of PD and other comorbidities did not relate to frailty ($P > 0.42$). Physical activity variables demonstrated a significant linear relationship with increasing frailty severity in non-PD (Table 3). Those physical activity variables that were significantly different between frailty phenotypes (Table 3) were entered into individual regression models for non-PD. Low step, counts, higher sedentary behaviour, reduced light activity and lower weekly self-reported energy expenditure accounted for 83.3% of the variance (R = 0.913; P = 0.002; Figures 2(a)–2(d), but no single variable in this model best-determined frailty (P = 0.108 to 0.226).

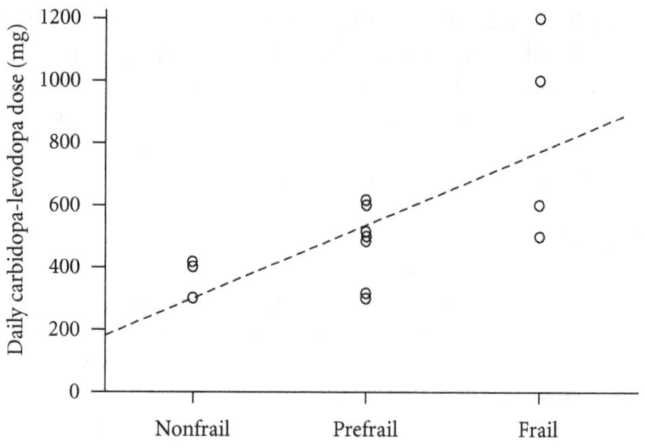

Figure 1: Relationship between frailty severity, measured by Cardiovascular Health Study frailty index, and daily carbidopa-levodopa dose (mg). Increased step count is positively correlated with greater frailty severity (r = 0.61) in females with PD. Females with PD are represented by the *open circles* and *dashed regression line*.

4. Discussion

This study examined the relationship between physical activity and frailty phenotype in community-dwelling females with PD and non-PD controls. Results of this study demonstrate physical activity (i.e., accelerometry counts and intensity, GPS, and self-reported) was not related to frailty phenotype in this sample group of females with PD; however, lower daily physical activity was associated with increased frailty severity in non-PD females. Current literature demonstrates physical inactivity as an important determinant of frailty phenotype [25], and persons with PD have reduced levels of accelerometry-assessed physical activity compared to non-PD controls [26]. This study suggests daily physical activity participation may not be the primary factor associated with frailty phenotype in females with PD. It is unclear from our cross-sectional data if a causal relationship exists between physical activity and frailty. However, results presented here support future longitudinal investigation into how PD progression impacts physical activity and how these changes in symptom expression and physical activity influence physical frailty.

4.1. Physical Activity: Not Related to Frailty Phenotype in PD. No relationship was demonstrated between daily physical activity and frailty phenotype in these females with PD. Although PD progression eventually debilitates motor performance, it is not likely to be the primary contributing factor to frailty in these females with PD. The results presented here do not necessarily exclude the contribution of physical activity to frailty, but rather suggest disease management may be a greater contributor to frailty. There is considerable variation in the manifestation of PD symptoms,

Table 1: Participant characteristics across frailty phenotypes in PD and non-PD females.

	PD			Non-PD		
	Nonfrail	Prefrail	Frail	Nonfrail	Prefrail	Frail
N	4	7	4	8	4	3
Age	69 ± 1	65 ± 10	63 ± 11	63 ± 8[ab]	79 ± 14[b]	90 ± 6
Body mass index (kg/m^2)	26.31 ± 5.6	22.95 ± 4.3	25.06 ± 4.3	23.20 ± 5.7	34.60 ± 5.4	32.49 ± 12.2
Number of medications	4.0 ± 2.0	2.9 ± 1.5	3.3 ± 2.6	1.3 ± 1.3	6.0 ± 4.2	5.3 ± 0.6
mg carbidopa-levodopa per day	366.67 ± 57.7	571.43 ± 340.2	825.00 ± 330.4			
carbidopa-levodopa only (N)	2	3	2			
carbidopa-levodopa + pram (N)	2	2	0			
carbidopa-levodopa + enta (N)	0	0	1			
carbidopa-levodopa + enta + pram (N)	0	1	1			
carbidopa-levodopa + aman + rop (N)	0	1	0			
Hoehn & Yahr disease severity	1.83 ± 0.8	1.86 ± 0.6	2.50 ± 0.4			

PD: Parkinson's disease, N: number, kg: kilogram, m: meter, mg: milligram, pram: pramipexole, enta: entacapone, aman, amantadine, and rop: ropinirole.
[a]Significantly different from prefrail.
[b]Significantly different from frail.

Table 2: Main effects on physical activity variables.

	PD	Non-PD	Nonfrail	Prefrail	Frail
Number	15	15	12	11	7
Total steps	3476 ± 2814	3731 ± 3827	5624 ± 3309[a]	3019 ± 3290	1636 ± 1599
% time spent sedentary	61.7 ± 14.1	60.9 ± 16.6	49.39 ± 9.5[a]	66.4 ± 14.6	71.9 ± 11.3
% time at light activity	32.2 ± 10.6	31.7 ± 10.6	39.4 ± 7.4[a]	28.6 ± 10.2	25.2 ± 8.2
MLTA questionnaire	3052.3 ± 1611.6[b]	2015.0 ± 1517.4	3045.0 ± 1096.2[a]	2826.4 ± 1790.4[a]	1196.1 ± 1493.7

Analysis adjusted for age.
%: percent, MLTA: Minnesota Leisure Time Activity, and PD: Parkinson's disease.
[a]Significantly different from frail, $P < 0.05$.
[b]Significantly different from non-PD, $P = 0.03$.

Table 3: The relationship of physical activity variables to frailty severity in non-PD females.

	ANOVA	Spearman correlation		Linear regression	
	Main effect (P)	Correlation coefficient (r)	Significance (P)	Beta coefficient (β)	Significance (P)
Accelerometer: total counts					
Total steps counts*	0.046	−0.79	0.001	1.113	0.202
Total activity counts	NS	−0.75	0.001		
Total activity time (min)	NS	−0.59	0.001		
Accelerometer: intensity					
% time spent sedentary*	0.002	0.84	0.000	2.602	0.110
% time at light activity*	0.012	−0.82	0.000	1.225	0.226
% time at MV activity	NS	−0.81	0.000		
GPS					
Total distance travelled (km)	NS	−0.63	0.012		
Average travel speed (km/h)	NS	−0.58	0.023		
Physical activity time (min)	NS	−0.54	0.036		
Self-reported activity					
MLTA questionnaire (kcal/week)*	0.007	−0.82	0.000	−0.386	0.108

%: percentage; GPS: global positioning system; h: hour; kcal: kilocalories; km: kilometers; MLTA: Minnesota Leisure Time Activity; min: minutes; MV: moderate-vigorous; PD: Parkinson's disease; NS: nonsignificant ($P > 0.05$).
*Significant main effects, therefore included in regression model.

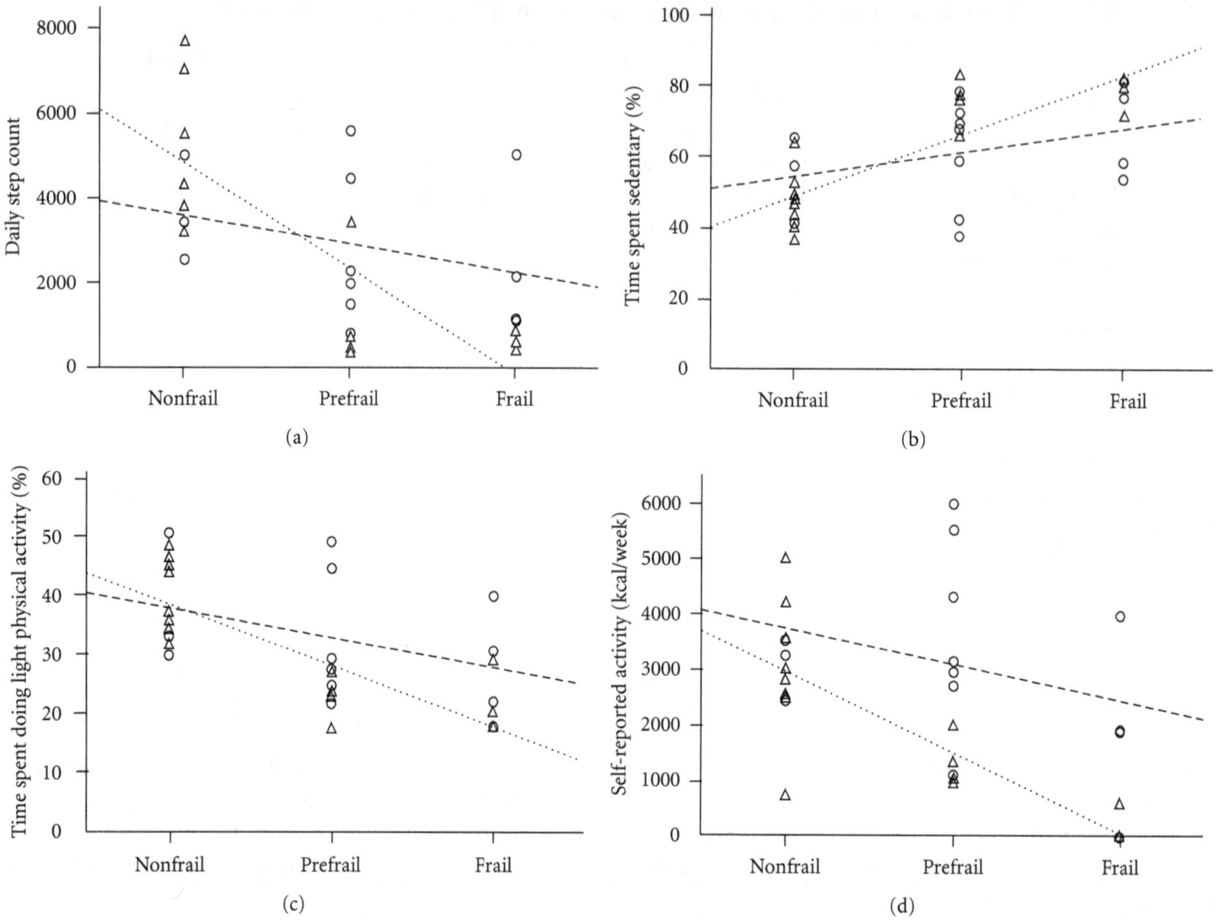

FIGURE 2: Relationship between frailty severity and: (a) daily step count. Total daily step count was negatively correlated with frailty severity ($r = -0.79$) in females without PD; (b) accumulated daily sedentary time. Sedentary time was positively correlated with frailty severity ($r = 0.84$) in females without PD; (c) accumulated light physical activity time. Light activity time was negatively correlated with frailty severity ($r = -0.82$) in females without PD; (d) self-reported leisure activity. Self-reported activity was negatively correlated with greater frailty severity ($r = -0.82$) in females without PD. Females with PD are represented by the *open circle* and *dashed regression line*; females without PD are represented by *the open triangle* and *dotted regression line.*

which necessitates further large-scale investigation into PD-related contributors to frailty over the disease course. During the first 10 years of the disease, symptoms such as akinesia and festinating gait may not have progressed to the point at which they inhibit physical activity participation, which was the case with these participants [27]. In the initial stages of the disease, slowness to execute day-to-day activities (i.e., bradykinesia) is more common, and this likely contributes to perceived exhaustion, which is a criterion for frailty. Thus, in community-dwelling persons with PD, self-reported exhaustion resulting from PD symptoms contributes to frailty [10], rather than reduced daily physical activity.

Results of this study indicate that although physical activity was not related to frailty in PD, females with PD self-reported greater leisure time activities compared to non-PD controls, regardless of frailty severity. This finding argues against previous research that states community-dwelling persons with PD have significantly less daily physical activity energy expenditure (measured using MLTA questionnaire) compared with controls, although the study sample included only males [28]. We speculate that increased self-reported leisure activity in these females with PD is due to the benefits of physical exercise being well recognized in the PD population to improve motor performance, functional and cognitive ability, safety, and confidence in ADL [27]. Persons living with PD are constantly encouraged to remain active despite disease-associated barriers (i.e., exhaustion) [29, 30]. Previous study demonstrated older adults with an increased risk of mortality, like persons with PD, adhere better to exercise programs compared to general community-dwelling older adults [31]. Therefore, we speculate that persons with PD may be involved in more physical activity and adhere better to exercise recommendations compared with community-dwelling counterparts because of PD-associated disease symptoms, regardless of frailty phenotype.

Unlike females with PD, physical activity influences frailty severity in community-dwelling females without PD. The importance of dedicating a greater percentage of daytime hours to light-intensity activities and decreasing sedentary time is highlighted in community-dwelling females.

Sedentary time was related to increased frailty in females without PD, likely through its influence on physiological decline (i.e., decreased fitness), leading to greater dependence [32]. The contribution of physical activity to frailty in females without PD may be attributed to reduced mobility, less activity intensity and restricted life-space (i.e., the spatial area a person moves through during daily life) [33, 34]. These physical and environmental challenges contribute to further reductions in physical activity and exacerbate declining functional reserves [35], encouraging transition to greater frailty severity. Remaining active during old age is important as sedentary lifestyle significantly increases risk of developing multiple chronic diseases and premature mortality [35]. Disease prevalence and functional impairment increases with age [36], which places the older adult at greater risk of frailty [5]. However, it is unclear whether age and age-related characteristics are associated with frailty in females with PD. This sample was randomly recruited from a population of females living independently in their own homes. Persons with PD seek institutional care sooner than non-PD counterparts [37], suggesting they may reach frailty sooner. Future longitudinal research may investigate onset of frailty in females with PD and follow frailty progression throughout the disease course. Also, further information on the contribution of physical activity to frailty onset and progression in PD is needed.

4.2. The Relationship between PD Management and Frailty. Accelerometers have been used in several research fields to monitor daily physical activity; monitoring of steps using waist-born accelerometers is feasible in PD populations and provides useful feedback on freezing (i.e., sudden inability to move, especially in the legs during walking), as well as long-term daily activity. Results of this study indicate that daily physical activity does not contribute to frailty phenotype in community-dwelling females with PD; however, daily carbidopa-levodopa dose was significantly related to frailty. Medication regimes for participants in this study included medications for the management of PD (i.e., carbidopa-levodopa, entacapone, pramipexole, amantadine, and ropinerole) and other conditions, such as anxiety/depression, blood pressure, migraine, muscle pain and inflammation, postmenopause symptoms, and difficulty sleeping. Multiple medication use in PD is associated with functional decline and high fall risk [38]; both of which are indicative of frailty. In addition, dopamine deficiency in PD may result in physical exhaustion [39], increasing ADL dependence risk for frailty. Therefore, the impact of PD medication regime on physical function and frailty requires further inquiry.

In addition to motor impairments, persons with PD face secondary symptoms that impact basic daily function, such as depression, cognitive impairments, and nonmotor symptoms that increase functional dependence through increased anxiety, social isolation, and confusion [40]. Cognition is considered an important component of frailty [41] and is also associated with adverse PD outcomes [40]. Cognitive function can be influenced by depression and physical decline, and females with PD report greater incidence of both compared with males [14]. Also, females with PD report greater symptom-related stress and sleep disturbances than males [42, 43]. The importance of these non-motor symptoms cannot be underestimated, however they are beyond the scope of this study. Future research should consider how PD symptoms (motor and non-motor), disease severity, duration, other comorbidities, polypharmacy, and age impact frailty severity in both males and females with PD.

4.3. Implications

4.3.1. Community-Dwelling Populations and Neurological Disorders. The progressive nature of PD and related symptoms such as bradykinesia and tremor causes persons with PD to seek long-term care earlier than the general older adult population [37]. Females with PD may be more vulnerable to frailty than persons without neurological disorder because of PD-related systems that exacerbate the frailty phenotype. Therefore, it is important to make an early identification of frailty in community dwelling persons, especially those with neurological disorder who express a frailty phenotype earlier than the general population.

4.3.2. Frailty Management. Physical inactivity is directly linked to declining physiological reserve capacity, defined as adaptive responses (i.e., heart rate, blood pressure, respiration) that enable us to perform tasks or overcome external stresses [44]. In persons with PD the complexity of symptom presentation results in a reduced adaptive capacity. These losses of adaptive capacity, related to aging or disease, lead to declining functional independence and are a determinant of frailty [25]. Comorbidities and clinical symptoms interact between frailty and PD making identification of frailty in persons with PD challenging to diagnose [11]. Few studies have examined how to accurately identify frailty in this population [45, 46]. Early identification of frailty in persons with PD is relevant since over half of older adults living independently in their own homes are at-risk for frailty and subsequent functional decline [6]. Due to the transitional nature of both frailty and PD, the majority of disease progression occurs long before the individual requires institutional care [47]. As PD severity increases, symptoms become aggravated, further exacerbating underlying frailty [46]. Awareness of frailty during the initial stages of PD development may contribute to improved management strategies that delay and/or reverse frailty factors and preserve functional independence [6]. This study demonstrated that frailty was related to decreased physical activity in community-dwelling non-PD, and symptom management in PD females. Knowledge gained from the current study can be used to inform effective strategies for identifying prefrailty in non-PD females. This information can be applied to the development and delivery of timely support that addresses age- and disease-associated declines in function. Preventing functional decline has important implications for healthcare resource use in PD and non-PD older adults, as well as reducing physical, emotional, social, and financial problems attributed to frailty [25].

Currently, there is little evidence on how PD specifically impacts females and contributes to increased risk of frailty. Greater risk of frailty may be a consequence of greater functional declines [10], distress, and cognitive impairment [41], all resulting in ADL dependence [8]. In females with PD, physical activity participation should be aimed at managing PD symptoms. Managing PD symptoms, through physical activity and medication, will incidentally contribute to frailty management. Emphasis, therefore, should be placed on managing frailty within the context of PD symptoms [11]. Further collaboration is crucial between neurological, geriatric practice, and physical therapy/rehabilitation in terms of frailty assessment, progression, and addressing complications resulting in declining physical activity that may culminate in frailty.

5. Conclusion

Physical activity influences frailty expression in older females without PD, surprisingly no relationship between physical activity and frailty was found in our sample of females with PD. In PD, disease management may better indicate frailty severity. Further study is warranted to establish how PD-associated characteristics (i.e., polypharmacy) contribute to frailty and how physical activity participation interplays with the complex progress of frailty within PD. This study suggests PD-associated symptoms motivate community-dwelling females with PD to engage in leisure-time physical activities. Considering its vast impact in the community and on healthcare resources, identification of early frailty and management of resulting disability remains a priority area for geriatric research. Ultimately, enabling older adults to remain physically active promotes independence in ADL and empowers positive aging, albeit it may not protect females with PD from becoming frail.

Acknowledgments

The authors would like to thank the participants for generously donating their time and contributing to this investigation. K. P. Roland is funded by the Canadian Institute of Health Research (CIHR) and Parkinson Society Canada's Psychosocial Doctoral Research Award.

References

[1] H. Bergman, F. Béland, S. Karunananthan, S. Hummel, D. Hogan, and C. Wolfson, "Development of a framework for understanding and studying frailty," *Gerontologie et Societe*, vol. 109, no. 2, pp. 15–29, 2004.

[2] L. L. Borges and R. L. Menezes, "Definitions and markers of frailty: a systematic review of literature," *Reviews in Clinical Gerontology*, vol. 21, no. 1, pp. 67–77, 2011.

[3] M. J. Levers, C. A. Estabrooks, and J. C. Ross Kerr, "Factors contributing to frailty: literature review," *Journal of Advanced Nursing*, vol. 56, no. 3, pp. 282–291, 2006.

[4] H. E. Whitson, J. L. Purser, and H. J. Cohen, "Frailty thy name is... Phrailty?" *Journals of Gerontology*, vol. 62, no. 7, pp. 728–730, 2007.

[5] L. P. Fried, C. M. Tangen, J. Walston et al., "Frailty in older adults: evidence for a phenotype," *Journals of Gerontology*, vol. 56, no. 3, pp. M146–M156, 2001.

[6] T. M. Gill, E. A. Gahbauer, H. G. Allore, and L. Han, "Transitions between frailty states among community-living older persons," *Archives of Internal Medicine*, vol. 166, no. 4, pp. 418–423, 2006.

[7] M. T. E. Puts, P. Lips, and D. J. H. Deeg, "Sex differences in the risk of frailty for mortality independent of disability and chronic diseases," *Journal of the American Geriatrics Society*, vol. 53, no. 1, pp. 40–47, 2005.

[8] S. G. Leveille, B. W. J. H. Penninx, D. Melzer, G. Izmirlian, and J. M. Guralnik, "Sex differences in the prevalence of mobility disability in old age: the dynamics of incidence, recovery, and mortality," *Journals of Gerontology*, vol. 55, no. 1, pp. S41–S50, 2000.

[9] A. B. Mitnitski, X. Song, and K. Rockwood, "The estimation of relative fitness and frailty in community-dwelling older adults using self-report data," *Journals of Gerontology*, vol. 59, no. 6, pp. M627–M632, 2004.

[10] K. P. Roland, J. M. Jakobi, C. Powell, and G. R. Jones, "Quality of life as a determinant of frailty phenotype in persons with Parkinson's disease," *Journal of the American Geriatrics Society*, vol. 60, no. 3, pp. 590–592, 2012.

[11] C. Powell, "Frailty and Parkinson's disease: theories and clinical implications," *Parkinsonism and Related Disorders*, vol. 14, no. 4, pp. 271–272, 2008.

[12] D. Twelves, K. S. M. Perkins, and C. Counsell, "Systematic review of incidence studies of Parkinson's disease," *Movement Disorders*, vol. 18, no. 1, pp. 19–31, 2003.

[13] L. M. Shulman, "Gender differences in Parkinson's disease," *Gender Medicine*, vol. 4, no. 1, pp. 8–18, 2007.

[14] Y. Baba, J. D. Putzke, N. R. Whaley, Z. K. Wszolek, and R. J. Uitti, "Gender and the Parkinson's disease phenotype," *Journal of Neurology*, vol. 252, no. 10, pp. 1201–1205, 2005.

[15] K. P. Roland, J. M. Jakobi, C. Powell, and G. R. Jones, "Factors related to functional independence in females with Parkinson's disease: a systematic review," *Maturitas*, vol. 69, no. 4, pp. 304–311, 2011.

[16] C. E. Garber and J. H. Friedman, "Effects of fatigue on physical activity and function in patients with Parkinson's disease," *Neurology*, vol. 60, no. 7, pp. 1119–1124, 2003.

[17] J. Grace, A. Mendelsohn, and J. H. Friedman, "A comparison of fatigue measures in Parkinson's disease," *Parkinsonism and Related Disorders*, vol. 13, no. 7, pp. 443–445, 2007.

[18] M. Nallegowda, U. Singh, G. Handa et al., "Role of sensory input and muscle strength in maintenance of balance, gait, and posture in Parkinson's disease: a pilot study," *American Journal of Physical Medicine and Rehabilitation*, vol. 83, no. 12, pp. 898–908, 2004.

[19] M. D. Rothman, L. Leo-Summers, and T. M. Gill, "Prognostic significance of potential frailty criteria," *Journal of the American Geriatrics Society*, vol. 56, no. 12, pp. 2211–2216, 2008.

[20] B. Dijkstra, Y. Kamsma, and W. Zijlstra, "Detection of gait and postures using a miniaturised triaxial accelerometer-based system: accuracy in community-dwelling older adults," *Age and Ageing*, vol. 39, no. 2, Article ID afp249, pp. 259–262, 2010.

[21] J. L. Copeland and D. W. Esliger, "Accelerometer assessment of physical activity in active, healthy older adults," *Journal of Aging and Physical Activity*, vol. 17, no. 1, pp. 17–30, 2009.

[22] S. C. Webber and M. M. Porter, "Monitoring mobility in older adults using global positioning system (GPS) watches and accelerometers: a feasibility study," *Journal of Aging and Physical Activity*, vol. 17, no. 4, pp. 455–467, 2009.

[23] K. Karnik and D. J. Mazzatti, "Review of tools and technologies to assess multi-system functional impairment and frailty," *Clinical Medicine: Geriatrics*, vol. 2009, no. 3, pp. 1–8, 2009.

[24] H. L. Taylor, D. R. Jacobs, and B. Schucker, "A questionnaire for the assessment of leisure time physical activities," *Journal of Chronic Diseases*, vol. 31, no. 12, pp. 741–755, 1978.

[25] T. M. Gill, D. I. Baker, M. Gottschalk, P. N. Peduzzi, H. Allore, and A. Byers, "A program to prevent functional decline in physically frail, elderly persons who live at home," *New England Journal of Medicine*, vol. 347, no. 14, pp. 1068–1074, 2002.

[26] M. Fujikane, S. Katayama, K. Hirata, and N. Yokota, "Objective measurement of motor activity in Parkinson's disease by actigraphy. Clinical assessment of akinesia," *Nippon Rinsho*, vol. 55, no. 1, pp. 153–157, 1997.

[27] M. E. Morris, "Movement disorders in people with parkinson disease: a model for physical therapy," *Physical Therapy*, vol. 80, no. 6, pp. 578–597, 2000.

[28] M. J. Toth, P. S. Fishman, and E. T. Poehlman, "Free-living daily energy expenditure in patients with Parkinson's disease," *Neurology*, vol. 48, no. 1, pp. 88–91, 1997.

[29] Parkinson Society Canada (PSC), "Exercise for people with Parkinson"," 2003, Retrieved from http://www.parkinson.ca/atf/cf/{9EBD08A9-7886-4B2D-A1C4-A131E7096BF8}/Exercise%20updated%20English%202010.pdf.

[30] C. Shaw, "Parkinson's disease exercise? Why not!," Vancouver Coastal Health, Catalogue # FM.490.P229.

[31] M. C. Morey, C. F. Pieper, G. M. Crowley, R. J. Sullivan, and C. M. Puglisi, "Exercise adherence and 10-year mortality in chronically Ill older adults," *Journal of the American Geriatrics Society*, vol. 50, no. 12, pp. 1929–1933, 2002.

[32] W. J. Chodzko-Zajko, D. N. Proctor, M. A. Fiatarone Singh et al., "Exercise and physical activity for older adults," *Medicine and Science in Sports and Exercise*, vol. 41, no. 7, pp. 1510–1530, 2009.

[33] N. Fallah, A. Mitnitski, S. D. Searle, E. A. Gahbauer, T. M. Gill, and K. Rockwood, "Transitions in frailty status in older adults in relation to mobility: a multistate modeling approach employing a deficit count," *Journal of the American Geriatrics Society*, vol. 59, no. 3, pp. 524–529, 2011.

[34] P. S. Baker, E. V. Bodner, and R. M. Allman, "Measuring life-space mobility in community-dwelling older adults," *Journal of the American Geriatrics Society*, vol. 51, no. 11, pp. 1610–1614, 2003.

[35] Q. L. Xue, L. P. Fried, T. A. Glass, A. Laffan, and P. H. M. Chaves, "Life-space constriction, development of frailty, and the competing risk of mortality: the women's health and aging study I," *American Journal of Epidemiology*, vol. 167, no. 2, pp. 240–248, 2008.

[36] K. Rockwood, R. A. Fox, P. Stolee, D. Robertson, and B. L. Beattie, "Frailty in elderly people: an evolving concept," *Canadian Medical Association Journal*, vol. 150, no. 4, pp. 489–495, 1994.

[37] D. Aarsland, J. P. Larsen, E. Tandberg, and K. Laake, "Predictors of nursing home placement in Parkinson's disease: a population-based, prospective study," *Journal of the American Geriatrics Society*, vol. 48, no. 8, pp. 938–942, 2000.

[38] A. Ashburn, E. Stack, R. M. Pickering, and C. D. Ward, "A community-dwelling sample of people with Parkinson's disease: characteristics of fallers and non-fallers," *Age and Ageing*, vol. 30, no. 1, pp. 47–52, 2001.

[39] J. S. Lou, G. Kearns, T. Benice, B. Oken, G. Sexton, and J. Nutt, "Levodopa improves physical fatigue in Parkinson's disease: a double-blind, placebo controlled, crossover study," *Movement Disorders*, vol. 18, no. 10, pp. 1108–1114, 2003.

[40] R. Shibley, H. J. Griffin, N. P. Quinn, and M. Jahanshahi, "Quality of life in Parkinson's disease: the relative importance of the symptoms," *Movement Disorders*, vol. 23, no. 10, pp. 1428–1434, 2008.

[41] J. A. Ávila-Funes, H. Amieva, P. Barberger-Gateau et al., "Cognitive impairment improves the predictive validity of the phenotype of frailty for adverse health outcomes: the three-city study," *Journal of the American Geriatrics Society*, vol. 57, no. 3, pp. 453–461, 2009.

[42] B. Scott, A. Borgman, H. Engler, B. Johnels, and S. M. Aquilonius, "Gender differences in Parkinson's disease symptom profile," *Acta Neurologica Scandinavica*, vol. 102, no. 1, pp. 37–43, 2000.

[43] M. C. Smith, H. Ellgring, and W. H. Oertel, "Sleep disturbances in Parkinson's disease patients and spouses," *Journal of the American Geriatrics Society*, vol. 45, no. 2, pp. 194–199, 1997.

[44] L. A. Lipsitz, "Physiological complexity, aging, and the path to frailty," *Science of Aging Knowledge Environment*, vol. 2004, no. 16, article pe16, 2004.

[45] N. N. Ahmed, S. J. Sherman, and D. VanWyck, "Frailty in Parkinson's disease and its clinical implications," *Parkinsonism and Related Disorders*, vol. 14, no. 4, pp. 334–337, 2008.

[46] F. Lauretani, M. Maggio, C. Silvestrini, A. Nardelli, M. Saccavini, and G. P. Ceda, "Parkinson's disease (PD) in the elderly: an example of geriatric syndrome (GS)?" *Archives of Gerontology and Geriatrics*, vol. 54, pp. 242–246, 2012.

[47] W. J. Mutch, A. Strudwick, S. K. Roy, and A. W. Downie, "Parkinson's disease: disability, review, and management," *British Medical Journal*, vol. 293, no. 6548, pp. 675–677, 1986.

14

Resistance Training and Older Adults with Type 2 Diabetes Mellitus: Strength of the Evidence

Nina Hovanec,[1] Anuradha Sawant,[2] Tom J. Overend,[2] Robert J. Petrella,[3] and Anthony A. Vandervoort[2]

[1] *Health and Rehabilitation Sciences Graduate Program, Western University, London, ON, Canada N6G 1H1*
[2] *School of Physical Therapy and Center for Physical Activity and Aging, Faculty of Health Sciences, Western University, London, ON, Canada N6G 1H1*
[3] *Department of Family Medicine, Western University, London, ON, Canada N6G 1H1*

Correspondence should be addressed to Anthony A. Vandervoort, vandervo@uwo.ca

Academic Editor: Bijan Najafi

Objective. This paper analyzes the effects of resistance training (RT) on metabolic, neuromuscular, and cardiovascular functions in older adults (mean age ≥ 65 years) with type 2 diabetes (T2DM). *Research Design and Methods.* A systematic review conducted by two reviewers of the published literature produced 3 records based on 2 randomized controlled trials that assessed the effect of RT on disease process measures and musculoskeletal/body composition measures. Statistical, Comprehensive Meta-Analysis (version 2) software was used to compute Hedge's g, and results were calculated using the random effects model to account for methodological differences amongst studies. *Results.* Largest effect of RT was seen on muscle strength; especially lower body strength, while the point estimate effect on body composition was small and not statistically significant. The cumulative point estimate for the T2DM disease process measures was moderate and statistically significant. *Conclusions.* RT generally had a positive effect on musculoskeletal, body composition, and T2DM disease processes measures, with tentative conclusions based on a low number of completed RCTs. Thus, more research is needed on such programs for older adults (≥65 years) with T2DM.

1. Introduction

Type 2 diabetes mellitus (T2DM) in older adults is an emerging epidemic [1]. (For the purpose of this paper, the term "older adults" refers to individuals who are at least 65 years old.) It is an age-prevalent metabolic disorder, characterized by insulin resistance with relative insulin deficiency [2, 3], with the highest prevalence found in individuals who are 80 years or older—an estimated number of 40 million is expected in the United States by the year 2050 [1].

Physical activity is considered to be a cornerstone of T2DM prevention and management [2, 4], and it is important to have accurate information for health care organizations to integrate into their knowledge management strategies [5]. Physical activity refers to "the expenditure of energy above that of resting by contraction of skeletal muscle to produce bodily movement," while exercise is "a type of physical activity that involves planned, structured and repetitive bodily movement performed for the purpose of improving physical fitness" [6, page 359]. Physical activity and exercise will be used interchangeably in this paper.

In terms of physical activity as a management method in populations living with T2DM, traditional focus has been given to aerobic training (AT) interventions [7, 8]. Aerobic training activates large muscle groups to perform activities such as swimming and running, increasing the function of the heart, lungs, and muscle mitochondria to meet the heightened oxygen demands, ultimately resulting in cardiorespiratory fitness improvements [9]. Over the past decade, interest has also emerged in conducting studies that assess the potential effect of resistance training (RT) interventions in older individuals with T2DM [10–12]. Resistance training activates the muscular system to generate force against a resistive load [4]; it can be performed by utilizing various exercise machines, lifting free-weights (e.g., dumbbells), or doing calisthenics such as situps, pushups, crunches, and lunges. If RT is performed regularly, where the weight lifted is increased to moderate (50% of 1RM

(1RM represents 1 Repetition Maximum, which refers to the maximum weight that a person can lift once)) and high levels of intensity (>75% 1RM), it often leads to increased muscle mass and improvements in muscular fitness [4, 13–15]. Muscular fitness refers both to muscle strength, the amount of force produced by a muscle, and muscle endurance, the ability of a muscle to "exert submaximal force for an extended period of time" [16, page 27].

Resistance training may be more appealing and feasible than AT for people with T2DM who are often overweight and sedentary [17], as well as for older adults, obese, and/or frail individuals [4, 12, 18]. With advanced age, there is a significant loss of muscle mass and strength, a phenomenon known as sarcopenia [19]. It has recently been indicated that older adults with T2DM tend to have greater muscle mass loss, worse muscle quality (defined as the amount of muscle strength per unit of regional muscle mass), reduced upper and lower body strength, greater visceral adipose content, as well as higher risk for functional decline and disability than their healthy, age-matched counterparts [20–24]. Resistance training might benefit older adults living with T2DM through muscle hypertrophy, enhanced muscle quality, strength gains for greater power development with more effective mobility function, and glycemic profile improvements [25].

Resistance training studies in populations with T2DM were not readily available prior to 1997 [4]. The first physical activity guidelines specifically designed for adults with T2DM were developed by the American College of Sports Medicine (ACSM) in the year 2000 [10]. As illustrated in Figure 1, a modified timeline first introduced by Hills and colleagues in 2010 [26], agencies such as the Canadian Diabetes Association (CDA), the American Diabetes Association (ADA), the Canadian Society for Exercise Physiology (CSEP), and ACSM now include RT recommendations within their physical activity guidelines [11, 27–37].

Due to the associated increases in blood pressure (BP) that may be harmful, there could be unsubstantiated apprehension in recommending RT, especially at higher intensities. The main concern is that these BP increases could lead to a stroke, myocardial ischemia, or retinal hemorrhage [4]. This may partially explain the historical dominance of AT interventions in populations living with T2DM. However, there is a lack of scientific evidence that RT actually increases any of the aforementioned risks, as no RT-related adverse events have been reported in studies where individuals with T2DM were assessed [4, 38]. Additionally, past researchers have suggested that RT may actually reduce BP levels [39–41]. Finally, there are precautions that can be employed to avoid potentially harmful side-effects of exercise, such as avoiding physical activity under certain circumstances (detailed by Gordon in 2002 [7]) and conducting appropriate preexercise screens and assessments [7, 35, 42].

Skeletal muscles are the largest postprandial glucose uptake and glycogen storage sites in the human body and as such are integral in maintaining glucose homeostasis. Resistance training may reverse or at least limit some of the aforementioned negative neuromuscular effects associated with aging and/or T2DM [43]. Previous meta-analyses have reported benefits of aerobic training, resistance training, or a combination of the two on reducing HbA1c levels, which signifies improved glycemic control [25, 38, 44–47]. A recent meta-analysis demonstrated that supervised aerobic or resistance training led to greater declines in HbA1c levels than exercise advice only [44]. However, no previous meta-analysis has assessed the effects of RT in older adults (≥65 years) with T2DM. At this time, the literature base may benefit from such a review, since older adults often experience detrimental neuromuscular and sensorimotor changes associated with aging (e.g., sarcopenia) placing them at an increased risk for mobility problems, injury from falls, and disability [21, 48]. Furthermore, T2DM is most common in older adults, who as a result of this disease often experience various comorbidities [49], further reducing their capacity to live independently (e.g., retinopathy, which may lead to blindness; peripheral neuropathy, which may lead to foot ulcers and amputations; nephropathy, which over time could result in renal failure, etc.). Thus, the purpose of this paper is to conduct a systematic review of the best available evidence, in order to assess the effect of RT on metabolic, neuromuscular, and cardiovascular functions in older adults with T2DM.

2. Methods

This meta-analysis utilized the PRISMA as a framework when selecting studies for inclusion in this paper [50]. This meta-analysis is not registered with any institution, such as the Cochrane Collaboration. The literature search was conducted until the end of August 2011, using electronic databases (Medline, EMBASE, AMED, PubMed, Scopus, CINAHL) that generated MESH terms based on the following keywords: resistance training, type 2 diabetes, and aged. The search terms were entered into the databases using the appropriate combinations of "OR" and "AND." In order for articles to be included in this paper, the following inclusion and exclusion criteria needed to be satisfied.

Inclusion Criteria

(i) RCTs.

(ii) Published between the years 2000 and 2011.

(iii) RT interventions or a combination of RT and other forms of intervention (e.g., flexibility, weight loss, standard care, etc.).

(iv) Participants with established T2DM.

(v) Participants' mean age ≥65 years.

Exclusion Criteria

(i) Participants with the presence of another chronic illness (e.g., cancer).

(ii) Non-English publications.

(iii) Studies reporting effect of RT in previously trained participants.

Table 1: Outcome measures.

Body composition measures	Musculoskeletal measures	Type 2 diabetes process measures
		Fasting glucose (mmol/L)
	Muscle strength (i) Upper body strength (ii) Lower body strength	Glycosylated hemoglobin (HbA1c) (%)
Whole body lean tissue mass (kg)	Muscle quality (defined as 1RM strength kg/unit lean body mass kg)	Blood pressure Serum/fasting insulin (pmol/L)
Whole body fat mass (kg)		
	Muscle fiber size (i) Type I cross sectional area (CSA) (μm^2) (ii) Type II CSA (μm^2)	Lipids (i) Total cholesterol (mmol/L) (ii) HDL cholesterol (mmol) (iii) Triglycerides (iv) Free fatty acids (FFAs) (μmol/L)

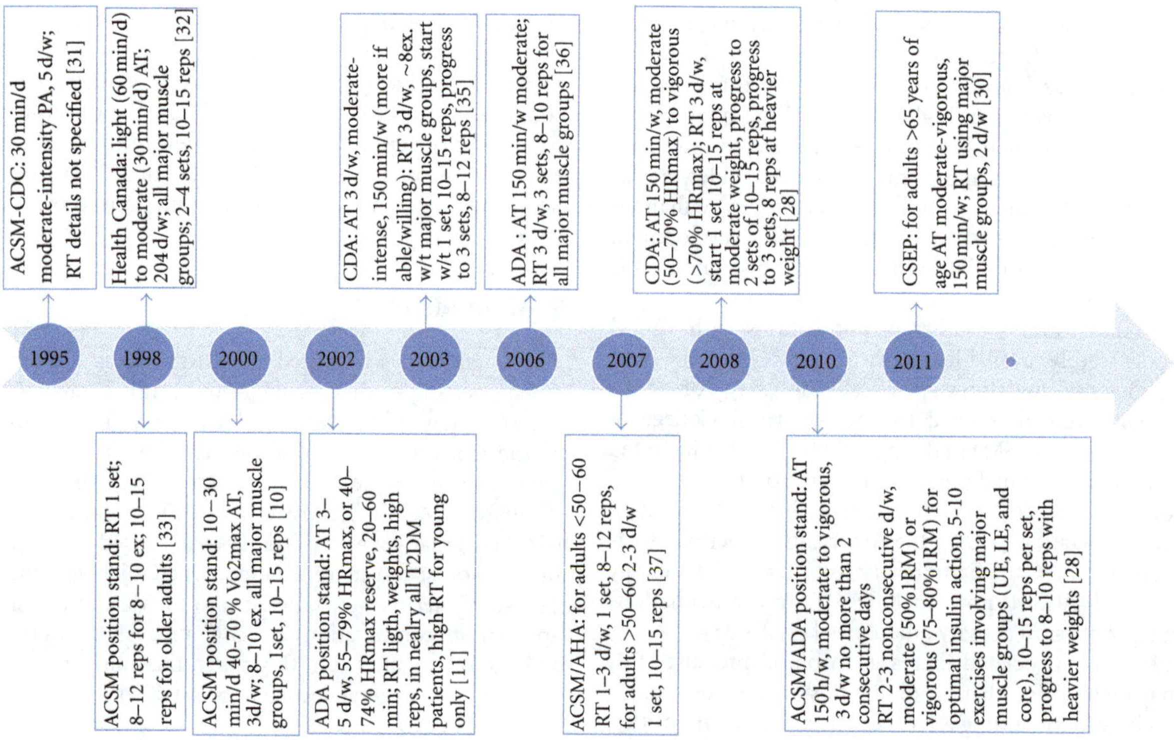

Figure 1: Chronological Timeline of PA Recommendations for T2DM from Various Professional Organizations [modified from [26]]. PHAC [Public Health Agency of Canada]; CSEP [Canadian Society for Exercise Physiology]; CDA [Canadian Diabetes Association]; ACSM [American College of Sports Medicine]; ADA [American Diabetes Association]; CDC [Centers for Disease Control and Prevention]; AHA [American Heart Association]. PA [Physical Activity]; RT [resistance training]; AT [aerobic training]; UE [upper extremity]; LE [lower extremity]; HR_{max} [maximum heart rate]; $VO_{2\,max}$ [maximal oxygen uptake/consumption]; d [days]; w [week]; w/t [with]; reps [repetitions]; ex [exercises]; h [hour]; min. [minute].

(iv) Studies reporting effect of RT on outcome measures not relevant to this paper (see Table 1 for all relevant outcome measures).

The aforementioned inclusion and exclusion criteria were developed in order to obtain the most recent (2000–2011), scientifically rigorous (RCTs) evidence on the specific effect of resistance training in older adults with type 2 diabetes. Various studies, review articles, and commentaries that did not satisfy the inclusion criteria were used to inform the introduction and the discussion sections of this paper. Furthermore, NH and AS independently reviewed and rated the articles and any differences were resolved by discussion or by comparison to the ratings provided on the PEDro website. To limit redundancy, Cohen's Kappa values were not calculated since there were no major disagreements between the authors (i.e., >95% agreement).

Outcome Measures. The primary outcome measures were grouped into three major areas including body composition, musculoskeletal, and type 2 diabetes disease process measures. Table 1 summarizes the major outcome headings and their respective measures.

Methodological Quality of the Studies. Internal validity of studies included in this paper was assessed using the PEDro

Table 2: Participant characteristics.

Source	Group (n)	Age (years)	Gender (M/F)	Whole body fat mass (kg)	BMI (kg/m^2)	Diabetes duration (years)	HbA1c (%)	Fasting glucose (mmol/L)	Fasting insulin (pmol/L)
*Brooks et al. [17]	Exercise 31	66 ± 11.1	10/21	35 ± 5.6	30.9 ± 6.1	8 ± 5.6	8.7 ± 5.6	8.79 ± 2.7	116 ± 167.4
Castaneda et al. [13]	Control 31	66 ± 5.6	19/12	33.7 ± 13.4	31.2 ± 5.6	11 ± 5.6	8.4 ± 1.7	9.85 ± 3.8	115 ± 176.9
Dunstan et al. [53]	Exercise 16	67.6 ± 5.2	10/6	33.1 ± 7.4	31.5 ± 3.7	7.6 ± 5.4	8.1 ± 1	9.5 ± 2.3	132.9 ± 63
	Control 13	66.5 ± 5.3	6/7	35.6 ± 6.8	32.5 ± 3.8	8.8 ± 7.9	7.5 ± 1.1	9.4 ± 2.1	101.9 ± 25.8

All measures are provided as means ± SD.
*Brooks et al. [17] and Castaneda et al. [13] included the same cohort of participants.

scale—a valid [51] and reliable [52] tool to evaluate study quality. Article ratings are included as PEDro scores listed in Table 3, while rating criteria are detailed in Table 5.

Statistical Analyses. Statistical software (Comprehensive Meta-Analysis—version 2) for meta-analysis of binary, continuous, and diagnostic data was used for computation of Hedge's g (a measure of effect size). Hedge's g values were used to assess the influence of strengthening exercises on body composition, musculoskeletal measures, and type 2 diabetes disease outcomes (previously summarized in Table 1). The effect sizes were interpreted as small, medium and large if they were 0.2, 0.5, and 0.8, respectively [54]. A 95% confidence interval was constructed around the point estimate of the effect size. Any standard errors that were reported by study authors were converted to standard deviations using the formula SD = $\sqrt{n} * \text{SE}$, where SD is the standard deviation, $\surd$ is the square root symbol, n refers to the sample size, $*$ represents the multiplication function, and SE is the standard error [55].

The statistical significance of the differences in the effects of RT on body composition, muscle quality, and strength along with moderator variables included for the effect on disease processes was computed by Page's L statistic with the use of PASW 18 statistical software to calculate the sum of squares (SS) between groups, as well as total SS. Page's L statistic was then calculated using the formula $L = [N - 1]r^2$, where N is the total number of effect sizes and r^2 is the product of $SS_{between}/SS_{total}$. (Further details regarding Page's L statistic can be found in [56]) When performing meta-analysis, the overall effect of an intervention can be influenced by use of particular outcome measures or intervention strategies. Page's L statistics was utilized to elucidate such differences in the current study.

The presence of heterogeneity among the moderator variables was evaluated by the Q statistic using a random effects model. The studies were considered heterogeneous if the P value of the Q statistic was <0.1, which has been proposed as the appropriate alternative to the conventional $P < 0.05$, when there is a low number of articles included in a review [57]. Publication bias was not assessed, since there were only three articles included, and any conclusions that are drawn from the results that emerge from this meta-analysis cannot be taken as definitive. The robustness of the findings was established based on the assessment of the effect size and its associated confidence intervals, rather than other methods, such as the calculation of Fail Safe N, which can lead to widely varied estimates [58]. The results reported were calculated using the random effects model, in order to account for methodological differences amongst studies. The statistical significance for the effect sizes' statistical tests (i.e., Hedge's g) was set at $P < 0.05$.

3. Results

Three [13, 17, 53] of the 446 citations were included in the final analysis (Figure 2). However, 2 of the citations [13, 17] are technically considered one study, since their findings are based on the same pool of participants, but they are both included in the meta-analysis since each of them provides relevant but different outcome measures. A total of 32 effect sizes, evaluating the effect of strength training on the disease process (20 effect sizes) and muscle quality (12 effect sizes), were extracted from the included studies. Participant and study characteristics are described in Tables 2 and 3 respectively.

3.1. Effect of RT on T2DM Disease Process Measures. Serum insulin [17, 53], HbA1c [17, 53], HDL [13, 53], LDL and total cholesterol [13, 53], fasting glucose [17, 53], and BP [13, 53] were analysed to evaluate the effect of RT on the disease process. The overall cumulative point estimate of this effect size was statistically significant (Hedge's $g = -0.246$; $P = 0.023$; 95% CI: -0.458, -0.034).

For individual variables, the effect of RT on BP (Hedge's $g = -0.540$; $P < 0.001$; CI: -0.832, -0.248), insulin (Hedge's $g = 0.505$; $P = 0.016$; CI: 0.094, 0.916), total cholesterol, and LDL cholesterol (Hedge's $g = 22120.464$, $P = 0.002$; CI: -0.760, -0.169) was statistically significant. However, the effect of RT on fasting glucose (Hedge's $g = -0.121$; $P = 0.559$; CI: -0.526, 0.284), HbA1c (Hedge's $g = -0.463$; $P = 0.145$; CI: -1.084, 0.159), and HDL cholesterol (Hedge's $g = 0.134$; $P = 0.517$; CI: -0.271, 0.539) was not as consistent between studies in terms of magnitude of improvement and fluctuations in control group. Also, the differences in effects of RT on fasting glucose, insulin, HBA1c, cholesterol, HDL, FFA, and BP were not statistically significant ($L(19) = 14.109$; $P > 0.05$).

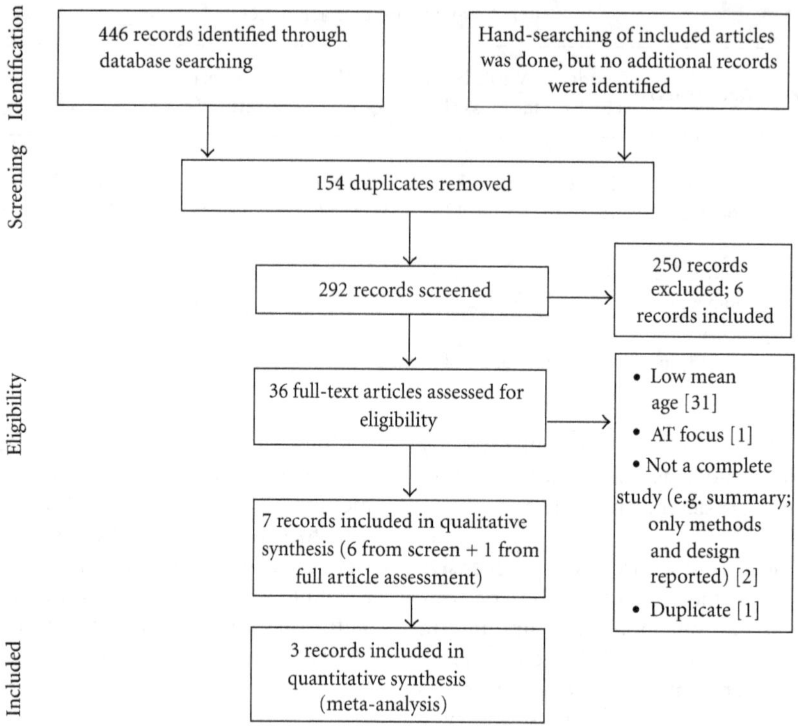

FIGURE 2: Study selection diagram [50] AT-aerobic training.

3.2. Effect of RT on Body Composition Measures. Lean body mass [17, 53] and fat body mass [53, 59] were analysed to evaluate the effect of RT on body composition. The cumulative point estimate effect of RT on body composition was small but not statistically significant (Hedge's $g = 0.199$; $P = 0.197$; CI: -0.103, 0.500). The effect of RT on lean body mass (Hedge's $g = 0.395$; $P = 0.220$; CI: -0.237, 1.028) was larger than on fat body mass (Hedge's $g = 0.066$; $P = 0.749$; CI: -0.339, 0.471), but neither was statistically significant.

3.3. Effect of RT on Musculoskeletal Measures. Whole body, lower and upper body muscles strength [13, 53], and muscle quality were analysed to evaluate the effect of RT on overall muscle strength and quality. The cumulative point estimate effect of RT on muscle strength (Hedge's $g = 1.05$; $P < 0.001$; 95% CI: 0.699, 1.404) and overall quality (Hedge's $g = 0.816$ $P = 0.008$; 95% CI: 0.216, 1.415) were large and statistically significant. The largest effect of RT was on lower body strength (Hedge's $g = 1.415$; $P < 0.001$; CI: 0.864, 1.967), followed by upper body strength (Hedge's $g = 0.974$; $P < 0.001$; CI: 0.453, 1.494), and both were statistically significant. The effect of RT on whole body strength was also large and statistically significant (Hedge's $g = 0.802$; $P = 0.002$; CI: 0.291, 1.313).

The effect of RT on muscle quality (Hedge's $g = 1.460$; $P < 0.001$; CI: 0.906, 2.015) was large and statistically significant. The differences in effect of RT on body composition, muscle quality, and strength were not statistically significant ($L(11) = 13.762$; $P > 0.05$). However, the CI ranges were wide for all measures (musculoskeletal, disease process, and body composition); as such any conclusion drawn based on the effect sizes and statistical significance needs to be considered with caution.

The heterogeneity (Q-values with their respective df and P values) for all moderator variables is summarized in Table 4. However, the number of studies included in the analysis is too small to infer definitive conclusions regarding heterogeneity.

4. Discussion

The purpose of this paper was to conduct a systematic review and meta-analysis of the currently available evidence, in order to assess the effect of resistance training in older adults with T2DM. The findings generally show that RT has an effect on the musculoskeletal system, disease process, and body composition to varying degrees (see Table 6 for a summary of the outcome measures, their respective effect sizes, and statistical significances). Overall, RT had the largest effect on the musculoskeletal measures, followed by disease process measures, while the smallest effect was seen on the body composition measures.

It is not surprising that RT had the largest effect on musculoskeletal measures, as it is a well-established mode of exercise to induce neuromuscular changes, such as increased muscle size and strength [15]. Specifically, findings from this analysis indicate that RT increases muscle strength and quality. These effects could be quite consequential for the investigated population, as aging and T2DM are linked with reduced muscle mass and strength, increased adiposity, and a sedentary lifestyle [12].

Although the underlying molecular causes of T2DM are unknown, it has been associated with obesity, visceral

TABLE 3: Study characteristics.

Study ID (reference number), PEDro score	Sample Size (n), intervention design	Intervention (duration, frequency, intensity, session duration, sets of reps, equipment: exercises)	Outcome measure (¥ P value)	Authors conclusion
*Brooks et al. [17] PEDro: 7	Exercise: $n = 31$ RT + SC Control: $n = 31$ SC	(i)16 weeks (ii) 3 d/week (iii) weeks 1–8: 60–80% of baseline 1RM; weeks 10–14: 70–80% of mid-study 1RM (iv) 45 min/session (5 min warmup; 5 min cooldown) (v) 3 sets of 8 reps (vi) 5 pneumatic machines: upper back, chest press, leg press, knee extension, and flexion	Whole-body lean tissue mass (0.04) Lower body muscle strength (<0.001) Upper body muscle strength (<0.001) Muscle quality (<0.001) Type I fiber CSA (0.04) Type II fiber CSA (0.04) HbA1c (<0.001) Fasting insulin (0.27) Fasting glucose (0.92) Whole body strength (0.0001)	16 weeks of RT resulted in musculoskeletal and metabolic improvements, and it is a mode of exercise worth considering as an adjunct to SC
*Castaneda et al. [13] PEDro: 6	Exercise: $n = 31$ RT + SC Control: $n = 31$ SC	(i) 16 weeks (ii) 3 d/week (iii) weeks 1–8: 60–80% of baseline 1RM; weeks 10–14: 70–80% of mid-study 1RM (iv) 45 min/session (5 min warmup; 5 min cooldown) (v) 3 sets of 8 reps (vi) 5 pneumatic machines: upper back, chest press, leg press, knee extension, and flexion	Whole body fat mass (0.26) Total cholesterol (0.59) LDL cholesterol (0.13) HDL cholesterol (0.46) Systolic BP (0.05) Diastolic BP (0.52)	RT was feasible among older adults with type 2 diabetes, and it resulted in improved metabolic control
Dunstan et al. [53] PEDro: 4	Exercise: $n = 16$ RT + WL Control: $n = 13$ WL	(i) 24 weeks (ii)3 d/week (iii) weeks 1-2: 50–60% 1RM; progress to: 75–85% 1RM (iv) 45 min/session (5 min warmup; 5 min cooldown) (v) 3 sets of 8–10 reps (minus abdominal curls) (vi) Free weights and multiple station weight machine; 9 exercises: bench press, leg extension, upright row, lateral pull down, standing leg curl with ankle weights, dumbbell seated shoulder press, dumbbell seated biceps curl, dumbbell biceps kickback, abdominal curls	Total cholesterol (N/A) LDL cholesterol (N/A) HDL cholesterol (N/A) HbA1c (<0.01) Fasting insulin (N/A) Fasting glucose (0.06) Systolic BP (<0.05) Diastolic BP (<0.05)	A 16-week progressive, high-intensity RT program was effective in improving glycemic control and muscle strength in older adults with T2DM

RT: resistance training; SC: standard care; d: days; min: minutes; sec: seconds; b/w: between; reps: repetitions; UE: upper extremity; LE: lower extremity; CSA: cross sectional area; HbA1c: glycosylated hemoglobin; WL: weight loss).
*Brooks et al. [17] and Castaneda et al. [13] include the same intervention and participants but different outcome measures.
¥ P value reported by the authors.

adiposity, and physical inactivity, which all contribute to an increased risk of developing cardiovascular disease and various disabilities [2, 23, 24]. As such, older adults with T2DM are placed at "double jeopardy" with regards to their health status, which greatly increases their dependence on health care services [1]. A large US-based, cross-sectional study illustrated this point when older adults (70–79 years) with and without T2DM were compared [1]. Various publications from this study showed that those with T2DM had lower muscle strength and quality [21], accelerated muscle loss (i.e., loss of knee extensor strength at a more rapid rate), and excessive muscle mass loss (i.e., greater loss in the amount of leg lean mass) when compared with healthy, age-matched counterparts [20, 22]. Reductions in muscle strength and quality have been linked to an increased risk of physical disability, such as mobility problems and falls [48]. Findings from the current meta-analysis suggest that muscle strength and quality improvements in older adults with T2DM could induce greater functional capacity and reduce the risk of disabilities. Furthermore, muscle quality and strength gains may result in greater physical activity participation in various populations [60–62], including older adults with T2DM [13], which could in turn improve this populations' overall health status by reducing negative disease outcomes.

In addition to improvements in muscle quality (the measure of strength per unit of muscle mass), one study

Table 4: Heterogeneity for moderator variables.

Variable	Q-value	df (Q)	P-value
All disease process measures	42.387	19	0.002
BP	2.171	3	0.538
Fasting glucose	0.364	1	0.546
Fasting insulin	0.181	2	0.913
HbA1c	3.099	2	0.212
HDL	0.055	1	0.814
Total cholesterol and LDL	3.079	3	0.380
All musculoskeletal measures	31.313	11	0.001
Muscle quality	8.184	4	0.085
Muscle strength	2.675	2	0.262
Body composition	3.256	3	0.354

that was included in this meta-analysis reported outcomes specifically regarding the cross-sectional area (CSA) of muscle fibers [17]. Although these outcome values could not be meta-analyzed since only one study included these measures, the fact that fiber hypertrophy resulted warrants further discussion. Brooks and colleagues showed that following a 16-week RT intervention the training group increased the CSA of type I and type II fibers, while the control group participants showed the opposite trend—a reduction in the CSA of both fiber types [17]. As well as strength gains leading to more effective force production, the increase in the CSA of muscle fibers, especially type I muscle fibers, might lead to a better delivery of oxygen through the greater capillary density and number of oxidative mitochondria [16]. In addition, these changes may improve the delivery of glucose from the blood to the muscle, while fiber hypertrophy may provide greater glycogen storage capacity within the muscles of individuals affected by T2DM and thus potentially improve insulin resistance [16, 17]. The hypothesis that muscle hypertrophy or larger muscle mass is associated with improved insulin sensitivity and glucose tolerance has previously been recognized [63].

A further elaboration may help to explain how RT might influence the interaction between the neuromuscular system and the underlying disease process of T2DM. Skeletal muscles represent the largest glucose deposition sites in the human body, which is negatively affected by insulin resistance—a defining feature of T2DM [64]. It has been suggested that people with T2DM have a defective insulin-dependent pathway, which is responsible for activating glucose transporters of the muscles to help move the glucose from the blood into the cells [65]. However, individuals with T2DM do not appear to have a flawed contraction-stimulated pathway for glucose transport [65]. For example, RT would induce a muscular contraction, in turn stimulating the translocation of the GLUT-4 (glucose transporter) to the tissue's cell membrane to dock and activate in order to accept the glucose molecules from the blood into the cell. Thus, glucose could enter the cell via this contraction-stimulated pathway even in individuals with T2DM whose insulin-dependent pathway is defective [65]. Furthermore, exercise has shown to increase GLUT4 expression in human skeletal muscle approximately two to four times, leading to improvements in glucose intolerance and insulin action [65–67]. This underlying mechanism may partially explain some of the effects of RT on the disease process outcomes in this meta-analysis.

Resistance training also had some effects on various markers of the disease process associated with T2DM, including HbA1c, BP, fasting insulin, fasting glucose, HDL, total and LDL cholesterol. For example, findings from this meta-analysis indicated a nonsignificant, medium-sized effect of RT on reducing HbA1c, with a wide CI range. This could be the result of low sample size and a few studies; all of the results of this meta-analysis should be considered with caution. Nevertheless, reduction of HbA1c is considered one of the most important markers for glucose control, and a small change or improvement in this marker may result in a significantly reduced risk of developing diabetic comorbidities. Findings from a prospective study might help illustrate this point further, as decreasing HbA1c by 1% could reduce the risk of any diabetes-related complication by 21% [68]. Although this paper cannot confidently conclude that RT can effectively reduce HbA1c levels in older adults with T2DM, a previous meta-analysis by Boulé and colleagues was able to illustrate that RT was equally effective as AT at improving glycemic control in middle-aged adults [25]. On the other hand, recently Jorge and colleagues compared RT, AT, combined AT and RT, and a control group that received standard care [39]. They did not find significant reductions in HbA1c within any of the exercise groups when compared with the control group [39]. However, all groups had small sample sizes and the control group might have improved their diet during the time of the intervention while their standard care medication also could have contributed to the small difference between groups. Previous researchers have demonstrated that, in addition to RT effectively reducing HbA1c levels, it can also increase glucose disposal and storage capacity, improve lipid, as well as cardiovascular disease risk profiles in adults with T2DM [69–71].

This meta-analysis also showed a moderate effect of RT on BP, and a small effect on total and LDL cholesterol. However, the effect of RT on body composition measures, including lean body mass and fat mass, was small and nonsignificant. The positive effect of RT on BP and cholesterol may be promising, since achieving lower BP with exercise is indicative of improved cardiovascular function, while a reduction in cholesterol levels, especially LDL, may help reduce the risk of micro- and macrovascular complications, such as atherosclerosis, stroke, and myocardial infarction [2]. Past researchers have also found positive changes of BP that might have been induced by RT [39, 40]. These findings may be of considerable value for those with T2DM who have a two- to fourfold greater risk of developing cardiovascular disease [72]; improvements in LDL cholesterol as well as BP could improve health outcomes for this group. Improved physical function could lead to a greater ability to participate in various physical activities safely and enjoyably and in turn reduce the sedentary behavior often found in individuals with T2DM. However, some researchers did not find that RT led to a reduction in BP [53], nor improvements in

TABLE 5: PEDro rating details.

Study ID (PEDro score)	Random allocation	Concealed allocation	Baseline comparability	Blind subjects	Blind therapists	Blind assessors	Adequate followup	Intention-to-treat analysis	Between-group comparisons	Point estimates and variability
Brooks et al. (7) [17]	Yes	No	Yes	No	No	Yes	Yes	Yes	Yes	Yes
Castaneda et al. (6) [13]	Yes	No	No	No	No	Yes	Yes	Yes	Yes	Yes
Dunstan et al. (4) [53]	Yes	No	Yes	No	No	No	No	No	Yes	Yes

TABLE 6: Summary of resistance training effect on outcome measures.

Outcome		Hedge's g	P value	Effect description (statistical significance)
Disease processes		$-0.271^{¥}$	0.008	Medium (significant)
BP (systolic/diastolic mmHg)		− 0.540	<0.001	Large (significant)
HbA1c (%)		−0.463	0.145	Medium (not significant)
Total and LDL cholesterol		−0.464	0.002	medium (significant)
Fasting glucose		−0.121	0.559	Small (not significant)
Fasting insulin		0.505	0.016	Medium (significant)
HDL cholesterol		0.134	0.517	Small (not significant)
Body composition		0.199	0.197	Small (not significant)
Lean body mass		0.395	0.220	Small (not significant)
Fat body mass		0.066	0.749	Small (not significant)
Muscle strength		1.05	<0.001	Large (significant)
Lower body muscle strength		1.415	<0.001	Large (significant)
Upper body muscle strength		0.974	<0.001	Large (significant)
Whole body muscle strength		0.802	0.002	Large (significant)
*Further muscle measures		Exercise	Control	P value
Quality	Baseline	61 ± 27.8	51 ± 22.3	<0.001
	Final	100 ± 33.4	48 ± 22.3	
Type I CSA (μm^2)	Baseline	4068 ± 1425.3	4546 ± 1503.3	0.04
	Final	4928 ± 2071.2	4381 ± 1692.6	
Type II CSA (μm^2)	Baseline	3885 ± 1547.8	4330 ± 1926.4	0.04
	Final	4605 ± 1575.7	4201 ± 1870.8	

BP-blood pressure; HbA1c: glycosylated hemoglobin; LDL: low density lipoprotein cholesterol; HDL: high-density lipoprotein cholesterol; CSA: cross sectional area.
¥ Negative values denote a decrease in the outcome measure (i.e., this is a positive effect, since a reduction in disease processes, such as lowered BP, LDL, and HBA1c, indicates an improvement in disease management).
*Further muscle measures were not entered into CMA; all values are means ± SE, taken from [17].

the LDL cholesterol levels following AT, RT, or combined training [25]. Further studies are needed in order to better understand the potential effect of RT on BP and cholesterol in people with T2DM [53].

The fact that body composition was not altered may be due to the short intervention durations, or it could be attributed to the low number of studies included in this meta-analysis. However, despite RT apparently not having an effect on the body composition of older adults with T2DM, their metabolic control could still be impacted by exercise alone, since Boulé et al. indicated that RT and/or AT can enhance insulin sensitivity and glycemic control even when the weight and/or body composition is unaltered [25]. Future studies are needed to confirm this claim for older adults with T2DM.

Although previous reviews indicate that RT can positively impact functional and metabolic changes in people with T2DM, this is the first meta-analysis that suggests that RT may benefit older adults (≥65 years) in the management of their disease. It is important to have accurate information for health care organizations to be able to integrate physical activity recommendations into their knowledge management strategies [5]. However, there are insufficient high quality studies (only 2 original RCTs, providing 3 records) that address the full impact of RT in older populations with T2DM. As such, confidence in conclusions based on the presented findings is limited. Furthermore, no study has included RT interventions with adults who were 80 years or older, despite this age group having the highest prevalence of T2DM [1]. Given the high prevalence and incidence of T2DM in geriatric populations [73], more research is needed to assess the potential benefits of RT for this age cohort. Also, some studies have suggested that there is an additive benefit from combining AT and RT exercises for adults with T2DM [9, 74, 75]. Future research should explore the effect of combined exercise training in populations who are at least 65 years old.

Finally, the importance of conducting appropriate preexercise screens prior to implementing an RT or any exercise intervention cannot be overlooked [7]. This is of particular interest when working with older/clinical populations who may have various complications and comorbidities, resulting in absolute or relative contraindications to physical activity detailed in [7, page 276] and elaborated further by other researchers [18, 49].

Measures that could provide additional insight into the benefits/risks of RT, such as muscle quality, fiber CSAs, changes in free fatty acid [17], and/or triglyceride concentrations [53], and medication reduction [13] were reported only in some papers and thus could not be meta-analyzed. As a result, a better understanding of the impact of RT in older adults with T2DM requires additional study.

5. Limitations

There are several limitations in this meta-analysis that are worth noting. Firstly, 68% of total participants from all three records are Hispanic. As such, the generalizability of the findings to different ethnic origins may be limited, due to the diversity of psychosocial and potentially genetic factors.

Secondly, using the terms physical activity and exercise interchangeably may have varying outcome implications. For instance, studies that focus on physical activity may report different outcomes and result in alternate findings when compared to studies using a targeted training approach with predefined aims.

Thirdly, the inclusion and exclusion criteria were developed to obtain the most relevant evidence for the population of older adults with type 2 diabetes, but with this strict criteria there is a risk that perhaps relevant studies that did not meet the specified inclusion requirements could have provided some additional insight for this paper.

Fourthly, there is a risk of having a confounding variable effect by including Dunstan et al. [53], since their RT intervention was combined with a weight loss component. Thus, it is not possible to have a definitive conclusion about the independent effect the RT intervention might have had if it was not combined with the weight loss component.

Despite these limitations, a rigorous approach has been undertaken to provide the first precise meta-analysis that assessed the currently available RCTs for RT effects on metabolic, musculoskeletal, and cardiovascular factors in adults 65 years or older with type 2 diabetes.

6. Conclusion

Although strong conclusions cannot be drawn from this meta-analysis, the potential role of RT to help older adults in the management of T2DM should be considered given the current trends in aging, obesity, and diabetes. In 2005, managing diabetes and its complications cost the Canadian acute healthcare system $5.6 billion [76], while in the US the current approximated annual cost is surpassing $134 billion dollars [1]. Also, these figures are excluding the personal costs endured by those with the disease and their families, associated with morbidity induced by various diabetic complications [1]. More recent statistics suggest that, factoring the cost of undiagnosed diabetes, prediabetes, and gestational diabetes, the total cost of diabetes in the US in 2007 totaled to $218 billion [77]. Considering that 26.9% of older adults in the US (approximately 10.9 million individuals) have diabetes [77], there ought to be specific and appropriately designed interventions for this cohort. Inclusion of RT in the management of T2DM has been recognized and supported by previous reviews [4, 12, 25, 47, 78, 79] and physical activity guidelines [27, 29, 34]. Future studies will help to confirm whether the metabolic benefits obtained with RT in younger populations could also positively impact older adults with T2DM, including the rapidly expanding population aged 80 years or more.

References

[1] S. R. Gambert and S. Pinkstaff, "Emerging epidemic: diabetes in older adults: demography, economic impact, and pathophysiology," *Diabetes Spectrum*, vol. 19, no. 4, pp. 221–228, 2006.

[2] R. I. G. Holt, C. S. Cockram, A. Flyvbjerg, and B. J. Goldstein, *Textbook of Diabetes*, Wiley-Blackwell, London, UK, 4th edition, 2010.

[3] "American Diabetes Association," Diabetes basics: Type 2., 2010, http://www.diabetes.org/diabetes-basics/type-2/?utm_source=WWW&utm_medium=DropDownDB&utm_content=Type2&utm_campaign=CON.

[4] R. J. Sigal, G. P. Kenny, D. H. Wasserman, and C. Castaneda-Sceppa, "Physical activity/exercise and type 2 diabetes," *Diabetes Care*, vol. 27, no. 10, pp. 2518–2539, 2004.

[5] A. Kothari, N. Hovanec, R. Hastie, and S. Sibbald, "Lessons from the business sector for successful knowledge management in health care: a systematic review," *BMC Health Services Research*, vol. 11, article 173, 2011.

[6] J. E. Yardley, A. Alberga, G. P. Kenny, and R. J. Sigal, "Lifestyle issues: exercise," in *Textbook of Diabetes*, R. I. G. Holt, C. S. Cockram, A. Flyvbjerg, and B. J. Goldstein, Eds., pp. 358–379, Wiley-Blackwell, London, UK, 4th edition, 2010.

[7] N. F. Gordon, "The exercise prescription," in *Handbook of Exercise in Diabetes*, pp. 269–288, American Diabetes Association, New York, NY, USA, 2nd edition, 2002.

[8] H. Wallberg-Henriksson, J. Rincon, and J. R. Zierath, "Exercise in the management of non-insulin-dependent diabetes mellitus," *Sports Medicine*, vol. 25, no. 1, pp. 25–35, 1998.

[9] A. Maiorana, G. O'Driscoll, C. Goodman, R. Taylor, and D. Green, "Combined aerobic and resistance exercise improves glycemic control and fitness in type 2 diabetes," *Diabetes Research and Clinical Practice*, vol. 56, no. 2, pp. 115–123, 2002.

[10] A. Albright, M. Franz, G. Hornsby et al., "ACSM position stand on exercise and type 2 diabetes," *Medicine and Science in Sports and Exercise*, vol. 32, no. 7, pp. 1345–1360, 2000.

[11] W. G. Hornsby and R. D. Chetlin, "Resistance training," in *Handbook of Exercise in Diabetes*, N. Ruderman, J. T. Devlin, S. H. Schneider, and A. Kriska, Eds., pp. 311–319, American Diabetes Association, New York, NY, USA, 2nd edition, 2002.

[12] K. A. Willey and M. A. Fiatarone Singh, "Battling insulin resistance in elderly obese people with type 2 diabetes: bring on the heavy weights," *Diabetes Care*, vol. 26, no. 5, pp. 1580–1588, 2003.

[13] C. Castaneda, J. E. Layne, L. Munoz-Orians et al., "A randomized controlled trial of resistance exercise training to improve glycemic control in older adults with type 2 diabetes," *Diabetes Care*, vol. 25, no. 12, pp. 2335–2341, 2002.

[14] D. W. Dunstan, R. M. Daly, N. Owen et al., "Home-based resistance training is not sufficient to maintain improved glycemic control following supervised training in older individuals with type 2 diabetes," *Diabetes Care*, vol. 28, no. 1, pp. 3–9, 2005.

[15] A. M. Swank and P. Hagerman, "Resistance-training strategies for individuals with type 2 diabetes," in *Resistance Training for Special Populations*, pp. 244–260, Delmar, Albany, NY, USA, 2010.

[16] J. L. Ivy, "Exercise physiology and adaptations to training," in *Handbook of Exercise in Diabetes*, J. T. Ruderman, S. H. Schneider, and A. Kriska, Eds., pp. 23–62, American Diabetes Association, New York, NY, USA, 2nd edition, 2002.

[17] N. Brooks, J. E. Layne, P. L. Gordon, R. Roubenoff, M. E. Nelson, and C. Castaneda-Sceppa, "Strength training improves muscle quality and insulin sensitivity in Hispanic older adults with type 2 diabetes," *International Journal of Medical Sciences*, vol. 4, no. 1, pp. 19–27, 2007.

[18] O. Theou, L. Stathokostas, K. P. Roland et al., "The effectiveness of exercise interventions for the management of frailty: a systematic review," *Journal of Aging Research*, vol. 2011, Article ID 569194, 2011.

[19] A. A. Vandervoort, "Aging of the human neuromuscular system," *Muscle and Nerve*, vol. 25, no. 1, pp. 17–25, 2002.

[20] W. P. Seok, B. H. Goodpaster, S. L. Jung et al., "Excessive loss of skeletal muscle mass in older adults with type 2 diabetes," *Diabetes Care*, vol. 32, no. 11, pp. 1993–1997, 2009.

[21] S. W. Park, B. H. Goodpaster, E. S. Strotmeyer et al., "Decreased muscle strength and quality in older adults with type 2 diabetes: the health, aging, and body composition study," *Diabetes*, vol. 55, no. 6, pp. 1813–1818, 2006.

[22] W. P. Seok, B. H. Goodpaster, E. S. Strotmeyer et al., "Accelerated loss of skeletal muscle strength in older adults with type 2 diabetes: the health, aging, and body composition study," *Diabetes Care*, vol. 30, no. 6, pp. 1507–1512, 2007.

[23] E. W. Gregg, C. M. Mangione, J. A. Cauley et al., "Diabetes and incidence of functional disability in older women," *Diabetes Care*, vol. 25, no. 1, pp. 61–67, 2002.

[24] E. W. Gregg, G. L. A. Beckles, D. F. Williamson et al., "Diabetes and physical disability among older U.S. Adults," *Diabetes Care*, vol. 23, no. 9, pp. 1272–1277, 2000.

[25] N. G. Boulé, E. Haddad, G. P. Kenny, G. A. Wells, and R. J. Sigal, "Effects of exercise on glycemic control and body mass in type 2 diabetes mellitus: a meta-analysis of controlled clinical trials," *Journal of the American Medical Association*, vol. 286, no. 10, pp. 1218–1227, 2001.

[26] A. P. Hills, S. P. Shultz, M. J. Soares et al., "Resistance training for obese, type 2 diabetic adults: a review of the evidence," *Obesity Reviews*, vol. 11, no. 10, pp. 740–749, 2010.

[27] American College of Sports Medicine and American College of Sports Medicine position stand, "Progression models in resistance training for healthy adults," *Medicine and Science in Sports and Exercise*, vol. 41, no. 3, pp. 687–708, 2009.

[28] S. R. Colberg, A. L. Albright, B. J. Blissmer et al., "Exercise and type 2 diabetes: American College of Sports Medicine and the American Diabetes Association: joint position statement," *Diabetes Care*, vol. 42, no. 12, pp. 2282–2303, 2010.

[29] Canadian Diabetes Assocation Clinicl Practice Guidelines Expert Committee, "Physical activity and diabetes," *Canadian Diabetes Journal*, vol. 32, supplement 1, pp. S37–S39, 2008.

[30] Canadian Society for Exercise Physiology, "Canadian physical activity guidelines for older adults-65 years & older," 2011, http://www.csep.ca/CMFiles/Guidelines/CSEP-InfoSheets-adults-ENG.pdf.

[31] R. R. Pate, M. Pratt, S. N. Blair et al., "Physical activity and public health: a recommendation from the Centers for Disease Control and Prevention and the American College of Sports Medicine," *Journal of the American Medical Association*, vol. 273, no. 5, pp. 402–407, 1995.

[32] Health Canada, Canada's Physical Activity Guide to Healthy Active Living, 1998.

[33] American College of Sports Medicine and American College of Sports Medicine Position Stand, "Exercise and physical activity for older adults," *Medicine and Science in Sports and Exercise*, vol. 30, no. 6, pp. 992–1008, 1998.

[34] American Diabetes Association, "Diabetes mellitus and exercise," *Diabetes Care*, vol. 25, supplement1, pp. S64–S68, 2002.

[35] Canadian Diabetes Association Clinical Practice Guidelines Expert Committee, "Physical activity and diabetes," *Canadian Journal of Diabetes*, vol. 27, pp. S24–S26, 2003.

[36] R. J. Sigal, G. P. Kenny, D. H. Wasserman, C. Castaneda-Sceppa, and R. D. White, "Physical activity/exercise and type 2 diabetes: a consensus statement from the American Diabetes Association," *Diabetes Care*, vol. 29, no. 6, pp. 1433–1438, 2006.

[37] W. L. Haskell, I. M. Lee, R. R. Pate et al., "Physical activity and public health: updated recommendation for adults from the American College of Sports Medicine and the American Heart Association," *Medicine and Science in Sports and Exercise*, vol. 39, no. 8, pp. 1423–1434, 2007.

[38] N. J. Snowling and W. G. Hopkins, "Effects of different modes of exercise training on glucose control and risk factors for complications in type 2 diabetic patients: a meta-analysis," *Diabetes Care*, vol. 29, no. 11, pp. 2518–2527, 2006.

[39] M. L. M. P. Jorge, V. N. de Oliveira, N. M. Resende et al., "The effects of aerobic, resistance, and combined exercise on metabolic control, inflammatory markers, adipocytokines, and muscle insulin signaling in patients with type 2 diabetes mellitus," *Metabolism*, vol. 60, no. 9, pp. 1244–1252, 2011.

[40] L. A. Gordon, E. Y. Morrison, D. A. McGrowder et al., "Effect of exercise therapy on lipid profile and oxidative stress indicators in patients with type 2 diabetes," *BMC Complementary and Alternative Medicine*, vol. 8, article 21, 2008.

[41] P. L. Gordon, E. Vannier, K. Hamada et al., "Resistance training alters cytokine gene expression in skeletal muscle of adults with type 2 diabetes," *International Journal of Immunopathology and Pharmacology*, vol. 19, no. 4, pp. 739–749, 2006.

[42] T. J. Overend, T. H. Versteegh, E. Thompson, T. B. Birmingham, and A. A. Vandervoort, "Cardiovascular stress associated with concentric and eccentric isokinetic exercise in young and

older adults," *Journals of Gerontology A*, vol. 55, no. 4, pp. B177–B182, 2000.

[43] N. K. LeBrasseur, K. Walsh, and Z. Arany, "Metabolic benefits of resistance training and fast glycolytic skeletal muscle," *American Journal of Physiology*, vol. 300, no. 1, pp. E3–E10, 2011.

[44] D. Umpierre, P. A. B. Ribeiro, C. K. Kramer et al., "Physical activity advice only or structured exercise training and association with HbA1c levels in type 2 diabetes: a systematic review and meta-analysis," *Journal of the American Medical Association*, vol. 305, no. 17, pp. 1790–1799, 2011.

[45] B. Strasser, U. Siebert, and W. Schobersberger, "Resistance training in the treatment of the metabolic syndrome: a systematic review and meta-analysis of the effect of resistance training on metabolic clustering in patients with abnormal glucose metabolism," *Sports Medicine*, vol. 40, no. 5, pp. 397–415, 2010.

[46] N. G. Boulé, G. P. Kenny, E. Haddad, G. A. Wells, and R. J. Sigal, "Meta-analysis of the effect of structured exercise training on cardiorespiratory fitness in Type 2 diabetes mellitus," *Diabetologia*, vol. 46, no. 8, pp. 1071–1081, 2003.

[47] D. E. Thomas, E. J. Elliott, and G. A. Naughton, "Exercise for type 2 diabetes mellitus," *Cochrane Database of Systematic Reviews*, vol. 3, Article ID CD002968, 2006.

[48] N. De Rekeneire, H. E. Resnick, A. V. Schwartz et al., "Diabetes is associated with subclinical functional limitation in nondisabled older individuals: the health, aging, and body composition study," *Diabetes Care*, vol. 26, no. 12, pp. 3257–3263, 2003.

[49] R. J. Petrella, K. Aizawa, K. Shoemaker et al., "Efficacy of a family practice-based lifestyle intervention program to increase physical activity and reduce clinical and physiological markers of vascular health in patients with high normal blood pressure and/or high normal blood glucose (SNAC): study protocol for a randomized controlled trial," *Trials*, vol. 12, article 45, 2011.

[50] D. Moher, A. Liberati, J. Tetzlaff, and D. G. Altman, "PRISMA Group. Preferred reporting items for systematic reviews and meta-analyses: the PRISMA statement," *PLoS Medicine*, vol. 6, no. 7, Article ID e1000097, 2009.

[51] N. A. de Morton, "The PEDro scale is a valid measure of the methodological quality of clinical trials: a demographic study," *Australian Journal of Physiotherapy*, vol. 55, no. 2, pp. 129–133, 2009.

[52] C. G. Maher, C. Sherrington, R. D. Herbert, A. M. Moseley, and M. Elkins, "Reliability of the PEDro scale for rating quality of randomized controlled trials," *Physical Therapy*, vol. 83, no. 8, pp. 713–721, 2003.

[53] D. W. Dunstan, R. M. Daly, N. Owen et al., "High-intensity resistance training improves glycemic control in older patients with type 2 diabetes," *Diabetes Care*, vol. 25, no. 10, pp. 1729–1736, 2002.

[54] J. Cohen, *Statistical Power Analysis for the Behavioral Sciences*, Academic Press, New York, NY, USA, 1969.

[55] J. P. T. Higgins and S. Green, "Cochrane Handbook for Systematic Reviews of Interventions," 2011, http://www.cochrane-handbook.org/.

[56] L. Li and W. R. Schucany, "Some properties of a test for concordance of two groups of rankings," *Biometrika*, vol. 62, no. 2, pp. 417–423, 1975.

[57] The Cochrane Collaboration, "Diversity and heterogeneity," 2002, http://www.cochrane-net.org/openlearning/html/mod13-3.htm.

[58] J. A. C. Sterne, M. Egger, and D. Moher, "Addressing reporting biases," in *Cochrane Handbook for Systematic Reviews of Interventions. Version 5.0.1*, J. P. T. Higgins and S. Green, Eds., chapter 10, 2008, 2008, http://www.cochrane-handbook.org/.

[59] F. Castaneda, J. E. Layne, and C. Castaneda, "Skeletal muscle sodium glucose co-transporters in older adults with type 2 diabetes undergoing resistance training," *International Journal of Medical Sciences*, vol. 3, no. 3, pp. 84–91, 2006.

[60] M. E. Nelson, M. A. Fiatarone, C. M. Morganti, I. Trice, R. A. Greenberg, and W. J. Evans, "Effects of high-intensity strength training on multiple risk factors for osteoporotic fractures: a randomized controlled trial," *Journal of the American Medical Association*, vol. 272, no. 24, pp. 1909–1914, 1994.

[61] M. A. Fiatarone, E. F. O'Neill, N. D. Ryan et al., "Exercise training and nutritional supplementation for physical frailty in very elderly people," *The New England Journal of Medicine*, vol. 330, no. 25, pp. 1769–1775, 1994.

[62] L. C. Rall and R. Roubenoff, "Body composition, metabolism, and resistance exercise in patients with rheumatoid arthritis," *Arthritis Care and Research*, vol. 9, no. 2, pp. 151–156, 1996.

[63] W. J. Miller, W. M. Sherman, and J. L. Ivy, "Effect of strength training on glucose tolerance and post-glucose insulin response," *Medicine and Science in Sports and Exercise*, vol. 16, no. 6, pp. 539–543, 1984.

[64] R. A. DeFronzo, E. Jacot, E. Jequier, E. Maeder, J. Wahren, and J. P. Felber, "The effect of insulin on the disposal of intravenous glucose. Results from indirect calorimetry and hepatic and femoral venous catheterization," *Diabetes*, vol. 30, no. 12, pp. 1000–1007, 1981.

[65] J. R. Zierath, A. Krook, and H. Wallberg-Henriksson, "Insulin action and insulin resistance in human skeletal muscle," *Diabetologia*, vol. 43, no. 7, pp. 821–835, 2000.

[66] V. A. Hughes, M. A. Fiatarone, R. A. Fielding et al., "Exercise increases muscle GLUT-4 levels and insulin action in subjects with impaired glucose tolerance," *American Journal of Physiology*, vol. 264, no. 6, part 1, pp. E855–E862, 1993.

[67] F. Dela, K. J. Mikines, M. von Linstow, N. H. Secher, and H. Galbo, "Effect of training on insulin-mediated glucose uptake in human muscle," *American Journal of Physiology*, vol. 263, no. 6, pp. E1134–E1143, 1992.

[68] I. M. Stratton, A. I. Adler, H. A. W. Neil et al., "Association of glycaemia with macrovascular and microvascular complications of type 2 diabetes (UKPDS 35): prospective observational study," *British Medical Journal*, vol. 321, no. 7258, pp. 405–412, 2000.

[69] M. K. Holten, M. Zacho, M. Gaster, C. Juel, J. F. P. Wojtaszewski, and F. Dela, "Strength training increases insulin-mediated glucose uptake, GLUT4 content, and insulin signaling in skeletal muscle in patients with type 2 diabetes," *Diabetes*, vol. 53, no. 2, pp. 294–305, 2004.

[70] A. Honkola, T. Forsén, and J. Eriksson, "Resistance training improves the metabolic profile in individuals with type 2 diabetes," *Acta Diabetologica*, vol. 34, no. 4, pp. 245–248, 1997.

[71] T. P. Wycherley, M. Noakes, P. M. Clifton, X. Cleanthous, J. B. Keogh, and G. D. Brinkworth, "A high-protein diet with resistance exercise training improves weight loss and body composition in overweight and obese patients with type 2 diabetes," *Diabetes Care*, vol. 33, no. 5, pp. 969–976, 2010.

[72] J. A. Beckman, M. A. Creager, and P. Libby, "Diabetes and atherosclerosis epidemiology, pathophysiology, and management," *Journal of the American Medical Association*, vol. 287, no. 19, pp. 2570–2581, 2002.

[73] M. Warren, "Physical activity: exercise prescription for the older adult with type 2 diabetes," *Topics in Geriatric Rehabilitation*, vol. 26, no. 3, pp. 221–232, 2010.
[74] T. S. Church, S. N. Blair, S. Cocreham et al., "Effects of aerobic and resistance training on hemoglobin A1c levels in patients with type 2 diabetes: a randomized controlled trial," *Journal of the American Medical Association*, vol. 304, no. 20, pp. 2253–2262, 2010.
[75] D. J. Cuff, G. S. Meneilly, A. Martin, A. Ignaszewski, H. D. Tildesley, and J. J. Frohlich, "Effective Exercise Modality to Reduce Insulin Resistance in Women With Type 2 Diabetes," *Diabetes Care*, vol. 26, no. 11, pp. 2977–2982, 2003.
[76] A. Ohinmaa, P. Jacobs, S. Simpson, and J. A. Johnson, "The projection of prevalence and cost of diabetes in Canada: 2000 to 2016," *Canadian Journal of Diabetes*, vol. 28, no. 2, pp. 1–8, 2004.
[77] American Diabetes Association, Diabetes basics: Diabetes Statistics, 2012, http://www.diabetes.org/diabetes-basics/diabetes-statistics/.
[78] S. F. E. Praet, R. A. M. Jonkers, G. Schep et al., "Long-standing, insulin-treated type 2 diabetes patients with complications respond well to short-term resistance and interval exercise training," *European Journal of Endocrinology*, vol. 158, no. 2, pp. 163–172, 2008.
[79] S. F. E. Praet and L. J. C. van Loon, "Exercise therapy in Type 2 diabetes," *Acta Diabetologica*, vol. 46, no. 4, pp. 263–278, 2009.

15

Could Some Geriatric Characteristics Hinder the Prescription of Anticoagulants in Atrial Fibrillation in the Elderly?

Paule Denoël,[1] Jacques Vanderstraeten,[2] Pierre Mols,[3] and Thierry Pepersack[4]

[1] *Emergency Service, Europe Hospital, 1040 Brussels, Belgium*
[2] *Centre de Recherche en Santé Environnementale et en Santé du Travail, Ecole de Santé Publique, Université Libre de Bruxelles, 1070 Brussels, Belgium*
[3] *Emergency Service, Saint-Pierre University Hospital, Université Libre de Bruxelles, 1000 Brussels, Belgium*
[4] *Department of Geriatrics, Erasme Hospital, Université Libre de Bruxelles, Lennik Street 808, 1070 Brussels, Belgium*

Correspondence should be addressed to Thierry Pepersack; thierry.pepersack@erasme.ulb.ac.be

Academic Editor: Simone Reppermund

Several studies have reported underprescription of anticoagulants in atrial fibrillation (AF). We conducted an observational study on 142 out of a total of 995 consecutive ≥75 years old patients presenting AF (14%) when admitted in an emergency unit of a general hospital, in search of geriatric characteristics that might be associated with the underprescription of anticoagulation therapy (mostly antivitamin K at the time of the study). The following data was collected from patients presenting AF: medical history including treatment and comorbidities, $CHADS_2$ score, ISAR scale (frailty), Lawton's scale (ADL), GDS scale (mood status), MUST (nutrition), and blood analysis (INR, kidney function, and albumin). Among those patients for who anticoagulation treatment was recommended (73%), only 61% were treated with it. In the group with anticoagulation therapy, the following characteristics were observed more often than in the group without such therapy: a recent (≤6 months) hospitalization and medical treatment including digoxin or based on >3 different drugs. Neither the value of the $CHADS_2$ score, nor the geriatric characteristics could be correlated with the presence or the absence of an anticoagulation therapy. More research is thus required to identify and clarify the relative importance of patient-, physician-, and health care system-related hurdles for the prescription of oral anticoagulation therapy in older patients with AF.

1. Introduction

Atrial fibrillation (AF) is the most frequent chronic arrhythmia in the elderly, affecting up to 10% of the population aged 80 and above. With the population aging, the burden of AF is expected to double over the next two generations, making this arrhythmia an increasingly important public health issue [1–4]. The risk of thromboembolic complications (stroke and systemic embolism) is high in AF, with the relative risk of ischemic stroke being evaluated to about five in AF without mitral valvular disease [5]. The indication of anticoagulation therapy with antivitamin K (AVK) for the prevention of thromboembolism in patients with AF is based on information derived from numerous well-designed and randomized control trials [6, 7].

Numerous studies have notably shown that long term anticoagulation treatment with AVK reduces the risk of ischemic stroke in patients with nonvalvular AF by about 68% [8, 9]. As a comparison, this reduction is only 22% for acetylsalicylic acid (ASA) at preventive doses (75 to 325 mg/day) [10, 11], with a hemorrhagic risk that is otherwise not lower than the one for AVK [12, 13].

In spite of current evidence of the benefits of anticoagulation therapy for AF in patients with moderate to high CHA_2DS_2-VASc risk scores [14, 15], AVK is underprescribed as highlighted in this study of the elderly (from here on defined as corresponding to the age of 75 and above).

While 50 to 60% of geriatric patients with AF should be treated with an AVK, only 15 to 44% are actually treated with it [16–18]. The studies evaluating possible hurdles to the prescription of AVK reveal three distinct types of obstacles: patient-, physician-, and health care system-related factors [18]. Physician-related difficulties reflect their misconception of the risk/benefit ratio of administering oral anticoagulation therapy. Within this category, we have identified three elements that may influence the prescriber. First, the personal experience of the prescriber such as a negative event with a patient (major gastrointestinal or cerebral bleeding) might discourage the prescription of AVK [16]. The second element is linked to the patients' own attributes. Some psychosocial factors may discourage the prescription of anticoagulants because of the concern of a higher risk of hemorrhagic complications [19] due to poor compliance. These factors are related to drug or alcohol abuse, psychiatric pathologies (schizophrenia, psychosis, major depression, etc.), underprivileged situations (patient isolated or without a fixed domicile) and/or a history of noncompliance. Other determining patients' attributes are the particulars of the geriatric patient, aged ≥75, and the specific risk of a potential fall, unjustifiably discouraging the prescription of AVK [16, 20–22], or inciting to target INR (international normalized ratio) levels that are below 2.0 [16, 20]. The third element of the misperception of the risk versus benefit ratio of AVK experienced by the prescriber is the constraints (INR control) and contingencies (food interactions, bleeding risk) of oral anticoagulation therapy [23, 24] and the complexity of keeping INR within the therapeutic range (2.0-3.0) [16, 18, 24, 25]. According to available data, INR remains within this range only 40 to 58% of time [26, 27].

The recipient's perception of the benefit versus risk ratio of AVK therapy also influences the agreement to submit to anticoagulation therapy. Well informed patients are more prone to accept the risk of such treatment [28]. One study reported that among those patients treated with AVK for AF, 48% did not understand the purpose of the treatment and 37% were not aware of their own risks of stroke [2]. The information provided to the patient also influences patient's decision to accept an AVK treatment [28]. Another study reported that the percentage of patients accepting AVK treatments varied between 30 and 87%, depending on the prescriber and the way he delivered such information about the treatment [29]. In general, patients appear to accept a lower benefit/risk ratio than the prescribers do [30, 31]. Finally, some health care system-related factors have also been identified as hindering AVK prescription in AF [18]; one example refers to the availability of a nearby laboratory for INR measurements [32].

It should be further investigated whether some geriatric characteristics or geriatric score could be predictive of the decision of the prescriber for anticoagulation in AF in the elderly. One study [33] compared some geriatric attributes of patients with AF who were given anticoagulants with those with AF who were not. This study was retroactive and was achieved in the geriatric unit of a general hospital. The following parameters were evaluated: $CHADS_2$ score, Katz score, Lawton scores (daily life activity), and various geriatric characteristics (cognitive, nutrition and mood status, and risk of fall). No difference could be observed between the two patients groups. Here, we suggest searching again for such predictive geriatric characteristics in patients ≥75 years old, this time in a prospective way, within the context of an emergency room while increasing the number of features to be investigated.

2. Objective

The aim of this study was to observe the prevalence of (nonvalvular) AF in consecutive geriatric patients admitted in an emergency room and to analyze the variables associated with such underprescription of anticoagulation therapy in patients with AF.

3. Methods

3.1. Design. This was an observational study. Consecutive eligible patients were assessed by the team in the emergency room under the supervision of one physician (first author).

3.2. Setting. The study took place in an emergency unit of a general hospital.

3.3. Patients. All consecutive patients ≥75 years old admitted between 27 May 2011 and 23 December 2012 in the emergency unit were assessed for the presence of (nonvalvular) AF. The total number of admitted patients as well as the number of the patients with AF was collected during the length of the study. The diagnosis of AF was based on the reading of a 12-lead-ECG. Patients with a history of paroxysmal AF were not enrolled in this study. Comprehensive assessment covered only those patients with AF irrespective of the presence or not of AVK (or low molecular weight heparin) therapy. Patients who were not able to answer the questionnaires of the comprehensive assessment were excluded and their number collated. Exclusion criteria were the following: language other than French, English or Dutch, aphasia, critical condition, and/or obvious cognitive disorders.

3.4. Comprehensive Assessment. The following items were systematically gathered and recorded.

(i) The cause of admission (general status alteration, fall, confusion, traumatism, dyspnea, precordium pain, stroke suspicion, pyrexia, and other).

(ii) A social evaluation stating the age, residency status (private home versus institution), living situation (alone or not), and presence (or absence) of a followup by a general practitioner.

(iii) The patient's medical history, with a special emphasis on previous history of stroke or transitory ischemic attack (TIA).

(iv) The medical treatment (drugs administrated to the patient before admission), with special attention to AVK therapy.

(v) The risk of an embolic stroke and related level of indication for anticoagulation therapy according to the $CHADS_2$ score [34].

(vi) The frailty of the patient, using the tool for *Identification of Senior at Risk* (ISAR) [35].

(vii) The level of daily activities (ADL) using the Lawton's scales [36], with special focus on the ability to manage medications.

(viii) The determination whether the patient had previous incidences of falling (≥1 fall within the 6 months before admission: named "faller") or not.

(ix) The probability of depression using the geriatric *depression* scale (GDS) [37].

(x) The nutritional status using the *Malnutrition Universal Screening Tool* (MUST) [38].

(xi) A polypathology and severity of the medical problems using the Charlson's comorbidity index [39].

(xii) The determination of the levels of serum urea, creatinine, albumin, and INR.

The dispatch of the patients were recorded (hospitalization or not). The use of the CHA_2DS_2-VASc instead of the $CHADS_2$ score would not have significantly changed the proportion of patients eligible for an anticoagulation therapy in our patient sample. We also choose not to determine the HAS-BLED score, because this score is hardly, if ever, used by general practitioners in our country; moreover, several criteria of this score (hypertension, stroke, and age) are also included in the $CHADS_2$ score and some (renal insufficiency, drugs) do not show any contraindication for AVK treatment.

3.5. Ethical Committee. All the research for this study met the criteria of the routine Good Clinical Practices. Data from the medical charts were collected anonymously in a database.

3.6. Statistics. Results were collected in a database on Microsoft's Excel and statistical analyses were performed using Stata 11.2 software (Lakeway Drive, Texas, United States). Results are means (±1 SD). Unpaired Student's *t*-test, comparing means and squared chi, was used to assess between group differences in proportion of variables. Univariate and multivariate logistic regression analyses were achieved in order to identify the variables that are associated with the anticoagulated status. A P value < 0.05 is considered as statistically significant.

4. Results

Between May 27th 2011 and December 23rd 2011, 1204 patients ≥75 years old were admitted at the emergency unit. Among those patients, 92 presented exclusion criteria and 117 were excluded because data collected was incomplete.

Among the 995 retained patients, 142 presented with atrial fibrillation (14%). Table 1 illustrates the characteristics of this group.

Among patients with AF for whom anticoagulation was recommended (73% of all patients), only 61% actually received anticoagulation therapy.

The main cause of their admission at the emergency room was "a deterioration of general status." Four percent of the patients were admitted for suspicion of a stroke and/or transient ischemic attack (TIA). None of those patients revealed a cerebral hemorrhage by brain CT-scan, and only 1 of those patients received AVK therapy (INR of 2.4 at the time of his admission).

Among those patients admitted after trauma (with or without a fall) and those admitted after a fall (30 patients, 15 receiving AVK therapy), only one patient presented a cerebral hemorrhage. This last patient had not received any AVK or aspirin therapy before admission.

In order to analyze geriatric characteristics potentially associated with the underprescription of AVK in AF, we compared geriatric characteristics, comorbidities, ISAR score, and drug treatment between patients receiving anticoagulation therapy and patient not receiving that therapy (Table 2): higher proportions of patients with recent (≤6 months) hospitalization, comedication with digoxin, and taking >3 different drugs were observed in the group receiving anticoagulation therapy than in the group not receiving it. All other parameters were not significantly different between these two groups. Comparing the percentages of patients receiving anticoagulation therapy according to the presence of digoxin in the admission treatment, we observed that 85% of the patients receiving this drug also received anticoagulation therapy, while only 55% of the patients without digoxin treatment received it ($P < 0.003$).

In univariate analysis, no geriatric characteristic was associated with the presence (or the absence) of anticoagulation therapy (Table 3). In multivariate analysis, only the presence of previous hospitalization within the last 6 months and the presence of digoxin treatment were factors associated with anticoagulation therapy (Table 4). The goodness-of-fit of this model remains significative, suggesting that those two factors were probably confounding.

5. Discussion

To the best of our knowledge, the present study is the first of its kind to address the issue of the variables associated with the underprescription of AVK in AF in the elderly, in a prospective way and in an emergency service. Out of a total of 995 geriatric subjects, the study covered 142 patients with AF. At first glance, one should notice factors which limit a potential generalization of the results. To begin, it concerned only a relatively small number of subjects in the context of their admission in the emergency service of a single, general, hospital that is situated in a neighborhood with a relatively high standard of living and where most patients have a suitable followup by their general practitioner. Secondly, the use of a questionnaire excluded patients with cognitive impairment (>4% of patients in the present study). Note that one cannot exclude that, in this study, slight confusion may have not been identified and may have been ascribed as "general status alteration." Also, as the collected data is quite subjective, the patient's answers might have been influenced by the attitude of the researcher. Finally, inclusion criteria could overestimate or underestimate the accurate proportion of patients with AF and known as such by their general practitioner. In our study, cases of paroxysmal AF (which

TABLE 1: Characteristics of the 142 old patients with AF.

	Mean (SD) or %	Median	Min	Max
% anticoagulation	61%			
AVK	50%			
LMWH	11%			
% aspirin alone	16%			
% association therapy				
Sintrom + aspirin	24%			
LMWH + aspirin	5%			
$CHADS_2$ (points)	2.4 (1.2)	2.0	1	5
% $CHADS_2 \geq 2$	73%			
Institution (long term care)	31%			
Number of classes of drugs	7.6 (3.2)	7.0	0	20
Ability to manage drug therapy				
Alone	51%			
Alone if prepared	33%			
Not possible	17%			
ISAR (points)	3.4 (1.7)	3	0	6
% ISAR ≥ 1	98%			
% ISAR ≥ 2	84%			
GDS (points)	0.8 (1.4)	0	0	4
% GDS > 1	33%			
% fallers < 6 months	34%			
% weight loss	34%			
% albumin < 3.5 g/100 mL	25%			
Hospitalizations	76%			

AVK: antivitamin K drug; LMWH: low molecular weight heparin; ISAR: identification of senior at risk; GDS: geriatric depression scale.

nevertheless need anticoagulation) could not be detected in the emergency room and some detected cases of AF might have been de novo or hitherto unknown paroxysmal AF.

Among all of the criteria analyzed in search of characteristics segregating patients who were anticoagulated from patients who were not, only three have been found. The first one is the condition of hospitalization within the 6 months that precede admission in the emergency room. Indeed, the proportion of anticoagulated patients is significantly higher in those who meet this criteria (52% versus 33%). A possible explanation is that hospitalization (whatever the reason) constitutes a prolonged period of medical observation which allows the detection of AF, including paroxysmal forms and the possibility to initiate anticoagulation in an easier way than in ambulatory practice. The second criterion is treatment with digoxin. Patients who were treated with this molecule were more often anticoagulated than subjects who were not (85% versus 55%). A possible explanation is that prescription of digoxin by the general practitioner attests his knowledge of the AF and/or of a closer monitoring of the patient. The third criterion is treatment with >3 different medications, with more such patients being anticoagulated (100% versus 89%). As for the digoxin, this could reflect closer monitoring by the physician.

On the basis of the referenced scores and scales, it was not possible to identify clearly any geriatric characteristic that could be associated with underprescription of AVK in AF. In other words and in accordance with the study by de Breucker et al. [33], no geriatric characteristic seems predictive of the decision by the physician to prescribe or not to prescribe anticoagulation in AF in the elderly. It can however not be excluded that such characteristic might be identified in a larger study. In the present study, 61% of patients with AF were anticoagulated, which is a higher share than the about 40% generally reported in medical literature [16–18]. A potential reason is the very large proportion of subjects included in the study (99%) which are monitored by a general practitioner. On the basis of the $CHADS_2$ score alone, 73% of the patients with AF should have been anticoagulated (score ≥ 2). Only 22% of anticoagulated patients had an INR between 2 and 3, which is much lower than the amount of 40 to 58% generally reported in literature [26, 27]. The enrollment of subjects in an emergency room (possibly unstable situation) may have underestimated the proportion of therapeutic INR in a stable situation. Of the 15 anticoagulated patients who were admitted for a trauma or a fall, no severe hemorrhage was diagnosed, even in patients with INR > 3 at the time of admission. Some observations may be made about comorbidities and comedications: 33% of patients with AF had heart failure and 60% had hypertension. This share is close to the one reported in the general geriatric population. Hypertension is known to be the most significant factor for AF in the elderly. 18% of patients with AF had previous history of stroke or TIA. In our subject pool, however, this

TABLE 2: Comparison of patients with AF according to their anticoagulation status.

(a) Geriatric characteristics

	Not anticoagulated		Anticoagulated		P
	n	Mean (SD) or %	n	Mean (SD) or %	
Institution (long term care)	56	37.5%	84	26.2%	0.155
Number of classes of drugs	54	6.5 (2.9)	86	8.2 (3.2)	**0.001**
Drug management ability	53	51%	80	50%	0.915
ISAR (points)	56	3.4 (1.7)	86	3.5 (1.6)	0.6173
% ISAR ≥ 1	56	95%	86	98%	0.338
% ISAR ≥ 2	56	82%	86	85%	0.665
GDS (points)	56	0.9 (1.4)	86	0.8 (1.4)	0.619
% GDS > 1	56	38%	86	30%	0.368
% patients who fell < 6 months	50	30%	77	36%	0.459
% weight loss	53	36%	78	32%	0.651
% albumin < 3.5 g/100 mL	47	26%	69	25%	0.913

(b) Comorbidities

	Not anticoagulated		Anticoagulated		P
	n	%	n	%	
% hospitalized < 6 months	52	33%	83	52%	**0.030**
Charlson (points)	54	2.4 (1.8)	83	2.6 (1.9)	0.525
Gastric ulcer	54	15%	84	19%	0.522
Liver	54	5%	84	9%	0.671
Hypertension	54	20%	84	25%	0.529
Myocardial infarction	54	13%	84	13%	0.982
COPD	54	13%	84	13%	0.982
Arteriopathy	54	11%	82	15%	0.553
Connectivitis	54	2%	84	2%	0.835
Cancer	54	24%	84	19%	0.053
HIV	54	0%	84	0%	—
Diabetes (not complicated)	56	9%	86	7%	0.671
Diabetes (complicated)	56	4%	86	3%	0.979
Hematological	54	7%	84	4%	0.316
		$CHADS_2$ score			
$CHADS_2$ (points)	56	2.3 (1.1)	86	2.44 (1.3)	0.557
% $CHADS_2$ ≥ 2	56	77%	86	70%	0.360
Congestive	54	28%	84	37%	0.267
Hypertension	54	67%	84	55%	0.165
Age	54	100%	84	100%	—
Diabetes	54	13%	84	11%	0.903
Stroke	54	15%	84	23%	0.284

(c) ISAR (identification of senior at risk).

	Not anticoagulated		Anticoagulated		P
	n	%	n	%	
>3 drugs	55	89%	86	100%	**0.002**
Need of help before admission	53	68%	80	64%	0.620
Need for help	53	45%	80	40%	0.546
Visual disorders	53	70%	79	75%	0.538

(c) Continued.

	Not anticoagulated		Anticoagulated		P
	n	%	n	%	
Memory disorders	52	50%	80	42%	0.398
Hospitalized < 6 months	52	33%	83	52%	**0.030**

(d) Drugs

	Not anticoagulated		Anticoagulated		P
	n	%	n	%	
Sintrom	54	0%	86	81%	0.000
LMWH	54	0%	86	19%	0.001
Antiaggregants	54	43%	86	20%	**0.004**
Digoxin	54	7%	86	20%	**0.003**
β Blockers	56	45%	86	57%	0.150
Flecainide	54	2%	86	1%	0.738
Ca-antagonists	54	20%	86	16%	0.230
IEC	54	35%	86	34%	0.723
Amiodarone	54	11%	86	22%	0.099
ARB	54	11%	86	10%	0.904
NSAI	54	2%	86	2%	0.851

TABLE 3: Univariate analysis of factors associated with the presence of anticoagulation (n = 142).

	Odds ratio (IC 95%)	P
Institution	0.59 (0.28–1.21)	0.155
% $CHADS_2 \geq 2$ points	0.69 (0.32–1.49)	0.359
% ISAR ≥ 1 point	2.37 (0.45–5.83)	0.338
% ISAR ≥ 2 points	1.12 (0.50–2.96)	0.664
% GDS > 1 point	0.72 (0.35–1.46)	0.368
% fallers < 6 months	1.33 (0.62–2.83)	0.459
% weight loss	0.84 (0.40–1.75)	0.651
% albumin < 3.5 mg/100 mL	0.95 (0.41–2.21)	0.913
% GFR < 40 mL/min	0.92 (0.35–2.41)	0.874

TABLE 4: Mutivariate analysis of factors associated with the presence of anticoagulation Logistic regression n = 135, Prob > χ^2 = 0.0005, and pseudo R^2 = 0.08.

	OR (IC 95%)	Err St	P
Hospitalization < 6 months	2.38 (1.12–5.04)	0.91	**0.023**
Digoxin therapy	5.24 (1.67–16.42)	3.05	**0.004**

Goodness-of-fit test: P = 0.0125.

previous history did not appear to influence the decision of the physician to prescribe anticoagulation. Such patients were not more often anticoagulated than others. This is in concordance with literature data on the influence of previous history of stroke on physician's decision to prescribe anticoagulation, with only the hemorrhagic type being known to exert an influence, by discouraging the prescription [1]. On the other hand, polymedication was systematic in our group of anticoagulated subjects: they all took at least 3 different medications, with an average of 7.

We have to recognize two limitations of our study that were due to the methodology used. Firstly, by excluding patients not able to answer the questionnaires of the comprehensive assessment, we couldn't study the impact of cognitive disorders. These are indeed often associated with underprescription of anticoagulation. Secondly, the recruitment in an emergency service required the use of a geriatric assessment that is less exhaustive than the classical "comprehensive geriatric assessment."

6. Conclusion

From this study of consecutive ≥75 years old patients with AF admitted in an emergency room and able to answer a questionnaire, no specific geriatric characteristic could be identified as significantly associated with, thus possibly predictive of, underprescription of AVK treatment. Only very few elements that reflect the influence of the quality of the monitoring on the probability for the patient to be actually anticoagulated could be noted. In accordance with available literature data, the present study confirms the underprescription of AVK in AF in the elderly and the lack of consideration for the $CHADS_2$ criteria. This study reports a very weak rate of INR in the therapeutic range, although with some reserves for its interpretation due to the design of study.

As already suggested, underprescription of anticoagulation in patients with AF is presumably due to complex interaction between patient-, physician-, and health care system-related factors [18], where the need, as well as the difficulty, of maintaining the INR level within the therapeutic range probably plays a major role. Could the new generations of oral anticoagulant (anti-Xa and anti-IIa) change this situation is a relevant question for the future.

Conflict of Interests

The authors declare that there is no conflict of interests regarding the publication of this paper.

Acknowledgment

Paule Denoël thanks the emergency team of the Europe Hospital, site St-Michel, for having actively participated in data collection which formed the basis for the present work.

References

[1] N. K. Choudhry, G. M. Anderson, A. Laupacis, D. Ross-Degnan, S.-L. T. Normand, and S. B. Soumerai, "Impact of adverse events on prescribing warfarin in patients with atrial fibrillation: matched pair analysis," *British Medical Journal*, vol. 332, no. 7534, pp. 141–145, 2006.

[2] A. Choudhury and G. Y. H. Lip, "How good is anticoagulation control in non-valvar atrial fibrillation? Observations on the elderly, ethnicity, patient perceptions, and understanding of AF thromboprophylaxis," *Heart*, vol. 91, no. 4, pp. 425–426, 2005.

[3] G. Y. Lip, S. Kamath, and R. G. Hart, "ABC of antithrombotic therapy: antithrombotic therapy for cerebrovascular disorders," *The British Medical Journal*, vol. 325, no. 7373, pp. 1161–1163, 2002.

[4] W. A. Wattigney, G. A. Mensah, and J. B. Croft, "Increasing trends in hospitalization for atrial fibrillation in the United States, 1985 through 1999 implications for primary prevention," *Circulation*, vol. 108, no. 6, pp. 711–716, 2003.

[5] T. J. Bungard, W. A. Ghali, K. K. Teo, F. A. McAlister, and R. T. Tsuyuki, "Why do patients with atrial fibrillation not receive warfarin?" *Archives of Internal Medicine*, vol. 160, no. 1, pp. 41–46, 2000.

[6] G. Y. H. Lip, H. F. Tse, and D. A. Lane, "Atrial fibrillation," *The Lancet*, vol. 379, no. 9816, pp. 648–661, 2012.

[7] A. B. Curtis, "Update on the clinical management of atrial fibrillation: guidelines and beyond," *Postgraduate Medicine*, vol. 123, no. 6, pp. 7–20, 2011.

[8] C. van Walraven, R. G. Hart, D. E. Singer et al., "Oral anticoagulants vs aspirin in nonvalvular atrial fibrillation: An individual patient meta-analysis," *Journal of the American Medical Association*, vol. 288, no. 19, pp. 2441–2448, 2002.

[9] H. Furusho, M. Takamura, S. Takata et al., "Current status of anticoagulation therapy for elderly atrial fibrillation patients in Japan: from Hokuriku atrial fibrillation trial," *Circulation Journal*, vol. 72, no. 12, pp. 2058–2061, 2008.

[10] "The efficacy of aspirin in patients with atrial fibrillation: analysis of pooled data from 3 randomized trials," *Archives of Internal Medicine*, vol. 157, no. 11, pp. 1237–1240, 1997.

[11] G. Y. Lip and H. S. Lim, "Atrial fibrillation and stroke prevention," *The Lancet Neurology*, vol. 6, no. 11, pp. 981–993, 2007.

[12] J. Mant, F. D. R. Hobbs, K. Fletcher et al., "Warfarin versus aspirin for stroke prevention in an elderly community population with atrial fibrillation (the Birmingham Atrial Fibrillation Treatment of the Aged Study, BAFTA): a randomised controlled trial," *The Lancet*, vol. 370, no. 9586, pp. 493–503, 2007.

[13] G. Y. Lip, R. Nieuwlaat, R. Pisters, D. A. Lane, and H. J. G. Crijns, "Refining clinical risk stratification for predicting stroke and thromboembolism in atrial fibrillation using a novel risk factor-based approach: the Euro Heart Survey on atrial fibrillation," *Chest*, vol. 137, no. 2, pp. 263–272, 2010.

[14] European Heart Rhythm Association, European Association for Cardio-Thoracic Surgery, and A. J. Camm, "Guidelines for the management of atrial fibrillation: the Task Force for the Management of Atrial Fibrillation of the European Society of Cardiology (ESC)," *European Heart Journal*, vol. 12, no. 10, pp. 1360–1420, 2010.

[15] B. F. Gage, A. D. Waterman, W. Shannon, M. Boechler, M. W. Rich, and M. J. Radford, "Validation of clinical classification schemes for predicting stroke: results from the National Registry of Atrial Fibrillation," *The Journal of the American Medical Association*, vol. 285, no. 22, pp. 2864–2870, 2001.

[16] R. J. Beyth, M. R. Antani, K. E. Covinsky et al., "Why isn't warfarin prescribed to patients with nonrheumatic atrial fibrillation?" *Journal of General Internal Medicine*, vol. 11, no. 12, pp. 721–728, 1996.

[17] N. Cohen, D. Almoznino-Sarafian, I. Alon et al., "Warfarin for stroke prevention still underused in atrial fibrillation: patterns of omission," *Stroke*, vol. 31, no. 6, pp. 1217–1222, 2000.

[18] S. Stewart, N. F. Murphy, A. Walker, A. McGuire, and J. J. McMurray, "Cost of an emerging epidemic: an economic analysis of atrial fibrillation in the UK," *Heart*, vol. 90, no. 3, pp. 286–292, 2004.

[19] D. P. Schauer, C. J. Moomaw, M. Wess, T. Webb, and M. H. Eckman, "Psychosocial risk factors for adverse outcomes in patients with nonvalvular atrial fibrillation receiving warfarin," *Journal of General Internal Medicine*, vol. 20, no. 12, pp. 1114–1119, 2005.

[20] L. M. Brass, H. M. Krumholz, J. M. Scinto, and M. Radford, "Warfarin use among patients with atrial fibrillation," *Stroke*, vol. 28, no. 12, pp. 2382–2389, 1997.

[21] M. A. Brodsky, J. G. Chun, P. J. Podrid, S. Douban, B. J. Allen, and R. Cygan, "Regional attitudes of generalists, specialists, and subspecialists about management of atrial fibrillation," *Archives of Internal Medicine*, vol. 156, no. 22, pp. 2553–2562, 1996.

[22] F. E. Munschauer, R. L. Priore, M. Hens, and A. Castilone, "Thromboembolism prophylaxis in chronic atrial fibrillation: practice patterns in community and tertiary-care hospitals," *Stroke*, vol. 28, no. 1, pp. 72–76, 1997.

[23] J. W. F. Mant, S. H. Richards, F. D. R. Hobbs et al., "Protocol for Birmingham Atrial Fibrillation Treatment of the Aged study (BAFTA): a randomised controlled trial of warfarin versus aspirin for stroke prevention in the management of atrial fibrillation in an elderly primary care population [ISRCTN89345269]," *BMC Cardiovascular Disorders*, vol. 3, article 9, 2003.

[24] D. C. McCrory, D. B. Matchar, G. Samsa, L. L. Sanders, and E. L. C. Pritchett, "Physician attitudes about anticoagulation for nonvalvular atrial fibrillation in the elderly," *Archives of Internal Medicine*, vol. 155, no. 3, pp. 277–281, 1995.

[25] M. Kutner, G. Nixon, and F. Silverstone, "Physicians' attitudes toward oral anticoagulants and antiplatelet agents for stroke prevention in elderly patients with atrial fibrillation," *Archives of Internal Medicine*, vol. 151, no. 10, pp. 1950–1953, 1991.

[26] J. H. Gurwitz, J. Monette, P. A. Rochon, M. A. Eckler, and J. Avorn, "Atrial fibrillation and stroke prevention with warfarin in the long- term care setting," *Archives of Internal Medicine*, vol. 157, no. 9, pp. 978–984, 1997.

[27] M. R. Patel, K. W. Mahaffey, J. Garg et al., "Rivaroxaban versus warfarin in nonvalvular atrial fibrillation," *The New England Journal of Medicine*, vol. 365, no. 10, pp. 883–891, 2011.

[28] G. C. Dantas, B. V. Thompson, J. A. Manson, C. S. Tracy, and R. E. G. Upshur, "Patients' perspectives on taking warfarin: qualitative study in family practice," *BMC Family Practice*, vol. 5, article 15, 9 pages, 2004.

[29] A. Laupacis and K. Sullivan, "Canadian atrial fibrillation anticoagulation study: were the patients subsequently treated with

warfarin?" *CMAJ : Canadian Medical Association journal*, vol. 154, no. 11, pp. 1669–1674, 1996.

[30] P. J. Devereaux, D. R. Anderson, M. J. Gardner et al., "Differences between perspectives of physicians and patients on anticoagulation in patients with atrial fibrillation: observational study," *The British Medical Journal*, vol. 323, no. 7323, pp. 1218–1221, 2001.

[31] M. Sudlow, R. Thomson, B. Thwaites, H. Rodgers, and R. A. Kenny, "Prevalence of atrial fibrillation and eligibility for anticoagulants in the community," *The Lancet*, vol. 352, no. 9135, pp. 1167–1171, 1998.

[32] R. Rozzini, T. Sabatini, M. Trabucchi, L. Kalra, I. Perez, and A. Melbourn, "Risk assessment and anticoagulation in atrial fibrillation in the elderly: malpractice or accuracy?" *Stroke*, vol. 30, no. 10, pp. 2239–2240, 1999.

[33] S. de Breucker, G. Herzog, and T. Pepersack, "Could geriatric characteristics explain the under-prescription of anticoagulation therapy for older patients admitted with atrial fibrillation? A retrospective observational study," *Drugs & Aging*, vol. 27, no. 10, pp. 807–813, 2010.

[34] G. Y. H. Lip, "Implications of the CHA_2DS_2-VASc and HAS-BLED scores for thromboprophylaxis in atrial fibrillation," *The American Journal of Medicine*, vol. 124, no. 2, pp. 111–114, 2011.

[35] J. McCusker, F. Bellavance, S. Cardin et al., "Screening for geriatric problems in the emergency department: reliability and validity," *Academic Emergency Medicine*, vol. 5, no. 9, pp. 883–893, 1998.

[36] M. P. Lawton and E. M. Brody, "Assessment of older people: self-maintaining and instrumental activities of daily living.," *Gerontologist*, vol. 9, no. 3, pp. 179–186, 1969.

[37] J. A. Yesavage, "Geriatric depression scale," *Psychopharmacology Bulletin*, vol. 24, no. 4, pp. 709–711, 1988.

[38] R. J. Stratton, A. Hackston, D. Longmore et al., "Malnutrition in hospital outpatients and inpatients: prevalence, concurrent validity and ease of use of the "malnutrition universal screening tool" ("MUST") for adults," *British Journal of Nutrition*, vol. 92, no. 5, pp. 799–808, 2004.

[39] J. Bernardini, S. Callen, L. Fried, and B. Piraino, "Inter-rater reliability and annual rescoring of the Charlson comorbidity index," *Advances in Peritoneal Dialysis. Conference on Peritoneal Dialysis*, vol. 20, pp. 125–127, 2004.

16

A Growing Troubling Triad: Diabetes, Aging, and Falls

Ryan T. Crews, Sai V. Yalla, Adam E. Fleischer, and Stephanie C. Wu

Center for Lower Extremity Ambulatory Research (CLEAR), Dr. William M. Scholl College of Podiatric Medicine, Rosalind Franklin University of Medicine and Science, 3333 Green Bay Road, North Chicago, IL 60064, USA

Correspondence should be addressed to Ryan T. Crews; ryan.crews@rosalindfranklin.edu

Academic Editor: Neil D. Reeves

There is a significant and troubling link between diabetes (DM) and falls in the elderly. Individuals with DM are prone to fall for reasons such as decreased sensorimotor function, musculoskeletal/neuromuscular deficits, foot and body pain, pharmacological complications, and specialty (offloading) footwear devices. Additionally, there is some concern that DM patients are prone to have more severe problems with falls than non-DM individuals. Fractures, poorer rehabilitation, and increased number of falls are all concerns. Fortunately, efforts to mitigate falls by DM patients show promise. A number of studies have shown that balance, strength, and gait training may be utilized to successfully reduce fall risk in this population. Furthermore, new technologies such as virtual reality proprioceptive training may be able to provide this reduced risk within a safe training environment.

1. Introduction

From 2000 to 2010 the elderly (65+ years) population in the USA has continued its upward trend, increasing by 5.25 million (15%) to a total of 40.26 million [1]. This amounts to 13% of the entire population [1]. Thanks to the aging baby boomers population, by the year 2050 the elderly population is expected to reach 88.5 million, which would represent 20% of the total population [2]. One of the greatest health challenges facing this population is falls. In 2000 there were a reported 10,300 fatal falls by the elderly in the USA that incurred $179 million in direct medical costs [3]. There were an additional 2.6 million medically treated falls that cost $19 billion in medical costs. Other western nations report similar significant burdens with the United Kingdom reporting £981 million (US $1.9 billion) in costs for falls in those 60 or more years old in 1999 [4], and in 2001 the annual cost of care attributable to falls in those 65 or older in Australia was $86.4 million (US $66.1 million) [5]. While the cause of falls is often multifactorial, diabetes mellitus (DM) has been shown to be a significant factor. The significance of the relationship between aging, DM, and falls has been highlighted by previous work that found the annual incidence of falls in elderly individuals with DM to be 39% [6]. This paper will review the association of fall occurrence and diabetes, the association of fall severity and diabetes, and efforts to limit diabetes associated risks for falls.

2. Association between Diabetes and Falls

Falls are a major concern for elderly adults with DM [7]. The high prevalence of falls in ambulatory elderly individuals with DM is well established with reported annual incidence rates of 39% in those over 65 years [6] and 35% in those over 55 years [8]. In addition to the reported high incidence of falls in this population, it has been established that DM individuals are at a higher risk for falls [9, 10]. There are a number of mechanisms by which DM may contribute to falls. Decreased sensorimotor function, musculoskeletal/neuromuscular deficits, foot and body pain, pharmacological complications, and specialty (offloading) footwear devices will be discussed.

3. Decreased Sensorimotor Function

Diabetic peripheral neuropathy (DPN) is common among the DM population, and its prevalence increases with age and duration of diabetes [11–13]. While a number of detrimental changes to the nervous system fall under the umbrella of

DPN, this section will focus on the most common type which is damage to the large nerve fibers that results in decreased sensorimotor function [14]. DPN patients with diminished plantar sensation on their feet have been observed to exhibit increased postural sway along with significant loss of postural control [15, 16]. Loss of proprioceptive feedback [17] during standing and walking in turn leads to increased risk of falls which is evident from a recent prospective cohort study on 9,249 women aged above 67 years where postural instability and DPN were observed to account for the largest percentage of the relationship between diabetes and falls [18]. Cross-sectional studies have also found a strong association between the development of DPN and falls. Among 21 DM patients over 55 years who reported at least one fall in the past year, MacGilchrist et al. found that 86% had peripheral neuropathy [8]. Furthermore, it has been shown that as DPN severity increases, performance on functional reach tests declines [19]. Thus, as DPN severity increases, there is a higher risk of falls occurring while completing reaching tasks in the standing position. While there are many risk factors that contribute to falls, DPN is definitely a significant contributor [20].

4. Musculoskeletal/Neuromuscular

Apart from DPN, lower physical activity, muscle strength, and poor postural control were also found to be among the significant risk factors that influence gait patterns and increased risk of falls among the DM population [21, 22]. Among the elderly population, postural control is an important factor to perform activities such as standing, sitting, walking, and reaching tasks [23–25]. Considering that the feet serve as the base supporting structure during these activities, the strength in lower extremity joints plays a vital role in establishing a strategy for postural stability [26]. Impaired postural control during static balance tests [27] as well as dynamic short whole body anterior translations of 1–4 mm in older patients with DM [28] increases the limitations at the base of support and in turn results in increased risk of falls.

In addition to the lack of sensorimotor function discussed previously, coordination of muscles for postural compensatory strategies is challenged in individuals with DPN. Najafi et al. [17] utilized a novel compensatory index for quantifying postural control strategy to compare strategies utilized by healthy young subjects to strategies of older DPN subjects. In comparison to the healthy young, the older DPN subjects had a significant 10% reduction in postural compensatory strategy. This was coupled with a 98% increase in postural sway. This difficulty in postural control coupled with an altered gait pattern [29] further increases the risk of falls in DPN patients.

Low plantar flexion strength has also been observed to be associated with increased center of mass (COM) displacement or sway among DM patients negatively affecting the maximum forward reach distance [24]. Accordingly, while studying ambulatory DM patients, Macgilchrit et al. found that ankle plantar flexion muscle strength was lower among fallers by 40% compared to nonfallers [8]. Reduced muscle strength has also been shown to result in reduced walking speeds [25, 30], and an increased double support phase of the gait cycle. Studies have shown increased double support time to be a significant factor for falls [31–33] especially in people with postural instability [34]. Individuals at high risk for falls likely adopt this increased double support strategy in order to limit the time during which they must maintain balance on a single limb. This further emphasizes the need for exercise training and developing a stable postural control strategy in DM patients to reduce the risk of falls.

5. Foot and Body Pain/Pharmacological Complications

While the majority of excess fall risk in patients with diabetes can be attributed to DPN sensorimotor decrements and aberrant neuromuscular control, it is important to recognize that other factors associated with diabetes (e.g., foot and body pain and the use of psychotropic medications and polypharmacy) can also contribute to a heightened fall risk profile.

Foot pain is another recognized risk factor for falls among community-dwelling older adults [35, 36]. Patients with diabetes frequently experience symptoms of painful polyneuropathy as the distal nerve fibers in the toes and foot begin to deteriorate. Similarly, patients with chronic disabilities encounter greater levels of chronic, generalized body pain [37, 38] which also places them at increased risk for recurrent falls [21]. This is because diabetic individuals suffering with chronic pain may be less capable of adhering to productive self-management practices like regular exercise [37] and have poorer mental health and physical functioning [38] which places them at increased risk for falls [35].

Diabetic patients that suffer with neuropathic pain are frequently managed with psychotropic and other central nervous system mediated medications. Amitriptyline and duloxetine hydrochloride, for example, are commonly used to treat the painful symptoms of diabetic neuropathy, the latter being one of only two FDA-approved medications for use in diabetic neuropathy. Psychotropic medications are frequently implicated in falls and nearly double an elderly adult's risk for experiencing a fall [39, 40] and having recurrent falls [21, 41]. Older adults suffering with diabetes are also more likely to be taking a greater number of prescription medications [21] and seem to be more sensitive to the effects of polypharmacy than their nondiabetic counterparts [40, 42]. Patients with diabetes start to experience an increased risk of falling with regimens involving just 4 or more prescription medications [42].

One of the hazards of managing diabetes is the increased risk for experiencing unexpectedly low blood glucose levels and symptomatic hypoglycemia. Hypoglycemic episodes can occur with oral hypoglycemic and/or insulin use and frequently result in a state of dizziness, confusion, and postural instability which increases ones' risk for a fall accident [43–46]. While the literature has been somewhat mixed regarding the extent to which the level of diabetes control influences fall risk [42, 47, 48], it remains clear that the medications associated with treating DM and its complications can contribute to increased fall risk.

6. Offloading Footwear

Footwear such as athletic shoes has been found to reduce fall risk in older adults [49, 50]. Within the DM population, foot ulcers are highly prevalent [51, 52] and often develop due to cumulatively high localized plantar pressure on their feet [53–55]. In order to reduce the risk of ulceration and also for treatment of ulcers, footwear that provides offloading of the localized stress is widely used [55–57]. Even though offloading footwear has not been directly associated with falls, some offloading devices have certainly been found to negatively affect postural stability [58, 59]. Of most concern are the casts and cast walkers used in the treatment of diabetic foot ulcers. These devices significantly restrict normal gait. In addition to being heavy, prohibiting ankle movement, prohibiting normal heel to toe progressive loading of the foot, and potentially decreasing proprioception, some offloading footwear also creates a limb length discrepancy [60]. Given the association of postural stability to fall risk [61], reduced postural stability due to offloading footwear will increase the risk of falls of those utilizing the footwear. Design modification for offloading footwear such as reduction in strut height and reduced weight has been suggested as a means to improve postural stability [62] which might in turn reduce fall risk.

7. Association of Fall Severity and Diabetes

In an editorial concerning complications of diabetes in elderly people, Gregg et al. noted that falls and fractures along with cognitive disorders, physical disability, and other geriatric syndromes may be as great a concern to older people with diabetes as the more traditionally recognized vascular complications [63]. Diabetes increases not only the risk of falls, but also the risk of fractures [64, 65]. Strotmeyer and coworkers found older adults with diabetes to be at higher fracture risk compared with nondiabetic adults with similar bone mineral density [65]. The literature suggests that the fracture risk point estimates described in type 1 diabetes are considerably higher than in type 2 diabetes [66]. However, increased fracture risk in longstanding type 2 diabetes is a paradoxical phenomenon because men and women with type 2 diabetes typically have normal to high bone mineral density [67–69]. Altered body composition and microvascular complications, including retinopathy, peripheral and autonomic neuropathy, hypoglycemia, and use of medications, particularly thiazolidinediones, are all related with increased risk of fractures in older adults with diabetes [7, 70].

In addition to a predisposition to fractures with falls, individuals with DM may be prone to poorer rehabilitation. In investigating rehabilitation following hip fracture, Semel et al. [71] found that patients with diabetes had worse outcomes. The authors noted that patients with diabetes had a worse length of stay efficiency (a measure of recovery per each day of hospital stay) compared with other patients. Similarly, when Liberman et al. compared 224 patients with diabetes to 738 patients without diabetes in a prospective cohort study, they found that patients with diabetes had a worse functional outcome following rehabilitation after hip fracture surgery [72]. Ekstrom and colleagues evaluated the health-related quality of life (HRQoL) after hip fractures and noted that patients with diabetes mellitus had more pain, comorbidities, and reduced health status preoperatively than patients without diabetes. The authors further noted that while there were no more medical complications among patients with diabetes during the first postoperative year, cardiac ($P = 0.023$) and renal failures ($P = 0.032$) were more frequent in patients with diabetes at 24 months.

One last factor to consider in the severity of falls is the occurrence of recurrent falls. Pijpers et al. compared the incidence of recurrent falls in older people with and without diabetes with a mean followup of 139 weeks and noted that 30.6% of the individuals with diabetes and 19.4% of the individuals without diabetes fell recurrently (incidence rate of 129.7 versus 77.4 per 1,000 persons-years, respectively, HR = 1.67 (95% CI: 1.11–2.51)) [21]. The authors noted that the greater number of medication, higher levels of pain, poorer self-perceived health, lower physical activity and grip strength, more limitations in activities of daily living, lower-extremity physical performance, and cognitive impairment may potentially increase the risk of recurrent falls, and these variables together accounted for 47% of the increased risk of recurrent falls associated with diabetes (adjusted HR = 1.30 (0.79–2.11)).

8. Combating DM-Related Fall Risks

A recent publication regarding falls of elderly people in long-term care facilities found that 49% of falls in this setting occurred while walking, 24% while standing, and 21% while either rising up or lowering oneself [73]. In studying daily physical activity patterns of DPN subjects with a mean age of 59 ± 8 years, it was found that each 24 hr day these subjects spend 13.5% of their time standing and 6.1% walking and performed 77 sit-to-stand postural transitions per day on average [74]. Therefore, unfortunately there are plenty of opportunities for elderly adults with DM to experience a fall. Accordingly, numerous investigations regarding improving balance, strength, and gait in order to reduce falls have been conducted [27, 30, 75–77].

Weekly balance training sessions with or without additional strength and/or gait training have been shown to reduce fall risk in DM patients [27, 30, 75, 76]. Positive outcomes have been found both in the broad perspective of DM patients in general [76] as well as specifically in DPN patients [30, 75]. What is more promising is that in a study comparing four groups (DM with fall history $n = 7$, DM without fall history $n = 9$, non-DM with fall history $n = 7$, non-DM without fall history $n = 14$), the greatest improvements were seen in DM patients with a history of falling [27]. One study to actually track fall occurrence following implementation of a strength and balance program for DPN patients did not show a reduction in falls compared to a DPN control group; however, there were several limitations to the study [77]. This was a secondary analysis of a study utilizing subjects with a somewhat low minimum age criteria of 50. Also the majority of the prescribed intervention was to be conducted at home without supervision. Only 8 training sessions were conducted with a physical therapist, all of which occurred during months 1–3. The first balance and strength assessments to occur after initiation of training did not occur until 6 months after study initiation. Finally no information was provided concerning compliance of exercise at home and only 45% of participants in the intervention group completed "more than half of the required study protocol elements (p. 1572)." In contrast, a study comparing home-based versus "center-based" balance and strength training for 107 community-dwelling adults (DM was not an inclusion criteria) referred for a falls prevention service found that the center-based service demonstrated significantly better results in preventing falls [78].

In addition to traditional balance and strength training, new technologies utilizing virtual reality may provide additional training methods with limited patient risk. It has been previously shown that DM patients either without or with minimum DPN demonstrate reduced toe-obstacle clearance with altered gait patterns during obstacle crossing [79]. In addition to increasing fall risk during daily living, training to improve clearance could be risky in that falls may occur during training sessions requiring subjects to step over obstacles. Recently an investigation validated a virtual reality protocol for assessing obstacle crossing while stepping in place [80]. The study showed that DPN participants had greater difficulty completing the virtual obstacle crossing. It is possible that this paradigm could be used as a minimal risk training program to improve real world obstacle crossing and subsequently reduce fall risk.

9. Conclusion

Falls in elderly individuals with DM are a significant burden to the healthcare system. A number of factors tied to DM predispose this population to a higher risk of falls. Additionally, the falls that this population suffers from have the potential to be more severe in terms of injuries sustained as well as the recovery process. Therefore much work is ongoing regarding the reduction of falls in this population. Numerous studies utilizing balance, strength, and/or gait training have demonstrated reduced fall risk for DM patients that undertook the training. More prospective work is needed regarding the long-term outcome of these interventions on actual fall prevention.

References

[1] C. A. Werner, *The Older Population: 2010*, in *2010 Census Briefs*, United States Census Bureau, 2011.

[2] G. K. Vincent and V. A. Velkoff, *THE NEXT FOUR DECADES The Older Population in the United States: 2010 to 2050*, in *Population Estimates and Projections*, United States Census Bureau, 2010.

[3] J. A. Stevens, P. S. Corso, E. A. Finkelstein, and T. R. Miller, "The costs of fatal and non-fatal falls among older adults," *Injury Prevention*, vol. 12, no. 5, pp. 290–295, 2006.

[4] P. Scuffham, S. Chaplin, and R. Legood, "Incidence and costs of unintentional falls in older people in the United Kingdom," *Journal of Epidemiology and Community Health*, vol. 57, no. 9, pp. 740–744, 2003.

[5] D. Hendrie, S. E. Hall, G. Arena, and M. Legge, "Health system costs of falls of older adults in Western Australia," *Australian Health Review*, vol. 28, no. 3, pp. 363–373, 2004.

[6] L. M. Tilling, K. Darawil, and M. Britton, "Falls as a complication of diabetes mellitus in older people," *Journal of Diabetes and Its Complications*, vol. 20, no. 3, pp. 158–162, 2006.

[7] K. S. Kim, S. K. Kim, K. M. Sung et al., "Management of type 2 diabetes mellitus in older adults," *Diabetes & Metabolism Journal*, vol. 36, no. 5, pp. 336–344, 2012.

[8] C. Macgilchrist, L. Paul, B. M. Ellis, T. E. Howe, B. Kennon, and J. Godwin, "Lower-limb risk factors for falls in people with diabetes mellitus," *Diabetic Medicine*, vol. 27, no. 2, pp. 162–168, 2010.

[9] P. P. Oliveira, S. Maria Fachin, J. Jozatti et al., "Comparative analysis of risk for falls in patients with and without type 2 diabetes mellitus," *Revista da Associação Médica Brasileira*, vol. 58, no. 2, pp. 234–239, 2012.

[10] A. V. Schwartz, T. A. Hillier, D. E. Sellmeyer et al., "Older women with diabetes have a higher risk of falls: a prospective study," *Diabetes Care*, vol. 25, no. 10, pp. 1749–1754, 2002.

[11] K. van Acker, D. Bouhassira, D. de Bacquer et al., "Prevalence and impact on quality of life of peripheral neuropathy with or without neuropathic pain in type 1 and type 2 diabetic patients attending hospital outpatients clinics," *Diabetes & Metabolism*, vol. 35, no. 3, pp. 206–213, 2009.

[12] M. J. Young, A. J. M. Boulton, A. F. Macleod, D. R. R. Williams, and P. H. Sonksen, "A multicentre study of the prevalence of diabetic peripheral neuropathy in the United Kingdom hospital clinic population," *Diabetologia*, vol. 36, no. 2, pp. 150–154, 1993.

[13] S. Tesfaye, L. K. Stevens, J. M. Stephenson et al., "Prevalence of diabetic peripheral neuropathy and its relation to glycaemic control and potential risk factors: the EURODIAB IDDM Complications Study," *Diabetologia*, vol. 39, no. 11, pp. 1377–1384, 1996.

[14] S. Tesfaye, "Diabetic Neuropathy," in *The Foot in Diabetes*, P. R. Cavanagh, A. J. M. Boulton, and G. Rayman, Eds., John Wiley & Sons, West Sussex, UK, 2006.

[15] B. Najafi, D. Horn, S. Marclay, R. T. Crews, S. Wu, and J. S. Wrobel, "Foot technology, part 1 of 2: assessing postural control and postural control strategy in diabetes patients using innovative and wearable technology," *Journal of Diabetes Science and Technology*, vol. 4, no. 4, pp. 780–791, 2010.

[16] H. B. Menz, S. R. Lord, R. St George, and R. C. Fitzpatrick, "Walking stability and sensorimotor function in older people with diabetic peripheral neuropathy," *Archives of Physical Medicine and Rehabilitation*, vol. 85, no. 2, pp. 245–252, 2004.

[17] B. Najafi, D. Horn, S. Marclay, R. T. Crews, S. Wu, and J. S. Wrobel, "Assessing postural control and postural control strategy in diabetes patients using innovative and wearable technology," *Journal of Diabetes Science and Technology*, vol. 4, no. 4, pp. 780–791, 2010.

[18] A. V. Schwartz, T. A. Hillier, D. E. Sellmeyer et al., "Older women with diabetes have a higher risk of falls: a prospective study," *Diabetes Care*, vol. 25, no. 10, pp. 1749–1754, 2002.

[19] S. I. Lin, Y. R. Chen, C. F. Liao, and C. W. Chou, "Association between sensorimotor function and forward reach in patients with diabetes," *Gait & Posture*, vol. 32, no. 4, pp. 581–585, 2010.

[20] J. K. Richardson and E. A. Hurvitz, "Peripheral neuropathy: a true risk factor for falls," *The Journals of Gerontology A*, vol. 50, no. 4, pp. M211–M215, 1995.

[21] E. Pijpers, I. Ferreira, R. T. de Jongh et al., "Older individuals with diabetes have an increased risk of recurrent falls: analysis of potential mediating factors: the Longitudinal Ageing Study Amsterdam," *Age Ageing*, vol. 41, no. 3, pp. 358–365, 2012.

[22] J. S. Wrobel, R. T. Crews, and J. E. Connolly, "Clinical factors associated with a conservative gait pattern in older male veterans with diabetes," *Journal of Foot and Ankle Research*, vol. 2, no. 1, article 11, 2009.

[23] M. E. Tinetti, M. Speechley, and S. F. Ginter, "Risk factors for falls among elderly persons living in the community," *The New England Journal of Medicine*, vol. 319, no. 26, pp. 1701–1707, 1988.

[24] S. I. Lin, Y. R. Chen, C. F. Liao, and C. W. Chou, "Association between sensorimotor function and forward reach in patients with diabetes," *Gait & Posture*, vol. 32, no. 4, pp. 581–585, 2010.

[25] P. P. Alvarenga, D. S. Pereira, and D. M. C. Anjos, "Functional mobility and executive function in elderly diabetics and non-diabetics," *Revista Brasileira de Fisioterapia*, vol. 14, no. 6, pp. 491–496, 2010.

[26] F. B. Horak, "Postural orientation and equilibrium: what do we need to know about neural control of balance to prevent falls?" *Age and Ageing*, vol. 35, supplement 2, pp. ii7–ii11, 2006.

[27] S. Morrison, S. R. Colberg, H. K. Parson et al., "Relation between risk of falling and postural sway complexity in diabetes," *Gait Posture*, vol. 35, no. 4, pp. 662–668, 2012.

[28] G. D. Fulk, C. J. Robinson, S. Mondal, C. M. Storey, and A. M. Hollister, "The effects of diabetes and/or peripheral neuropathy in detecting short postural perturbations in mature adults," *Journal of NeuroEngineering and Rehabilitation*, vol. 7, no. 1, article 44, 2010.

[29] J. S. Wrobel and B. Najafi, "Foot technology, part 1 of 2: diabetic foot biomechanics and gait dysfunction," *Journal of Diabetes Science and Technology*, vol. 4, no. 4, pp. 833–845, 2010.

[30] L. Allet, S. Armand, R. A. de Bie et al., "The gait and balance of patients with diabetes can be improved: a randomised controlled trial," *Diabetologia*, vol. 53, no. 3, pp. 458–466, 2010.

[31] E. Nordin, R. Moe-Nilssen, A. Ramnemark, and L. Lundin-Olsson, "Changes in step-width during dual-task walking predicts falls," *Gait & Posture*, vol. 32, no. 1, pp. 92–97, 2010.

[32] D. A. Winter, A. E. Patla, J. S. Frank, and S. E. Walt, "Biomechanical walking pattern changes in the fit and healthy elderly," *Physical Therapy*, vol. 70, no. 6, pp. 340–347, 1990.

[33] S. M. Friedman, B. Munoz, S. K. West, G. S. Rubin, and L. P. Fried, "Falls and fear of falling: which comes first? A longitudinal prediction model suggests strategies for primary and secondary prevention," *Journal of the American Geriatrics Society*, vol. 50, no. 8, pp. 1329–1335, 2002.

[34] L. Allet, S. Armand, R. A. de Bie et al., "Clinical factors associated with gait alterations in diabetic patients," *Diabetic Medicine*, vol. 26, no. 10, pp. 1003–1009, 2009.

[35] S. G. Leveille, J. Bean, K. Bandeen-Roche, R. Jones, M. Hochberg, and J. M. Guralnik, "Musculoskeletal pain and risk for falls in older disabled women living in the community," *Journal of the American Geriatrics Society*, vol. 50, no. 4, pp. 671–678, 2002.

[36] A. Gabell, M. A. Simons, and U. S. L. Nayak, "Falls in the healthy elderly: predisposing causes," *Ergonomics*, vol. 28, no. 7, pp. 965–975, 1985.

[37] S. L. Krein, M. Heisler, J. D. Piette, F. Makki, and E. A. Kerr, "The effect of chronic pain on diabetes patients' self-management," *Diabetes Care*, vol. 28, no. 1, pp. 65–70, 2005.

[38] M. J. Bair, E. J. Brizendine, R. T. Ackermann, C. Shen, K. Kroenke, and D. G. Marrero, "Prevalence of pain and association with quality of life, depression and glycaemic control in patients with diabetes," *Diabetic Medicine*, vol. 27, no. 5, pp. 578–584, 2010.

[39] R. M. Leipzig, R. G. Cumming, and M. E. Tinetti, "Drugs and falls in older people: a systematic review and meta-analysis: I. Psychotropic drugs," *Journal of the American Geriatrics Society*, vol. 47, no. 1, pp. 30–39, 1999.

[40] A. J. Campbell, M. J. Borrie, and G. F. Spears, "Risk factors for falls in a community-based prospective study of people 70 years and older," *Journals of Gerontology*, vol. 44, no. 4, pp. M112–M117, 1989.

[41] H. Luukinen, K. Koski, P. Laippala, and S. L. Kivela, "Predictors for recurrent falls among the home-dwelling elderly," *Scandinavian Journal of Primary Health Care*, vol. 13, no. 4, pp. 294–299, 1995.

[42] E. S. Huang, A. J. Karter, K. K. Danielson, E. M. Warton, and A. T. Ahmed, "The association between the number of prescription medications and incident falls in a multi-ethnic population of adult type-2 diabetes patients: the diabetes and aging study," *Journal of General Internal Medicine*, vol. 25, no. 2, pp. 141–146, 2010.

[43] J. M. Nelson, K. Dufraux, and P. F. Cook, "The relationship between glycemic control and falls in older adults," *Journal of the American Geriatrics Society*, vol. 55, no. 12, pp. 2041–2044, 2007.

[44] S. S. Johnston, C. Conner, M. Aagren et al., "Association between hypoglycaemic events and fall-related fractures in Medicare-covered patients with type 2 diabetes," *Diabetes, Obesity and Metabolism*, vol. 14, no. 7, pp. 634–643, 2012.

[45] A. V. Schwartz, E. Vittinghoff, D. E. Sellmeyer et al., "Diabetes-related complications, glycemic control, and falls in older adults," *Diabetes Care*, vol. 31, no. 3, pp. 391–396, 2008.

[46] J. E. Signorovitch, D. Macaulay, M. Diener et al., "Hypoglycaemia and accident risk in people with type 2 diabetes mellitus treated with non-insulinantidiabetes drugs," *Diabetes, Obesity and Metabolism*. In press.

[47] D. K. Miller, L.-Y. Lily Lui, F. E. Kaiser et al., "Reported and measured physical functioning in older inner-city diabetic African Americans," *The Journals of Gerontology A*, vol. 54, no. 5, pp. M230–M236, 1999.

[48] A. V. Schwartz, K. L. Margolis, D. E. Sellmeyer et al., "Intensive glycemic control is not associated with fractures or falls in the ACCORD randomized trial," *Diabetes Care*, vol. 35, no. 7, pp. 1525–1531, 2012.

[49] H. B. Menz, M. E. Morris, and S. R. Lord, "Footwear characteristics and risk of indoor and outdoor falls in older people," *Gerontology*, vol. 52, no. 3, pp. 174–180, 2006.

[50] J. L. Kelsey, E. Procter-Gray, U. S. D. T. Nguyenb, W. Li, D. P. Kiel, and M. T. Hannan, "Footwear and falls in the home among older individuals in the MOBILIZE Boston study," *Footwear Science*, vol. 2, no. 3, pp. 123–129, 2010.

[51] S. Kumar, H. A. Ashe, L. N. Parnell et al., "The prevalence of foot ulceration and its correlates in type 2 diabetic patients: a population-based study," *Diabetic Medicine*, vol. 11, no. 5, pp. 480–484, 2009.

[52] D. J. Margolis, D. S. Malay, O. J. Hoffstad et al., "Prevalence of diabetes, diabetic foot ulcer, and lower extremity amputation among Medicare beneficiaries, 2006 to 2008: data

Points #1," in *Data Points Publication Series*, Agency for Healthcare Research and Quality, Rockville, Md, USA, 2011, http://www.ncbi.nlm.nih.gov/books/NBK63602/.

[53] A. Veves, H. J. Murray, M. J. Young, and A. J. M. Boulton, "The risk of foot ulceration in diabetic patients with high foot pressure: a prospective study," *Diabetologia*, vol. 35, no. 7, pp. 660–663, 1992.

[54] L. A. Lavery, S. A. Vela, D. C. Lavery, and T. L. Quebedeaux, "Reducing dynamic foot pressures in high-risk diabetic subjects with foot ulcerations: a comparison of treatments," *Diabetes Care*, vol. 19, no. 8, pp. 818–821, 1996.

[55] S. C. Wu, R. T. Crews, and D. G. Armstrong, "The pivotal role of offloading in the management of neuropathic foot ulceration," *Current Diabetes Reports*, vol. 5, no. 6, pp. 423–429, 2005.

[56] A. J. M. Boulton, "Pressure and the diabetic foot: clinical science and offloading techniques," *The American Journal of Surgery*, vol. 187, no. 5, supplement 1, pp. S17–S24, 2004.

[57] P. R. Cavanagh, B. A. Lipsky, A. W. Bradbury, and G. Botek, "Treatment for diabetic foot ulcers," *The Lancet*, vol. 366, no. 9498, pp. 1725–1735, 2005.

[58] R. van Deursen, "Footwear for the neuropathic patient: offloading and stability," *Diabetes/Metabolism Research and Reviews*, vol. 24, no. supplement 1, pp. S96–S100, 2008.

[59] L. A. Lavery, J. G. Fleishli, T. J. Laughlin, S. A. Vela, D. C. Lavery, and D. G. Armstrong, "Is postural instability exacerbated by offloading devices in high risk diabetics with foot ulcers?" *Ostomy Wound Management*, vol. 44, no. 1, pp. 26–34, 1998.

[60] M. EI-Nahas, H. M. Gawish, M. M. Tarshoby et al., "Effect of simulated leg length discrepancy on plantar pressure distribution in diabetic patients with neuropathic foot ulceration," *Journal of Wound Care*, vol. 20, no. 10, pp. 473–477, 2011.

[61] S. R. Lord, P. N. Sambrook, C. Gilbert et al., "Postural stability, falls and fractures in the elderly: results from the Dubbo Osteoporosis Epidemiology Study," *The Medical Journal of Australia*, vol. 160, no. 11, pp. 684–688, 1994.

[62] R. T. Crews, F. Sayeed, and B. Najafi, "Impact of strut height on offloading capacity of removable cast walkers," *Clinical Biomechanics*, vol. 27, no. 7, pp. 725–730, 2012.

[63] E. W. Gregg, M. M. Engelgau, and V. Narayan, "Complications of diabetes in elderly people," *British Medical Journal*, vol. 325, no. 7370, pp. 916–917, 2002.

[64] W. Ekstrom, A. N. Al-Ani, M. Sääf et al., "Health related quality of life, reoperation rate and function in patients with diabetes mellitus and hip fracture—a 2 year follow-up study," *Injury*. In press.

[65] E. S. Strotmeyer, J. A. Cauley, A. V. Schwartz et al., "Nontraumatic fracture risk with diabetes mellitus and impaired fasting glucose in older white and black adults: the health, aging, and body composition study," *Archives of Internal Medicine*, vol. 165, no. 14, pp. 1612–1617, 2005.

[66] J. E. Compston, N. B. Watts, R. Chapurlat et al., "Obesity is not protective against fracture in postmenopausal women: GLOW," *The American Journal of Medicine*, vol. 124, no. 11, pp. 1043–1050, 2011.

[67] P. L. A. van Daele, R. P. Stolk, H. Burger et al., "Bone density in non-insulin-dependent diabetes mellitus. The Rotterdam Study," *Annals of Internal Medicine*, vol. 122, no. 6, pp. 409–414, 1995.

[68] V. Rakic, W. A. Davis, S. A. P. Chubb, F. M. A. Islam, R. L. Prince, and T. M. E. Davis, "Bone mineral density and its determinants in diabetes: the Fremantle Diabetes Study," *Diabetologia*, vol. 49, no. 5, pp. 863–871, 2006.

[69] A. Räkel, O. Sheehy, E. Rahme, and J. LeLorier, "Osteoporosis among patients with type 1 and type 2 diabetes," *Diabetes & Metabolism*, vol. 34, no. 3, pp. 193–205, 2008.

[70] A. C. dos Santos, M. Roberto Cucê Nobre, A. Nussbacher et al., "Predictors of the risk of falls among elderly with chronic atrial fibrillation," *Clinics*, vol. 67, no. 4, pp. 305–311, 2012.

[71] J. Semel, J. M. Gray, H. J. Ahn, H. Nasr, and J. J. Chen, "Predictors of outcome following hip fracture rehabilitation," *PM & R*, vol. 2, no. 9, pp. 799–805, 2010.

[72] D. Lieberman, M. Friger, and D. Lieberman, "Rehabilitation outcome following hip fracture surgery in elderly diabetics: a prospective cohort study of 224 patients," *Disability and Rehabilitation*, vol. 29, no. 4, pp. 339–345, 2007.

[73] S. N. Robinovitch, F. Feldman, Y. Yang et al., "Video capture of the circumstances of falls in elderly people residing in long-term care: an observational study," *The Lancet*, vol. 381, no. 9860, pp. 47–54, 2012.

[74] B. Najafi, R. T. Crews, and J. S. Wrobel, "Importance of time spent standing for those at risk of diabetic foot ulceration," *Diabetes Care*, vol. 33, no. 11, pp. 2448–2450, 2010.

[75] H. Salsabili, F. Bahrpeyma, B. Forogh et al., "Dynamic stability training improves standing balance control in neuropathic patients with type 2 diabetes," *Journal of Rehabilitation Research and Development*, vol. 48, no. 7, pp. 775–786, 2011.

[76] S. Morrison, S. R. Colberg, M. Mariano, H. K. Parson, and A. I. Vinik, "Balance training reduces falls risk in older individuals with type 2 diabetes," *Diabetes Care*, vol. 33, no. 4, pp. 748–750, 2010.

[77] R. L. Kruse, J. W. Lemaster, and R. W. Madsen, "Fall and balance outcomes after an intervention to promote leg strength, balance, and walking in people with diabetic peripheral neuropathy: "feet first" randomized controlled trial," *Physical Therapy*, vol. 90, no. 11, pp. 1568–1579, 2010.

[78] T. A. Comans, S. G. Brauer, and T. P. Haines, "Randomized trial of domiciliary versus center-based rehabilitation: which is more effective in reducing falls and improving quality of life in older fallers?" *Journals of Gerontology A*, vol. 65, no. 6, pp. 672–679, 2010.

[79] M. W. Liu, W. C. Hsu, T. W. Lu, H. L. Chen, and H. C. Liu, "Patients with type II diabetes mellitus display reduced toe-obstacle clearance with altered gait patterns during obstacle-crossing," *Gait & Posture*, vol. 31, no. 1, pp. 93–99, 2010.

[80] G. Grewal, R. Sayeeda, S. Yescheka et al., "Virtualizing the assessment: a novel pragmatic paradigm to evaluate lower extremity joint perception in diabetes," *Gerontology*, vol. 58, no. 5, pp. 463–471, 2012.

17

An Online Platform to Support the Network of Caregivers of People with Dementia

April B. C. G. Boessen, Renée Verwey, Saskia Duymelinck, and Erik van Rossum

Centre of Expertise for Innovative Care and Technology (EIZT), Zuyd University of Applied Sciences, Heerlen, Netherlands

Correspondence should be addressed to Renée Verwey; renee.verwey@zuyd.nl

Academic Editor: Elke Bromberg

Increasing numbers of persons with dementia (PWD) augment the pressure on dementia care, especially informal care. Care technology can support the network of PWD. We tested the usability and perceived value of an online platform that aims to support the communication and collaboration between family and professional caregivers of PWD. A mixed methods design was used for this pilot study, including semistructured interviews, a postal questionnaire, and monitoring of log data. Seven family and thirty-two professional caregivers involved with four PWD participated during a 10-week period. Overall, the results indicate that the platform is easy to use and valuable for both family and professional caregivers. They felt better informed and prepared regarding the situation of the PWD and felt supported by the more direct lines of communication within the network. Also, a broadening and deepening of the relationship between family and professional caregivers was experienced. Although connecting care organizations' record systems with the platform and an active contribution of all care professionals involved (e.g., general practitioners and those working at day care units) were suggested for optimal use of the platform, family and professional caregivers positively valued the platform for improving the efficiency and ease of communication and collaboration.

1. Introduction

Worldwide, the number of persons with dementia (PWD) is 47.5 million [1], of which 260,000 are living in the Netherlands [2]. Due to aging of the population, the Dutch number of PWD is expected to increase to more than half a million in 2040 [3]. This increase, as well as changes in healthcare policy towards aging in place, has a substantial impact on dementia care. For example, as elderly people, including PWD, are supposed to live longer in their home environments, psychogeriatric care in nursing homes is focused on people with advanced stages of dementia [3]. Thus, dementia care transfers from the formal (professional) to the informal (family) network of caregivers. Currently, 70% of PWD in the Netherlands live at home, of which approximately 60% reside with a partner or other family members [4]. Family caregivers residing with the PWD experience the highest burden [5]. PWD without a partner are dependent on their children, friends, and neighbours; however, not all PWD have such social networks. The Dutch Health Care Inspectorate is concerned about the neglect of PWD without a widespread social network and the overburden of the family caregivers involved [6]. Therefore, the challenge is to strengthen the network of caregivers of PWD in such a way that collaboration between formal and informal caregivers is optimally supported.

Care technology can support these networks [3]. Technologies such as sensors or GPS systems support family caregivers, increase their perceived safety, and have the potential to increase the autonomy of PWD and their ability to live independently [7–9]. Other technology-driven interventions are being developed to inform caregivers of PWD alongside behavioural change support [10]. Despite the availability of such technologies, the use of care technology is still limited in daily practice [11, 12]. Technologies are often directed at specific target groups, for example, either the formal or informal network, however, not at both [12]. In addition, different disciplines of professional caregivers use their own record systems, which fragmentizes information supply. Furthermore, professionals are often insufficiently informed about the possibilities of care technology and find it difficult to incorporate such technologies into their daily work routines [11].

Most importantly, problems are encountered in adjusting technologies to the needs and wishes of end users [13]. Verwey et al. [14] investigated the needs of family and professional caregivers in their support for PWD and the possible role of technology therein. Family caregivers specifically stated the need for good information regarding dementia and contact with fellow family caregivers [14]. Professional caregivers primarily experienced problems in sharing information regarding the situation of the PWD (e.g., changes in medication, weight, and hospitalization). They also stated that they needed clarity on the roles and responsibilities of everyone involved with the PWD. A comprehensive record system, available for all persons involved, would be helpful [14]. Based on the possible advantages of care technology in meeting these needs, an online platform was developed to support collaboration and communication between family and professional caregivers of PWD. We tested the usability and perceived value of this platform by family and professional caregivers of PWD in a pilot study.

2. Materials and Methods

2.1. Design. An iterative, user-centred design method was applied for the development of the online platform [13]. In this subsequent pilot study, a mixed methods design including semistructured interviews, a postal questionnaire, and monitoring of log data was used to evaluate the usability and perceived value of the platform [15]. The study was approved by the medical ethical committee of Zuyderland-Zuyd (15-N-207).

2.2. Participants. Participants in this study were family and professional caregivers of PWD. Professional caregivers of two community care organizations in Limburg, The Netherlands, recruited family caregivers of four PWD. Purposeful sampling was used in this recruitment [15], aimed at sufficient heterogeneity in the sample regarding relationship to the PWD (partner, child, etc.), residing with the PWD or not, stage of dementia, and the number of persons involved in the network of the PWD. Furthermore, family caregivers were only included when they had a sufficient level of experience with technologies such as smartphones and tablets. All professional caregivers involved with the four selected PWD were recruited, even those who were not working within the abovementioned home care organizations, such as general practitioners (GPs) and physiotherapists.

2.3. Materials. Two care organizations and four ICT companies integrated their services in an online platform, based on the standard product of one of the companies. This product is an easy-to-use platform with individually tailored Cubes™ (i.e., applications) that access a range of services [16]. Services of the other companies were a video conferencing tool [17] and a tool to share care activities among (family) caregivers [18]. At the start of the study, the integrated platform consisted of standard Cubes (e.g., "Contacts/Clients," "Messaging," and "Calendar"), Cubes for care related information (e.g., "Info Dementia," a care record called "Care Notebook," "ShareCare," and "Medication plan/reminder"), and, only for family caregivers, Cubes for entertainment ("Radio," "YouTube," and "My Games"). After four weeks, a "Videocall" service was added to the platform of both family and professional caregivers. An example of the platform Cubes for family caregivers is shown in Figure 1. Participants gained access to the platform via personal login codes and could individually rearrange, add, or delete Cubes according to their personal wishes.

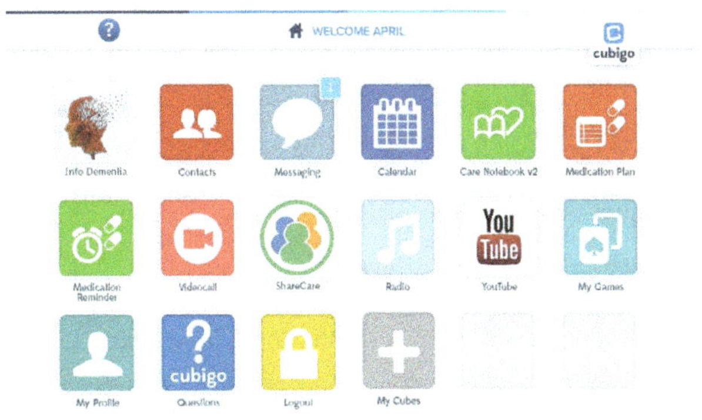

FIGURE 1: Platform Cubes for family caregivers.

2.4. Procedure. Selected family and professional caregivers received information letters on the study, including an informed consent form, which they signed before the start of the study. Prior to the start of the study, all participants received 2 h of instruction about the use of the platform. Family caregivers were instructed by the researchers and professional caregivers by an employee of the company that provided the standard platform. Furthermore, all primary family caregivers received a tablet for use during the study. Participants were also informed about the possibility of continuing to use the platform after the study.

2.5. Measurements. A 10-week test period took place from February to April 2016. During this period, the use of the platform was monitored by quantitative log data (i.e., clicks per Cube). Researchers did not have access to the contents of messages or the care record. The usability of the platform was measured by the Post-Study System Usability Questionnaire (PSSUQ) at the end of the test period. The PSSUQ is a validated, 19-item questionnaire that measures perceived user satisfaction with products or systems [19]. The 19 items of the questionnaire are divided over three subscales: system usefulness (8 items), information quality (7 items), and interface quality (4 items). All items were answered by using a 7-point Likert scale ranging from 1 (strongly disagree) to 7 (strongly agree). Higher scores indicate higher acceptance and usability. Furthermore, after 4 and 10 weeks, family caregivers were interviewed for approximately 1 h in their homes or another preferred location about the usability and

TABLE 1: Topic lists of interviews with caregivers.

Family caregivers	Professional caregivers
Actual use: frequency, duration, Cubes	Actual use: frequency, duration, Cubes
Usability: efficiency, information, interface, possibilities	Usability: efficiency, information, interface, possibilities
Key experiences: positive/negative	Key experiences: positive/negative
Support by professional caregivers	Collaboration with family caregivers (frequency and content of communication, sharing care)
Communication with family or professional caregivers	Collaboration with other professional caregivers (frequency and content of communication, sharing care)
Collaboration/sharing care	Care registration
Future use	Use at organizational levels
Finances/costs	Finances/costs

TABLE 2: Participant characteristics.

	Family caregivers (n = 7)	Professional caregivers (n = 32)
Mean age (SD)	59.2 (17.6)	44.6 (16.5)
Gender: female	5	29
Mean number of persons involved per client (SD)	1.75 (0.5)	9 (3.7)
Position in network	Daughter (n = 5) Son (n = 1) Partner (n = 1)	Nurse (n = 23) Case manager (n = 4) General practitioner (n = 1) Physiotherapist (n = 1) Day care professional (n = 1) Domestic worker (n = 1) Care farm worker (n = 1)
Technology experience*: mean (SD)	3.7 (0.5)	3.1 (1.1)

*Scores varied from 1 (no technology experience) to 5 (excellent technology experience).

perceived value of the platform. Professional caregivers were interviewed after 10 weeks. The development of the topic lists (Table 1) was based on the guidelines of the Dutch Institute for Healthcare Improvement [20]. During the interviews, family and professional caregivers were also asked to rate their technology experience on a 5-point Likert scale ranging from 1 (no technology experience) to 5 (excellent technology experience). Family and professional caregivers reported their experiences on feedback forms during the study as well.

2.6. Data Analyses. The semistructured interviews with family and professional caregivers were recorded and transcribed manually. These qualitative data, together with data from the feedback forms, were separately analysed by two researchers (AB, RV) using Nvivo (version 11) and based on the directed content analysis according to Hsieh and Shannon [21]. The initial coding scheme was determined on the basis of the Unified Theory of Acceptance and Use of Technology (UTAUT) model and was established by a consensus between the two researchers [22]. This model outlines seven main constructs that have a direct impact on behavioural intent and use of technology (performance expectancy, effort expectancy, social influence, facilitating conditions, hedonic motivation, price value, and habit). If necessary, initial codes were removed, integrated, or separated. General themes emerged, which were summarized. Data from the PSSUQ questionnaire were analysed using descriptive statistics and t-tests in SPSS (version 23), and log data were analysed using Excel 2016.

3. Results

In total, 7 family caregivers and 32 professional caregivers participated in this study. These participants were involved in the care of four PWD. Participant characteristics are shown in Table 2.

3.1. Use of the Platform Based on Log Data. Only a few Cubes were frequently used by both family and professional caregivers. Mean clicks per user of the five most frequently used Cubes are shown in Figure 2. The care record and message Cubes were most frequently used by both groups of caregivers. Use of these Cubes was three to four times higher for family caregivers compared with professionals. Clicks per user per week (not shown) indicated that use of these Cubes by family caregivers was the highest in the second half of the study, whereas the use of these Cubes was the highest in the first weeks and stabilized afterwards for professionals. In contrast to these Cubes, use of "Contacts" was much lower among family caregivers, but comparable to its use among professionals. Both family and professional caregivers

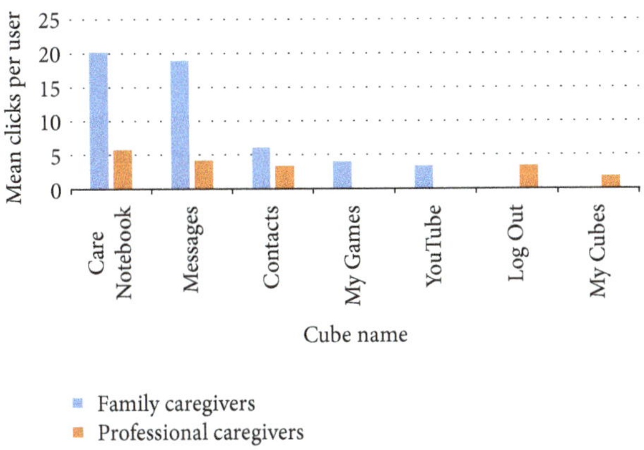

FIGURE 2: Mean clicks per user of the five most frequently used Cubes.

used "Contacts" mainly at the start of the study. Family caregivers also used the Cubes "YouTube" and "My Games" (only with a peak in one of the weeks). Among professional caregivers, "Log Out" and "My Cubes" were in the top five of most frequently used Cubes. Follow-up log data showed that 71% of family caregivers and 31% of professional caregivers continued using the platform for up to 10 weeks after the test period and a similar proportion of family caregivers and 15% of professional caregivers continued using it for up to 20 weeks after the test period.

3.2. Use of the Platform Based on Interviews. Most family caregivers reported daily use of the platform, usually on a laptop or tablet. Professionals reported using the platform on a weekly basis or more frequently if needed in view of the complexity of the client's situation. They preferred using a tablet or smartphone. With "use of the platform," both groups mainly referred to its care record and message functions. These were perceived as the most important Cubes to communicate with others: *"Via the care record and message functions, I share information about the situation of my partner and reach every person involved" (network 2, son, 63 years).* Some family caregivers mentioned using the Cubes "Calendar" and "Info Dementia" in the beginning, but this was not continued in most cases. Most of the other Cubes were perceived as unnecessary or their functions were not understood by both family and professional caregivers: *"I did not use the medication reminder. I did not understand what to do with it. Is it a kind of alarm? Or is it only useful if the client has access to the platform as well?" (network 4, daughter, 56 years).*

3.3. Usability Measured by the PSSUQ. Usability of the platform was rated with an average score of approximately 6 per item (data not shown) as well as per subscale (Table 3). Only a mean score of 3.3 for the item "The platform gave error messages that clearly told me how to fix problems" (system usability subscale) was relatively low. On average, family caregivers scored this item with a 2.0 and professionals caregivers with a 3.4. Scores between family and professional

TABLE 3: Mean scores* of family and professional caregivers per subscale of the PSSUQ.

	Family caregivers	Professional caregivers
System usefulness		
N	7	19
Mean (SD)	6,07	6,15
Information quality		
N	6	19
Mean (SD)	5,55	5,87
Interface quality		
N	5	18
Mean (SD)	6,31	6,05

Scores varied from 1 (strongly disagree) to 7 (strongly agree).

caregivers significantly differed for only one item on the system usability subscale: "It was simple to use this platform" (χ^2 (2, n = 26) = 5.085, p = 0.034), which professionals rated more positively (mean of 6,4) than family caregivers (mean of 5,7).

3.4. Perceived Value Based on Interviews. Overall, both family and professional caregivers were optimistic about the use of the platform. Soon after the start, participants indicated that they would like to continue using the platform after the study. Family caregivers felt that they were more easily and quickly informed about the situation of the PWD: *"On the days that I am not able to visit my father, I now know someone else did and the platform makes it able to read what this person discussed or undertook with my father or noticed about him. In the current situation, this person would never call to inform me" (network 3, daughter, 38 years).* Professionals perceived shorter communication lines with other professionals as well as family caregivers and therefore could take action more quickly. This was mainly seen as an advantage for more complex cases, where communication was essential. Due to this improved information provision, family caregivers felt calmer and more prepared before or without visiting the PWD. Professionals added that they had an overview of the network involved with a particular client: *"The advantage of the platform is that we as professionals are more aware of situations that occur regarding the client and of the persons involved with this client" (network 4, community nurse, 65 years).* Furthermore, family caregivers felt supported by the direct communications lines with professionals and their increased involvement. Professionals also perceived a broadening and deepening of the relationship with family caregivers: *"I think the relationships with families of clients have broadened in a certain way. There is more involvement and understanding of the situation on both sides" (network 1, nurse, 54 years).* This increased involvement was recognized by the fact that professionals reported using the platform outside working hours or at home. Family caregivers reported that it was sometimes difficult to discuss problems with others in the presence of the PWD. Therefore, they were optimistic about the possibility of using the platform to communicate about the PWD without causing commotion or confusion for the PWD.

3.5. Suggestions for Improvement Based on Interviews. Both family and professional caregivers advised limiting the number of Cubes, so that only Cubes with added value for family and professional caregivers would be available: *"The platform is a system with lots of different services of which I think not all are necessary. Keep it simple!" (network 4, daughter, 59 years).* A challenge for professionals was that they had to continue using their current record systems, while reporting similar information in the care record of the platform. For them, the ideal situation would be a connection between the care organizations system and the platform. Family caregivers thought that professionals could have used the platform more frequently, although they mentioned that the dual recording was a possible reason for their disappointing frequency of use: *"The double records that professionals had to write might have discouraged them from using the platform more often" (network 2, son, 63 years).* Along these lines, some family caregivers mentioned that they had to take the first step in using the platform, although they thought that professionals could have taken this initiative as well. However, when the lines of communication were established, communication was initiated both ways. For optimal information provision and thus use of the platform, both family and professional caregivers thought it was essential to include every person involved in the care of the PWD: *"Every person who visits the client could provide important information to this online network, even an alert domestic worker who might notice the client's falls" (network 4, physiotherapist, 56 years).* Furthermore, some technical issues of the platform arose, such as starting problems (e.g., white screen) and a high battery consumption of the application on smartphones.

4. Discussion

The results of this pilot study show that family and professional caregivers of PWD find the online platform easy to use and valuable. They indicated that the platform supported better information provision regarding the situation of the PWD, shortened communication lines within a caregiver network, and improved the involvement and commitment of caregivers towards each other and the PWD. Actual use of the platform appeared to be mainly restricted to the communication and care registration functionalities. Important suggestions for optimal use were connecting care organizations' record systems with those of the platform (to prevent dual recording) and active contributions of all caregivers involved (e.g., GPs and those working at day care units).

A previous needs assessment study among family and professional caregivers of PWD identified needs regarding care of PWD, which primarily concerned needs for better information provision, contact with fellow family caregivers, and a comprehensive record systems for all persons involved [14]. Participating family and professional caregivers welcomed the deployment of an online platform in meeting these needs. In this study, the technological feasibility of such an online platform is shown, as well as its perceived value among family and professionals caregivers. Other studies aimed at technological support of caregivers of PWD mainly focus on caregiver burden. Technology platforms and telecommunication or Internet-based platforms indicated a reduction of this burden [23–25]. In line with these results, we found that caregivers valued the platform for shortening communication lines between caregivers and improving caregiver involvement, which both may contribute to reducing perceived caregiver burden.

Today, many technological (care) platforms with diverse contents are being developed, which results in fragmentation as well as confusion for caregivers [26]. Different care organizations and companies develop their own platforms separately, whereas the functionalities of these platforms have many similarities. Users must log on to too many different systems. The platform in this study was developed as a response to this fragmentation with the aim of integrating various services and products so that end users would have access to various functionalities via one platform. Family and professional caregivers in this study only seem to feel a need for those functionalities supporting communication and joint care registration (and only if an active contribution of all caregivers involved would be guaranteed). This is in line with previous studies reporting that the value of (assistive) technologies mainly lies in functionalities that facilitate care coordination or communication between family and/or professional caregivers [25, 27, 28]. Although today's technological possibilities in care settings are far reaching (e.g., remote care and video calls), networks of caregivers do not really seem to miss such possibilities. Possible reasons for the limited use of some functionalities of the platform in this study might be a mismatch between family and professional caregivers' needs and technology requirements of the platform or insufficient instructions to participants regarding the use of the different functionalities of the platform. Another important factor that hampered the integration of services is that different care professionals (e.g., nurses, GPs, and physiotherapists) use different client registration systems. GPs experience the lack of possibilities to connect or integrate different applications as one of the most important constraints to the exchange of patient-related information [29]. This inability to integrate applications entails double recording of information, which seems to have influenced the frequency or content of use by the professionals in this study. Professional caregivers involved therefore advised making connections with the different record systems they use within the care registration functionality of the platform.

A strength of the study was the user-centred approach. This approach supports a feel of ownership of the final product among participants. The collaboration with the networks of the PWD resulted in a higher consumer satisfaction and could lead to a smoother implementation of the product [30]. With regard to the methodology, data triangulation increased the credibility and confirmability of this study [31]. As professional caregivers recruited family caregivers, this may have introduced some selection bias. They may have selected mainly family caregivers who were enthusiastic and willing to use the platform (e.g., early adopters or early majority) [32]. Furthermore, they only selected PWD who received care within the care organizations, although the platform might also be useful for networks of PWD with little or no professional care involved. Since this was a pilot study, we believe that the impact of these impediments upon the results was limited. The experiences of participants in this study, regardless of their early adopter status or the care situation of the PWD, show the potential of the platform.

Before technologies such as the platform in this study can be implemented on a large scale, further robust demonstration of its application should be investigated. Testing the usefulness and perceived value of the platform with a small group of caregivers, as we did in this study, is one of several steps in the iterative user-centred design process [13]. Although the results are promising and the number of participating caregivers per network supporting the PWD was high, the number of networks studied should be increased to obtain a better view on the platform's feasibility and generalizability of the results. To realize the potential of this online platform for family and professional caregivers, a number of issues should be addressed in a feasibility study. For example, how do family and professional caregivers experience an online instead of face-to-face introduction to the platform (due to time and resource restraints) and how do professional caregivers use and value the platform in case of their involvement with more than one PWD and his or her family caregivers? Therefore, we initiated a feasibility study in which the impact and potential limiting and facilitating factors for using the platform are investigated in a larger group of family and professional caregivers.

5. Conclusion

We showed the technological feasibility of an online platform that integrates various functionalities or applications. The results of this pilot study are promising for future use of the online platform. Use of the online platform was accepted and valued by family and professional caregivers as a result of perceived improvements in communication and collaboration regarding the care of the PWD. However, the results should still be tested on a larger scale.

Conflicts of Interest

The authors declare that there are no conflicts of interest regarding the publication of this paper.

Acknowledgments

The authors would like to thank the participants for their time and interest in the study. Furthermore, the authors acknowledge the contributions of the four companies, Sananet, Cubigo, Simac, and ZoemEurope, and the two care organizations, MeanderGroep and Proteion, involved in this study.

References

[1] World Health Organization, "10 facts on dementia, Geneva," 2015, http://www.who.int/features/factfiles/dementia/en/.

[2] The Dutch Alzheimer Society, "Amersfoort: The Dutch Alzheimer Society," 2016, https://www.alzheimer-nederland.nl/informatie.

[3] The Netherlands Federation of University Medical Centres/The Dutch Alzheimer Society/VUmc Alzheimer Centre and The Hague: ZonMw, "Deltaplan Dementia 2012–2020," 2012, http://www.neurodegenerationresearch.eu/wp-content/uploads/2014/08/rapport-deltaplan-dementie.pdf.

[4] J. Peeters, W. Werkman, and A. L. Francke, *Family Caregivers about Network and Municipality Support: Dementiamonitor Informal Care 2013*, NIVEL, Utrecht, The Netherlands, 2014.

[5] J. Peeters, W. Werkman, and A. L. Francke, *Dementiamonitor Informal Care: Problems, Healthcare Needs, Healthcare Utilization and Judgements by Family Caregivers*, NIVEL, Utrecht, The Netherlands, 2012.

[6] R. Van Diemen-Steenvoorde, *Organization Care Network of Community Dwelling People with Dementia Promising, Yet Some Parts Are Still at Risk*, The Health Care Inspectorate (IGZ), Utrecht, The Netherlands, 2013.

[7] A. Olsson, M. Engström, K. Skovdahl, and C. Lampic, "My, your and our needs for safety and security: Relatives' reflections on using information and communication technology in dementia care," *Scandinavian Journal of Caring Sciences*, vol. 26, no. 1, pp. 104–112, 2012.

[8] A. M. Pot, B. M. Willemse, and S. Horjus, "A pilot study on the use of tracking technology: Feasibility, acceptability, and benefits for people in early stages of dementia and their informal caregivers," *Aging and Mental Health*, vol. 16, no. 1, pp. 127–134, 2012.

[9] M. Mokhtari, H. Aloulou, T. Tiberghien, J. Biswas, D. Racoceanu, and P. Yap, "New trends to support independence in persons with mild dementia - A mini-review," *Gerontology*, vol. 58, no. 6, pp. 554–563, 2012.

[10] K. M. Godwin, W. L. Mills, J. A. Anderson, and M. E. Kunik, "Technology-driven interventions for caregivers of persons with dementia: A systematic review," *American Journal of Alzheimer's Disease and other Dementias*, vol. 28, no. 3, pp. 216–222, 2013.

[11] L. van Doninck, V. van Cooten, and L. Neven, "Zorgtechnologie voor ouderen," *Geroñ*, vol. 18, no. 1, pp. 29–32, 2016.

[12] J. Krijgsman, J. Peeters, A. Burghouts, A. Brabers, J. De Jong, T. Moll et al., "Between the spark and the flame: eHealth-monitor 2015," The Hague: Nictiz, 2015 http://www.nivel.nl/sites/default/files/bestanden/eHealth_monitor_2015.pdf.

[13] S. G. S. Shah and I. Robinson, "User involvement in healthcare technology development and assessment: structured literature review," *International Journal of Health Care Quality Assurance Incorporating Leadership in Health Services*, vol. 19, no. 6-7, pp. 500–515, 2006.

[14] R. Verwey, M. Van Berlo, S. Duymelinck, S. Willard, and E. van Rossum, "Development of an online platform to support the network of caregivers of people with dementia," *Studies in Health Technology and Informatics*, vol. 225, pp. 567–571, 2016.

[15] D. F. Polit and C. T. Beck, *Nursing Research: Principles and Methods*, Lippincott Williams & Wilkins, Philadelphia, Pa, USA, 2004.

[16] L. Van Der Elst, "Cubigo promotes independent living," *ILYA*, vol. 23, pp. 12–14, 2016.

[17] ZoemEurope, 2016, http://www.zoemeurope.eu/.

[18] S. Vermeulen, "Sharing care via the internet," *Denkbeeld*, vol. 22, no. 1, pp. 26–28, 2010.

[19] J. R. Lewis, "Psychometric evaluation of the PSSUQ using data from five years of usability studies," *International Journal of Human-Computer Interaction*, vol. 14, no. 3-4, pp. 463–488, 2002.

[20] Dutch Institute for Healthcare Improvement (CBO), *Guideline for Focus Group Research*, CBO, Utrecht, The Netherlands, 2004.

[21] H. F. Hsieh and S. E. Shannon, "Three approaches to qualitative content analysis," *Qualitative Health Research*, vol. 15, no. 9, pp. 1277–1288, 2005.

[22] V. Venkatesch, J. Y. L. Thong, and X. Xu, "Consumer acceptance and use of information technology: extending the unified theory of acceptance and use of technology," *MIS Quarterly*, vol. 36, no. 1, pp. 157–178, 2012.

[23] S. Finkel, S. J. Czaja, R. Schulz, Z. Martinovich, C. Harris, and D. Pezzuto, "E-care: A telecommunications technology intervention for family caregivers of dementia patients," *American Journal of Geriatric Psychiatry*, vol. 15, no. 5, pp. 443–448, 2007.

[24] M. Torkamani, L. McDonald, I. S. Aguayo, C. Kanios, M.-N. Katsanou, and L. Madeley, "A randomized controlled pilot study to evaluate a technology platform for the assisted living of people with dementia and their carers," *Journal of Affective Disorders*, vol. 41, no. 2, pp. 515–523, 2014.

[25] E. Marziali and L. J. Garcia, "Dementia caregivers' responses to 2 internet-based intervention programs," *American Journal of Alzheimer's Disease and other Dementias*, vol. 26, no. 1, pp. 36–43, 2011.

[26] T. Otte-Trojel, A. de Bont, M. Aspria et al., "Developing patient portals in a fragmented healthcare system," *International Journal of Medical Informatics*, vol. 84, no. 10, pp. 835–846, 2015.

[27] S. J. Czaja and M. P. Rubert, "Telecommunications technology as an aid to family caregivers of persons with dementia," *Psychosomatic Medicine*, vol. 64, no. 3, pp. 469–476, 2002.

[28] S. Dang, N. Remon, J. Harris et al., "Care coordination assisted by technology for multiethnic caregivers of persons with dementia: A pilot clinical demonstration project on caregiver burden and depression," *Journal of Telemedicine and Telecare*, vol. 14, no. 8, pp. 443–447, 2008.

[29] J. Krijgsman, I. Swinkels, B. van Lettow, J. De Jong, K. Out, and R. Friele, *More than Technique: ehealth Monitor 2016*, Nictiz and NIVEL, The Hague, The Netherlands, 2016.

[30] J. Preece, Y. Rogers, and H. Sharp, *Interaction Design: beyond Human-Computer Interaction*, John Wiley & Sons, Inc., New York, NY, USA, 2002.

[31] D. Mortelmans, *Manual Qualitative Research Methods*, Acco, Leuven, Belgium, 2007.

[32] E. M. Rogers, *Diffusion of Innovations*, The Free Press, New York, NY, USA, 1995.

18

Diagnosis and Prognosis of Prostate Cancer from Circulating Matrix Metalloproteinases and Inhibitors

William Khalil El-Chaer,[1] Clayton Franco Moraes,[1,2] and Otávio Toledo Nóbrega[1]

[1]*University of Brasília (UnB), 70910-900 Brasília, DF, Brazil*
[2]*Catholic University of Brasília (UCB-DF), 71966-700 Brasília, DF, Brazil*

Correspondence should be addressed to Otávio Toledo Nóbrega; otnobrega@gmail.com

Academic Editor: Carmela R. Balistreri

Although prostate cancer (PCa) is the sixth most common type of neoplasm in the world and the second in prevalence among men (10% of all cases), there is shortage of studies focused on primary prevention of the disorder as well as little understanding on its pathophysiology. Currently, the PCa screening tools are the prostate specific antigen (PSA) dosage conjugated to rectal examination and confirmed by prostate biopsy. Despite the name, the PSA presents reduced specificity, being necessary the identification of new biomarkers that allow an earlier and more precise diagnosis and even better prognosis. Several studies have associated matrix metalloproteinases (MMPs) and their tissue inhibitors (TIMPs) to PCa tumorigenesis and metastasis. Most of the studies so far have been carried out by investigating in situ expression of the metalloproteinases, either by transcriptional measures or by immunohistochemistry with biopsy or postoperative tissue. Investigations in human plasma and serum are scarce, and a bibliographical search resulted in 17 studies which are presented and interpreted herein. This narrative review discusses their settings and findings along with aspects related to circulating metalloproteinases as potential biomarkers for diagnosis or prognosis of the prostatic malignancy, expressing the authors' reticent view on their applicability due to the poor quality of evidence available.

1. Introduction

Statistics worldwide indicate that prostate cancer (PCa) has high prevalence and lethality, with three-quarters of cases among 65-year-oldsters [1]. Serum prostate specific antigen (PSA) levels are measured for early detection, staging, and monitoring despite not being a specific marker for PCa, rising in cases of prostatitis or benign prostatic hyperplasia (BPH) [2, 3].

Biochemical evidence indicates that serum proteinases, namely, matrix metalloproteinases (MMPs), play key roles in the pathophysiology of this malignancy. MMPs are zinc- or calcium-dependent endopeptidases that degrade various components of extracellular matrix, mainly collagen, elastin, laminin, fibronectin, and proteoglycans, being involved in tumorigenesis and metastasis to favor migration of tumor cells besides being proangiogenic [3].

Twenty-four MMPs have been identified, including collagenases (MMP-1, 8, 13, and 18), gelatinases (MMP-2 and 9), stromelysins (MMP-3 and 10), matrilisins (MMP-7 and 26), and membrane-type MMPs (MMP-14, 15, 16, 17, 24, and 25), among other types. They are found in all tissues and in plasma, being secreted mostly as pro-MMPs activated by the urokinase-plasminogen/plasmin system of cell membranes. In parallel and with regulatory and antagonistic action, four tissue inhibitors of MMPs (TIMPs) were described: TIMP-1, 2, 3, and 4. Hyperexpression of TIMP-1, 2 and 3 normally accompanies the course of tumor growth [2].

Studies performed so far on MMPs/TIMPs to assess risk for PCa seem to yield inconclusive results, with data on specificity and sensitivity being scarce. In this context, this minireview aimed at identifying studies that correlated circulating MMPs and TIMPs with PCa, focusing on reports that aimed at having them tested as serum/plasma

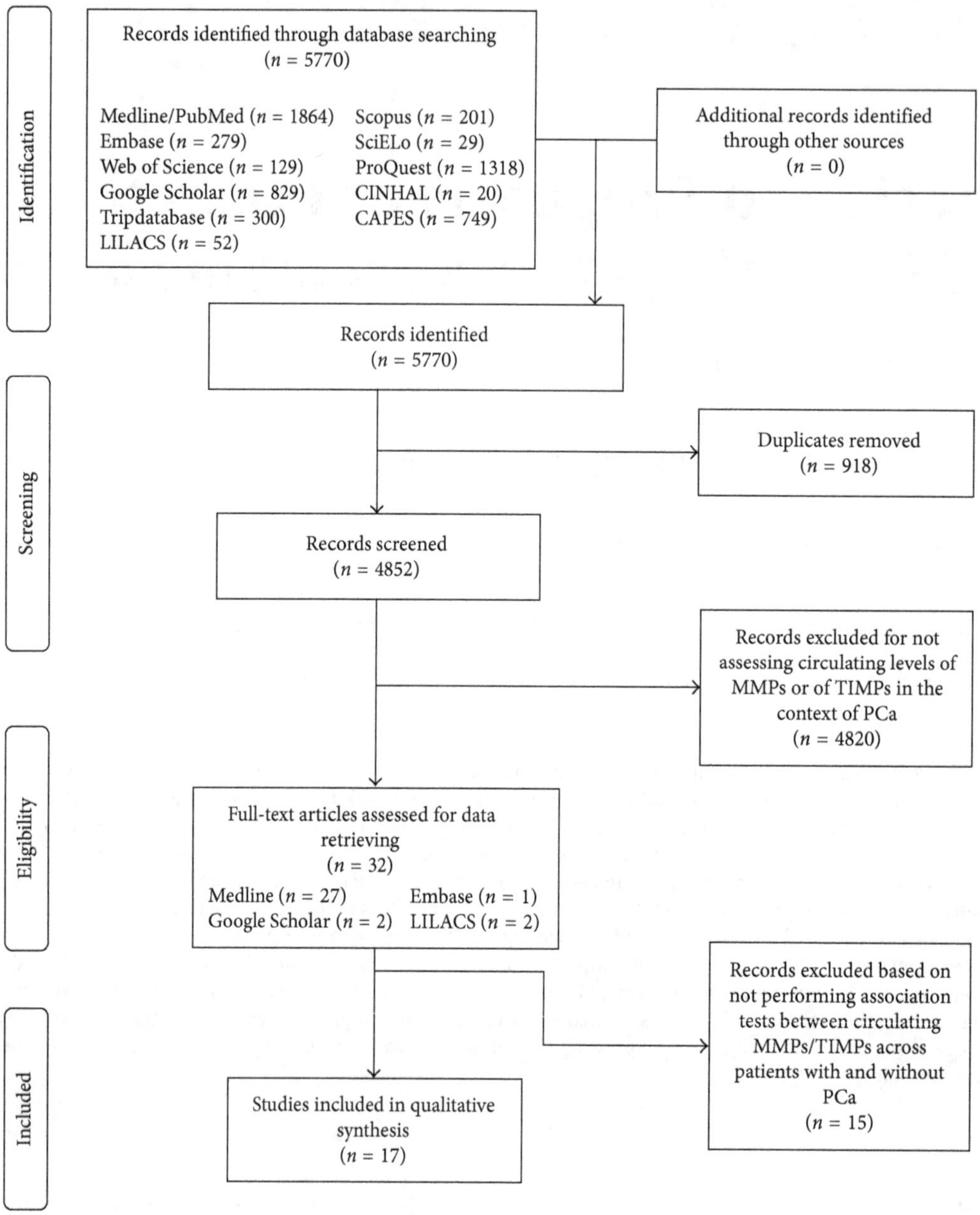

FIGURE 1: Rationale of the selection of articles.

biomarkers and describing accuracy scores, when available. A bibliographic survey was carried out in February and March 2017, using the following key words: metalloproteinases OR inhibitors of metalloproteinases OR MMPs OR TIMPs AND prostate cancer. The following quantitative studies were identified in the following primary databases: CINAHL, 20; EMBASE, 141; Google Scholar, 500; Library COCHRANE, 0; LILACS, 52; MEDLINE, 1859; SCOPUS, 201; and Web of Science, 129, and also in the following secondary sources of information: CAPES theses and dissertations database, 749; SCIELO, 29; PROQUEST, 1318; and Tripdatabase, 295. This search, after excluding replicates, produced a total of 17 reports addressing association of plasma/serum MMPs and/or TIMPs with PCa (Figure 1), which were obtained, analyzed, and systematized as depicted in Table 1.

There is a higher prevalence of studies on MMP-2 and MMP-9. In 1998, Gohji et al. [20] accumulated evidence of the correlation between the higher serum levels of MMP-2 and tumor extension. The authors measured MMP-2 by ELISA in the serum of 98 PCa patients, with 76 BPH carriers and 70 healthy men. Serum levels of MMP-2 were significantly higher in the PCa group than in the healthy and BPH counterparts and even higher in patients with metastatic PCa. In line, Kanoh et al. [19] measured by ELISA serum MMP-2 and PSA levels of 51 PCa patients and of 39 BPH carriers. The result consisted of increasing serum levels of both along with disease progression. Very high values of MMP-2 (>950 ng/ml) and PSA (>300 ng/ml) were observed when bone metastases was observed. Those authors advocate that MMP-2 can be coupled to PSA for prognostic purposes in PCa.

Table 1: Summary of the 17 articles revised.

Authors and title	Objective of the study	Design	Material and sample	Analysis method	Conclusion
Baker et al. [4]	To measure serum levels of collagenases, stromelysins, and TIMP-1 and 2 in patients with PCa, before treatment and 6 and 12 months after starting.	Prospective cohort	Test: serum of 19 individuals with metastatic PCa and 16 with PCa without metastases. Control: 21 patients with rheumatoid arthritis and 57 healthy subjects without rheumatoid arthritis.	ELISA	Increase of collagenases and TIMP-1 in patients with metastatic PCa compared to those without metastases and in the former in relation to the control group with or without rheumatoid arthritis. Reduction of TIMP-1 and collagenase levels 6 months after treatment. After 12 months, the levels of collagenases remained low; however, those of TIMP-1 returned to pretreatment values.
Bonaldi et al. [5]	To dose e-cadherin and MMP-13 at the diagnosis of PCa and three and six months after treatment, comparing with the control group.	Prospective cohort	Test: plasma (EDTA) of 29 PCa patients. Control: 10 healthy men with PSA <1.5 ng/ml.	ELISA	No difference between mean MMP-13 values among test and control groups at any test period.
Castellano et al. [6]	To compare levels of osteopontin (OPN), MMP-2, MMP-9, and TIMP-1.	Cross-sectional	Test: plasma (heparin) of 96 patients with PCa. Control: 92 individuals with BPH and 125 healthy subjects.	ELISA	Differences of MMP-9 and TIMP-1 (but not MMP-2) between groups; significant increase of MMP-9 and reduction of TIMP-1 in the CaP group relative to the healthy and BPH control; decreased serum levels of MMP-9 six months after radical prostatectomy.
Cicco et al. [7]	Correlate preoperative serum levels of 6 markers (including MMPs-2 and 9 and TIMPs-1 and 2) with tumor staging, Gleason score, and disease-free survival.	Cross-sectional	Serum of 162 PCa carriers for MMP-2 and 9 and plasma (EDTA) for TIMP-1 and 2.	ELISA	Patients with serum levels of MMP-2 < 206 ng/ml had a higher risk of PCa progression.
Gong et al. [8]	To compare TIMP-1 levels of castrated metastatic PCa patients with noncastrated (responsive to androgen ablation therapy).	Descriptive	Test: serum of 39 castrated metastatic PCa patients. Control: 24 noncastrated metastatic PCa patients.	ELISA	Higher TIMP-1 serum levels in castrated PCa patients.
Incorvaia et al. [9]	To compare levels of MMP-2 and 9 in individuals with PCa with bone metastases in relation to healthy individuals.	Cohort	Test: plasma (EDTA) of 35 patients with breast cancer and 44 with PCa with bone metastases. Control: 57 healthy patients.	ELISA	MMP-2 and MMP-9 significantly higher in PCa patients with bone metastases than in the control group.
Jung et al. [10]	To compare levels of MMP-1, MMP-3, and TIMP-1 as well as the MMP-1/TIMP-1 ratio of subjects with metastatic PCa and with nonmetastatic PCa.	Cross-sectional	Plasma (heparin) of 47 patients with prostate cancer, 29 with no metastasis (T2, 3pN0M0), and 18 with metastasis (T2, 3, 4pN1, 2M1). Control: 35 healthy subjects and 29 with BPH.	ELISA	Mean MMP-1 and TIMP-1 scores were significantly higher in the metastatic PCa group than in the nonmetastatic PCa, BPH, and healthy subjects groups. 10 of the 18 patients with metastatic PCa presented high levels of TIMP-1.

TABLE 1: Continued.

Authors and title	Objective of the study	Design	Material and sample	Analysis method	Conclusion
Morgia et al. [11]	To measure plasma levels of MMPs-2, 9, and 13 of TIMP-1, and of the enzymatic activity of MMPs-2 and 9 in patients with metastatic PCa, nonmetastatic PCa, BPH, and healthy, at diagnosis and 90 days after starting treatment.	Cohort	Plasma (heparin) of 40 patients with prostate cancer, 20 with no metastasis and 20 with metastasis. Control: 20 healthy patients and 20 with BPH.	ELISA	Plasma levels of MMP-2, 9, and 13 higher at diagnosis in the PCa group with metastasis than in the other groups, with reduction after treatment. Decreased TIMP-1 in the PCa group with metastasis in relation to the healthy group but without significant difference between groups.
Oh et al. [12]	To evaluate TIMP-1 as a predictor of survival in castrated PCa patients.	Survival study	Test: plasma (EDTA) of 362 castrated PCa patients; sample was divided into two groups: one with 60 (pilot group) individuals with a follow-up time of 5.8 years and the other with 302 (primary group) participants followed by 6.6 years.	ELISA	Lower survival rates among individuals with higher levels of TIMP-1 in both groups.
Prior et al. [13]	To determine sensitivity, specificity, and predictive values for MMP-2 as a biomarker for PCa.	Diagnostic study	Test: serum of 34 PCa patients. Control: 79 patients without PCa.	ELISA	Increased levels of MMP-2 among subjects with PCa compared to the group without PCa. Sensitivity: 24.1%; specificity: 78.6%; PPV: 31.8%; NPV: 71.4%. Cutoff of 718.36 ng/ml (mean level of MMP-2 in those without PCa).
González Rodríguez et al. [14]	To dose MMP-9 in patients who underwent prostate biopsy.	Cross-sectional	Test: serum of 32 patients with positive biopsy (PCa group). Control: 58 patients with negative biopsy.	ELISA	No difference in MMP-9 levels between groups.
Salminen et al. [15]	To evaluate the prognostic value of MMP-2 and MMP-9 in PCa with and without bone metastasis, comparing with ALP and PSA.	Cross-sectional and prognostic	Test: serum of 35 individuals with PCa with bone metastasis. Control: 49 individuals with PCa without bone metastasis.	ELISA	No differences in MMP-2 and 9 levels between groups. MMP-2 and 9 presented low accuracy for the diagnosis of bone metastasis in PCa and were not associated with survival.
Szarvas et al. [16]	To compare serum levels of MMP-7 in PCa patients with and without metastasis and to assess its prognostic value.	Cross-sectional and prognostic	Test: serum of 93 individuals with localized PCa and 13 PCa cases with bone metastasis. Control: 19 healthy individuals.	ELISA	Higher serum levels of MMP-7 in PCa patients with distant metastasis; specificity of 69% and sensitivity of 92% for detection of metastasis.
Zhang et al. [17]	To search mRNA and enzymatic activity of MMP-2 and 9 in prostatic tissue and serum of PCa patients (with and without metastasis) comparing with BPH and healthy group.	Cross-sectional	Test: serum of 15 PCa patients with metastasis and 10 without metastasis. Control: 26 BPH patients and 20 healthy.	RT-PCR and zymography	Increased expression and enzymatic activity of MMP-9 compared to the other groups.

Table 1: Continued.

Authors and title	Objective of the study	Design	Material and sample	Analysis method	Conclusion
Gil-Ugarteburu et al. [18]	To correlate the 1562C/T polymorphism of the MMP-9 gene with its plasma levels.	Prospective cohort	Test: plasma (heparin) of 90 patients submitted to prostatic biopsy with positive results for PCa. Control: 135 with negative biopsy for PCa.	ELISA	No correlation between the gene polymorphism and plasma concentration of MMP-9.
Kanoh et al. [19]	To correlate the serum levels of MMP-2 and PSA with the different stages of PCa.	Cross-sectional	Test: serum of 51 PCa patients. Control: serum of 39 BPH.	ELISA	MMP-2 and PSA levels associated with metastatic PCa; higher levels of MMP-2 (>950 ng/ml) and PSA (>300 ng/ml) in PCa with bone metastasis.
Gohji et al. [20]	To compare MMP-2 levels between individuals with and without PCa.	Cross-sectional	Test: serum of 98 individuals with PCa without previous treatment. Control: serum of 76 individuals with BPH and 70 healthy.	ELISA	Higher levels of MMP-2 in the PCa than in the control group.

BPH = benign prostate hyperplasia; MMP = matrix metalloproteinase; NPV = negative predictive value; PCa = prostate cancer; PPV = positive predictive value; TIMP = tissue inhibitor of metalloproteinase.

In this same sense, the study by Morgia et al. [11] investigated the use of MMPs as circulating biomarkers for the diagnosis and prognosis of PCa. Levels of MMP-2, 9, and 13 were significantly higher among PCa patients than in healthy or HPB subjects. The authors concluded that serum MMPs can be used as adjuvant biomarkers (combined with PSA) for the diagnosis (MMP-13) and prognosis (MMP-2 and MMP-9) of PCa. In addition, Prior et al. [13] also measured MMP-2 (and others, including PSA) in serum (and urine) of 113 men, stating that MMP-2 assessed in combination with PSA increases sensitivity for the diagnosis of PCa.

Likewise, Zhang et al. [17] investigated enzyme activity by zymography of MMPs-2, among others, in the serum of healthy men (n = 20), with BPH (n = 26), with localized PCa (n = 10), and with metastatic PCa (n = 15). The results indicated significant differences in enzyme activity between groups for MMP-9 but not for MMP-2. Thus, unlike previous studies, it was concluded that only serum levels of MMP-9 would be correlated with the presence of malignancy and metastases.

Incorvaia et al. [9] measured serum MMP-2 and 9 in patients with breast and prostate cancer, with and without bone metastases. Regarding PCa, both MMPs were significantly higher in patients with PCa compared to control subjects, but being indistinguishable between subjects with and without bone metastases, conversely to Kanoh et al. Therefore, it was concluded that MMPs (mainly MMP-2) display low accuracy for the diagnosis of bone metastatic PCa. Salminem et al. [15] obtained the same conclusions as Incorvaia et al. [9] on the accuracy of MMP-2 and 9 in the diagnosis of bone metastatic PCa, compared to the accuracy of PSA and alkaline phosphatase, contraindicating the testing of these MMPs for diagnostic purpose. Likewise, MMP-9 was the target of Gil-Ugarteburu et al. [18], which correlated MMP-9 plasma concentrations of 235 patients (measured by ELISA) with the 1562C/T polymorphism of the promoter region of the gene. Among the findings, the authors did not identify differences in the circulating concentrations of MMP-9 in the derived subgroups or any correlation with the polymorphism investigated.

In contrast, Castellano et al. [6] evidenced that serum levels of MMP-9 and its activator, osteopontin, declined significantly 6 months after prostatectomy. They also identified a correlation between serum MMP-9 and PSA and Gleason staging values. De Cicco et al. [7] quantified MMP-2, MMP-9, TIMP-1, and TIMP-2 among other molecules in the plasma of 162 men diagnosed with PCa, having found only a significant association between low MMP-2 values (less than 206 ng/ml) and an worsened disease progression (corrected HR = 1.7 and CI = 95%).

González Rodrigues et al. [14] found unsatisfactory results when serum MMP-9 was determined by ELISA in 100 patients with indication for prostate biopsy (prospective cohort study). Of these, 32 were diagnosed with PCa with 52% classified with Gleason greater than or equal to 7. No significant difference in MMP-9 levels was found between groups with PCa and benign or uncertain histological results. No association was found between MMP-9 levels and PSA or Gleason scores.

Concerning other varieties of MMPs, Jung et al. in 1997 [10] performed ELISA assessments for plasma MMP-1, 3, and TIMP-1 on 19 nonmetastatic PCa, 18 metastatic, and 29 HPB patients, along with 35 healthy men. No difference was found in the MMP-1 means across groups. The mean concentration of MMP-3 and TIMP-1 in metastatic patients was significantly higher than in the other groups, with 10 out of the 18 metastatic cases displaying remarkably high levels of TIMP-1. They concluded that TIMP-1 can be correlated with the PCa condition. Previously, Baker et al. [4] also found higher levels of TIMP-1 (but not TIMP-2) in patients with PCa.

Serum MMP-7 was investigated by Szarvas et al. [16] using ELISA in 93 patients with focal PCa at the preoperative stage, along with 13 patients with bone metastases and 19 normal individuals. No statistically significant difference was found between PCa carriers and normal individuals. However, MMP-7 levels were significantly elevated in patients with metastatic PCa compared to focal counterparts, with specificity and sensitivity of 69 and 92%, respectively, when a cutoff point of 3.7 ng/ml was adopted.

Plasma TIMP-1 was also the subject of Oh et al. [12] in a cohort study with mean follow-up of 6.6 years. Based on 362 samples from hormone-resistant and castrated patients with metastatic PCa, patients with higher levels of plasma TIMP-1 had the lowest survival (19 versus 43 months). Values of PSA, alkaline phosphatase, and Gleason scores were also considered. Plasma TIMP-1 was shown as the best predictor of survival in patients with these characteristics and independently of other classic markers.

Bonaldi et al. [5] correlated serum levels of e-cadherin and MMP-13 on PCa patients with serum levels of total PSA, free PSA, total testosterone, and clinical evolution, measured before onset of treatment as well as three and six months afterwards. The same was done in a parallel control group. At baseline, e-cadherin titers were lower in the PCa group than in the control group while for MMP-13, differences were not noticed. With treatment, authors identified only positive correlation between PSA and e-cadherin levels in the third month of treatment. Gong et al. [8] compared circulating TIMP-1 in hormone-resistant PCa patients who underwent orchiectomy with patients responsive to hormone therapy. In the first group, plasma TIMP-1 was significantly higher.

Thus, with regard to MMPs as circulating biomarkers to diagnose and monitor PCa, we conclude that very few studies were conducted in this matter, having rendered contradictory and inconclusive data. Nonetheless, the premise of differential levels in circulating MMPs among PCa patients for a diagnostic purpose seems worth investigating in light of evidence already existent for other neoplastic entities [21], with emphasis on what concerns MMP-2, 7, and 9 and TIMP-1 in the opinion of the authors of this minireview.

Although having reviewed seventeen scientific papers, it was not possible to meta-analyze results due to methodological heterogeneities and poor description of central tendency scores. Only five articles reported mean values for the plasma/serum markers assessed, three of which for MMP-2 and MMP-9 while the others for MMP-7 and TIMP-1 each. Specificity and sensitivity were only described in 1 study [13].

Considering that the current screening diagnosis, based on serum PSA dosage and rectal examination, has a limited accuracy (mainly specificity) for differentiation of PCa from other prostatic diseases and considering the fragility of the results pointed out in this review, more studies with the aim of confirming (or excluding) MMPs and TIMPs as elective biomarkers for PCa should be welcomed, either for diagnosis, prognosis, or therapeutic referral.

Authors' Contributions

William Khalil El-Chaer executed the bibliographical research and systematized the data obtained. William Khalil El-Chaer and Otávio Toledo Nóbrega analyzed and interpreted results as well as prepared the original manuscript. Clayton Franco Moraes critically revised the manuscript.

Acknowledgments

The research was supported with grants from CNPq (no. 445692/2014) and FAPDF (193.001.240/2016), with a fellowship for productivity in research to O.T. Nóbrega (CNPq).

References

[1] Epidemiology: epidemic rates of cancer incidence in Latin America," *Nature Reviews Clinical Oncology*, vol. 10, no. 6, p. 304, 2013.

[2] R. Visse and H. Nagase, "Matrix metalloproteinases and tissue inhibitors of metalloproteinases: structure function, and biochemistry," *Circulation Research*, vol. 92, no. 8, pp. 827–839, 2003.

[3] E. I. Deryugina and J. P. Quigley, "Matrix metalloproteinases and tumor metastasis," *Cancer and Metastasis Reviews*, vol. 25, no. 1, pp. 9–34, 2006.

[4] A. H. Baker, D. R. Edwards, and G. Murphy, "Metalloproteinase inhibitors: biological actions and therapeutic opportunities," *Journal of Cell Science*, vol. 115, no. 19, pp. 3719–3727, 2002.

[5] C. M. Bonaldi, L. A. Azzalis, V. B. Junqueira et al., "Plasma levels of E-cadherin and MMP-13 in prostate cancer patients: correlation with PSA, testosterone and pathological parameters," *Tumori Journal*, vol. 101, no. 2, pp. 185–188, 2015.

[6] G. Castellano, G. Malaponte, M. C. Mazzarino et al., "Activation of osteopontin/matrix metalloproteinaes-9 pathway correlates with prostate cancer progression," *Clinical Cancer Research*, vol. 14, no. 22, pp. 7470–7480, 2008.

[7] C. De Cicco, L. Ravasi, L. Zorzino et al., "Circulating levels of VCAM and MMP-2 may help identify patients with more aggressive prostate cancer," *Current Cancer Drug Targets*, vol. 8, no. 3, pp. 199–206, 2008.

[8] Y. Gong, U. D. Chippada-Venkata, M. D. Galsky, J. Huang, and W. K. Oh, "Elevated circulating tissue inhibitor of metalloproteinase 1 (TIMP-1) levels are associated with neuroendocrine differentiation in castration resistant prostate cancer," *The Prostate*, vol. 75, no. 6, pp. 616–627, 2015.

[9] L. Incorvaia, G. Badalamenti, G. Rini et al., "MMP-2, MMP-9 and activin A blood levels in patients with breast cancer or prostate cancer metastatic to the bone," *Anticancer Research*, vol. 27, pp. 1519–1525, 2007.

[10] K. Jung, L. Nowak, M. Lein, F. Priem, D. Schnorr, and S. A. Loening, "Matrix metalloproteinases 1 and 3, tissue inhibitor of metalloproteinase-1 and the complex of metalloproteinase-1/tissue inhibitor in plasma of patients with prostate cancer," *International Journal of Cancer*, vol. 74, no. 2, pp. 220–223, 1997.

[11] G. Morgia, M. Falsaperla, G. Malaponte et al., "Matrix metalloproteinases as diagnostic (MMP-13) and prognostic (MMP-2, MMP-9) markers of prostate cancer," *Urological Research*, vol. 33, no. 1, pp. 44–50, 2005.

[12] W. K. Oh, R. Vargas, S. Jacobus et al., "Elevated plasma tissue inhibitor of metalloproteinase-1 levels predict decreased survival in castration-resistant prostate cancer patients," *Cancer*, vol. 117, no. 3, pp. 517–525, 2011.

[13] C. Prior, F. Guillen-Grima, J. E. Robles et al., "Use of a combination of biomarkers in serum and urine to improve detection of prostate cancer," *World Journal of Urology*, vol. 28, no. 6, pp. 681–686, 2010.

[14] I. González Rodríguez, M. Rivas del Fresno, R. Gil Ugarteburu et al., "Expresión de metaloproteasa de matriz 9 en el cáncer de próstata: experiencia preliminar," *Archivos Españoles de Urología*, vol. 63, no. 2, pp. 119–124, 2010.

[15] E. K. Salminen, M. J. Kallioinen, M. A. Ala-Houala et al., "Survival markers related to bone metastases in prostate cancer," *Anticancer Research*, vol. 26, pp. 4879–4884, 2006.

[16] T. Szarvas, M. Becker, F. VomDorp et al., "Elevated serum matrix metalloproteinase 7 levels predict poor prognosis after radical prostatectomy," *International Journal of Cancer*, vol. 128, no. 6, pp. 1486–1492, 2011.

[17] L. Zhang, J. Shi, J. Feng, H. Klocker, C. Lee, and J. Zhang, "Type IV collagenase (matrix metalloproteinase-2 and -9) in prostate cancer," *Prostate Cancer and Prostatic Diseases*, vol. 7, no. 4, pp. 327–332, 2004.

[18] I. G. R. Gil-Ugarteburu, M. Rivas del Fresno, P. Benito García, A. Fenández Somoano, and A. Tardón García, "Plasmatic variations of metalloproteinase 9 (MMP-9) due to functional polymorphism in prostate cancer," *Urology*, vol. 80, no. 3, p. S276, 2012.

[19] Y. Kanoh, T. Akahoshi, T. Ohara et al., "Expression of matrix metalloproteinase-2 and prostate-specific antigen in localized and metastatic prostate cancer," *Anticancer Research*, vol. 22, no. 3, p. 1813, 2002.

[20] K. Gohji, N. Fujimoto, I. Hara et al., "Serum matrix metalloproteinase-2 and its density in men with prostate cancer as a new predictor of disease extension," *International Journal of Cancer*, vol. 79, no. 1, pp. 96–101, 1998.

[21] F. L. Fonseca, B. C. A. Alves, L. A. Azzalis, and T. M. Belardo, "Matrix metalloproteases as biomarkers of disease," *Methods in Molecular Biology*, vol. 1579, pp. 299–311, 2017.

19

Patient-Reported and Performance Outcomes Significantly Improved in Elderly Patients with Vestibular Impairment following Rehabilitation

Daniel Héctor Verdecchia,[1,2] **Agustina Maria Monzón**,[1] **Valentina Urbina Jaimes**,[2] **Fernando Rocha Oliveira**,[3] **Laércio da Silva Paiva**,[4] **and Tatiana Dias de Carvalho**[1]

[1]*Departamento de Ciencias de la Salud, Kinesiología y Fisiatría, Universidad Nacional de La Matanza, San Justo, Buenos Aires, Argentina*
[2]*Área de Rehabilitación Vestibular, Universidad Maimónides, Ciudad Autónoma de Buenos Aires, Buenos Aires, Argentina*
[3]*Departamento de Epidemiologia, Faculdade de Saúde Pública da Universidade de São Paulo, São Paulo, SP, Brazil*
[4]*Laboratório de Epidemiologia e Análise de Dados, Departamento de Saúde da Coletividade, Faculdade de Medicina do ABC, Santo André, SP, Brazil*

Correspondence should be addressed to Tatiana Dias de Carvalho; carvalho.td1@gmail.com

Academic Editor: Jean-Francois Grosset

Objective. To describe the results of a vestibular rehabilitation (VR) program in the timed up and go (TUG), gait speed (GS), and dizziness handicap inventory (DHI) scores for elderly vestibular patients in a developing country. *Methods.* Descriptive study with retrospective data collected from the clinical records of vestibular patients. The following information was recorded: sex, age, type of vestibular disorder, DHI score, and performance in TUG and GS, before and after participation in a VR program taking place from January 1 to August 30, 2017. The VR program consisted of 10 twice weekly sessions in the clinic and daily exercises at the patient's home. We used Student's t-test for paired and Wilcoxon's test according to the data distribution. The level of significance was 5%. *Results.* Data from 57 patients (49 females; 78 ± 5.8 years old) were used. There were statistically significant differences in TUG (12.52 versus 11.56), GS (0.81 versus 0.90 m/s), DHI total handicap (46 versus 24), physical (14 versus 8), emotional (14 versus 6), and functional (18 versus 12) domains. *Conclusion.* The functional outcome measures reported, including TUG, gait speed, and DHI, reflect statistically significant improvements in elderly patients after vestibular rehabilitation; the DHI improvements are clinically relevant.

1. Introduction

Patients with dysfunction in the vestibular system often complain of dizziness, balance impairments, and visual or gaze disturbances [1, 2]. In particular, dizziness is one of the most important single symptoms with a negative influence on well-being in old age [1]. While barriers to determining true prevalence and incidence exist due to differences in diagnosing and reporting, a previous survey showed that about 35% of people over 40 have experienced a vestibular disorder, a problem that can significantly impair the quality of life [2–4]. This dysfunction may be due to a disease-related pathology or trauma (surgical intervention) and can be located in the central (brain) or peripheral (inner ear) portions of the vestibular system.

One of the treatment options for vestibular disorders (unilateral and bilateral vestibular hypofunction and central or mixed vestibular disorders) is vestibular rehabilitation (VR). This consists of an individualized exercise program which has been developed to address the deficits identified during the physical therapy evaluation and which has been shown to be an effective treatment for patients with dizziness and balance disorders [5]. Currently, this program includes compensatory responses, adaptation for visual-vestibular interaction, substitution and postural control exercises, fall prevention, (re)conditioning activities, and functional/occupational retraining [6].

The objective of the VR program is to encourage compensation after peripheral and central vestibular disorders, thus reducing symptoms of dizziness and vertigo and the risk of falls, while increasing confidence in equilibrium and encouraging the return to activities of daily living [5, 7]. The efficacy of vestibular rehabilitation can be evaluated using performance-based outcome measures such as gait speed (GS), timed up and go (TUG) [8], and patient-reported outcome measures such as the dizziness handicap inventory (DHI) [9–11]. The outcome measures are simple, easy, and quick to administer in a clinical setting. There is moderate to strong evidence to support the use of vestibular rehabilitation for persons with peripheral unilateral vestibular disorders [5, 12]. Information is still lacking, however, on the population that suffers from peripheral and central vestibular disorders and the effects of VR programs, especially in developing countries.

Another major problem in elderly populations, one which is not a hypofunction but rather a mechanical disorder, is benign paroxysmal positional vertigo (BPPV). This is believed to be one of the most common causes of vertigo [13] and can be present at any age but is most common among people in their 6th and 7th decades [14]. BPPV is caused by free otoconia dislodged from the utricular macula that have entered the semicircular canal, where they provoke an inappropriate flow of endolymph whenever the head is rotated in the plane of the affected canal [15]. Residual dizziness (RD) is a common condition in patients with idiopathic BPPV, which starts in the first episode, even after quick resolution with repositioning maneuvers. Early treatment of BPPV is advisable for preventing RD, especially in anxious and elderly patients [16].

For BPPV, there is considerable evidence to support the use of repositioning maneuvers at the outset and also to show that vestibular rehabilitation should be incorporated in the long term as a preventative measure or to promote functional recovery or both [6]. A recent clinical practice guideline concluded that a clinician may offer VR in the treatment of BPPV for patients with additional impairments and that this can result in prevention of falls and an improved return of natural balance function [17]. A recent systematic review [18] found that there is an urgent need for more research conducted in low-middle-income environments. Here in our country, we have not found any studies evaluating VR or describing its impact on functional test results (TUG and GS). The objective of this study, then, is to describe the outcomes of a vestibular rehabilitation program on the timed up and go, gait speed, and dizziness handicap inventory scores for elderly vestibular patients in a developing country.

2. Methods

2.1. Study Design and Population. This is a descriptive study with retrospective data collected from the clinical records of vestibular patients aged 65 years or older at a vestibular rehabilitation clinic located in an urban middle-income environment. The following information was recorded: sex, age, type of vestibular disorder, DHI score, and performance in TUG and GS, before and after their participation in a vestibular rehabilitation program taking place from January 1 to August 30, 2017.

Patients were referred by otolaryngologists. In those cases where the prescription did not contain a specific diagnosis, an experienced physiotherapist evaluated each subject by means of a battery of clinical oculomotor (ocular alignment and tests of Skew, ocular range of motion, smooth pursuit, volitional saccades, and vergence) and vestibular tests (vestibulo-ocular reflex cancellation test (VORc), head impulse test, head shaking test, or mastoid vibration test), thus ensuring that the disorder was primarily of the vestibular origin. The patients who gave positive results in the clinical vestibular tests were included in the study [19].

Incomplete records, failure to complete the rehabilitation program and other neurologic conditions (Parkinson's disease, multiple sclerosis, stroke, and others) were the criteria for exclusion. People without a specific diagnosis who had central signs during the physiotherapist's evaluation were referred to a neurologist, and patients who only suffered from BPPV without residual symptoms were not included in a VR program, thus no data from functional tests were found in the clinical history of these two groups of patients (incomplete records).

Both the rehabilitation clinic and the patients signed consent forms authorizing all procedures, which was carried out in accordance with the Code of Ethics of the World Medical Association (Declaration of Helsinki) and authorized by the local ethics committee.

2.2. Vestibular Rehabilitation Program. The VR program consisted of 10 twice weekly sessions in the rehabilitation clinic and daily exercises at the patient's home. It was based on the treatment protocol published in Binetti et al. [7] and Verdecchia et al. [20], with adaptation exercises and/or habituation and/or substitution exercises determined and adapted in accordance with an assessment of the patient. Subjects received vestibular and balance rehabilitation provided by three physical therapists with specialized training in the treatment of balance and vestibular disorders.

The vestibulo-ocular and oculomotor exercises included X1 and X2 viewing paradigm (near and far) with periods of stimulation 1 to 2 minutes long (3–5 times daily for a total of 20–40 minutes per day). Oculomotor training for patients with bilateral vestibular hypofunction included two cards exercises (visualization of 2 targets) and remembered target (1 target), designed to challenge saccadic movements and gaze shifting [12]. The vestibulospinal exercises included static balance with progressive reduction of the support base, eyes open and closed, and firm to soft surface. The dynamic balance and gait tasks included walking with head and body turns, velocity changes, and walking with progressively narrower base of support.

Patients who suffered from BPPV with residual symptoms (imbalance and dizziness) were treated with repositioning maneuvers before they were included in a customized VR program based on a functional evaluation of each patient [3, 17]. Some non-BPPV patients with dizziness provoked by their own head or body movement were prescribed habituation exercises based on the results of the 16 movements in the motion sensitivity quotient (MSQ) [21]. The movements chosen for habituation were performed as follows: four repetitions four times a day, until the exercises did not generate any symptoms for 48 h, at which time they were suspended.

In addition, all the subjects performed adaptation exercises for the vestibulo-ocular and vestibulospinal reflexes, three to five times a day in their homes, for a total stimulus time of 20 to 40 minutes daily.

2.3. Timed Up and Go. Subjects were asked to complete 3 trials of the TUG. For this, they were given verbal instructions to stand up from a seated position on a chair, walk 3 m as quickly and as safely as possible, cross a line marked on the floor, turn around, walk back, and sit down. The stopwatch was started on the word "go" and stopped when the subject'is back came into contact with the chairback after sitting down. The TUG time was measured in seconds (sec). One practice trial was given, and the score discarded. Two scored trials were then performed, and the average of these scores was used for this study [22]. Those subjects who used an assistive device when walking in the community were asked to use that device [23]. Whitney el al. [24] found that a TUG cutoff of 11.1 seconds appeared to display the best balance between sensitivity (80%) and predictive positive value (46%) in patients with vestibular dysfunction. They concluded that the sensitivity of the TUG test for fall prediction was 80%, and the specificity was 56% in patients who scored greater than 11.1 seconds on the test. People who scored greater than 11.1 seconds on the TUG were 5 times (p = 0.001) more likely to have reported a fall in the previous 6 months.

2.4. Gait Speed. To evaluate the usual gait speed, we used the timed 10-meter walk test. Each patient was instructed to walk 10 meters at a comfortable and normal pace (3 trials). Only the middle 6 meters section was timed to eliminate the effects of acceleration and deceleration. A certified examiner started the timing when the subject's first foot crossed the "start" line and stopped timing when his/her last foot crossed the "finish" line. Walking speed (in meter/second, or m/s) was calculated as walking distance (20 ft = 6.10 m) divided by time (in seconds), and the average of the 3 trials was registered [25, 26]. Older persons with gait speed slower than 1 m/s (equal to or more than 6 seconds to walk 6 m) should be considered at high risk of adverse health outcomes [27].

2.5. Dizziness Handicap Inventory. The DHI is a 25-item tool used to help the patient rate their self-perception of handicap from dizziness [9]. It is subdivided into functional (36 points), emotional (36 points), and physical domains (28 points) and ranges from zero (no perceived handicap) to 100 (the maximum perceived handicap) [10]. We decided to use the Argentine version of this questionnaire [28], which is a reliable and valid tool for quantifying self-perceived handicap resulting from vertigo, dizziness, or unsteadiness and has high internal consistency ($\alpha = 0.87$) and very high test-retest reliability for the total DHI score (intraclass correlation coefficient: 0.98) and its domains.

2.6. Statistical Analysis. We have carried out a descriptive analysis of the data. The characteristics of the population are presented by absolute and relative frequency, and the quantitative variables are presented by measures of central tendency and dispersion in accordance with the normality test (Shapiro–Wilk test). To analyze the tests and perception of impairment before and after the rehabilitation program, we used Student's t-test for paired and Wilcoxon's test in accordance with the data distribution. The level of significance was 5%. The statistical program used was the Stata 12.0 version.

3. Results

We have evaluated 76 clinical records. Of these, 19 were excluded because of incomplete information and failure to complete the rehabilitation program. Data from 57 patients (49 females; 78 ± 5.8 years old) with vestibular disorders were used. Unilateral vestibular hypofunction and BPPV had a higher prevalence with 29 (50.88%) and 12 (21.05%) of the cases, respectively. Table 1 presents the population characteristics.

The median improvement in the total DHI score was about 22 points after VR (a change >18 points meets the minimally clinically important difference (MCID) for the vestibular population). The median total DHI score before VR was 46 (CI 95% 37.13–56.86) and after, 24 (CI 95% 18.00–36.86), demonstrating improvements after VR (Wilcoxon signed rank, $p < 0.001$). In the analyses of pre- and post-VR median DHI points, a decrease and a consequent improvement were observed in all domains: emotional (pre-VR 14 (CI 95% 10.00–18.00), post-VR 6 (CI 95% 4.00–10.00), and Wilcoxon-signed rank test $p < 0.0001$), functional (pre-VR 18 (CI 95% 16.00–20.00), post-VR 12 (CI 95% 8.00–14.00), and Wilcoxon-signed rank test $p < 0.0001$) and physical (pre-VR 14 (CI 95% 12.00–18.00), post-VR 8 (CI 95% 4.00–10.00), and Wilcoxon-signed rank test $p < 0.0001$). Figure 1 shows the results of total DHI and its respective domains, pre- and postvestibular rehabilitation program.

The mean gait speed increased by 0.09 m/sec after VR. Mean values obtained before and after VR were 0.81 m/sec (SD: 0.21) *y* and 0.90 m/sec (SD: 0.19), respectively (Student's t-test, $p < 0.001$).

Following VR, the median TUG decreased by 0.96 sec. In the analysis of pre- and post-VR TUG results, the medians were 12.52 (CI 95% 11.33–13.15) and 11.56 (CI 95% 10.58–12.08), respectively (Wilcoxon-signed rank test, $p < 0.001$).

4. Discussion

Our study shows that there were statistically significant differences in timed up and go, gait speed and dizziness handicap inventory values after a VR program. Patients were predominantly female, and the most common diagnosis was unilateral vestibular hypofunction.

This type of disorder affects both sexes, and since there is evidence suggesting that the patient's sex may not impact rehabilitation outcomes, a VR program can be offered to males and females with the expectation of similar outcomes [12].

While Jung et al. [29] and Moreira Bittar et al. [30] have noted that age is not a significant factor in the response rate to vestibular exercises, Smith-Wheelock et al. [31] have reported that older patients required modifications in therapy due to increased risk for falls. In the same study, more of the patients in the older group required supervised therapy compared to the younger group. However, the only significant difference noted for older than 65 years was in the length of time required to maximize the benefit from therapy.

As for diagnoses, our findings coincide with a previous study [32]. Vestibular rehabilitation is also indicated for the most common type of vestibular disorders in this study: unilateral vestibular hypofunction (regardless of whether it is on the left or right side). Bayat et al. [33] found no significant differences in VR outcomes between men and women or those with right- or left-side lesions ($p > 0.05$). Tee and Chee [34] reported that individuals with stable unilateral peripheral vestibular loss with incomplete central compensation benefited the most from a VR program, but the treatment strategies are different for unilateral and bilateral dysfunction [5].

BPPV is the most widely recognized vestibular disorder [5] and is characterized by vertigo of short duration after a change in the position of an individual's head with respect to gravity and with symptoms typically lasting less than one minute [5, 35]. Our study included 12 patients with unilateral posterior BPPV who presented with residual dizziness and unsteadiness after successful canalith repositioning procedures (CRPs). While there is reason to believe that habituation exercises cannot replace CRPs in the initial treatment of BPPV, adaptation and habituation exercises can nevertheless serve as adjuvant therapy for selected patients with BPPV [17]. BPPV can be associated with significant residual complaints of generalized dizziness (abnormal motion sensitivities not associated with provocation of nystagmus) and definable abnormal postural control with heightened fall risk even after CRP has successfully resolved paroxysmal positional nystagmus [36, 37]. There is a statistically significant increased risk for persistent postural abnormalities in the elderly in general where multifactorial comorbid impairments may be present [38]. A randomized controlled trial (RCT) showed that subjects with BPPV who were treated with CRP and additional VR exercises had significantly improved measures of overall gait stability when compared with those who had received isolated CRP (Epley maneuver) for their BPPV [39].

A limitation of our study is that the results were obtained from patients with different disorders and have not been classified accordingly. However, there is promising evidence that suggests that VR improves symptoms and can reduce falls in persons with a variety of vestibular conditions [5]. In the present study, results show statistically significant differences in TUG, GS, and DHI values, indicating improvement in the patients' performance and reported outcomes after a VR program, thus demonstrating the effectiveness of such intervention even in a developing country.

Table 1: Population characteristics.

Variables	n	%
Gender		
Female	49	85.96
Male	8	14.04
Diagnoses		
Unilateral vestibular hypofunction (UVH)	29	50.88
Benign paroxysmal positional vertigo (BPPV)	12	21.05
Nonspecific diagnosis	6	10.53
Multisensory dizziness syndrome	5	8.78
Bilateral vestibular hypofunction	3	5.26
Mixed vestibular disorder	1	1.75
Central vestibulopathy	1	1.75
Classification of diagnosis		
Peripheral	50	87.72
Central	6	10.53
Mixed	1	1.75

Our results for TUG are different from the study of Gill-Body et al. [40], whose values were greater than ours. Their results were unilateral vestibular hypofunction 19.5 (5.72), range 12.67–39.0, $n = 34$; bilateral vestibular hypofunction 23.33 (11.66), range 12.74–52.01, $n = 44$. This difference was probably due to the fact that they used a modified version of the TUG.

After the VR program, an increase was observed in GS and a decrease in TUG scores. This corroborated the previous studies [16, 41, 42] demonstrating that after a VR program, patients with vestibular disorders usually walk faster [43, 44]. Gait speed has been considered an important indicator of patient health, regardless of the diagnosis [45]. Indeed, it has been observed in another study that older adults with impaired semicircular canal function had slower gait compared to adults with intact function [46]. However, there is no published evidence of minimal detectable change (MDC) in the gait speed tests (GSTs) or in the TUG for vestibular patients. Although a number of authors have published studies with MDC values in other patient populations and these values range from 0.08 to 0.19 m/sec in GS [47–49] and from 1.10 to 4.00 sec in TUG [50–53], these populations were different from vestibular patients and consequently we can't be sure that they are suitable for our purposes here. Studies on vestibular populations are necessary. In our study, the difference found in the pre- and post-RV TUG scores was statistically significant but failed to reach the lowest MDCs already published with reference to other populations. The TUG values in our study were similar to those found in patients with mild DHI (TUG 12 ± 3 sec) and moderate DHI (TUG 11 ± 4 sec) in Whitney et al. [10].

With regard to patients' perception of impairment at the completion of the VR program, there were statistically

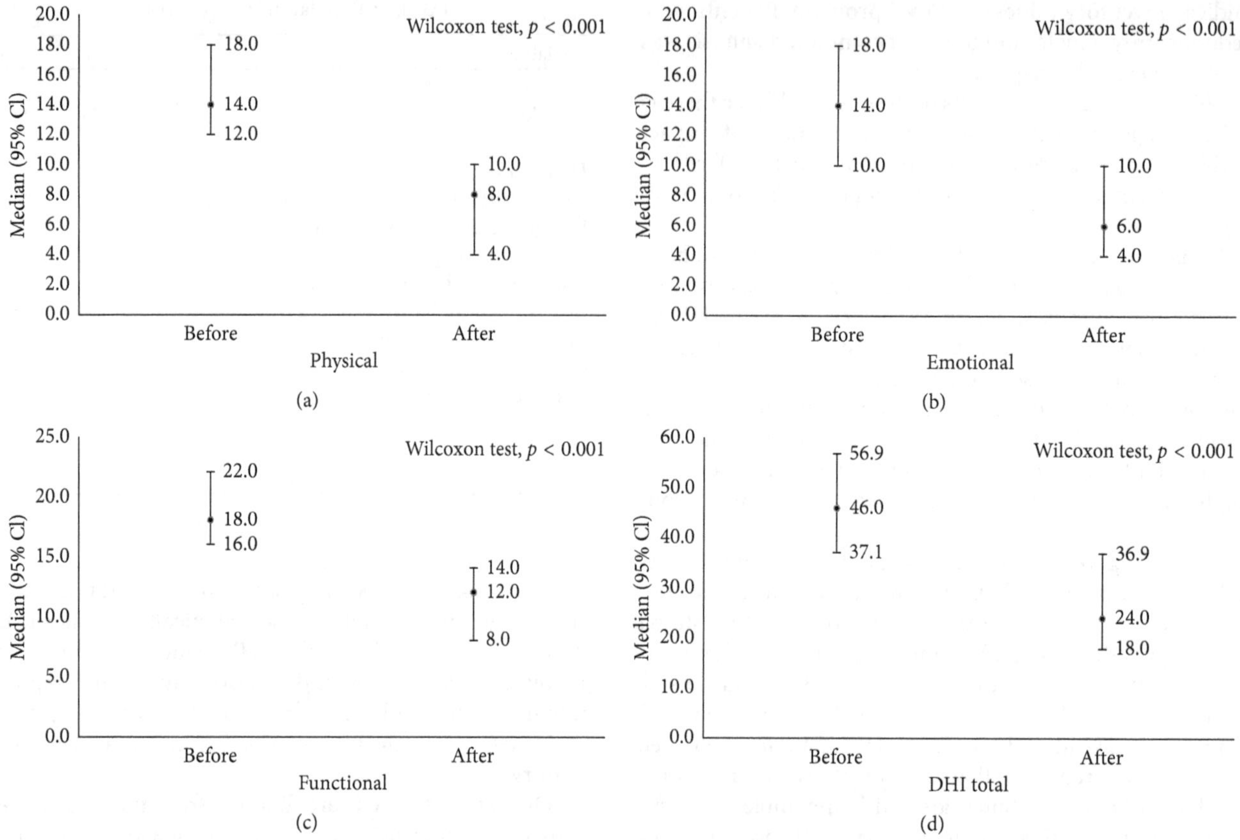

FIGURE 1: DHI total and respective domains and pre- and postvestibular rehabilitation program.

significant differences in total and functional DHI as well as in the emotional and physical domains. Whitney et al. [10] categorized the DHI scores into mild handicap (0–30), moderate handicap (31–60), and severe handicap (61–100); therefore, higher scores on the DHI indicate greater handicap. Using this classification, our results indicate that patients progressed from moderate to mild handicap. The TUG and gait speed values reported by Whitney et al. [10] were similar to ours (TUG and GS in mild DHI: 12 ± 3 and 1.02 ± 0.2; in moderate DHI: 11 ± 4 and 1.04 ± 0.2; in severe DHI: 14 ± 5 and 0.9 ± 0.2). This study was also similar to ours in that the functional test results from a group of 85 patients with vestibular disorders (peripheral and central) were analyzed without being broken down into subgroups. The reduction we found in the posttreatment score was superior to the 18-point minimum clinically important difference (MCID) published by Jacobson et al. [9]. These results of DHI coincide with the study of Humphriss et al. [32] and also with one study carried out in our country in which statistically significant reductions in DHI values were observed after VR [20]. These authors analyzed differences in the self-perception of impairment, the risk of falls, and gaze stability in patients with chronic unilateral vestibular hypofunction before and after VR with complementary Wii® therapy. Unlike the present study, there was no evaluation of the TUG or the GS; however, they also found an improvement in DHI scores.

Taken together, our results point to the importance of VR programs, regardless of the diagnosis of vestibular disorders. The rehabilitation program in this study consisted of exercises of adaptation and/or habituation and/or substitution, depending on each patient, twice a week in the rehabilitation clinic, and daily at the patient's home [7, 20]. Clinical practice guidelines for vestibular hypofunction suggest that the number of visits may need to be varied in accordance with comorbidities that can affect movement and psychological functioning [12].

The frequency, duration of optimal treatment, and total number of visits for the best results from physical therapy are as yet unknown. Knowledge on the effects of VR programs in developing countries is still incipient. In our country, this is one of the few studies carried out so far that evaluates the benefits of this type of care and the first to describe the effects of a VR program on TUG and gait speed in older people. Further studies are needed to observe the effects of this treatment in other Latin American countries in order to facilitate the dissemination of VR in the region and to compare performance in functional tests and self-perception of impairment in these countries. It should be noted that the results of this study were reported after the completion of a VR program in South America, which shows that in developing countries there are physical therapists who have been trained to carry out vestibular evaluation and exercise protocols. The cultural, economic, and social differences among environments with low, middle, and high incomes and their impact on the outcomes of VR have to date not been reported. We may hypothesize that these differences could change the results of a rehabilitation process and must be studied.

This study has some other limitations. The sample was one of convenience, and while it represented a wide range in function and cognition, all of the participants were from an urban area and may not be representative of all older people in the same area. We did not have information on the patients' socioeconomics and educational level, factors which may have affected performance. The testing sessions were not conducted in conditions of privacy, so the influence of other older adults or staff in the room may have affected performance. Although there were more females than males in our study, we do not believe that this influenced our results since a recent guideline [12] affirms that a VR program should be offered to males and females with the expectation of similar outcomes. Another limitation is the retrospective design. However, the patient records were all from a specialized VR clinic which used a uniform procedure for the evaluation and treatment of all its patients, and the outcome measures were obtained by the same experienced physical therapist, that is, the therapist who took the measurement for a specific patient was always the same, thus increasing the reliability of the measurement.

Some of our participants had a nonspecific diagnosis (such as dizziness or vertiginous syndrome). In these cases, an experienced physiotherapist assessed each subject with clinical vestibular tests [22].

Randomized controlled trial evidence for the efficacy of customized VR is available elsewhere, as already described. The present study demonstrates the effectiveness of VR where it has been successfully applied in a common clinical context in an urban middle-income environment. The study results are relevant to function and quality of life in elderly patients; yet, more research is needed to assess the effects of vestibular rehabilitation on quality of life and frequency of falls.

5. Conclusion

The functional outcome measures reported, including TUG, gait speed, and DHI, reflect statistically significant improvements in elderly patients after vestibular rehabilitation; the DHI improvements are clinically relevant.

Conflicts of Interest

The authors declare no potential conflicts of interest with respect to the research, authorship, and/or publication of this article.

References

[1] A. Grimby and U. Rosenhall, "Health-related quality of life and dizziness in old age," *Gerontology*, vol. 41, no. 5, pp. 286–298, 1995.

[2] J. Burzynski, S. Sulway, and J. A. Rutka, "Vestibular rehabilitation: review of indications, treatments, advances, and limitations," *Current Otorhinolaryngology Reports*, vol. 5, no. 3, pp. 160–166, 2017.

[3] M. N. McDonnell and S. L. Hillier, "Vestibular rehabilitation for unilateral peripheral vestibular dysfunction," *Cochrane Database of Systematic Reviews*, vol. 1, article CD005397, 2015.

[4] Y. Agrawal, J. P. Carey, C. C. Della Santina, M. C. Schubert, and L. B. Minor, "Disorders of balance and vestibular function in US adults: data from the National Health and Nutrition Examination Survey, 2001–2004," *Archives of Internal Medicine*, vol. 169, no. 10, pp. 938–944, 2009.

[5] S. Whitney, A. Alghwiri, and A. Alghadir, "An overview of vestibular rehabilitation," *Handbook of Clinical Neurology*, vol. 137, pp. 187–205, 2016.

[6] S. Hillier and M. N. McDonnell, "Is vestibular rehabilitation effective in improving dizziness and function after unilateral peripheral vestibular hypofunction? An abridged version of a Cochrane review," *European Journal of Physical and Rehabilitation Medicine*, vol. 52, no. 4, pp. 541–556, 2016.

[7] A. C. Binetti, A. X. Varela, D. L. Lucarelli, and D. H. Verdecchia, "Unilateral head impulses training in uncompensated vestibular hypofunction," *Case Reports in Otolaryngology*, vol. 2017, Article ID 2145173, 6 pages, 2017.

[8] O. A. Donoghue, G. M. Savva, H. Cronin, R. A. Kenny, and N. F. Horgan, "Using timed up and go and usual gait speed to predict incident disability in daily activities among community-dwelling adults aged 65 and older," *Archives of Physical Medicine and Rehabilitation*, vol. 95, no. 1, pp. 1954–1961, 2014.

[9] G. P. Jacobson and C. W. Newman, "The development of the dizziness handicap inventory," *Archives of Otolaryngology–Head and Neck Surgery*, vol. 116, no. 4, pp. 424–427, 1990.

[10] S. L. Whitney, D. M. Wrisley, K. E. Brown, and J. M. Furman, "Is perception of handicap related to functional performance in persons with vestibular dysfunction?," *Otology & Neurotology*, vol. 25, no. 2, pp. 139–143, 2004.

[11] D. Podsiadlo and S. Richardson, "The Timed "Up & Go": a test of basic functional mobility for frail elderly persons," *Journal of the American Geriatrics Society*, vol. 39, no. 2, pp. 142–148, 1991.

[12] C. D. Hall, S. D. Herdman, S. L. Whitney et al., "Vestibular rehabilitation for peripheral vestibular hypofunction: an evidence-based clinical practice guideline: from the American Physical Therapy Association Neurology Section," *Journal of Neurologic Physical Therapy*, vol. 40, no. 2, pp. 124–155, 2016.

[13] D. Nuti, G. Agus, M. Barbieri, and D. Passali, "The management of horizontal-canal paroxysmal positional vertigo," *Acta Otolaryngologica*, vol. 118, pp. 455–460, 1998.

[14] M. Hilton and D. Pinder, "Benign paroxysmal positional vertigo," *BMJ*, vol. 326, no. 7391, p. 673, 2003.

[15] T. Brandt and S. Steddin, "Current view of the mechanisms of benign paroxysmal positioning vertigo: cupulolithiasis or canalolithiasis?," *Journal of Vestibular Research*, vol. 3, pp. 373–382, 1993.

[16] M. Faralli, R. Lapenna, G. Giommetti, C. Pellegrino, and G. Ricci, "Residual dizziness after the first BPPV episode: role of otolithic function and of a delayed diagnosis," *European Annals of Otorhinolaryngology*, vol. 273, no. 10, pp. 3157–3165, 2016.

[17] N. Bhattacharyya, S. P. Gubbels, S. R. Schwartz et al., "Clinical practice guideline: benign paroxysmal positional vertigo (update)," *Otolaryngology–Head and Neck Surgery*, vol. 156, no. 3, pp. S1–S47, 2017.

[18] A. D. Furlan, E. Irvin, C. Munhall et al., "Rehabilitation service models for people with physical and/or mental disability living in low- and middle-income countries: a systematic review," *Journal of Rehabilitation Medicine*, vol. 50, no. 6, pp. 487–498, 2018.

[19] E. Dannenbaum, G. Chilingaryan, and J. Fung, "Visual vertigo analogue scale: an assessment questionnaire for visual vertigo," *Journal of Vestibular Research*, vol. 21, no. 3, pp. 153–159, 2011.

[20] D. H. Verdecchia, M. Mendoza, F. Sanguineti, and A. C. Binetti, "Outcomes after vestibular rehabilitation and Wii® therapy in patients with chronic unilateral vestibular hypofunction," *Acta Otorrinolaringológica Española*, vol. 65, no. 6, pp. 339–345, 2014.

[21] M. Smith-Wheelock, N. Shepard, and S. Telian, "Physical therapy program for vestibular rehabilitation," *American Journal of Otology*, vol. 12, no. 3, pp. 297–301, 1991.

[22] T. Steffen, T. Hacker, and L. Mollinger, "Age-and gender-related test performance in community-dwelling elderly people: Six-Minute Walk Test, Berg Balance Scale, Timed Up & Go Test, and gait speeds," *Physical Therapy*, vol. 82, no. 2, pp. 128–137, 2002.

[23] A. Shumway-Cook, S. Brauer, and M. Woollacott, "Predicting the probability for falls in community-dwelling older adults using the Timed Up & Go Test," *Physical Therapy*, vol. 80, no. 9, pp. 896–903, 2000.

[24] S. L. Whitney, G. F. Marchetti, A. Schade, and D. M. Wrisley, "The sensitivity and specificity of the Timed "Up & Go" and the Dynamic Gait Index for self-reported falls in persons with vestibular disorders," *Journal of Vestibular Research*, vol. 14, no. 5, pp. 397–409, 2004.

[25] S. L. Wolf, PA. Catlin, K. Gage, K. Gurucharri, R. Robertson, and K. Stephen, "Establishing the reliability and validity of measurements of walking time using the Emory Functional Ambulation Profile," *Physical Therapy*, vol. 79, no. 12, pp. 1122–1133, 1999.

[26] Y. J. Xie, E. Y. Liu, E. R. Anson, and Y. Agrawal, "Age-related imbalance is associated with slower walking speed: an analysis from the National Health and Nutrition Examination Survey," *Journal of Geriatric Physical Therapy*, vol. 40, no. 4, pp. 183–189, 2017.

[27] M. Cesari, S. B. Kritchevsky, B. W. Penninx et al., "Prognostic value of usual gait speed in well-functioning older people–results from the health, aging and body composition study," *Journal of the American Geriatrics Society*, vol. 53, no. 10, pp. 1675–1680, 2005.

[28] B. Caldara, A. I. Asenzo, G. Brusotti Paglia et al., "Adaptación cultural y validación del Dizziness Handicap Inventory: versión argentina," *Acta Otorrinolaringológica Española*, vol. 63, no. 2, pp. 106–114, 2012.

[29] J. Y. Jung, J. S Kim, P. S. Chung, S. H. Woo, and C. K. Rhee, "Effect of vestibular rehabilitation on dizziness in the elderly," *American Journal of Otolaryngology*, vol. 30, no. 5, pp. 295–299, 2009.

[30] R. S. Moreira Bittar, L. Simoceli, M. E. Bovino Pedalini, and M. A. Bottino, "The treatment of diseases related to balance disorders in the elderly and the effectiveness of vestibular rehabilitation," *Brazilian Journal of Otorhinolaryngology*, vol. 73, no. 3, pp. 295–298, 2007.

[31] M. Smith-Wheelock, N. T. Shepard, S. A. Telian, and T. Boismier, "Balance retraining therapy in the elderly," in *Proceedings of Otolaryngic Cherry Blossom Conference, Clinical Otolaryngologic Care of the Geriatric Patient*, vol. 71–80BC Decker Inc., Washington, DC, USA, 1992.

[32] R. L. Humphriss, D. M. Baguley, S. Peerman, T. E. Mitchell, and D. A. Moffat, "Clinical outcomes of vestibular rehabilitation," *Physiotherapy*, vol. 87, no. 7, pp. 368–373, 2001.

[33] A. Bayat, A. Pourbakht, N. Sak, Z. Zainun, S. Nikakhlagh, and G. Mirmomeni, "Vestibular rehabilitation outcomes in the elderly with chronic vestibular dysfunction," *Iranian Red Crescent Medical Journal*, vol. 14, no. 11, pp. 705–708, 2012.

[34] L. H. Tee and N. W Chee, "Vestibular rehabilitation therapy for the dizzy patient," *Annals of the Academy of Medicine of Singapore*, vol. 34, no. 4, pp. 289–294, 2005.

[35] M. Von Brevern, A. Radtke, F. Lezius et al., "Epidemiology of benign paroxysmal positional vertigo: a population based study," *Journal of Neurology, Neurosurgery, and Psychiatry*, vol. 78, no. 7, pp. 710–715, 2007.

[36] S. Di Girolamo, G. Paludetti, G. Briglia, A. Cosenza, R. Santarelli, and W. Di Nardo, "Postural control in benign paroxysmal positional vertigo before and after recovery," *Acta Otorrinolaringologica*, vol. 118, no. 3, pp. 289–293, 1998.

[37] P. B. Giacomini, M. Alessandrini, and A. Magrini, "Long-term postural abnormalities in benign paroxysmal positional vertigo," *ORL; Journal for Otorhinolaryngology and Its Related Specialties*, vol. 64, no. 4, pp. 237–241, 2002.

[38] P. J. Blatt, G. A. Georgakakis, S. J. Herdman, R. Clendaniel, and R. Tusa, "The effect of the canalith repositioning maneuver on resolving postural instability in patients with benign paroxysmal positional vertigo," *American Journal of Otolaryngology*, vol. 21, no. 3, pp. 356–363, 2000.

[39] W. C. Chang, Y. R Yang, L. C. Hsu, C. M. Chern, and R. Y. Wang, "Balance improvement in patients with benign paroxysmal positional vertigo," *Clinical Rehabilitation*, vol. 22, no. 4, pp. 338–347, 2008.

[40] K. M. Gill-Body, M. Beninato, and D. E. Krebs, "Relationship among balance impairments, functional performance, and disability in people with peripheral vestibular hypofunction," *Physical Therapy*, vol. 80, no. 8, pp. 748–758, 2000.

[41] K. A. Alahmari, P. J. Sparto, G. F. Marchetti, M. S. Redfern, J. M. Furman, and S. L. Whitney, "Comparison of virtual reality based therapy with customized vestibular physical therapy for the treatment of vestibular disorders," *IEEE Transactions on Neural Systems and Rehabilitation Engineering*, vol. 22, no. 2, pp. 389–399, 2014.

[42] Y. Saman, D. E. Bamiou, L. Murdin et al., "Balance, falls risk, and related disability in untreated vestibular schwannoma patients," *Journal of Neurological Surgery Part B: Skull Base*, vol. 75, no. 5, pp. 332–338, 2014.

[43] S. A. Arnold, A. M. Stewart, H. M. Moor, R. C. Karl, and J. C. Reneker, "The effectiveness of vestibular rehabilitation interventions in treating unilateral peripheral vestibular disorders: a systematic review," *Physiotherapy Research International*, vol. 22, no. 3, p. e1635, 2017.

[44] N. A. Ricci, M. C. Aratani, H. H. Caovilla, and F. F. Gananca, "Effects of vestibular rehabilitation on balance control in older people with chronic dizziness: a randomized clinical trial," *American Journal of Physical Medicine & Rehabilitation*, vol. 95, no. 4, pp. 256–269, 2016.

[45] S. Studenski, S. Perera, K. Patel et al., "Gait speed and survival in older adults," *JAMA*, vol. 305, no. 1, pp. 50–58, 2011.

[46] Y. Agrawal, M. Davalos-Bichara, M. G. Zuniga, and J. P. Carey, "Head impulse test abnormalities and influence on gait speed and falls in older individuals," *Otology & Neurotology*, vol. 34, no. 9, pp. 1729–1735, 2013.

[47] K. M. Palombaro, R. L. Craik, K. K. Mangione, and J. D. Tomlinson, "Determining meaningful changes in gait

speed after hip fracture," *Physical Therapy*, vol. 86, no. 6, pp. 809–816, 2006.

[48] S. Perera, S. H. Mody, R. C. Woodman, and S. A. Studenski, "Meaningful change and responsiveness in common physical performance measures in older adults," *Journal of the American Geriatrics Society*, vol. 54, no. 5, pp. 743–749, 2006.

[49] K. K. Mangione, R. L. Craik, A. A. McCormick et al., "Detectable changes in physical performance measures in elderly African Americans," *Physical Therapy*, vol. 90, no. 6, pp. 921–927, 2010.

[50] S. L. Huang, C. L. Hsieh, R. M. Wu, C. H. Tai, C. H. Lin, and W. S. Lu, "Minimal detectable change of the Timed "Up & Go" Test and the Dynamic Gait Index in people with Parkinson disease," *Physical Therapy*, vol. 91, no. 1, pp. 114–121, 2001.

[51] J. D. Ries, J. L. Echternach, L. Nof, and M. Gagnon Blodgett, "Test-retest reliability and minimal detectable change scores for the Timed "Up & Go" Test, the Six-Minute Walk Test, and gait speed in people with Alzheimer disease," *Physical Therapy*, vol. 89, no. 6, pp. 569–579, 2009.

[52] E. Yuksel, S. Kalkan, S. Cekmece, B. Unver, and V. Karatosun, "Assessing minimal detectable changes and test-retest reliability of the Timed Up and Go Test and the 2-Minute Walk Test in patients with total knee arthroplasty," *Journal of Arthroplasty*, vol. 32, no. 2, pp. 426–430, 2017.

[53] A. Alghadir, S. Anwer, and J. M. Brismée, "The reliability and minimal detectable change of Timed Up and Go test in individuals with grade 1–3 knee osteoarthritis," *BMC Musculoskeletal Disorders*, vol. 16, no. 174, 2015.

20

Polypharmacy among Underserved Older African American Adults

Mohsen Bazargan,[1,2] James Smith,[1] Masoud Movassaghi,[2] David Martins,[1,2] Hamed Yazdanshenas,[1,2] Seyede Salehe Mortazavi,[3] and Gail Orum[1,4]

[1]*Charles R. Drew University of Medicine and Science (CDU), Los Angeles, CA, USA*
[2]*University of California, Los Angeles (UCLA), Los Angeles, CA, USA*
[3]*Mental Health Research Center, Tehran Institute of Psychiatry, School of Behavioral Sciences and Mental Health, Iran University of Medical Sciences, Tehran, Iran*
[4]*Keck Graduate Institute, School of Pharmacy, Claremont, CA, USA*

Correspondence should be addressed to Mohsen Bazargan; mohsenbazargan@cdrewu.edu

Academic Editor: F. R. Ferraro

The purpose of the present study was to examine correlates of polypharmacy among underserved community-dwelling older African American adults. *Methods.* This study recruited 400 underserved older African Americans adults living in South Los Angeles. The structured face-to-face interviews collected data on participants' characteristics and elicited data pertaining to the type, frequency, dosage, and indications of all medications used by participants. *Results.* Seventy-five and thirty percent of participants take at least five and ten medications per day, respectively. Thirty-eight percent of participants received prescription medications from at least three providers. Inappropriate drug use occurred among seventy percent of the participants. Multivariate analysis showed that number of providers was the strongest correlate of polypharmacy. Moreover, data show that gender, comorbidity, and potentially inappropriate medication use are other major correlates of polypharmacy. *Conclusions.* This study shows a high rate of polypharmacy and potentially inappropriate medication use among underserved older African American adults. We documented strong associations between polypharmacy and use of potentially inappropriate medications, comorbidities, and having multiple providers. Polypharmacy and potentially inappropriate medications may be attributed to poor coordination and management of medications among providers and pharmacists. There is an urgent need to develop innovative and effective strategies to reduce inappropriate polypharmacy and potentially inappropriate medication in underserved elderly minority populations.

1. Introduction

Almost 72% of elderly Medicare beneficiaries have at least two medical chronic conditions, and 39% suffer from four or more chronic conditions [1]. Every year, Medicare beneficiaries with five or more chronic conditions see an average of thirteen physicians each and fill over fifty prescriptions [2]. Proper treatment of many medical conditions requires the use of medications that can be misused, abused, and/or lead to dependency. A recent study using the National Health and Nutrition Examination Survey (1988–2010) shows that, between 1988 and 2010, the median number of prescription medications (Rx) used among adults aged 65 and older doubled from 2 to 4, and the proportion taking at least 5 medications tripled from 12.8% to 39% [3].

Older persons with multiple chronic conditions often receive duplicate testing, conflicting treatment advice, and prescriptions that are contraindicated [4, 5]. Polypharmacy is a major problem that contributes to costs, adverse drug events, confusion, compliance issues, management errors, hospitalization, and premature mortality among the elderly [6–16]. Research has shown that those taking numerous medications have a higher likelihood of emergency room visits and hospitalizations [17, 18]. A recent study documented that older people who took multiple medications faced an increased risk of frailty and death, and for older individuals who took a higher number of medicines, each additional medicine incurred a 22% increase in the risk of transitioning from a state of robust health to dying over the three-year study period [19]. Despite awareness of polypharmacy and its potential consequences in older patients, polypharmacy remains widespread [20]. While Rx use increased dramatically within the last decade, studies also indicate that polypharmacy in the United States continues to increase and is affecting 33% to 60% of patients, and that multiple medication use is associated with a host of undesirable outcomes, including adverse drug reactions, geriatric syndromes, and poor adherence [7].

African Americans, compared to whites, are disproportionally affected by chronic medical conditions for which multiple prescriptions and treatments are required [21]. Almost 47% of elderly African American Medicare beneficiaries suffer from at least four chronic conditions, compared to 38% of their non-Hispanic white counterparts [1]. While underserved elderly African Americans have high-risk profiles for increased morbidity and disability, generally they receive less aggressive treatment and are less likely to be prescribed newer, more effective and simplified medication combinations [22–26]. Therefore, lack of access to combined and simpler medication regimens among underserved older African American adults likely results in the use of a higher number of older, generic medications with more complex dosing regimens. Indeed, systematic reviews of studies confirmed that simpler, less frequent dosing regimens resulted in better medication adherence across a variety of therapeutic classes [27].

Lack of equitable access to Rx among elderly African Americans, compared to their white counterparts, was noted two decades ago [28] yet remains a major concern [29]. Recent National data show that older African Americans are more likely to report not having a *"regular care provider"* or a *"regular place of care"* (noncoordinated care) than their white counterparts [30], which is associated with inappropriate use of Rx prescribed by multiple providers. Despite the introduction of a Medicare outpatient prescription drug benefit in January 2006, the longstanding Rx access gaps between elderly African Americans and whites remain unchanged, with three times as many elderly African American beneficiaries (18%) going without prescribed medication compared to white beneficiaries (6%) [31].

In summary, national studies show that race/ethnicity is associated with polypharmacy variation in middle age and older adults [32]. Indeed, polypharmacy, a common and important problem related to drug use, occurs subsequent to this multimorbidity in the elderly in all populations [33], however; there is a significant need for additional research to reduce the burden of medication mismanagement and polypharmacy among underserved older African American adults.

The goal of this study is to describe characteristics of underserved older African American adults engaging in polypharmacy. We defined polypharmacy merely based on the number of medications used by participants. Polypharmacy is characterized as the use of multiple medications for the treatment of a single, or several, coexisting diseases [33]. Additionally, correlates of medication use, including demographic characteristics, smoking status, alcohol use, number of providers (physicians and pharmacies), severity of pain, and number of potentially inappropriate medications (PIM) for older adults, are examined.

2. Methods

Details of the study design have been previously described [34]. In brief, data were collected between 2013 and 2014 from 400 community-dwelling, underserved, older adult, self-identified African Americans from 16 predominantly African American churches located in Service Planning Area 6 (SPA 6) of Los Angeles (LA) County. LA County has the largest population of any county in the nation. More than 1.3 million of the 10.3 million residents who live in LA County are 65 years and older [35]. A Service Planning Area, or SPA, is a specific geographic region within LA County. Due to the large size of LA County (4,300 square miles), it has been divided into 8 geographic areas [36]. These distinct regions allow the Department of Public Health to develop and provide more relevant public health and clinical services targeted to the specific health needs of the residents in these different areas. We specifically selected SPA 6 because the vast majority of elderly living in SPA 6 are African American (49%).

In addition to posting flyers announcing the proposed project at respective churches, the coordinator of this project assisted church leaders to convene pre- or post-Sunday sermon meetings to introduce the program project to the parishioners. Participants were encouraged to consider the potential benefits of this project to society. They were told that the information they provide may contribute to improving minority senior population health outcomes. In addition, they received a $20 remuneration fee. Two coauthors of this study, both trained physicians, conducted the face-to-face interviews in a private room at participating sites. Less than 5% (n = 19) of individuals who were approached refused to participate. Written informed consent was obtained from participants. This study was approved by the Charles R. Drew University of Medicine and Science Institutional Review Board.

2.1. Measurement

2.1.1. Medication Use. Medication use was assessed by the drug inventory method. Participants were asked to bring all over-the-counter and prescription medications that they had taken in the two weeks prior to the interview. The interviewer transcribed from the container label the name of the medication, strength of the drug, expiration date, instructions, special warnings, providers' information, and so on.

2.1.2. Potentially Inappropriate Medication (PIM) on Beers' List. The Beers list identifies medications and types of medications that are "potentially inappropriate" for older people. Using the 2012 American Geriatrics Society revised Beers Criteria [37], we documented the number of PIM use for each participant.

2.1.3. Severity of Pain. Pain was measured using the revised version of Short-Form McGill Pain Questionnaire-2 (SF-MPQ-2) [38, 39]. Participants completed the SF-MPQ-2 by rating the extent to which they experienced each of 22 pain descriptors in the past week using an 11-point numeric rating scale (0 = "none" to 10 = "worst possible"). Severe pain was defined according to the World Health Organization scale, which was 7 to 10 on the 11-point numeric rating scale [40].

2.1.4. Comorbidity. Participants self-reported "Yes" or "No" to a list of medical conditions, such as arthritis, back pain, kidney disease, stroke, and hypertension.

2.1.5. Number of Providers and Copayment for Rx. Participants were asked if any copayment is required to fill a prescription. Number and description of pharmacies and providers used by participants were recorded from the label of medication containers.

2.1.6. Smoking Status and Alcohol Use. Smoking status and alcohol use were computed from self-reporting during the past year. Smoking status was categorized into three groups: current, former, and never smoked. In addition, alcohol use was categorized based on number of drinks per day (none, 1-2, and ≥ 3 drinks per day).

2.1.7. Statistical Analysis. Descriptive statistics were used to measure the frequency, mean, and standard deviation of all variables. Furthermore, we used the chi-square test to examine associations between medication used and demographic characteristics, comorbidities, and medication complications. In addition, multiple logistic regression was employed to examine the correlates of using medications (use of ≥ 5 medications versus fewer), adjusting for demographic characteristics and other relevant characteristics. We utilized a p value < 0.05 to identify statistically significant differences. To avoid multicollinearity, a diagnostic test was performed in multivariate analysis to examine intercorrelation among independent variables.

3. Results

3.1. Characteristics of Sample. This sample included 400 African American individuals who were between the ages of 65 to 94 years (Mean 73.5 ± 7). More than 21% were 80 years of age or older. One out of four participants reported having no high school diploma. Almost 65% of participants were women. Only 20% of the sample were currently married or lived with a companion. Table 1 reports the percentage of self-reported chronic conditions among our sample. In all, the number of reported chronic illnesses ranged from zero to seventeen, with the average at just over five (5.2 ± 3.01). Nineteen percent of participants reported at least eight chronic conditions. Over 85% reported that they have been diagnosed with hypertension. One out of four individuals who were diagnosed with hypertension was using at least three antihypertensive agents from different classes. Almost 37% of participants were diagnosed with diabetes mellitus. Three out of four reported visiting more than one type of physician. Only 8% of respondents did not have a regular or primary care provider. Participants reported having an average of 6.71 scheduled physician visits within the past twelve months (range: 0 to 24; SD: 5.4). Thirty-eight percent of participants received Rx from at least three providers. Furthermore, the medication containers showed that 28% of participants used at least two pharmacies to fill their prescriptions.

Participants were taking an average of 5.7 (range: 0 to 18; SD: 3.02) prescription drugs. Twenty-three percent were using at least eight medications, whereas 37% and 40% of participants were taking five to seven and zero to four prescription medications, respectively. In addition, participants were taking an average of 1.25 over-the-counter medications. Using the 2012 American Geriatrics Society revised Beers Criteria [37], our data show that 27% and 43% of participants used at least one medication that was classified as "Avoid" and "Use Conditionally," respectively. The most common drugs in the "Avoid" group were nifedipine 6% (24), diphenhydramine 3% (13), glyburide 2% (8), lorazepam 2% (8), cyclobenzaprine 2% (7), diazepam 2% (7), and digoxin hydroxyzine 2% (7).

3.2. Bivariate Correlates of Polypharmacy. Table 1 reports bivariate correlates of medication use with all other variables. The number of medications used was divided into two categories: "0–4" and "≥ 5" medications. Eight out of twelve variables were significantly associated with the number of medications used. This table reports that the proportions of older adults on 0–4 and ≥ 5 medications were 25% and 75%, respectively. Compared with those taking 0–4 medications, persons taking ≥ 5 medications were more likely to be women, 70–79 years of age, former smokers, visiting two or more providers, filling their prescriptions in different pharmacies, diagnosed with a higher number of comorbidities, suffering from a higher level of pain, and used a higher number of PIMs.

3.3. Multivariate Correlates of Medication Use. Table 2 reports the result of multiple logistic regression, adjusting for demographic characteristics including age, gender, education, and marital status. This table reports adjusted odd ratios (OR) between independent variables and two categories of medications used ("0–4" and "≥ 5" medications). Four variables were significantly associated with the use of medications. Adjusting for demographic characteristics and other related variables, number of providers was the strongest correlate of excessive use of medications. The odds of being in the group of survey respondents who used ≥5 medications were almost seven times (OR = 6.67; CI: 2.82–15.71) higher among individuals who received medical care from multiple providers. Participants with one or at least two PIMs were 2.24 (CI: 1.17–4.30) and 4.6 (CI: 2.10–10.04) times more likely to use ≥ 5 medications than their counterparts with no PIMs, respectively. Moreover, when demographic characteristics and other variables were adjusted, participants who were diagnosed with 4–7 or ≥8 comorbidities were 3.2 (CI: 1.72–5.94) and 6.11 (CI: 2.02–18.50) times more likely than their counterparts with less than ≤ 3 comorbidities to use ≥ 5

TABLE 1: Characteristics of study sample by high versus low medication use ($N = 400$).

Characteristic of sample	N (%)	Groups of medication users		p Value
		0–4 N (%) 100 (25)	≥5 N (%) 300 (75)	
Gender				
Female	259 (65)	50 (19)	209 (81)	0.001
Male	141 (35)	50 (36)	91 (65)	
Age				
65–69	135 (34)	47 (35)	88 (65)	0.002
70–79	180 (45)	31 (17)	149 (83)	
≥80	85 (21)	22 (26)	63 (74)	
Education				
No high school diploma	99 (25)	19 (19)	80 (81)	0.078
High school diploma	301 (75)	81 (27)	220 (73)	
Marital status				
Married/living with partner	78 (20)	17 (22)	61 (78)	0.283
Not married	322 (80)	83 (26)	239 (74)	
Copayment for RX				
No	83 (21)	27 (33)	56 (67)	0.075
Yes	317 (79)	73 (23)	244 (77)	
Number of providers				
1-2	247 (62)	92 (37)	155 (63)	0.001
≥3	153 (38)	8 (5)	145 (95)	
Number of pharmacies				
1	287 (72)	82 (29)	205 (71)	0.009
≥2	113 (28)	18 (16)	95 (84)	
Number of Comorbidity				
≤3	128 (32)	60 (47)	68 (53)	0.001
4–7	195 (49)	34 (17)	161 (83)	
≥8	77 (19)	6 (8)	71 (92)	
Smoking status				
Current	81 (20)	14 (17)	67 (83)	0.001
Former	64 (16)	28 (44)	36 (56)	
Never	255 (64)	58 (23)	197 (77)	
Alcohol use (drinks per day)				
None	291 (73)	70 (24)	221 (76)	0.404
1-2	71 (18)	22 (31)	49 (69)	
≥3	38 (9)	8 (21)	30 (79)	
Number of PIM				
None	122 (31)	54 (44)	68 (56)	0.001
One	143 (36)	31 (112)	112 (78)	
≥2	135 (34)	15 (11)	120 (89)	
Level of pain				
None-mild	114 (29)	46 (40)	68 (60)	0.001
Moderate	84 (21)	22 (26)	62 (74)	
Severe	202 (50)	32 (16)	170 (84)	

TABLE 2: Multivariate logistic analysis of correlates of use of high versus low medication use ($N = 400$).

Independent variables	OR (95% CI)	p
Gender		
Female	2.36 (1.26–4.42)	0.007
Male	1	
Age		
65–69	0.69 (0.30–1.57)	0.067
70–79	1.53 (0.69–3.41)	0.374
≥80	1	0.297
Education		
No high school diploma	1.71 (0.82–3.56)	0.151
High school diploma	1	
Marital status		
Not married	2.21 (0.99–4.857)	0.501
Married/living with partner	1	
Copayment for RX		
No	1.14 (0.55–2.34)	0.725
Yes	1	
Number of providers		
1-2	1	0.001
≥3	6.67 (2.82–15.71)	
Number of pharmacies		
1	1	0.620
≥2	1.52 (0.73–3.17)	
Number of comorbidity		
≤3	1	0.001
4–7	3.20 (1.72–5.94)	0.001
≥8	6.11 (2.02–18.50)	0.064
Smoking status		
Never	1	0.852
Current	1.08 (0.49–2.38)	0.028
Former	0.38 (0.16–0.90)	0.338
Alcohol use (drinks per day)		
None	1	0.572
1-2	0.80 (0.37–1.74)	0.227
≥3	1.98 (0.65–6.01)	0.000
Number of PIM		
None	1	0.015
One	2.24 (1.17–4.30)	0.001
≥2	4.60 (2.10–10.04)	0.221
Level of pain		
None-mild	1	0.892
Moderate	0.95 (0.44–2.05)	0.136
Severe	1.70 (0.85–3.41)	
−2 log likelihood	303.6	
Nagelkerke R-square	0.454	
Percentage of correctly predicted outcome	82%	

medications, respectively. Finally, gender was the only demographic variable that was associated with polypharmacy. The odds of being in the group of survey participants who used ≥ 5 medications were 2.36 (CI: 2.36–4.42) times higher among women than their male counterparts.

4. Discussion

We documented that polypharmacy remains an important issue among underserved older African American adults. The National Health and Nutrition Examination Survey

(NHANES) shows 39% (CI: 35.8, 42.3) of older adults aged 65 years and older are taking ≥ 5 medications [3], whereas our data show 75% of participants currently taking ≥ 5 medications and 30% taking ≥ 10 medications. The high rate of polypharmacy documented in our study may reflect the compromised level of care for the senior population residing in SPA 6 of LA County. Home to over one million residents, SPA 6 is disproportionately harmed by health disparities compared to the rest of LA County [41].

A recent systematic review and meta-analysis of 25 studies targeting older adults with polypharmacy (≥ 4 drugs) found no convincing evidence that the strategies assessed in these studies were effective in reducing polypharmacy or had an impact on clinically relevant endpoints [42]. Even though interventional strategies employed in these studies were complex, it is unclear yet how to best organize and implement them to achieve a reduction of inappropriate polypharmacy [42]. Additional investigational and interventional studies are needed to offer practical solutions to reduce polypharmacy, PIM use, and other medication related complications.

Our study echoes previous research that shows that one of the important correlates of inappropriate prescription medication use in older patients is the number of prescribed medications [43–46]. Our data show that 70% of the sample used at least one medication classified as potentially inappropriate by the 2012 Beers Criteria. Additionally, 27% and 43% of the participants used at least one medication classified as "Avoid" and "Use Conditionally" by the 2012 Beers Criteria, respectively. Analyzing the 2006–2010 Medical Expenditure Panel Survey (MEPS), Davidoff and her colleagues documented that almost 43% of older adults with Rx had at least one medication fill that met the board definition of 2012 Beers Criteria [47]. Therefore, the number of PIMs used among our sample of African American older adults is higher than national averages reported by Davidoff and her colleagues.

Our study suggests that having multiple comorbidities and multiple providers (physicians and pharmacists) may be additional independent risk factors for polypharmacy. More than 28% of our sample of underserved, older African Americans used multiple pharmacies. The multivariate analysis of our data shows that when controlling for PIM, having multiple providers remains a significant correlate of polypharmacy. Switching between providers and pharmacies may exacerbate communication among patients, pharmacists, and physicians, increasing the risk of PIM and polypharmacy. Other researchers documented that filling prescriptions at multiple pharmacies is associated with lower medication adherence across multiple chronic medications and a greater likelihood of drug-drug interactions in concurrent pharmacy users [48]. Therefore, pharmacists serving older adults in underserved communities need to be aware that their patients may be using multiple pharmacies, especially those with multiple providers and comorbidities, as well as those who may get some of their prescriptions filled at the pharmacy of free clinics.

Another finding of this study that needs additional attention is that older African American women in our sample are more likely to use a higher number of medications than their male counterparts. Our data show that 65% and 81% of men and women are taking ≥ 5 medications, respectively. In addition, 35% of women participating in this study were taking at least 10 medications. Furthermore, African American women in our sample are more likely than their male counterparts to use medications categorized as "potentially inappropriate" by the Beers Criteria (31% versus 19%); to use medication with drug-drug interactions (56% versus 47%); to use multiple providers (73% versus 62%); and have more than three chronic conditions (63% versus 71%). However, using multivariate analysis, even after all the above-mentioned variables and other demographic characteristics were controlled for, women are still more likely to use a higher number of medications that men.

It is imperative to mention several limitations of this study. First, this study used a cross-sectional study design, which allowed us to collect data at a single point in time. Second, African Americans who participated in this study were selected from local churches that may be different than non-church attenders and this may introduce a selection bias. Third, the assumption is made that participants brought in all of the medication vials that they used within two weeks prior to the interviews. Lack of access to participants' medical or pharmacy records limits our ability to validate this assumption. In addition, participants were asked to bring medications used within the last two weeks; these may exclude medications dosed monthly or old medications patients find when they have a cold, and so on. However, several attempts were made prior to the face-to-face interviews to ensure that participants would follow the instructions and bring all their medications with them. Finally, our sample was generated from an underserved, urban African American community; the results of this study may not be generalizable to all African American older adults.

5. Conclusion

This study shows a high rate of polypharmacy and PIM use among our sample of underserved older African American adults residing in South Los Angeles. We documented a strong association between polypharmacy and PIM use, comorbidities, and having multiple providers. Exacerbation of these issues may be attributed to poor coordination and management of medications among providers and pharmacists. Therefore, there is a need to develop more innovative and effective strategies to reduce inappropriate polypharmacy [42]. Home-based, community-patient-centered, multidisciplinary approaches that connect local, community-based pharmacists with patients and their providers may be a promising approach. While a few researchers have suggested a multidisciplinary approach that coordinates medication use of older adults by providing both physicians and pharmacists with the ability to view online the prescription histories of patients [49], Lancaster and colleagues suggest that home-based, multidisciplinary assessments and reconciliation activities on an ongoing basis are needed to prevent medication related complications [50]. A Swedish study among older adults indicated that when reconciliation activities are mandated by law, the number of prescribed drugs and the extent of inappropriate drug therapy decreased significantly [51]. Regardless, patient and provider barriers to polypharmacy are numerous, and resources must be made available to facilitate deliberate yet judicious deprescribing among this segment of our population that needs it the most.

Conflicts of Interest

There are no conflicts of interest. In addition, there is no financial support or relationships that may pose conflicts of interest.

Authors' Contributions

All authors have contributed significantly and they all are in agreement with the content of the manuscript. They all approved the manuscript and this submission.

Acknowledgments

This study was supported by the Center for Medicare and Medicaid Services (CMS) Grant 1/0CMS030458 to Charles R. Drew University of Medicine and Science (PI: Mohsen Bazargan). Drs. James Smith and Yazdanshenas are scholars supported by the Clinical Research Education and Career Development (CRECD), Phase II Grant # "R25MD007610," NIH-NIMHD. Additionally, Dr. Bazargan was supported by the NIH-NIMHD under Award nos. "U54MD008149; U54MD007598; and 2P20MD000182."

References

[1] K. A. Lochner and C. S. Cox, "Prevalence of multiple chronic conditions among Medicare beneficiaries, United States, 2010," *Preventing Chronic Disease*, vol. 10, p. E61, 2013.

[2] Partnership for Solutions, "Better Lives for People with Chronic Conditions," 2006, http://www.partnershipforsolutions.org.

[3] C. J. Charlesworth, E. Smit, D. S. H. Lee, F. Alramadhan, and M. C. Odden, "Polypharmacy among adults aged 65 years and older in the United States: 1988–2010," *Journals of Gerontology Series A*, vol. 70, no. 8, pp. 989–995, 2015.

[4] K. Johnell and I. Klarin, "The relationship between number of drugs and potential drug-drug interactions in the elderly: a study of over 600 000 elderly patients from the Swedish prescribed drug register," *Drug Safety*, vol. 30, no. 10, pp. 911–918, 2007.

[5] E. S. Huang, "Appropriate application of evidence to the care of elderly patients with diabetes," *Current Diabetes Reviews*, vol. 3, no. 4, pp. 260–263, 2007.

[6] B. D. Hayes, W. Klein-Schwartz, and F. Barrueto Jr., "Polypharmacy and the Geriatric Patient," *Clinics in Geriatric Medicine*, vol. 23, no. 2, pp. 371–390, 2007.

[7] E. R. Hajjar, A. C. Cafiero, and J. T. Hanlon, "Polypharmacy in elderly patients," *The American Journal of Geriatric Pharmacotherapy*, vol. 5, no. 4, pp. 345–351, 2007.

[8] E. Astrand, B. Åstrand, K. Antonov, and G. Petersson, "Potential drug interactions during a three-decade study period: a cross-sectional study of a prescription register [erratum appears in Eur J Clin Pharmacol. 2007 Nov;63(11):1095]," *European Journal of Clinical Pharmacology*, vol. 63, no. 9, pp. 851–859, 2007.

[9] J. T. Hanlon, C. F. Pieper, E. R. Hajjar et al., "Incidence and predictors of all and preventable adverse drug reactions in frail elderly persons after hospital stay," *Journals of Gerontology Series A*, vol. 61, no. 5, pp. 511–515, 2006.

[10] D. A. Gorard, "Escalating polypharmacy," *An International Journal of Medicine*, vol. 99, no. 11, pp. 797–800, 2006.

[11] K. T. Cannon, M. M. Choi, and M. A. Zuniga, "Potentially inappropriate medication use in elderly patients receiving home health care: a retrospective data analysis," *American Journal Geriatric Pharmacotherapy*, vol. 4, no. 2, pp. 134–143, 2006.

[12] M. I. Baena, M. J. Faus, P. C. Fajardo et al., "Medicine-related problems resulting in emergency department visits," *European Journal of Clinical Pharmacology*, vol. 62, no. 5, pp. 387–393, 2006.

[13] M. M. Fulton and E. R. Allen, "Polypharmacy in the elderly: a literature review," *Journal of the American Academy of Nurse Practitioners*, vol. 17, no. 4, pp. 123–132, 2005.

[14] N. H. Ballentine, "Polypharmacy in the elderly: maximizing benefit, minimizing harm," *Critical Care Nursing Quarterly*, vol. 31, no. 1, pp. 40–45, 2008.

[15] M. I. Rossi, A. Young, R. Maher et al., "Polypharmacy and health beliefs in older outpatients," *American Journal Geriatric Pharmacotherapy*, vol. 5, no. 4, pp. 317–323, 2007.

[16] J. C. Milton and S. H. D. Jackson, "Inappropriate polypharmacy: reducing the burden of multiple medication," *Clinical Medicine*, vol. 7, no. 5, pp. 514–517, 2007.

[17] J. H. Flaherty, H. M. Perry III, G. S. Lynchard, and J. E. Morley, "Polypharmacy and hospitalization among older home care patients," *Journals of Gerontology Series A*, vol. 55, no. 10, pp. M554-M559, 2000.

[18] G. Onder, C. Pedone, F. Landi et al., "Adverse drug reactions as cause of hospital admissions: results from the Italian group of pharmacoepidemiology in the elderly (GIFA)," *Journal of the American Geriatrics Society*, vol. 50, no. 12, pp. 1962–1968, 2002.

[19] K. M. Jamsen, J. S. Bell, S. N. Hilmer et al., "Effects of changes in number of medications and drug burden index exposure on transitions between frailty states and death: the concord health and ageing in men project cohort study," *Journal of the American Geriatrics Society*, vol. 64, no. 1, pp. 89–95, 2016.

[20] L. L. Dwyer, B. Han, D. A. Woodwell, and E. A. Rechtsteiner, "Polypharmacy in nursing home residents in the United States: results of the 2004 National Nursing Home Survey," *American Journal Geriatric Pharmacotherapy*, vol. 8, no. 1, pp. 63–72, 2010.

[21] W. Rosamond, K. Flegal, K. Furie et al., "Heart disease and stroke statistics—2008 update: a report from the american heart association statistics committee and stroke statistics subcommittee," *Circulation*, vol. 117, no. 4, pp. e25-e146, 2008.

[22] J. Wang, I. H. Zuckerman, N. A. Miller, F. T. Shaya, J. M. Noel, and C. D. Mullins, "Utilizing new prescription drugs: disparities among non-Hispanic whites, non-Hispanic blacks, and Hispanic whites," *Health Services Research*, vol. 42, no. 4, pp. 1499–1519, 2007.

[23] D. P. Schauer, J. A. Johnston, C. J. Moomaw, M. Wess, and M. H. Eckman, "Racial disparities in the filling of warfarin prescriptions for nonvalvular atrial fibrillation," *American Journal of the Medical Sciences*, vol. 333, no. 2, pp. 67–73, 2007.

[24] T. L. Mark, K. J. Axelsen, L. Mucha, and Y. Sadkova, "Racial differences in switching, augmentation, and titration of lipid-lowering agents by Medicare/Medicaid dual-eligible patients," *American Journal of Managed Care*, vol. 13, no. 3, 2007.

[25] J. Wang, J. M. Noel, I. H. Zuckerman, N. A. Miller, F. T. Shaya, and C. D. Mullins, "Disparities in access to essential new prescription drugs between non-Hispanic whites, non-Hispanic blacks, and Hispanic whites," *Medical Care Research & Review*, vol. 63, no. 6, pp. 742–763, 2006.

[26] J. F. Farley, R. R. Cline, and K. Gupta, "Racial variations in antiresorptive medication use: results from the 2000 Medical Expenditure Panel Survey (MEPS)," *Osteoporosis International*, vol. 17, no. 3, pp. 395–404, 2006.

[27] A. J. Claxton, J. Cramer, and C. Pierce, "A systematic review of the associations between dose regimens and medication compliance," *Clinical Therapeutics*, vol. 23, no. 8, pp. 1296–1310, 2001.

[28] G. G. Fillenbaum, R. D. Horner, J. T. Hanlon, L. R. Landerman, D. V. Dawson, and H. J. Cohen, "Factors predicting change in prescription and nonprescription drug use in a community-residing black and white elderly population," *Journal of Clinical Epidemiology*, vol. 49, no. 5, pp. 587–593, 1996.

[29] M. Hussein, T. M. Waters, C. F. Chang, J. E. Bailey, L. M. Brown, and D. K. Solomon, "Impact of medicare part D on racial disparities in adherence to cardiovascular medications among the elderly," *Medical Care Research and Review*, vol. 73, no. 4, pp. 410–436, 2016.

[30] C. A. Okoro, T. W. Strine, S. L. Young, L. S. Balluz, and A. H. Mokdad, "Access to health care among older adults and receipt of preventive services. Results from the Behavioral Risk Factor Surveillance System, 2002," *Preventive Medicine*, vol. 40, no. 3, pp. 337–343, 2005.

[31] J. D. Reschovsky and L. E. Felland, "Access to prescription drugs for Medicare beneficiaries," *Tracking Report*, no. 23, pp. 1–4, 2009.

[32] W. Cashion, W. McClellan, G. Howard et al., "Geographic region and racial variations in polypharmacy in the United States," *Annals of Epidemiology*, vol. 25, no. 6, pp. 433–438, 2015.

[33] S. S. Mortazavi, M. Shati, A. Keshtkar, S. K. Malakouti, M. Bazargan, and S. Assari, "Defining polypharmacy in the elderly: a systematic review protocol," *BMJ Open*, vol. 6, no. 3, Article ID e010989, 2016.

[34] H. Yazdanshenas, M. Bazargan, J. Smith, D. Martins, H. Motahari, and G. Orum, "Pain treatment of underserved older african americans," *Journal of the American Geriatrics Society*, vol. 64, no. 10, pp. 2116–2121, 2016.

[35] Department of Finance, "Population Projections (Baseline 2016)," 2017, http://www.dof.ca.gov/Forecasting/Demographics/Projectionsdocuments/P_PressRelease.pdf.

[36] County of Los Angels, "SPA 6 South Area—LA County Department of Public Health," http://publichealth.lacounty.gov/chs/spa6/index.htm.

[37] American Geriatrics Society, "American Geriatrics Society updated Beers Criteria for potentially inappropriate medication use in older adults," *Journal of the American Geriatrics Society*, vol. 60, no. 4, pp. 616–631, 2012.

[38] R. Melzack, "The short-form McGill pain questionnaire," *Pain*, vol. 30, no. 2, pp. 191–197, 1987.

[39] R. H. Dworkin, D. C. Turk, D. A. Revicki et al., "Development and initial validation of an expanded and revised version of the short-form mcgill pain questionnaire (SF-MPQ-2)," *Pain*, vol. 144, no. 1-2, pp. 35–42, 2009.

[40] World Health Organization, 2015, http://www.who.int/cancer/palliative/painladder/en/.

[41] Los Angeles County Department of Public Health and Office of Health Assessment and Epidemiology, "Key Indicators of Health by service Planning Area," March 2013.

[42] T. Johansson, M. E. Abuzahra, S. Keller et al., "Impact of strategies to reduce polypharmacy on clinically relevant endpoints: a systematic review and meta-analysis," *British Journal of Clinical Pharmacology*, pp. 532–548, 2016.

[43] E. Tommelein, E. Mehuys, I. Van Tongelen et al., "Community pharmacists' evaluation of potentially inappropriate prescribing in older community-dwelling patients with polypharmacy: observational research based on the GheOP(3)S tool," *Journal of Public Health*, 2016.

[44] K. Hudhra, M. García-Caballos, E. Casado-Fernandez, B. Jucja, D. Shabani, and A. Bueno-Cavanillas, "Polypharmacy and potentially inappropriate prescriptions identified by Beers and STOPP criteria in co-morbid older patients at hospital discharge," *Journal of Evaluation in Clinical Practice*, vol. 22, no. 2, pp. 189–193, 2016.

[45] B. Clyne, J. A. Cooper, C. M. Hughes, T. Fahey, and S. M. Smith, "'Potentially inappropriate or specifically appropriate?' Qualitative evaluation of general practitioners views on prescribing, polypharmacy and potentially inappropriate prescribing in older people," *BMC Family Practice*, vol. 17, no. 1, p. 109, 2016.

[46] G. Nightingale, E. Hajjar, K. Swartz, J. Andrel-Sendecki, and A. Chapman, "Evaluation of a pharmacist-led medication assessment used to identify prevalence of and associations with polypharmacy and potentially inappropriate medication use among ambulatory senior adults with cancer," *Journal of Clinical Oncology*, vol. 33, no. 13, pp. 1453–1459, 2015.

[47] A. J. Davidoff, G. E. Miller, E. M. Sarpong, E. Yang, N. Brandt, and D. M. Fick, "Prevalence of potentially inappropriate medication use in older adults using the 2012 beers criteria," *Journal of the American Geriatrics Society*, vol. 63, no. 3, pp. 486–500, 2015.

[48] Z. A. Marcum, J. Driessen, C. T. Thorpe, W. F. Gellad, and J. M. Donohue, "Effect of multiple pharmacy use on medication adherence and drug-drug interactions in older adults with medicare part D," *Journal of the American Geriatrics Society*, vol. 62, no. 2, pp. 244–252, 2014.

[49] A. B. Jena, D. Goldman, L. Weaver, and P. Karaca-Mandic, "Opioid prescribing by multiple providers in Medicare: retrospective observational study of insurance claims," *British Medical Journal*, vol. 348, 2014, Article ID: g1393.

[50] R. Lancaster, K. D. Marek, L. D. Bub, and F. Stetzer, "Medication regimens of frail older adults after discharge from home healthcare," *Home Healthcare Nurse*, vol. 32, no. 9, pp. 536–542, 2014.

[51] B. Hovstadius, G. Petersson, L. Hellström, and L. Ericson, "Trends in inappropriate drug therapy prescription in the elderly in Sweden from 2006 to 2013: assessment using national indicators," *Drugs and Aging*, vol. 31, no. 5, pp. 379–386, 2014.

21

Participant Perspectives of Cognitive Rehabilitation for Type 2 Diabetes: Expectations and Impact

Heather E. Cuevas, Alexa K. Stuifbergen, and Catherine Ward

School of Nursing, The University of Texas at Austin, 1710 Red River, Austin, TX 78701, USA

Correspondence should be addressed to Heather E. Cuevas; hcuevas@mail.nur.utexas.edu

Academic Editor: Barbara Shukitt-Hale

Purpose. To describe the experiences of people with type 2 diabetes who have completed a comprehensive cognitive rehabilitation intervention. *Method.* Nineteen participants with type 2 diabetes enrolled in an 8-week intervention consisting of 4 educational classes to learn strategies to improve cognitive function and an online training program at home to practice cognitively stimulating activities. Two focus groups were conducted as part of a study designed to assess the feasibility of the comprehensive cognitive rehabilitation intervention. *Results.* Three main themes were identified in the qualitative data: (1) expectations of cognitive change; (2) use of cognitive strategies; and (3) effect on diabetes self-management. Participants shared valuable insight into how their experiences with the intervention changed and how they viewed diabetes. *Conclusions.* While the participants did not initially tie their cognitive complaints to diabetes, they were able to show how and why they might use cognitive strategies to improve diabetes self-management activities. By adapting those strategies for diabetes, quality of life can improve as well as potentially glycemic control.

1. Introduction

Older adults with type 2 diabetes (T2DM) are at higher risk for dementia than those without T2DM, and once cognitive problems have been diagnosed, there is a potential for faster progression of cognitive decline [1]. Additionally, cognitive decline may begin early in T2DM's development since a diagnosis of T2DM at midlife is associated with about a 20% greater deterioration in cognitive function over 20 years than for those without T2DM [2]. Attention has been paid to changes in cognitive function in the context of diabetes, but few studies have examined how cognitive function affects diabetes self-management [3, 4]. This is unfortunate because if the ability to complete self-management activities such as dietary management, physical activity, and glucose self-monitoring is altered, then interventions to educate patients may not be successful.

Prior examinations have addressed self-management activities, but focused on only one aspect of diabetes self-management and/or one cognitive domain and have had limited inclusion of underrepresented minority populations [5, 6]. Preliminary investigations have demonstrated connections between lower levels of perceived cognitive function (memory and executive function) and diabetes self-management adherence, but testing of cognitive rehabilitation interventions in diabetes is a novel and understudied focus.

The National Academy of Neuropsychology (NAN) has stated that aspects of effective cognitive rehabilitation include teaching both compensatory skills and brain retraining [7]. Practice and repetition (online computer training) can strengthen skills (e.g., memory, attention, and executive function), and these improvements can be translated into more complex functional behaviors through integration with compensatory strategies that are taught in person [8]. Comprehensive cognitive rehabilitation interventions in other chronic conditions have been shown to be effective in improving function in daily life, but this has not been demonstrated in diabetes [9–12].

Due to this gap, a comprehensive cognitive rehabilitation intervention was developed, and 19 people with T2DM were invited to participate. This project was built on prior work examining the relationships of perceived memory, cognitive ability, and T2DM self-management [13]. One of the aims of the study was to determine the acceptability of this type of intervention in this population. Cognitive training can give individuals a greater sense of control over cognitive changes as well as have a beneficial effect on quality of life [14]. Therefore, central to understanding if these types of investigations will be effective is to explore the experiences of participants who have taken part in comprehensive cognitive rehabilitation interventions.

The purpose of this paper was to describe and focus specifically on the perceptions of people with T2DM in a cognitive rehabilitation intervention in order to refine it for testing in a randomized controlled trial with a larger sample. Qualitative studies have examined participant perceptions of comprehensive cognitive rehabilitation interventions in other chronic conditions. Haesner et al. [15] found that 60 older adults, both with and without mild cognitive impairment, who took part in an computer-based cognitive rehabilitation intervention expressed interest in regular, long-term use of the cognitive training platform that included both social ("chat") and mental ("brain training" exercises) features and emphasized that the content of the exercises should have a connection to their daily activities.

In a metasynthesis of qualitative research on perceptions of people participating in group-based cognitive rehabilitation, das Nair et al. [16] found that cognitive rehabilitation was associated with increased confidence, self-awareness, and learning of new skills and strategies to compensate for deficits. Additionally, they found that those changes had a positive impact on daily life in personal and professional spheres [16]. das Nair and Lincoln [17] also found that participation in a cognitive rehabilitation intervention improved insight and awareness of memory problems, knowledge, and use of memory aids as well as improved mood and assertiveness. Participants also reported an altered perspective of life that helped them deal with their problems [17]. These themes have been echoed in other analyses of cognitive rehabilitation programs [18–20]. However, qualitative examinations of cognitive rehabilitation interventions for those with type 2 diabetes have not been done. Further research is needed in light of the effect the interventions have on confidence and acquisition of new skills—concepts that are strongly linked to self-management of type 2 diabetes [21].

2. Methodology

2.1. Design. This qualitative descriptive study was part of a project (Clinical Trials Registration NCT03221452) to adapt a comprehensive cognitive rehabilitation intervention originally designed for multiple sclerosis for people with T2DM. The primary aim of the main study was to adapt and test the feasibility of the intervention in a population (people with T2DM) for which it was not originally designed.

The intervention consisted of 4 2-hour educational sessions held every other week to teach compensatory cognitive strategies. Participants were also asked to complete 45 minutes of an online brain-training program three times a week at home. All class sessions emphasized maximizing cognitive function first and then addressed the interrelated effects of improved cognition on self-management skills and improved glycemic control on cognition. Each class session followed the same basic format: (a) introduction/revisiting content from the prior class and answering questions; (b) review of progress on computer exercises prescribed in the previous class; (c) practice of cognitive strategies in the class; (d) content on weekly topic; and (e) closure—prescribed computer training and cognitive strategy assignments for the upcoming week. Discussion on how to use this information in day-to-day self-management activities was also included. Participants received notebooks with class content to support what was taught in each session. Table 1 includes a description of each of the classes.

For both the feasibility study and the qualitative substudy, university ethics approval was obtained, and all study participants provided written informed consent.

2.2. Participants. Participants were 40 to 70 years old with T2DM living in Central Texas. Demographics are described in Table 2. All participants from the main study were invited to participate in the qualitative substudy.

2.3. Data Collection. A trained facilitator, who was not involved in the intervention delivery, completed 2 focus groups of approximately 45 minutes each with 11 participants in one group and 8 participants in the other. The focus groups took place after the last class session of the intervention. Focus group participants were asked about their experiences in the program and cognitive strategies they found most useful as well as motivation and self-efficacy related to use of the cognitive strategies (Table 3). The focus group facilitator took extensive notes and audio-recorded the sessions. The audio recordings were transcribed verbatim. All data were deidentified, and numbers were used to differentiate participant responses (e.g., Participant 1 said...).

2.4. Data Analysis. Since this study used a qualitative descriptive design, Miles, Huberman, and Saldana's recommendations for content analysis were employed to review and code the transcripts [22]. In a qualitative descriptive inquiry, little inference is applied to explain information in everyday language so the codes and themes are derived from the data rather than from a theoretical framework [23]. Additionally, conventional content analysis is used to describe a phenomenon when existing research is limited [24]. This approach allows categories to emerge from the data and to use terms that reflect the participants' frameworks and are meaningful to them.

First, the data were read repeatedly to obtain a sense of the whole; next, the data were read word-for-word, highlighting the text that appeared to capture key thoughts and concepts; codes were then derived from the key concepts; and the codes were categorized according to their relationships and linked and grouped into meaningful clusters [22]. A second member of the research team separately coded the transcripts using the themes from the initial

Table 1: Class content.

	Class content
Week 1	(i) Understanding T2DM, symptoms, complications, and medications. (ii) Understanding how cognitive function is related to T2DM. (iii) Orientation to computer training. (iv) Discussing effective strategies to facilitate better communication with health-care providers, for example, understanding instructions or recommendations from health-care providers. (v) Strategies to enhance attention and problem solving.
Week 3	(i) Strategies to enhance memory. (ii) Addressing resources and barriers to self-management (e.g., planning ahead for meals and organizing medications) that take into account elements of executive functioning. (iii) Visuospatial skills required for blood glucose self-monitoring.
Week 5	(i) Addressing ADA dietary recommendations and how they can benefit cognitive health. (ii) Discussion of favorite recipes, more healthy food preparation, eating out, and emphasis on portion control. (iii) Acknowledging and appreciating stress associated with diabetes and cognitive issues. (iv) Providing resources for mental health-care services. (v) Strategies to manage stress.
Week 8	(i) Addressing ADA activity recommendations and benefits of following the guidelines on cognitive function. (ii) Discussion of practical ways to increase activity. (iii) Review of cognitive skills/training and the potential impact on self-management skills including blood glucose monitoring, medication adherence, diet, and exercise. (iv) Addressing resources and barriers to maintaining cognitive function.

Table 2: Participant characteristics.

Characteristic	*n*	Range	%	M (SD)
Age in years	19	40–70	—	55.1 (10.9)
Hemoglobin A1C	19	5.4–12	—	8.3 (1.8)
Length of time with T2DM in years	19	2–21	—	7.1 (4.8)
Hispanic	10	—	52.6	—
Non-Hispanic White	6	—	31.6	—
African American	3	—	15.8	—
Female	11	—	57.9	—

T2DM, type 2 diabetes; M, mean; SD, standard deviation.

coding. Agreement between the two coders was 90%. In the case of disagreements, the items were discussed, and the section of the text was either placed in a different coding category or a new code was created from similar themes. During coding, notes were made on the procedures, analysis, and reflections on the emerging themes.

3. Results

Three main themes were found to describe participants' experiences: (1) expectations of cognitive change; (2) use of cognitive strategies; and (3) effect on diabetes self-management (Table 4). The themes span the participants' experiences with cognitive issues and diabetes self-management from prior to the intervention, during the intervention, and after the intervention was completed.

3.1. Expectations of Cognitive Change. Participants were asked to describe how they felt the class sessions and computer training met their expectations as well as their thoughts on what could be changed to make the intervention better. None of the participants expected to have "major improvements in brain function." Instead, most felt they would be able to learn strategies and put them into practice and improvement would take time that extended beyond taking part in the intervention. Even though most participants did not complete the full time requested for the computer training (averaged 106 minutes out of a requested 135 minutes per week), they had a strong interest in the classes and recommended a continued focus on teaching cognitive strategies "to make life easier." Several participants said they did not know what to expect from the classes because they had problems obtaining information about cognitive function and diabetes from other sources; for example, "I feel like I was not sure what kinds of questions to ask in the class. No one has ever talked to me before about how diabetes could change how well I think."

The source and type of information that came from the intervention played a role in what they expected would help their cognition. All said they appreciated clarification on popular "brain games" and information on currently available evidence regarding what the games did and did not do. Some stated this was contrary to the information presented by the press and advertising. One participant commented, "It's hard to know what I need to do when the information and advertising is misleading. And I get that there's still more research that's needed. There's so much out that trying to sell me things. It helped to have someone in health care clear it up for us." Participants also appreciated explanations of the causes of cognitive problems. Some felt changes in cognitive function were a "slippery slope" to Alzheimer's disease and that nothing could be done to prevent that progress. Because of this, they believed there was no need to make their health-care providers aware of cognitive issues. However, due to the information provided in the intervention, they realized there might be ways to maximize their cognitive function. They now had questions for their health-care providers such as checking for vitamin B12 deficiency related to metformin use or tests that would be useful in investigating other causes of cognitive problems.

All expected to "learn cognitive strategies from each other and share ideas" and preferred a group format. They were split on if the classes should be online (via a program like Skype) or in person in a clinic setting. Regardless of the method, the sharing of strategies to assist cognitive function was a prominent concept brought to light by almost all of the participants. For example, one woman stated, "I wasn't sure what would work and what wouldn't. I didn't anticipate that most people had tried different things, and I want to continue talking about this with others."

TABLE 3: Focus group guide.

Cognitive strategies used	Intervention content	Effect of the intervention
What strategies did you try?	What was the most useful thing you learned?	Why did you choose to take part in this project?
Why did you choose those particular strategies?	What could be changed about the classes to make them better?	Have you talked with your health care provider about cognitive issues? How will you approach the topic of cognitive function with your health care provider in the future?
What was difficult?	How did the online sessions go?	What did you know about cognitive rehabilitation before the intervention? Have your ideas about it changed? If so, how?
What worked well?	How will you use the information you learned in the future?	How do you think participating in this project will affect the way you manage diabetes?

TABLE 4: Exemplar quotes.

Themes	Quotes
Expectations of cognitive change	"I wanted my brain to change in a better way. And I think this may be one way to do it. It takes a lot of work, but I think with exercise, diet, paying attention to my sugar and practicing strategies, I can at least help my brain not get worse." "I'm glad to do something like this. I see ads on TV all the time for vitamins for my brain, but I don't know what works. This helps a lot and makes me think better. I like sharing with other people what I work and then I can go to my doctor too and talk about what I've been doing."
Use of cognitive strategies	"I had no idea I could do things to help my brain. Not all the cognitive strategies are things I've been able to do, but I feel like I'm making small changes and they are super useful." "I think the computer training was fun, but I like working on the cognitive strategies better. I spent more time on making lists and stopping to think things through than on video games."
Effect on diabetes self-management	"I'm more motivated to work on my diabetes now. I feel like I can do things that will help both my brain and my diabetes at the same time." "I realized that setting small goals will help diabetes and thinking about how adding may be 15 minutes of exercise here and there does a lot—it makes me feel better, it helps my sugar, and it can help me think better."

3.2. Use of Cognitive Strategies. Most of the participants talked about the difficulties of living with diabetes and perceived cognitive problems. Some were aware of cognitive strategies before the intervention but had not tried them because they felt like "this was just a normal part of getting old." Others had no prior knowledge of cognitive strategies. All participants tried at least 3 strategies during the 8-week period. Some used a combination of strategies for single tasks. For example, one participant described strategies she used in preparing meals for her family, "It takes a lot. If I think of everything I have to do all at once, I know I forget things. So I now I make a list of groceries and then I quit checking my phone while I'm at [grocery store]." This demonstrated use of planning ahead, list making, and limiting multitasking—all strategies that were discussed in the session on boosting attention. Others were concerned with slow speed of processing and mentioned they would "stay quiet because people will think I'm stupid if I can't come up with an answer quickly." One person said he started asking people to let him read an item in question (he was a customer service representative). This gave him more time to process the information as well as let him review the concepts discussed.

Challenges of using cognitive strategies were also elucidated, and barriers of initiating planned activities such as an exercise program were prominent findings. For example, "I have every intention to exercise. I make time in my schedule, but something always comes up." Goal setting assisted with those problems, but a few felt it was not enough: "I need more than just writing down one goal. Sometimes I never look at it again."

Difficulties in changing habits were noted. Lack of time, lack of "discipline," and other priorities were barriers to use the online computer training. Another said that "one more thing is being asked of me and I do not know if I can do any more." Motivation to use the strategies included encouragement from health-care providers. For example, "When I see my physician, she tells me to keep trying to be healthy and to keep us the good work." Or "I realized that if I don't want to get worse diabetes then I have to take control of my sugars. But I can't always remember what I need to do next. These classes helped me figure out ways to think about what I'm doing and then make a list or set my phone alarm. It's motivation to be think in better ways so my diabetes can be better. . .and my diabetes nurse can help me."

Most had a sense of achievement even with small changes such as making lists. They felt the intervention helped increase their "mental abilities" and flexibility with cognitive strategy plans. Others said some of the at-home assignments were too easy and recommended having them increase in difficulty as they progressed through the program. Some wanted more guidance and practice with "real-life" situations that could occur in self-management and suggested text messaging as a way to communicate with the intervention facilitator.

3.3. Impact on Diabetes Self-Management. The groups consistently stressed the effect of cognitive problems had on diabetes self-management. Many said, "I forget too easily" or "I have problems planning, I can't think that far ahead." Most were appreciative of the information related to cognitive changes in diabetes and said the information lessened their concerns fear of Alzheimer's disease.

The cognitive strategies were also felt to be useful in assisting with diabetes self-management, and while some felt the intervention did not have a direct effect on their actual glucose readings, it gave them a greater sense of control and self-efficacy. However, two participants shared their glucose records with the focus group. They believed the cognitive strategies they employed such as list making, avoiding multitasking, and setting specific goals helped with diabetes self-management and improved their glycemic control. One said the meditation practice taught in a session helped to "decrease my anxiety and let me think more clearly about what I needed to do that day. I think anxiety was a big piece of what was keeping me from working on my diabetes and I didn't realize it before." This sentiment was echoed by 3 others in the group, and they recommended more emphasis on practices such as meditation and deep breathing to help improve focus and decrease the anxiety they associated with diabetes management.

Many described how the intervention helped them look at diabetes self-management through a different lens and think more broadly about the ways good self-management could improve glucose, cholesterol, blood pressure, and cognitive function. Some described the intervention as having short-term and long-term outcomes. Short-term outcomes were related to specific tasks such as the online games and weekly practice of cognitive strategies. The long-term aims were related to more general changes, for example, improving A1C values and "keeping my brain healthy for a longer time." One participant said it this way: "The shorter goals were things that I knew I needed to do, but I had to keep in mind that they were for a bigger purpose. I need to keep doing these things and make them habits so I can be healthier." Another said: "This isn't the solution to all my diabetes and thinking problems. But it's a good foundation course that I think underlies a lot of other approaches to getting me to work more on thinking better and keeping my glucose controlled."

4. Discussion

4.1. Summary. Diabetes is a serious chronic illness that has implications for multiple facets of a person's health, including cognitive function. The theme of "impact on diabetes" emphasizes participants' experiences with self-management in light of any perceived cognitive problems. Participants often described not meeting the self-management standards that were set for them (by themselves or by their health-care provider) and felt that anything they could do to improve cognitive function would also help with diabetes self-management. The relationship of perceived cognitive function and diabetes self-management has been seen in the recent literature [13, 25] and suggests perceived executive function and memory capabilities are significantly associated with diabetes self-management adherence. Other studies have also found that self-management and glycemic outcomes are even worse when screening for cognitive dysfunction is delayed despite complaints of cognitive problems [26]. This indicates a positive relationship and involvement with health-care professionals are essential [27]. However, like this group of participants, many people attribute the changes in cognitive function to "old age" or to "natural processes" and are misinformed about activities that can support cognitive health—both within and outside of the context of diabetes—such as diet, exercise, and blood pressure control. Based on this study's findings, Table 5 lists recommended features for cognitive rehabilitation interventions, which are discussed in more detail below.

4.2. Expectations of Cognitive Change. Participants in comprehensive cognitive rehabilitation interventions have shown improvement on neuropsychological tests and have reported the interventions' cognitive strategies that improved their ability to function in daily life [12, 28–30]. Therefore, testing interventions of this type shows promise for people with diabetes. As results of this study demonstrate, many people with T2DM are unaware of not only the interventions that may benefit cognitive function, but also lack information on the effect diabetes can have on cognitive function.

This issue highlights a need for increased education and counseling on diabetes self-management, the risk of cognitive dysfunction, and the expected benefits of cognitive rehabilitation. The use of tested interventions is important due to the marketing efforts of certain "brain games" which consumers may interpret as cures for cognitive problems or that games will definitively prevent diseases such as Alzheimer's. Using an educational approach that incorporates goal setting along with practice of realistic, practical activities allows people to manage their expectations and empower them to increase adherence to their diabetes self-management plan. Furthermore, heightened understanding of the persons' experiences with these interventions may further increase the capacity of health-care providers to address questions patients do not know to ask and improve the probability that they receive accurate, evidence-based recommendations.

In this study, one person stopped participating after one class. He felt that the class was not going to give him the type of progress he wanted (he wanted something that would "work faster"). This is in line with behavior change theory that finds interventions are discontinued when expectations do not match results [31]. In cases such as this, it may be helpful to emphasize the aspects of the intervention that improve both global cognition and glycemic control, such as physical exercise. Stressing the potentially additive benefits of a multimodal approach may improve retention as well as outcomes [32].

4.3. Use of Cognitive Strategies. Consistent with previous research [9, 28, 29], the most common barriers for using the strategies learned in the intervention were time and low

Table 5: Recommended cognitive rehabilitation intervention features.

Themes	Intervention features
Expectations of cognitive change	(i) Include education on diabetes self-management, cognitive dysfunction, and expected/realistic benefits of cognitive rehabilitation. (ii) Use a group format to increase sharing of information related to strategies that may or may not work. (iii) Teach participants to ask questions of their health-care providers regarding cognitive function and diabetes.
Use of cognitive strategies	(i) Relate cognitive strategies to everyday activities and/or diabetes self-management tasks. (ii) Consider one-on-one training or more frequent contact with a health-care provider familiar with cognitive rehabilitation to facilitate use of online games. (iii) Incorporate motivational interviewing techniques to increase adherence and decrease anxiety.
Effect on diabetes self-management	(i) Include feedback from a class facilitator to enhance motivation to complete homework items. (ii) Include participants in goal setting using real-world situations as examples. (iii) Emphasize the potential benefits of cognitive rehabilitation on both diabetes and cognitive function. (iv) Explore alternatives such as providing class instruction via an online meeting format to reduce travel/time burden.

motivation. A meta-analysis of adherence in cognitive rehabilitation studies showed adherence to the interventions ranged from 62% to 67% [33], but in this study, most participants did not fulfill the full time requested for the online computer training. Some felt the exercises were not making a difference and wanted to focus on the "useful hands-on strategies" instead. Indeed, most of the participants felt their time was better spent practicing the cognitive strategies taught in the class. Participants also said that life events (work and family demands) sometimes caused them to miss practicing the weeks' activities. But most indicated that they tried to make up the time or practice the strategies at a later time. Some participants were initially frustrated with the online portion of the intervention due to difficulty or confusion with the instructions, which lowered motivation levels. They felt the time on the online training reported by the program was inaccurate and did not account for the time spent reading directions and trying to understand how to play the games.

In the future, it may be beneficial to have one-on-one training with a facilitator to help them overcome those initial problems. It is also possible that contact with a health-care provider who has "prescribed" cognitive rehabilitation may decrease anxiety and motivate patients to meet the recommended practice times [34–36]. Motivational interviewing strategies have been effective in increasing adherence to cognitive rehabilitation interventions in other chronic conditions [37–39] and could be useful in diabetes. By integrating motivational interviewing principles into the intervention, intervention facilitators can investigate and address any ambivalence or emotional factors participants may have and possibly increase adherence.

4.4. Impact on Diabetes Self-Management. Baseline adherence to diabetes self-management activities was low, and the focus group results show that knowledge was a barrier to diabetes self-management changes. This again highlights the need for public health information regarding diabetes and cognitive health. The risks are there, but it is something that may or may not be discussed with health-care providers. Incorrect information can have an impact of whether or not to make lifestyle changes. Health-care professionals are often the contact point for clarifying health information and are an essential source for those concerned about cognitive problems in the context of diabetes self-management.

Participants frequently mentioned goal setting as one helpful strategy, but they wanted guidance from health-care professionals in setting and monitoring goals. This has implications for adherence since goal setting has been shown to be a part of effective diabetes self-management and cognitive rehabilitation [40, 41]. The selection of goals by participants can create more meaning, maximize outcomes, and increase adherence. For example, Rodakowski et al. [42] found that older adults with mild cognitive impairment in a cognitive rehabilitation program valued self-selection of exercise goals. Additionally, Lie et al. [43] and D. B. Reuben and M. E. Tinetti [44] found that combining a goal-directed diabetes eHealth intervention with face-to-face consultations had potential to increase motivation and adherence. The results here indicate goal setting using "real-world" situations was critical and added to diabetes self-management adherence.

Participants feared developing dementia and worsening of any perceived cognitive problems. These findings are consistent with Kim et al. [45] who found in their investigation of glucose variability and cognitive function that a majority of their participants had the same worries. In this project, feedback from the class facilitator and other participants was clearly a motivator for trying new cognitive strategies and completing the brain-training homework. But while feedback indicated that the social component of the intervention was valuable to discuss common self-management concerns, the intervention required time and sometimes time off from work. The authors believe this was the main problem with recruitment and retention. It was challenging to recruit participants, and it took 8 weeks to enroll the first participant. At that point, modifications were made to the class schedule to change it from weekly classes over 8 weeks to 4 classes every other week for 8 weeks.

Alternatives to the intervention format suggested by the focus groups included online/virtually based classes or phone conferencing to reduce the time and travel burden.

Studies have demonstrated that diabetes self-management education can be effectively delivered via technology such as online conferencing and can be effective in improving both physiologic and behavioral outcomes [46]. Patients who have gone through such programs have reported more satisfaction with access to the provider as well as decreasing the time and travel burden associated with attending classes [47]. However, the research on cognitive rehabilitation using distance learning format is sparse in the context of chronic illnesses. A meta-analysis in 2014 showed distance learning alone did not produce improvement. Improvements were only seen in those people who were supervised by a trainer in 1 to 3 sessions per week [48]. The authors of the meta-analysis also noted that the findings were only specific to healthy older adults and may not apply to those who already have chronic illness, and future research should explore these methods [48]. In this project, the social contact supported self-management behavior change and discussion with other participants that provided aspects of role modeling that should be included in future iterations of the intervention.

4.4.1. Limitations. One of the aims of this study was to test the acceptability of a comprehensive cognitive rehabilitation intervention for people with T2DM. While a good description of the perceptions of the intervention was obtained from the participants, there are several limitations. The first is that the results are limited by convenience sampling. It is possible that purposive sampling would give a broader range of views than what was found in this project. Also participation may reflect motivation for behavioral change that may not be present in the general population with perceived cognitive problems and/or diabetes. However, this is the first study, to our knowledge, examining a comprehensive cognitive rehabilitation intervention to deal with both conditions.

4.4.2. Clinical Implications. While participants in this project did not originally tie their cognitive concerns to diabetes, they showed how and why they used cognitive strategies to enhance diabetes self-management activities by the end of the intervention. Currently, there are no standardized treatment recommendations for cognitive function in the context of diabetes, but the results here demonstrate that comprehensive cognitive rehabilitation interventions may be promising. In adapting the strategies for diabetes, there is a potential for improved quality of life. Future research needs to identify barriers to cognitive activities and strategy use, such as the time and emotional factors found here, which may be important to assist in self-management and therefore glycemic control.

Conflicts of Interest

The authors report no conflicts of interest.

Acknowledgments

This work was supported by the Center for Transdisciplinary Collaborative Research in Self-Management Science at the University of Texas at Austin (TCRSS; P30, NR015335: PI Kim). The authors would also like to thank the participants for their time and willingness to share their perspectives on diabetes and cognitive function.

References

[1] G. J. Biessels, M. W. J. Strachan, F. L. J. Visseren, L. J. Kappelee, and R. A. Whitmer, "Dementia and cognitive decline in type 2 diabetes and prediabetic stages: towards targeted interventions," *The Lancet Diabetes and Endocrinology*, vol. 2, no. 3, pp. 246–255, 2014.

[2] E. R. Mayeda, M. N. Haan, K. Yaffe, A. K. Kanaya, and J. Neuhaus, "Does type 2 diabetes increase rate of cognitive decline in older Mexican Americans?," *Alzheimer Disease and Associated Disorders*, vol. 29, no. 1, pp. 206–212, 2015.

[3] P. K. Gatlin and K. C. Insel, "Severity of type 2 diabetes, cognitive function, and self-care," *Biological Research For Nursing*, vol. 17, no. 5, pp. 540–548, 2014.

[4] S. Primozic, R. Tavcar, M. Avbelj, M. Z. Dernovsek, and M. M. Oblak, "Specific cognitive abilities are associated with diabetes self-management behavior among patients with type 2 diabetes," *Diabetes Research and Clinical Practice*, vol. 95, no. 1, pp. 48–54, 2012.

[5] C. J. Camp, K. Fox, M. J. Skrainer, V. Antenucci, and J. Haberman, "Creating effective self-management for older adults with type 2 diabetes and cognitive impairment," *Advances in Aging Research*, vol. 4, no. 2, pp. 33–41, 2015.

[6] V. Whitelock, A. Nouwen, K. Houben et al., "Does neurocognitive training have the potential to improve dietary self-care in type 2 diabetes? Study protocol of a double-blind randomized controlled trial," *BMC Nutrition*, vol. 1, no. 11, 2017.

[7] National Academy of Neuropsychology, *Cognitive Rehabilitation: Official Statement of the National Academy of Neuropsychology*, 2002, https://www.nanonline.org/docs/PAIC/PDFs/NANPositionCogRehab.pdf.

[8] P. D. Bamidis, A. B. Vivas, C. Styliadis et al., "A review of physical and cognitive interventions in aging," *Neuroscience & Biobehavioral Reviews*, vol. 44, pp. 206–220, 2014.

[9] D. Von Ah, J. S. Carpenter, A. Saykin et al., "Advanced cognitive training for breast cancer survivors: a randomized controlled trial," *Breast Cancer Research and Treatment*, vol. 135, no. 3, pp. 799–809, 2012.

[10] S. J. Pressler, B. Therrien, P. L. Riley et al., "Nurse-enhanced memory intervention in heart failure: the MEMOIR study," *Journal of Cardiac Failure*, vol. 17, pp. 832–843, 2011.

[11] D. E. Bredesen, "Reversal of cognitive decline: a novel therapeutic program," *Aging*, vol. 6, no. 9, pp. 707–717, 2014.

[12] G. W. Rebok, K. Ball, L. T. Guey et al., "Ten-year effect of the advanced cognitive training for independent and vital elderly cognitive training trial on cognition and everyday functioning in older adults," *Journal of the American Geriatrics Society*, vol. 62, no. 1, pp. 16–24, 2014.

[13] H. Cuevas and A. Stuifbergen, "Perceived cognitive deficits are associated with diabetes self-management in a multiethnic sample," *Journal of Diabetes and Metabolic Disorders*, vol. 16, no. 1, p. 7, 2017.

[14] R. F. Buckley, M. M. Saling, I. Frommann, S. Wolfsgruber, and M. Wagner, "Subjective cognitive decline from a phenomenological perspective: a review of the qualitative literature," *Journal of Alzheimer's Disease*, vol. 48, no. s1, pp. S125–S140, 2015.

[15] M. Haesner, J. L. O'Sullivan, M. Govercin, and E. Steinhagen-Thiessen, "Requirements of older adults for a daily use of an internet-based cognitive training platform," *Informatics for Health and Social Care*, vol. 40, no. 2, pp. 138–153, 2015.

[16] R. das Nair, K. J. Martin, and E. J. Sinclair, "A meta-synthesis of qualitative research on perceptions of people with long-term neurological conditions about group-based memory rehabilitation," *Neuropsychological Rehabilitation*, vol. 25, no. 4, pp. 479–502, 2015.

[17] R. das Nair and N. B. Lincoln, "The effectiveness of memory rehabilitation following neurological disabilities: a qualitative inquiry of patient perspectives," *Neuropsychological Rehabilitation*, vol. 23, no. 4, pp. 528–545, 2013.

[18] S. E. McEwen, H. J. Polatajko, J. A. Davis, M. Huijbregts, and J. D. Ryan, ""There's a real plan here, and I am responsible for that plan": participant experiences with novel cognitive-based treatment approach for adults living with chronic stroke," *Diability and Rehabilitation*, vol. 32, no. 7, pp. 541–550, 2010.

[19] A. Mantynen, E. Rosti-Otajarvi, K. Koivisto, A. Lilja, H. Huhtala, and P. Hamalainen, "Neuropsychological rehabilitation does not improve cognitive performance but reduces perceived cognitive deficits in patients with multiple sclerosis: a randomized, controlled, multi-centre trial," *Multiple Sclerosis Journal*, vol. 20, no. 1, pp. 99–107, 2014.

[20] I. Moebs, S. Gee, M. Miyahara, H. Paton, and M. Croucher, "Perceptions of a cognitive rehabilitation group by older people living with cognitive impairment and their caregivers: a qualitative interview study," *Dementia*, vol. 16, no. 4, pp. 513–522, 2017.

[21] S. A. Brown, A. A. Garcia, A. Brown et al., "Biobehavioral determinants of glycemic control in type 2 diabetes: a systematic review and meta-analysis," *Patient Education & Counseling*, vol. 99, no. 10, pp. 1558–1567, 2016.

[22] M. S. Miles, A. M. Huberman, and J. Saldana, *Qualitative Data Analysis: A Methods Sourcebook*, SAGE, Thousand Oaks, CA, USA, 3rd edition, 2014.

[23] M. Sandelowski, "What's in a name? Qualitative descriptive revisited," *Research in Nursing and Health*, vol. 33, pp. 77–84, 2010.

[24] S. Sullivan-Bolyai, C. Boya, and D. Harper, "Developing and refining intervention in persons with health disparities: the use of qualitative description," *Nursing Outlook*, vol. 53, no. 3, pp. 127–133, 2005.

[25] H. E. Cuevas, A. K. Stuifbergen, S. A. Brown, and J. L. Rock, "Thinking about cognitive function: perceptions of cognitive changes in people with type 2 diabetes," *The Diabetes Educator*, vol. 43, no. 5, pp. 486–494, 2017.

[26] R. D. Romo, M. I. Wallhagen, L. Yourman et al., "Perceptions of successful aging among diverse elders with late-life disability," *The Gerontologist*, vol. 53, no. 6, pp. 939–949, 2012.

[27] A. Solomon, M. Kivipelto, and S. Hilkka, "Prevention of Alzheimer's disease: moving backward through the lifespan," *Journal of Alzheimer's Disease*, vol. 33, no. s1, pp. S465–S469, 2013.

[28] G. E. Smith, P. Housen, K. Yaffe et al., "A cognitive training program based on principles of brain plasticity: results from the improvement in memory with plasticity-based adaptive cognitive training (IMPACT) study," *Journal of the American Geriatrics Society*, vol. 57, pp. 594–603, 2009.

[29] H. Becker, A. M. Henneghan, D. L. Volker, and S. Q. Mikan, "A pilot study of a cognitive-behavioral intervention for breast cancer survivors," *Oncology Nursing Forum*, vol. 44, pp. 255–264, 2017.

[30] A. K. Stuifbergen, H. Becker, F. Perez, J. Morrison, V. Kullberg, and A. Todd, "A randomized controlled trial of a cognitive rehabilitation intervention for persons with multiple sclerosis," *Clinical Rehabilitation*, vol. 26, no. 10, pp. 882–893, 2012.

[31] E. M. Di Battista, R. M. Bracken, J. W. Stephens et al., "Workplace delivery of a dietician-led cardiovascular disease and type 2 diabetes prevention programme: a qualitative study of participants' experiences in the context of Basic Needs Theory," *Nutrition Bulletin*, vol. 42, no. 4, pp. 309–320, 2017.

[32] P. D. Bamidis, P. Fissler, S. G. Papageorgiou et al., "Gains in cognition through combined cognitive and physical training: the role of training dosage and severity of neurocognitive disorder," *Frontiers in Aging Neuroscience*, vol. 7, p. 152, 2015.

[33] J. Hunsley and C. M. Lee, "Research-informed benchmarks for psychological treatments: efficacy studies, effectiveness studies, and beyond," *Professional Psychology: Research and Practice*, vol. 38, no. 1, pp. 21–33, 2007.

[34] T. M. Cruickshank, J. A. Thompson, J. F. Dominguea et al., "The effect of multidisciplinary rehabilitation on brain structure and cognition in Huntington's disease: an exploratory study," *Brain and Behavior*, vol. 5, no. 2, article e00312, 2015.

[35] J. D. Morrison and L. Mayer, "Physical activity and cognitive function in adults with multiple sclerosis: an integrative review," *Disability and Rehabilitation*, vol. 39, no. 19, pp. 1909–1920, 2017.

[36] M. Semkova and E. Ahern, "Online neurocognitive remediation therapy to improve cognition in community-living individuals with a history of depression: a pilot study," *Internet Interventions*, vol. 9, pp. 7–14, 2017.

[37] J. M. Fiszdon, M. M. Kurtz, J. Choi, M. D. Bell, and S. Martino, "Motivational interviewing to increase cognitive rehabilitation adherence in schizophrenia," *Schizophrenia Bulletin*, vol. 42, no. 2, pp. 327–334, 2016.

[38] J. Choi and E. W. Twamley, "Cognitive rehabilitation therapies for Alzheimer's disease: a review of methods to improve treatment engagement and self-efficacy," *Neuropsychology Review*, vol. 23, no. 1, pp. 48–62, 2013.

[39] K. T. Hanssen, A. G. Beiske, N. I. Landro, D. Hofoss, and E. Hessen, "Cognitive rehabilitation in multiple sclerosis: a randomized controlled trial," *Acta Neurologica Scandinavica*, vol. 133, no. 1, pp. 30–40, 2016.

[40] C. K. Miller and J. Bauman, "Goal setting: an integral component of effective diabetes," *Current Diabetes Reports*, vol. 14, no. 8, p. 509, 2014.

[41] B. Regan, Y. Wells, M. Farrrow, P. O'Halloran, and B. Workman, "MAXCOG—Maximizing cognition: a randomized controlled trial of the efficacy of goal-oriented cognitive rehabilitation for people with mild cognitive impairment and early Alzheimer disease," *American Journal of Geriatric Psychiatry*, vol. 25, no. 3, pp. 258–269, 2017.

[42] J. Rodakowski, A. M. Becker, and K. W. Golias, "Activity-based goals generated by older adults with mild cognitive impairment," *OTJR: Occupation, Participation and Health*, vol. 38, no. 2, pp. 84–88, 2018.

[43] S. S. Lie, B. Karlsen, E. R. Oord, M. Graue, and B. Oftedal, "Dropout from an eHealth intervention for adults with type 2 diabetes: a qualitative study," *Journal of Medical Internet Research*, vol. 19, no. 5, p. e187, 2017.

[44] D. B. Reuben and M. E. Tinetti, "Goal-oriented patient care—an alternative health outcomes paradigm," *New England Journal of Medicine*, vol. 366, pp. 777–779, 2012.

[45] C. Kim, J. H. Sohn, M. U. Jang et al., "Association between visit-to-visit glucose variability and cognitive function in aged type 2 diabetic patients: a cross-sectional study," *PLoS One*, vol. 10, no. 7, Article ID e0132118, 2015.

[46] American Diabetes Association, "10. Older adults: table 10.1," *Diabetes Care*, vol. 39, no. 1, pp. S81–S85, 2016.

[47] G. Horigan, M. Davies, F. Findlay-White, D. Chaney, and V. Coates, "Reasons why patients referred to diabetes education programmes choose not to attend: a systematic review," *Diabetic Medicine*, vol. 34, pp. 14–26, 2017.

[48] A. Lampit, H. Hallock, and M. Valenzuela, "Computerized cognitive training in cognitively healthy older adults: a systematic review and meta-analysis of effect modifiers," *PLoS Medicine*, vol. 11, no. 11, article e1001756, 2014.

22

The Development of a Design and Construction Process Protocol to Support the Home Modification Process Delivered by Occupational Therapists

Rachel Russell,[1] **Marcus Ormerod**,[2] **and Rita Newton**[3]

[1]*School of Health Sciences, The University of Salford, Salford M6 6PU, UK*
[2]*School of the Built Environment, The University of Salford, Salford M5 4WT, UK*
[3]*School of Health Sciences, The University of Manchester, Manchester M13 9PL, UK*

Correspondence should be addressed to Rachel Russell; r.c.russell@salford.ac.uk

Academic Editor: F. R. Ferraro

Modifying the home environments of older people as they age in place is a well-established health and social care intervention. Using design and construction methods to redress any imbalance caused by the ageing process or disability within the home environment, occupational therapists are seen as the experts in this field of practice. However, the process used by occupational therapists when modifying home environments has been criticised for being disorganised and not founded on theoretical principles and concepts underpinning the profession. To address this issue, research was conducted to develop a design and construction process protocol specifically for home modifications. A three-stage approach was taken for the analysis of qualitative data generated from an online survey, completed by 135 occupational therapists in the UK. Using both the existing occupational therapy intervention process model and the design and construction process protocol as the theoretical frameworks, a 4-phase, 9-subphase design and construction process protocol for home modifications was developed. Overall, the study is innovative in developing the first process protocol for home modifications, potentially providing occupational therapists with a systematic and effective approach to the design and delivery of home modification services for older and disabled people.

1. Introduction

Current government policy within the UK [1] is encouraging the design and construction industry to build new mainstream housing that supports people to successfully age in place and to reduce the architectural barriers previous design standards have caused since the majority of older and disabled people live in homes that are not designed to meet their needs [2–4]. However, current policy recognises the social and economic benefits of enabling older and disabled people to remain in their own homes by making it a statutory obligation [5, 6] for the assessment and provision of social care services to achieve this. Home modifications are one such service. Whilst home modifications can involve the removal of hazardous features, such as worn rugs, or changing the behaviour in how activities of daily living are performed [7], home modification services in the UK focus on providing "structural changes to a person's home so they can continue to live and move, or be moved, safely" (p. 410) [8]. Occupational therapists make an important contribution to the home modification process, as their professional skills in "problem solving, enablement, prevention and environmental adaptations" (p. 11) [9] are being used to help health and social care departments within local authorities deliver their legislative responsibilities for the assessment and provision of home modifications for older and disabled people.

Despite the perceived positive role of the occupational therapist in this field of practice [10] and the fact that home modifications improve the health and well-being of older people [11–13], evidence suggests that some home modifications fail to meet the client's needs [14–16] and expectations [10] and that failing to involve the client (who is usually the older person but may also be the caregiver or relative) in the decision-making process is a further cause of dissatisfaction

[17, 18]. Questions have also been raised about the complexity and coordination of the home modification process because of the number of agencies and professionals involved [19–21], with the use of the analogy of a "patchwork of services," which are relatively "unplanned and uncoordinated" in nature (p. 4) [20].

It is further suggested that people's experience of the process and satisfaction with the home modification would improve if occupational therapists had a greater understanding of their role [20, 22, 23], and the lack of available guidance and standardised assessment tools is seen as a contributing factor [16, 21, 22, 24]. This issue is further exacerbated by a lack of design and construction knowledge [8, 20, 25], leading to occupational therapists making the assumption that the modification process is simple [26]. Interestingly, evidence suggests that occupational therapists want a more standardised approach to the whole modification process [21] and that the profession should consider ways to amalgamate the occupational therapy process into the wider design and construction process [22, 23, 27]. Thus, given that occupational therapists use the principles of design and construction in interventions involving modifying the home environment in their everyday practice, the aim of this study was to develop an occupational therapy design and construction protocol for modifying home environments.

2. Learning from the Design and Construction Industry

Interestingly, in the 1990s, the UK design and construction industry faced similar criticisms to those discussed above, and three key factors were identified [28]. The first factor is the difficult nature of coordinating a building project requiring the careful planning, management, and coordination of a number of phases and subphases [28] and coordinating a large number of highly specialised professional groups who do not typically work alongside each other and only have a broad understanding of each other's role [29]. The second factor is the flow of information through the various sequential phases of the process [28] such that it was seen as important that each professional group understood the value of information they produced to the other professionals involved in the project and that they were aware of what information needed to flow through to the next phase and also the timing of their information such that subsequent phases were not delayed [30]. Thirdly, the involvement of end users was identified, thus ensuring that information necessary to design and construct a building to meet their needs and requirements was appropriately captured throughout the project [31, 32]. These criticisms led to the development of the generic design and construction process protocol (GDCPP) [33]. In describing the process, Cooper et al. [34] explain that the GDCPP breaks down the design and construction process into four phases, and within each phase, there are subphases; each phase and each subphase are associated with specific actions, and these actions are linked to different elements of design and construction. Each phase should be complete before moving on to the next phase. Whilst there have been no longitudinal follow-up studies investigating the long-term benefits gained from using the GDCPP, it is reported [35] that the case study sites involved in the original research continued to use the GDCPP after the formal research project was concluded.

3. The Need for an Occupational Therapy Design and Construction Process Protocol

When providing interventions, the College of Occupational Therapy states that "any advice or intervention provided should be based upon the most recent evidence available, best practice, or local/national guidelines and protocol" (p. 17) [36]. The occupational therapy profession has a number of generic process frameworks [37–39], and as with the design and construction industry, these processes help occupational therapists to structure the evaluation, diagnosis, treatment, and reevaluation phases of therapy. However, the occupational therapy process is generic and applied to the full range of interventions such that there is no published process which makes visible the process required for housing modifications. This should be a concern for the profession as practitioners have an ethical and professional requirement to make visible their practice such that they can demonstrate that the interventions they are providing are effective and that the person receiving the intervention is able to understand and consent to all aspects of the treatment that they are receiving [40, 41].

The assessment for, and the identification of, what home modifications are required is a complex part of occupational therapy practice, and practitioners use conceptual models as "an organising tool" to help structure and "make sense" of this process (p. 57) [42]. There is general agreement in the literature [42–44] that the Person Environment Occupation (PEO) models are the most relevant conceptual model to practitioners in this field of practice. However, there has been criticism that the traditional PEO models [45–47] do not fully capture the concepts occupational therapists require to guide effective home modification practice [48]. The Occupational Therapy Intervention Process Model [38] is used in the research reported here, and as such, these criticisms are addressed in three key ways. Firstly, the OTIPM [38] uses similar terms associated with the built environment literature such as "required space," "required tools," and "required actions" and similar terms used in the built environment [49] when describing the space, equipment, and objects people use to perform an activity. Secondly, unlike other PEO models [49], the OTIPM separately operationalises the process for delivering interventions. Thirdly, as with GDCPP [34], the OTIPM [38] encourages occupational therapists not to proceed to the next phase of the process until they have all the necessary information to continue, thereby reducing the risk of planning ineffective interventions.

Despite the professional [41] and ethical requirements [40] to make visible the core reasoning skills and process used within occupational therapy professional practice within the UK, there are concerns [50, 51] that very few research studies have evaluated or attempted to describe the home modification process and make visible the practice involved. Protocols have been used successfully to improve the interventions provided by occupational therapists, for example, to improve the clinical reasoning of novice practitioners using a specific assessment to identify appropriate interventions to reduce upper limb hypertonia [52]. The purpose of this study, therefore, is to develop an occupational therapy design and construction process protocol specifically for home modifications because protocols "... help clinicians focus on what is important, specify intervention procedures, delineate the theoretical rationale behind treatment, and contribute to the evolution of the intervention by explicating the reasoning process necessary to solve clinical dilemmas" (p. 712) [53].

4. Methodology

A survey strategy [54] was used for this study so that the home modification processes used by occupational therapists could be understood by analysing the situation in which occupational therapists undertake the process of modifying the home environment. The specific technique used to collect the survey data was an online questionnaire, as this approach provides an effective method of generating knowledge and the most efficient way of delivering the survey to a larger sample of respondents [54].

The questionnaires were designed to include both open and closed questions, capturing quantitative data about respondent attitudes and experience of the home modification process and qualitative data to capture fact-based information. Respondents were asked to consider their answers in relation to bathroom modifications as they are the most common modification [55]. A pilot study involving five experienced occupational therapists was conducted [56] to ensure the validity and reliability of the data generated, as well as ensuring that the questions could be understood by the respondents.

For the main study, purposeful sampling was chosen as an effective way to identify a sample of respondents with specific attributes necessary to generate data [57]. Inclusion criteria, alongside the rationale, are presented in Table 1. The online questionnaire was advertised through the UK College of Occupational Therapy monthly e-newsletter to all members (approximately 250 members) of the specialist section for housing. Whilst 232 questionnaires were received, only 135 met the inclusion criteria. Reasons for exclusion included the following:

(1) Respondent retired from practice

(2) Respondent worked outside of the UK

(3) Respondent not a qualified occupational therapist

(4) Respondent's main role no longer involved using home modifications as an intervention

Data analysis involved three separate stages. Firstly, a directed content analysis technique was used. Directed content analysis is a useful form of thematic analysis when validating or extending a conceptual theoretical framework, such as the occupational therapy process [58]. The OTIPM [38] acted as a theoretical framework to analyse the data. Data generated from the question "describe your role in the process of designing a bathroom modification" were downloaded into NVivo 10. Using the software, each statement from individual respondents was read and reread. Once familiar with the range of statements, the initial coding of the data involved separating the response statements into individual activities or actions performed by the respondents in their role and matching responses to one of the three phases of the OTIPM [38]. These three phases of the OTIPM [38] became the separate themes for this step of the data analysis. When using a directed content analysis, [59] states that it is important to "remember to stay grounded in the data and remain open to the possibility that, ultimately, the data and the framework may be incompatible" [59]. Therefore, codes not matched to one of the three themes were reviewed.

Table 1: Respondent inclusion criteria.

Inclusion criteria	Rationale for criteria
Occupational therapy	The study is interested in occupational therapy and the use of home modifications
Involved in using home modifications as an intervention	For respondents to be able to comment of the home modification process, they need to have relevant knowledge of using this as an intervention
UK-based	Different countries use different terms for describing concepts within occupational therapy, so UK knowledge was important

The second stage of the data analysis involved conceptualising the activities and actions of the respondents during the main phases of the occupational therapy process, as a home modification process. NVivo 10 software was used to produce four separate code books. Each book represented one of the themes identified from Step 1 of the directed content analysis and contained the data coded under each theme. Once familiar with the content of each book, activities and actions in each code book were matched with similar actions and activities in each of the 10 subphases of the GDCPP [33]. As with the previous stage of analysis, thematic codes not matched to the subphases were reviewed at the end of the process. The outcome of this stage of the analysis was a 4-phase, 10-subphase process used by the occupational therapist to design and construct home modification.

A third stage of the analysis was required to create an embryonic home modification process protocol framework. An iterative approach was required to generate the protocol, and a brief description of this process is given below. A framework was developed; along the top of the framework, the headings were used from the 4 phases and 10 subphases of the occupational therapy design and construction process. Running down the far left-hand side were the following principles taken from the GDCPP [33]:

(i) Description of the phase

(ii) Key question

(iii) Action needed at each phase

(iv) Outcome of the phase

Then, using the actions and activities described by respondents in the code books generated at the second stage of the data analysis, the framework was populated. Gaps in the framework were populated by referring to *An Occupational Therapist's Guide to Home Modification Practice* [60] and the researcher's knowledge of this field of practice. To improve the trustworthiness of the data included in the framework, the principal researcher was challenged by 2 researchers not involved in this stage of the data analysis and adjustments were made accordingly.

4.1. Step 1 Findings. During the thematic analysis, it became evident that an additional phase not captured by the OTIPM [38] existed within the codes. This additional phase occurred between the assessment and the goal setting phase and the intervention phase. Because the respondents performed a number of actions or tasks that were not associated with the initial assessment of occupational need and the setting of goals for the intervention, nor were they related to the intervention itself. Instead, respondents performed a series of activities associated with planning the intervention; thus, the term "intervention planning phase" was developed to code these responses into a theme.

As an intervention, the home modification is not installed by the occupational therapist; however, from the responses, it was evident that a number of occupational therapy practitioners were involved in supporting the installation of the modification. Firstly, their support appeared to be essential for ensuring the health and safety of the person, for example, making the builder aware of any medical conditions which could be exacerbated by the construction methods being used to install the modification, for instance, dust exacerbating the person's respiratory condition. Secondly, some of the respondents ($n = 13$) indicated that they were involved in giving advice on the position of equipment or in purchasing specialist equipment to be installed as part of the modification. Thirdly, some respondents ($n = 9$) indicated that they had a role in providing the person with emotional support during the installation or acted as an intermediary if issues arose between the person and the builder. Therefore, using the term "intervention implementation" makes distinct that the invention is not the final installed modification alone; it involves a series of activities the occupational therapist is involved with during the phase of installing the intervention. Table 2 presents examples of responses coded under each of the phases of the OTIPM.

4.2. Step 2 Findings. In Step 2 of the data analysis, NVivo 10 software was used to produce four separate code books. Each book represented one of the themes identified from Step 1 of the analysis and contained responses coded under each theme. Thematic analysis was initially attempted by looking for similarities between activities in the four main phases of the GDCPP [33]. However, it became apparent that the activities within the four main phases of the GDCPP [33] were not congruent with the activities within the four main phases of the OTIPM [38]. To overcome this issue, the activities were coded using the descriptions of the subphase of the GDCPP [33] looking for similarities in the responses in each of the four code books.

Using the abovementioned approach to the analysis, it became evident that two additional phases not captured by the GDCPP [33] existed in the responses. These two subphases occurred between subphases 1 and 2 of the GDCPP [33]. In these phases, respondents indicated a number of actions or tasks involved in analysing how the person was performing the activity in the existing environment as well as professionally reasoning what the person required in the final design. The themes "conduct an occupational performance analysis to identify the person(s) PET requirements" and "develop occupational-focused home modification goals and PET based on the person's PET requirements" were developed to capture these codes. Similarly, there were three activities described in the GDCPP [33] where no similar activity could be found in the code books; thus, no data were coded under the following themes:

(i) Outline feasibility

(ii) Outline conceptual design

(iii) Production information

The findings of this analysis are presented in Table 3 with example of responses.

To be able to compare the subphases of the GDCPP [33] and the subphases of the home modification process, the results are displayed in Table 4. The four main phases of the GDCPP [33] were differentiated by colour. By doing this, it became evident where the lack of congruence occurs between the four main phases of the GDCPP [33] and the four main phases of the home modification process. As the aim of this stage of the analysis was to conceptualise the occupational therapy practice as a design and construction process, it was necessary to resolve the issue with the lack of congruence between the four main phases so that parallels between the four main phases of the GDCPP [33] and the OTIPM [38] could be visualised, as illustrated in Table 4.

5. The Development of the Home Modification Process Protocol

Step 3 involved the development of a single framework based on the GDCPP [33] and the OTIPM [38]. Across the top of the framework, the 9 subphases developed from Step 2 of the analysis of the data were used to label the headings of individual columns. Populating the framework with content was an iterative process. NVivo 10 software was used to create a code book for each individual subphase of the home modification process, with each book containing the written responses coded under each of the subphases. The GDCPP Book [33] and the OTIPM Manual [38] guided the development of the content for the description of each phase, key questions needing to be asked at each subphase, and the outcome of each subphase. As such, the framework has nine subphases (0 to 8), and each of these is presented separately.

5.1. Subphase 0. Subphase 0, shown in Table 5, has used the GDCPP principle that a prospective client may not want to proceed with a project following an initial discussion of their need with the building professional such that the purpose of this subphase is to gather data on what has prompted the person to contact the service and whether involvement from an occupational therapist will improve the person's health and well-being.

TABLE 2: Example of responses for the main phases of the OTIPM [38].

Main phase of the OTIPM [38]	Direct quote taken from different respondents
Assessment and goal setting	"Assessing with the person what their needs are in relation to home environment" (R2) "My role firstly involves an OT assessment which takes into account the goals of the individual as regards achieving the best bathroom facility for them and/or their care requirements" (R48) "Carry out an assessment of need, and if the assessed need results in the provision of a bathroom adaptation, would proceed to the next phase of the adaptation process" (R63)
Intervention planning	"I work with the client and technician to agree on the best possible layout to meet a person's long-term needs. This is a joint agreement with client OT, technician and builders all giving input. However, it is my role to advice on installations that may be beneficial and that the client is not aware of existing" (R3) "Following a functional assessment of needs, my role is to design and plan the layout and facilities in the bathroom to meet the individual's current to long-term needs" (R14) "Using a plan see if intended adaptation fits exploring options, i.e., shape dimensions how the client intends to use it" (R42)
Intervention implementation	"Remaining available through alterations, for site visits and answering questions as and when they arise" (R10) "Communicating any special needs (e.g. re dust inhalation) to surveyor/contractor" (R56) "Availability for consultation during the building work" (R72)
Reevaluation	"When work completed to ensure modifications are safe for client, that the work specified has been completed to a high standard and to ensure client completely happy. If not, to assist client to ensure all changes are made to ensure clients safety and ability to enjoy their new facility. Finally, there is a key role in evaluating the provision with the client and or care staff" (R6) "Visiting tenant once work completed to check suitability, demonstrate use of shower and other equipment and to check the adaptations meet the need" (R24)

TABLE 3: Example responses for each of the subphases of the home modification process.

Subphase	Example of responses
Demonstrate an occupational need within the person-centred performance context	"Identifying what problems exist and either what the relevant parties wish to achieve or providing information of what can be achieved (within public funding but with acknowledgement of what is available outside of public funding)" (R83)
Conceptualise the occupation need as identified by the person	"A thorough understanding of persons aspirations and their needs/wishes" (R6)
Conduct an occupational performance analysis to identify the person(s) PET requirements	"Do an initial assessment of the person and their environment looking at their functional ability and/or the needs of their carer" (R46)
Develop collaborative goal(s) and identify person, environment, and task (PET) requirements for the home modification	"Following the assessment OT recommendations discussed with the person" (R72)
Conduct substantive feasibility study for achieving the PET requirement (including funding route)	"I work with the client and technician to agree on the best possible layout to meet a person's long-term needs. This is a joint agreement with client OT, technician and builders all giving input. However, it is my role to advice on installations that may be beneficial and that the client is not aware of existing" (R3)
Obtain agreement on the full detailed design of the home modification	"Approval from service user then written options proposal, specification and CAD diagrams" (R8)
Coordinate and support procurement of the occupation-focused home modification	"Referral to District Council or RSL for DFG/minor works funding" (R100)
Construct the occupation-focused home modification	"Once work is on site, deal with any queries regarding change of layout due to unforeseen problems" (R57)
Conduct site visit to check the operation and maintenance of the occupational-focused home modification	"When work completed to ensure modifications are safe for client, that the work specified has been completed to a high standard and to ensure client completely happy. If not, to assist client to ensure all changes are made to ensure clients safety and ability to enjoy their new facility" (R6)

A further principle of the GDCPP [33] is that the project manager is aware of which professionals should be involved in the process and when. Thus, taking this concept and the OTIPM [38] concept of identifying who else is involved in the person's situation, subphase 0 gathers data on who the practitioner may need to involve in later subphases of the process.

Subphase 0 has also captured the OTIPM [38] concept of making the person aware of the limitations within the practitioner's field of practice. It appeared to be important to

TABLE 4: Conceptualising the occupational therapy home modification process as a design and construction process.

Main phase of the GDCPP [33]	Subphase	Terms used in the GDCPP [33]	Activity themes generated from coding	Subphase of the home modification process	Main phase of the OTIPM [33]
Preproject	0	Demonstrating the need	Demonstrate an occupational need within the person-centred performance context	0	Evaluation
	1	Conception of need	Conceptualise the need as identified by the person	1	
	2	Outline of feasibility	Conduct an occupational performance analysis to identify the person(s) PET requirements	2	
Preproject	3	Substantive feasibility study	Develop collaborative goal(s) by identifying the detailed PET design requirement for the home modification	3	Modification planning
	4	Outline conceptual design	Conduct substantive feasibility study for achieving the PET specification (including funding route)	4	
Preconstruction	5	Full conceptual design	Obtain agreement on the full detailed design of the home modifications	5	Modification planning
Preconstruction	6	Coordinate design, procurement, and full financial authority	Coordinate and support procurement of the occupation-focused home modification	6	Modification implementation
Construction	7	Production information	Coordinate and support procurement of the occupation-focused home modification	6	Modification implementation
Construction	8	Construction	Construct the occupation-focused home modification	7	Modification implementation
After completion	9	Operation and maintenance	Conduct site visit to check the operation and maintenance of the occupational-focused home modification	8	Reevaluation

ask this question at this phase, given the theme in the literature and the data gathered from respondents, on the influence departmental policies and resources have on the role of the practitioner.

As the GDCPP [33] is concerned with ensuring that all information is available to support the next phase of the process, the outcome subphase 0 also ensures that the practitioner has all relevant information for the next phase, in particular that the person has given consent. As consent to an assessment is an ethical and professional requirement, it appeared appropriate to include it in this phase so that when the person is first visited, they have already consented to a visit and the start of the assessment process.

5.2. Subphase 1. Subphase 1, shown in Table 6, captures the values the OTIPM [33] places on collaborative practice through the occupational therapy process such that the person, in collaboration with the practitioner, identifies the occupation(s) impacting upon their health and well-being.

Since the literature was critical of occupational therapists focusing on safety and function and identifying the need based on eligibility criteria, the outcome of subphase 1 assists the practitioner to identify what occupation they need to observe in the next subphase of the process. This reflects ethical practice, as the person is not arbitrarily made to perform unnecessary activities based on home-grown assessments designed to focus on safety and independence or what can or cannot be funded by the practice setting. Instead, the influence of funding arrangements is considered in subphase 4 and the feasibility study. Similarly, as the practitioner builds a collaborative relationship with the person and new data provide insights into the person's situation, subphase 1 ensures that due consideration is given to the appropriateness of the intervention in providing the person with the appropriate solution to improve their health and well-being.

5.3. Subphase 2. Subphase 2, shown in Table 7, has been influenced by the OTIPM [38] description of how practitioners should analyse occupational performance and participation since it is recommended that the practitioner should initially observe the person performing or participating in the occupation, identifying the strengths and weaknesses in the person's performance. Once the practitioner has these data, the OTIPM [38] describes how the practitioner can then analyse the cause of the problem based on the transaction of the person, environment, and task. This is a two-pronged approach to analysing performance and participation because it prevents the occupational therapist making assumptions about the cause of the problem. The conceptual model developed as part of the OTIPM [38] guides the type of person, environment, and occupation data the practitioner needs to collect. It should

Table 5: Subphase 0 of home modification process protocol.

Assessment phase	Subphase 0
Description	Demonstrate an occupational need within the person-centred performance context
Key questions	What is the situation that has prompted contact with the occupational therapist/service? Is an occupation-focused home modification intervention appropriate for the situation? Is the person aware of the limitation in this practice setting? Should a home modification approach be taken?
Action	Identity the context of the situation Identify who (persons) is involved in the situation Identify the tasks involved in the situation Identify how resources and other limitations within the practice setting may affect the situation Identify how a collaborative relationship with the occupational therapist/service could impact on the situation
Outcomes	Referral accepted/declined Key referral (situational) information documented Person(s) aware of limitations within the OT's field of practice, that is, funding criteria for home modification Consent to assessment documented

Table 6: Subphase 1 of home modification process protocol.

Assessment phase	Subphase 1
Description	Conceptualise the occupational need as identified by the person(s)
Key questions	What is the reported occupation(s) the person(s) needs/wants to address through an occupation-focused home modification? Should a home modification approach be taken?
Action	Identify the specific occupation(s) the person(s) wants/needs/has to do Identify the person(s) occupational priorities Identify occupations that cannot be addressed through occupation-focused home modification intervention
Outcome	Identify the person(s) occupational priorities Provide advice including referral to alternative services

be noted that the OTIPM [38] uses the term "task" and not "occupation" in the conceptual model, thereby acknowledging that a practitioner does not objectively observe an occupation; they observe the task part of the transaction between the person and the environment. This is because only the person can experience an occupation, since it only has meaning and value to them.

Table 7: Subphase 2 of home modification process protocol.

Assessment phase	Subphase 2
Description	Identify the person, environment, and task elements impacting on occupational performance
Key questions	How does the transaction between the person, environment, and task (PET) factors impact on occupational performance? Should a home modification approach be taken?
Action	Identify the actions, within the occupation(s), the person(s) does not perform effectively Identify actions, within the occupation(s), the person(s) does perform effectively Identify the elements of the person, environment, and task (PET) [38] that are affecting the person(s) occupational performance
Outcomes	Occupational performance analysis completed and effective and ineffective elements of performance documented PET element(s) causing effective or ineffective occupational performance documented PET information needed to support subphase 4 documented Provide advice including referral to alternative services

5.4. Subphase 3. Goals are an important part of the occupational therapy process since they provide the benchmark on which the occupational therapist and person establish if the intervention has been successful. Thus, the purpose of subphase 3, shown in Table 8, is to identify those goals. Given that one of the principles of the GDCPP [33] is to collect data relevant for the success of later subphases, subphase 3 makes the distinction as to how the modification is improving health and well-being and whether it is being designed to restore, maintain, or acquire performance/participation in the person's occupation. Thus, this question prompts the practitioner to consider what impact this decision would have on the final subphase of the process.

5.5. Subphase 4. The purpose of subphase 4, shown in Table 9, is to conduct a feasibility study to identify how the home can be modified to improve the person's performance or participation in the occupation for which it was necessary to ensure that the protocol could accommodate a range of regional, policy, and regulatory differences between practice settings. To achieve this, the principles of the GDCPP [33] were used to develop the question of how contextual issues within the practice setting will influence the choice of design. Similarly, it was important to ensure that design decisions were made explicit to the person and documented, thus overcoming the difficulty of people not always being aware as to why certain decisions have been made.

TABLE 8: Subphase 3 of home modification process protocol.

Intervention planning phase	Subphase 3
Description	Develop collaborative goal(s) to identify the detailed PET design requirement for the home modification
Key questions	Is the person(s) goal(s) for the modification to restore their occupational performance/participation? maintain their occupational performance/participation? develop their skills or role to perform or participate in a new occupation? What are the detailed PET design requirements for achieving the collaborative goals? Should a home modification approach be taken?
Actions	Identify, with the person(s), if the goals for the home modification are restoring their occupational performance/participation? maintaining their occupational performance/participation? developing their skills or role to perform or participate in a new occupation? Identify, with the person(s), how the abovementioned approach will impact on the evaluation phases Identify the specific "person factors/body functions" design requirements Identify the specific "environmental" design requirements Identify the specific "task" design requirements Identify any occupations(s) that cannot be addressed through an occupation-focused home modification
Outcomes	Person(s) has collaborated on the goals of the home modification Goals for home modification documented PET design requirements to achieve the goal(s) documented Reablement, rehabilitation, and/or training requirements following the completion of the home modification documented

TABLE 9: Subphase 4 of home modification process protocol.

Intervention planning phase	Subphase 4
Description	Conduct a substantive feasibility study for achieving the PET requirements (including funding route)
Key questions	What design options are there for meeting the PET requirements? What other factors in the person's occupational context will affect the choice of design solutions? Does the design proposal meet the PET requirements outlined in subphase 3? Should a home modification approach be taken?
Actions	Identify that the design has addressed all the requirements identified in subphase 3 Identify that the design meets any other occupational performance context requirements Identify any practice setting contextual issues that will influence the person(s) choice of design solution Identify any potential built environment issues, in the existing space, that will impact on the PET requirements being accommodated Identify funding requirements for the home modification
Outcomes	Professional reasoning on the modification design solution process Document any issues related to the practice setting or built environment that prevent the optimum design solution being provided The specification related to space, space layout, and tools documented

TABLE 10: Subphase 5 of home modification process protocol.

Intervention planning phase	Subphase 5
Description	Obtain agreement on the full detailed design and specification of the home modification
Key questions	Does the full detailed design provide the solution to address the occupational performance requirements of the person? Do the detailed design plans and specifications provide the person with the information they need to give informed consent? Should a home modification approach be taken?
Actions	Ensure that the person(s) understands how the design solution addresses their occupational performance requirements Identify how any unmet requirements will impact on the occupational performance of the modification Confirm that the person(s) agrees to proceed with the design solution
Outcomes	Informed consent documented

5.6. Subphase 5. The development of the content from subphase 5, shown in Table 10, arose from the professional and ethical requirement of practitioners needing to ensure that the person has a full understanding of the intervention so that they are able to give informed consent to proceed with the intervention, and the questions make overt the need for the person to have a full understanding of the design before giving informed consent to proceed with the intervention.

One of the principles of the GDCPP [33] is that it provides an audit trail of the reason why decisions were made at particular subphases of the process. Thus, subphase 5 enables the occupational therapist and person to be accountable for the decisions made during the process, and it makes the information readily available if the outcomes of this subphase, or other subphases, are called into question.

TABLE 11: Subphase 6 of home modification process protocol.

Intervention implementation phase	Subphase 6
Description	Coordinate and support procurement of the occupation-focused home modification
Key questions	What information and action are required to procure the home modification? Has all the information been obtained for the builder/contractor/others to construct the home modification?
Actions	Identify and communicate information required for the procurement of the home modification Identity and communicate the information required for the builder/contractor/others to proceed with the construction of the home modification Identify and communicate what ongoing support will be required of the occupational therapist/service during construction phase
Outcomes	Funding application/support completed Plans, specifications, product information, and health and safety information provided to the builder and/or those involved in construction of the modification Agree with person and builder support being provided by the occupational therapist during construction

5.7. *Subphase 6.* As with subphase 5, it was necessary to allow the questions to reflect the different ways modifications are funded and for the building professionals to have appropriate information to help them understand why the specific layout and requirement contained in the design plan are important in achieving the person's goals. Therefore, subphase 6, Table 11, places a duty on the occupational therapist to provide this information, thereby improving communication. Also, at subphase 6, the occupational therapist is no longer given the option to consider if a home modification approach should be taken because issues that could make a home modification inappropriate would have been identified by the person and occupational therapist earlier in the process.

5.8. *Subphase 7.* By using the principles of the GDCPP [33], subphase 7, shown in Table 12, reflects the tasks identified by respondents in the questionnaire, where their involvement was required to ensure that the person and builder were both supported during the physical construction phase of the modification.

Subphase 7 also ensures that the practitioner provides any specialist equipment that is required once the modification is installed and which could prevent the final modification from being used immediately by the person if not provided.

5.9. *Subphase 8.* Subphase 8, shown in Table 13, is an important part of the occupational therapy design and construction process. The content of subphase 8 was influenced by the requirement a number of respondents identified in ensuring that the standard of workmanship met the standards expected from the housing authority. In the GDCPP [33], the final subphase ensures that the building is handed over ensuring that the end users have an understanding of how the building operates and needs to be maintained; thus, this section ensures that the person has

TABLE 12: Subphase 7 of home modification process protocol.

Intervention implementation phase	Subphase 7
Description	Construct the home modification
Key questions	Is the appropriate support being provided to the person(s) and building professional during the construction phase of the home modification?
Actions	Provide ongoing support during the construction of the home modification Provide and/or supply tools not part of the construction process Provide advice on final positioning of tools
Outcomes	Modification completed

TABLE 13: Subphase 8 of home modification process protocol.

Evaluation phase	Subphase 8
Description	Conduct site visit to check the operation and maintenance of the occupation-focused home modification
Key questions	Is the home modification operating in the way it is intended to? Does the home modification perform in the way that achieves the goals and requirements identified in subphase 3? What can we learn from the process?
Actions	Provide reablement, rehabilitation, and/or training to enable the use of the modification Conduct reevaluation following completion of the home modification and compare with subphase 2 Provide training on the maintenance of the home modification Complete professional evaluation of the intervention and what can be learned
Outcomes	Complete and document the reablement, rehabilitation, and/or training provided Person(s) provided with information and documentation needed to manage the home modification Person(s) satisfied with the performance of the modification. Feedback documented Occupational therapist satisfied with the performance of the modification completed. Outcome documented Modification resolves the occupational need identified in subphase 3. Case closed

a similar understanding in terms of the modification. To capture concepts associated with the OTIPM process [38] and the occupational therapy process in general, the questions and outcomes of subphase 8 reflect the need to evaluate whether the goals identified in the earlier subphases have been achieved. Also, subphase 8 provides opportunity for the occupational therapist to reflect on their practice.

6. Discussion

As a problem-solving profession, the occupational therapy process provides the logical route that the practitioner should follow in order to provide effective interventions [61] such that practitioners are able to operationalise their professional practice [62]. From the findings of Step 1 of the data analysis, it appears that the occupational therapy process was assisting respondents to articulate their role in home modifications. For example, the quotes from R6 and R56, presented in "Findings" (although their answers differed considerably in terms of the detail provided by each respondent) still provide evidence of assessment, goal setting, and intervention phases, and in the case of R6, an evaluation phase.

The thematic analysis also raised theoretical challenges about what constitutes an intervention? The intervention has been traditionally viewed as the completed home modification [8, 63]. However, it is the skills and knowledge of the occupational therapist during all aspects of the occupational therapy process that are essential in the final design and performance of the modification, and this raises the question as to whether the occupational therapy profession should place greater emphasis on the *process* being the intervention rather than the *completed modification*. Indeed, if the process becomes the intervention, then it would be more evident as to what the intervention is and what training is required to gain the skills to carry out the intervention. By developing outcome measures that evaluate the process as the intervention, it also allows practitioners to identify which phases of the intervention were more or less effective and how the process has contributed to the person's health and well-being.

It has been possible to use the OTIPM [38] and GDCPP [33] to describe the occupational therapy process used by respondents in this area of practice. However, the outcome of this does not reflect the actual practice described by respondents, and it appears to differ in one important way, namely, the way respondents combine departmental processes with the occupational therapy process. As an example, it can be seen that respondent R29 using both phrases that are associated with the occupational therapy process (words in red) and the phrases that seem to suggest the influence of the systems, structures, and policies within the respondent's practice setting (words in blue).

> *As an OT I complete an overview assessment with the service user in their home environment to identify their needs. To address these assessed needs (according to the FACS criteria), I may be required to provide adaptive equipment and in some cases recommend adaptations. If adaptations are required, I complete a referral for DFG for adaptations which, following my Manager's approval, is forwarded to the District Council & HIA or Housing Association to begin the DFG process. I provide technical diagrams and guidelines for the adaptations to ensure they can best meet the client's needs as well as completing joint site visits with technical officers if required. Once the modification is complete, I am involved with signing off the work. I am also responsible, if relevant, to obtain quotes.* (R29)

The actions of respondent R29 may not directly lead to a poorly designed modification, but previous findings [64–66] have noted how departmental policies enacted by occupational therapists have been associated with dissatisfaction with the modification. Thus, this finding raises the question as to whether practitioners are aware of how departmental structures and guidance influence their professional practice and the design options presented to the person. Again, this is an important question to answer, given the professional and ethical responsibility professionals have in ensuring that the intervention they provide has been fully explained and explored with the person, so the occupational therapist needs to be able to describe to the person how the intervention they are providing is being influenced by the practice setting.

Another important finding from the second stage of the analysis was the use of the term "assessment of need" in which respondents used their professional reasoning skills to identify occupations (activity) the person is having difficulty performing or participating in, identifying and analysing why the person is having difficulty, and analysing and identifying if a home modification will address the occupational need. From the data collected, it is not possible to establish whether in everyday practice respondents make a distinction between the different types of professional reasoning necessary to support each aspect involved in the "assessment of need" and what the consequence might be if they do not make the distinction. However, given that one principle of the GDCPP [33] is to ensure that, where possible, a subphase does not progress to the next phase until the outcome of the previous phase is achieved, the research suggests that occupational therapists are prematurely progressing through the process without all relevant data being collected and analysing as to how it might impact on the subsequent phases. If this is the case, then a process protocol for home modifications may reduce the risk of this occurring.

7. Conclusion

The purpose of the study was to develop a home modification process protocol by conceptualising the occupational therapy practice involved in home modifications as a design and construction process, and a number of conclusions can be drawn. Firstly, with data from the questionnaire and guided by the OTIPM [38], it was possible to both visualise and describe this process. Whilst interventions involving home modifications can be described through the occupational therapy process, it was interesting to note that practitioners have an important role in planning the design of the intervention. Furthermore, the term "intervention implementation" better describes the involvement of the occupational therapist as they are not directly responsible for the installation of the intervention themselves. Thus, the term "intervention implementation" acknowledges that installing a home modification is a dynamic process and one that the practitioner works with building professionals to achieve.

Secondly, by using the occupational therapy process for home modifications, it was then possible to use the GDCPP [33] to conceptualise the process as a home modification as four main phases based on the OTIPM [38] and 9 subphases based on the GDCPP [33]. Thirdly, using the principles of the GDCPP [33], it was possible to create a framework for the protocol, and by using an iterative process, it was possible to populate the content of this framework, which then became the home modification process protocol. This iterative process was an important part of developing the protocol because it allowed for the development of the content based on a conceptual model of practice and for issues identified in the literature to be addressed. Thus, the home modification process protocol potentially should

(1) provide a systematic approach to the process of modifying the home;
(2) ensure that ethical and professional practice is followed by enabling occupational therapists to verbalise and visualise their role in the process; reduce the complexity of the current process by identifying the key questions, actions, and outcome of each phase;
(3) improve the effectiveness and efficiency of practice by ensuring that practitioners collect the right information, at the right time;
(4) ensure that the person has choice and control through their involvement in all phases of the process;
(5) guide professional reasoning based on a conceptual model of practice;
(6) ensure consistency of occupational therapy practice by accommodating regional, legislative, and regulatory differences between practice settings;
(7) ensure that financial constraints and other contextual issues within practice become a design consideration and not a barrier for accessing funding for a modification.

Whilst home modifiications have been a traditional area of practice for occupational therapists, the home modification process protocol is the first time this practice been described as an occupational therapy design and constuction process. Through the development of the protocol, there is the potential to address the professional [50, 51] and ethical need [40, 41] for practitioners to better understand the intervention they are providing and to be able to express their role in the design and construction of a home modification.

Importantly, this study has also raised the question as to what is the "intervention" within home modification practice? In the literature, the intervention appears to be the installed modification, and outcome measures designed to evaluate the intervention tend to be focused on how the installed modification has improved the person's performance in the occupation. However, the findings from this research have shown that each phase of the protocol is important because the outcomes from each phase can ultimately influence the final performance of, and satisfaction with, the modification. Therefore, this raises the question as to whether the home modification process is what practitioners should be defining as their intervention?

Crucially, the necessary skills and knowledge to design and construct a home modification are not taught in detail or depth at undergraduate level within occupational therapy education. Once qualified, there are training opportunities for practitioners, but these tend to be based on the knowledge and skills required to design a particular type of modification or to design a modification for a particular health condition or disability. Building the necessary knowledge of the design and construction process should therefore be reviewed within undergraduate education.

Finally, there is a need to consider how the home modification process protocol could be implemented beyond England, which was the boundary of the research reported here. Home modification is a complex area of practice, and there is a need to find ways to implement systematic assessment, intervention, and evaluation strategies within occupational therapy practice [67] The challenge for further research is that it is difficult for the process to be standardised as each country provides and funds home modifications in different ways as well as design standards and regulations also being different in each country [68].

Conflicts of Interest

The authors declare that there are no conflicts of interest regarding the publication of this paper.

Acknowledgments

This study is based on a doctoral thesis, which was supported by the UK Engineering and Physical Sciences Research Council, "Russell, R.C., 2016. The development of a design and construction process protocol to support occupational therapists in delivering effective home modifications, Doctoral Thesis, University of Salford, UK" [69].

References

[1] HAPPI, *Housing Our Ageing Population Panel for Innovation*, Home and Communities Agency, London, UK, 2009, https://www.gov.uk/government/uploads/system/uploads/attachment_data/file/378171/happi_final_report_-_031209.pdf.

[2] Care and Repair, "Making the case," 2016, http://careandrepair-england.org.uk/wp-content/uploads/2014/12/Making-the-Case-final.pdf.

[3] Papworth Trust, "Housing and the care crisis," 2016, http://www.papworthtrust.org.uk/campaigns/housing-and-the-care-crisis.

[4] Later Life in the United Kingdom, 2016, http://www.ageuk.org.uk/Documents/EN-GB/Factsheets/Later_Life_UK_factsheet.pdf?dtrk=true.

[5] The Care Act, 2014, http://www.legislation.gov.uk/ukpga/2014/23/contents/enacted.
[6] Housing Grants, Construction and Regeneration Act, 1996, http://www.legislation.gov.uk/ukpga/1996/53/contents.
[7] J. Pynoos, B. A. Steinman, A. Q. Do Nguyen, and M. ressette, "Assessing and adapting the home environment to reduce falls and meet the changing capacity of older adults," *Journal of Housing for the Elderly*, vol. 26, no. 1-3, pp. 137–155, 2012.
[8] C. Bridges, "Home modification: occupational as the basis for effective practice," in *Occupational Therapy and Physical Dysfunction: Enabling Occupation*, M. Curtin, M. Molineux, and J. Supyk-Mellson, Eds., Churchill Livingston, London, UK, 2010.
[9] J. Riley, S. Whitcombe, and C. Vincent, *Occupational Therapy in Adult Social Care in England: Sustaining a High Quality Workforce for the Future*, Department of Health, London, UK, 2008.
[10] C. Nord, P. Eakin, P. Astley, and A. R. Atkinson, "An exploration of communication between clients and professionals in the design of home adaptations," *British Journal of Occupational Therapy*, vol. 72, no. 5, pp. 197–204, 2009.
[11] S. Stark, A. Landsbaum, J. L. Palmer et al., "Client-centred home modifications improve daily activity performance of older adults," *Canadian Journal of Occupational Therapy*, vol. 76, no. 1, pp. 235–245, 2009.
[12] E. Hwang, L. Cummings, A. Sixsmith, and J. Sixsmith, "Impacts of home modifications on aging-in-place," *Journal of Housing for the Elderly*, vol. 25, no. 3, pp. 246–257, 2011.
[13] K. Johansson, "Have they done what they should? Moral reasoning in the context of translating older persons' everyday problems into eligible needs for home modification services," *Medical Anthropology Quarterly*, vol. 27, no. 3, pp. 414–433, 2013.
[14] S. I. Klein, L. Rosage, and G. Shaw, "The role of occupational therapists in home modification programs at an area agency on aging," *Occupational Therapy Geriatrics*, vol. 16, no. 3-4, pp. 19–37, 2000.
[15] F. Heywood, *Money Well Spent: The Effectiveness and Value of Housing Adaptations*, The Policy Press, Bristol, UK, 2001.
[16] A. Fange and S. Iwarsson, "Changes in accessibility and usability in housing: an exploration of the housing adaptation process," *Occupational Therapy International*, vol. 12, no. 1, pp. 44–59, 2005.
[17] B. Sapey, "Disabling homes: a study of the housing needs of disabled people in Cornwall," *Disability & Society*, vol. 10, no. 1, pp. 71–86, 1995.
[18] A. Nocon and N. Pleace, ""Until disabled people get consulted...": the role of occupational therapy in meeting housing needs," *British Journal of Occupational Therapy*, vol. 60, no. 3, pp. 115–122, 1997.
[19] J. Adams, "Adapting for community care, Part 1," *British Journal of Occupational Therapy*, vol. 59, no. 3, pp. 115–118, 1996.
[20] J. Pynoos, M. Tabbarah, J. Angelelli, and M. Demiere, "Improving the delivery of home modifications," *Technology and Disability*, vol. 8, no. 1, pp. 3–14, 1998.
[21] A. Fänge and S. D. Ivanoff, "The home is the hub of health in very old age: findings from the ENABLE-AGE Project," *Archives of Gerontology and Geriatrics*, vol. 48, no. 3, pp. 340–345, 2009.
[22] K. Forsyth and E. Hamilton, "Social services occupational therapists' view of practice and integration with health: a survey," *British Journal of Occupational Therapy*, vol. 71, no. 2, pp. 64–71, 2008.
[23] J. Grisbrooke and S. Scott, "Moving into housing: experiences of developing specialist occupational therapy posts in local authority housing departments," *British Journal of Occupational Therapy*, vol. 72, no. 1, pp. 29–36, 2009.
[24] C. Picking and H. Pain, "Home adaptations: user perspectives on the role of professionals," *British Journal of Occupational Therapy*, vol. 66, no. 1, pp. 2–8, 2003.
[25] E. Steinfeld and J. Maisel, *Universal Design: Creating Inclusive Environments*, John Wiley & Sons, Hoboken, NJ, USA, 2012.
[26] L. Milikan, *Summary Bulletin: Environmental Assessment and Modification for Australian Occupational Therapists*, University of New South Wales, Kensington, NSW, Australia, 2012.
[27] J. Pynoos and J. Sanford, "New tools for better home modifications," *The Case Manager*, vol. 13, no. 1, pp. 67–70, 2002.
[28] J. Egan, *Rethinking Construction, Construction Task Force Report for Department of the Environment*, Transport and the Regions, HMSO, London, UK, 1998.
[29] F. E. Gould and N. E. Joyce, *Construction Project Management*, Prentice-Hall, London, UK, 2009.
[30] L. Koskela, G. HowelL, G. Ballard, and I. Tommelein, *The Foundations of Lean Construction. Design and Construction: Building in Value*, Butterworth-Heinemann, Oxford, UK, 2002.
[31] P. Tzortzopoulos, R. Cooper, P. Chan, and M. Kagioglou, "Clients' activities at the design front-end," *Design Studies*, vol. 27, no. 6, pp. 657–683, 2006.
[32] P. Christiansson, K. Svidt, K. B. Sørensen, and U. Dybro, "User participation in the building process," *Journal of Information Technology in Construction*, vol. 16, pp. 309–334, 2011.
[33] R. Cooper, M. Kagioglou, G. Aouad, J. Hinks, M. Sexton, and D. Sheath, "The development of a generic design and construction process," in *Proceedings of the European Conference Product Data Technology Days 1998*, Building Research Establishment, Watford, UK, March 1998.
[34] R. Cooper, G. Aouad, A. Lee, S. WU, A. Fleming, and M. Kagioglou, *Process Management in Design and Construction*, Wiley, London, UK, 2008.
[35] M. Kagioglou, R. Cooper, G. Aouad, and M. Sexton, "Rethinking construction: the generic design and construction process protocol," *Engineering Construction and Architectural Management*, vol. 7, no. 2, pp. 141–153, 2000.
[36] College of Occupational Therapists, *Occupational Therapy Guidance on Parkinson's Disease*, College of Occupational Therapists, London, UK, 2010.
[37] J. Creek, *Occupational Therapy Defined as a Complex Intervention*, College of Occupational Therapists, London, UK, 2003.
[38] A. Fisher, *Occupational Therapy Intervention Process Model: A Model for Planning and Implementing Top-Down, Client Centered and Occupation Based Interventions*, Three Star Press Inc., Fort Collins, CO, USA, 2009.
[39] J. C. Rogers, "Occupation reasoning," in *Occupational Therapy and Physical Dysfunction*, M. Curtin, M. Molineux, and J. A. Supyk-Mellson, Eds., Churchill Livingstone, London, UK, 2010.
[40] College of Occupational Therapists, *Code of Ethics and Professional Conduct*, College of Occupational Therapists, London, UK, 2015, https://www.cot.co.uk/sites/default/files/publications/public/CODE-OF-ETHICS-2015.pdf.
[41] Health Care Professional Council, *Standards of Conduct, Performance and Ethics*, Health and Care Professions Council, London, UK, 2013.
[42] S. Davis, *Rehabilitation: The Use of Theories and Models in Practice*, Elsevier Health Sciences, London, UK, 2006.
[43] S. Stark, "Home modifications that enable occupational performance," in *Using Environments to Enable Occupational*

Performance, L. Letts, P. Rigby, and D. Stewart, Eds., Slack Inc., Thorofare, NJ, USA, 2003.

[44] B. Tanner, "History and future of home modification services," in *An Occupational Therapist's Guide to Home Modification Practice*, E. Ainsworth and D. de Jonge, Eds., pp. 67–83, Slack Incorporated, Thorofare, NJ, USA, 2011.

[45] M. Law, "The person-environment-occupation model: a transactive approach to occupational performance," *Canadian Journal of Occupational Therapy*, vol. 63, no. 1, pp. 9–23, 1996.

[46] C. Christiansen and C. Baum, *Occupational Therapy: Enabling Function and Well-Being*, Slack Inc., Thorofare, NJ, USA, 2nd edition, 1997.

[47] E. Townsend, S. Stanton, M. Law et al., *Enabling Occupation: An Occupational Therapy Perspective*, CAOT Publications ACE, Ottawa, ON, Canada, 2002.

[48] J. Rousseau, L. Potvin, E. Dutil, and P. Falta, "Understanding the issue of home adaptation: searching for a conceptual framework," *Occupational Therapy in Health Care*, vol. 14, no. 1, pp. 27–37, 2002.

[49] T. W. Kim, R. Rajagopal, M. Fischer, and C. Kam, "A knowledge-based framework for automated space-use analysis," *Automation in Construction*, vol. 32, pp. 165–176, 2013.

[50] K. Johansson, L. Borell, and M. Lilja, "Older persons' navigation through the service system towards home modification resources," *Scandinavian Journal of Occupational Therapy*, vol. 16, no. 4, pp. 227–237, 2009.

[51] L. M. Clemson and K. E. Laver, "Active ageing and occupational therapy align," *Australian Occupational Therapy Journal*, vol. 61, no. 3, pp. 204–207, 2014.

[52] K. Kuipers and J. W. Grice, "The structure of novice and expert occupational therapists' clinical reasoning before and after exposure to a domain-specific protocol," *Australian Occupational Therapy Journal*, vol. 56, no. 6, pp. 418–427, 2009.

[53] E. I. Blanche, D. Fogelberg, J. Diaz, M. Carlson, and F. Clark, "Manualization of occupational therapy interventions: illustrations from the pressure ulcer prevention research program," *American Journal of Occupational Therapy*, vol. 65, no. 6, pp. 711–719, 2011.

[54] C. Robson, *Real World Research: A Resource for Social Scientists and Practitioner-Researchers*, Wiley, Oxford, UK, 2002.

[55] J. Adams and J. Grisbrooke, "The use of level access showers 12 months after installation," *British Journal of Therapy and Rehabilitation*, vol. 5, no. 10, pp. 504–510, 1998.

[56] K. Forsyth, F. Kviz, and G. Kielhofner, "Survey research design," in *Research in Occupational Therapy: Methods of Inquiry for Enhancing Practice*, G. Kielhofner, Ed., pp. 91–109, Davis Company, Philadelphia, PA, USA, 2006.

[57] G. Kielhofner, *Research in Occupational Therapy Methods of Inquiry for Enhancing Practice*, F. A. Davis, Philadelphia, PA, USA, 2006.

[58] H. F. Hsieh and S. E. Shannon, "Three approaches to qualitative content analysis," *Qualitative Health Research*, vol. 15, no. 9, pp. 1277–1288, 2005.

[59] B. C. Evans, D. W. Coon, and E. Ume, "Use of theoretical frameworks as a pragmatic guide for mixed methods studies a methodological necessity?," *Journal of Mixed Methods Research*, vol. 5, no. 4, pp. 276–292, 2011.

[60] E. Ainsworth and D. de Jonge, *An Occupational Therapist's Guide to Home Modification Practice*, Slack Incorporated, Thorofare, NJ, UK, 2010.

[61] E. A. S. Duncan, *Foundations for Practice in Occupational Therapy*, Churchill Livingstone, London, UK, 2011.

[62] M. J. Turpin and M. K. Iwama, *Using Occupational Therapy Models in Practice: A Fieldguide*, Elsevier Health Sciences, Atlanta, GA, USA, 2011.

[63] J. A. Sanford, *Universal Design as a Rehabilitation Strategy: Design for the Ages*, Springer Publishing Company, New York, NY, USA, 2012.

[64] F. Heywood, "Understanding needs: a starting point for quality," *Housing Studies*, vol. 19, no. 5, pp. 709–726, 2004.

[65] D. Sakellariou, "Towards the construction of a nicer life: subjectivity and the logic of choice," *Anthropology in Action*, vol. 22, no. 1, pp. 46–55, 2015.

[66] D. Sakellariou, "Home modifications and ways of living well," *Medical Anthropology*, vol. 34, no. 5, pp. 456–469, 2015.

[67] A. M. Fänge, K. Lindberg, and S. Iwarsson, "Housing adaptations from the perspectives of Swedish occupational therapists," *Scandinavian Journal of Occupational Therapy*, vol. 20, no. 3, pp. 228–240, 2013.

[68] S. Iwarsson, "Housing adaptations and home modifications," in *International Handbook of Occupational Therapy Interventions*, Springer, New York, NY, USA, 2015.

[69] R. Russell, "The development of a design and construction process protocol to support occupational therapists in delivering effective home modifications," Unpublished award thesis, University of Salford, Salford, UK, 2016, https://portal.salford.ac.uk/+CSCO+00756767633A2F2F686676652E666E79736265712E6E702E6878++/40013/3/Rachel%20Russell%201.pdf.

23

Impact of Polypharmacy on the Rehabilitation Outcome of Japanese Stroke Patients in the Convalescent Rehabilitation Ward

Eiji Kose,[1] Riku Maruyama,[1] Susumu Okazoe,[2] and Hiroyuki Hayashi[1]

[1] *Department of Pharmacotherapy, School of Pharmacy, Nihon University, Chiba, Japan*
[2] *Department of Pharmacy, Sagami Rehabilitation Hospital, Kanagawa, Japan*

Correspondence should be addressed to Eiji Kose; kose.eiji@nihon-u.ac.jp

Academic Editor: Arshad Jahangir

Background. A risk factor associated with stroke onset is chronic kidney disease (CKD). To prevent stroke reoccurrence, it is necessary to strictly manage blood pressure, lipids, and plasma glucose. Therefore, some cases are forced to polypharmacy, elderly patients in particular. Polypharmacy often leads to adverse drug reactions and has the potential to negatively affect the rehabilitation of stroke patients. The aim of the present study was to investigate the effects of polypharmacy using a functional independence measure (FIM). *Methods*. A total of 144 stroke patients with CKD were included in the present analysis. We divided stroke patients into those taking six or more drugs (polypharmacy group) and those taking less than six drugs (nonpolypharmacy group) upon admission. Patient background features, laboratory data, and FIM scores were compared. *Results*. FIM-Motor (FIM-M) efficiency, age, and diabetes mellitus were positively associated with polypharmacy. FIM-M efficiency in the polypharmacy group was significantly lower than in the nonpolypharmacy group. *Conclusion*. Polypharmacy interferes with the effect of rehabilitation in stroke patients with CKD. Pharmacists and doctors should make efforts to optimize medications to be able to respond to the outcome of each patient.

1. Introduction

Stroke is the fourth leading cause of death in Japan and ranks number one in terms of required nursing care. While the number of deaths due to a stroke has been decreasing, according to a study group of the Ministry of Health, Labour, and Welfare, the prevalence of stroke and associated nursing care will continue to increase until 2025. Even if appropriate treatment after stroke onset increases patient survival, there are cases in which some neurological disorders such as allopathy or motility disorder and high-order function disorders such as aphasia or memory impairment remain. In such cases, the role of the convalescent rehabilitation ward is to lead patients into social rehabilitation by improving their activities of daily living (ADL). There is an expectation that the demand for rehabilitation will continue to grow as the prevalence of strokes continues to increase.

One risk factor associated with stroke onset is chronic kidney disease (CKD), according to the 2015 Japanese guidelines for the management of strokes and national and international epidemiological studies [1–5]. Furthermore, the Fukuoka Stroke Registry reported that 32.1% of patients hospitalized for a stroke also had CKD [6]. In Japan, 30% of men and 40% of women aged over 65 years are CKD patients [7]. The number of CKD patients in Japan is approximately 13,300,000 and continues to increase [8]. Lifestyle-related diseases such as hypertension, dyslipidemia, and diabetes mellitus have been implicated in the development and progression of CKD. CKD management is extremely important, because it is a risk factor not only for end-stage renal failure, but also for coronary artery diseases such as myocardial infarction or stroke [2, 9].

For CKD patients, strict management of their blood pressure, lipids, and plasma glucose is required in order to prevent a stroke reoccurrence [1]. As a consequence, some patients are forced to polypharmacy. Elderly patients often experience adverse drug reactions due to polypharmacy because their decrease in organ function is associated with the metabolism of multiple drugs [10, 11]. Therefore, we consider that there is a possibility that polypharmacy may negatively affect the rehabilitation outcome of stroke patients in the convalescent rehabilitation wards. Previous studies have reported the intervention of a nutritional support team or stroke subtype associated with the functional independence measure (FIM), which is an evaluation index of ADL [12, 13]. However, few reports exist on the influence of drugs on FIM. Therefore, we investigated the effects of drugs on FIM in stroke patients with CKD.

2. Materials and Methods

2.1. Subjects. Among the 244 stroke patients with CKD who were discharged from Sagami Rehabilitation Hospital between January 2013 and July 2014, 144 patients were included in the present study. The frequency of adverse drug reactions rapidly increases when six or more drugs are prescribed to elderly people aged over 65 years [14]. Therefore, it is desirable to reduce the number of drugs to five or less in order to reduce the likelihood of adverse drug reactions. Thus, we defined a combination of at least six or more drugs as polypharmacy. We divided stroke patients into those taking six or more drugs (polypharmacy group) and those taking less than six drugs (nonpolypharmacy group) upon admission. In addition, CKD stage was classified according to the Japanese Society of Nephrology Evidence-based Clinical Practice Guideline for CKD 2013.

2.2. Investigation Items. We examined the following parameters to elucidate any differences between the polypharmacy and nonpolypharmacy groups: patient gender, age, body mass index, days from stroke onset to admission, length of stay, number of drugs upon admission, number of complications, medical history (e.g., hypertension, diabetes mellitus, dyslipidemia, cardiovascular disease, dementia, and epilepsy), FIM score on admission and at discharge [total (FIM-T), motor (FIM-M), and cognitive (FIM-C) items], and FIM efficiency. Laboratory data included albumin (Alb), serum creatinine (Scr), creatinine clearance (Ccr), estimated glomerular filtration rate (eGFR), glycosylated hemoglobin (HbA1c), fasting plasma glucose level (FPG), total cholesterol (T-Cho), total lymphocyte count (TLC), and white blood cell (WBC) count. We assessed these data upon admission to a convalescent rehabilitation ward. Drug data included the use of antihypertensive, antidiabetic, antihyperlipidemic, bisphosphonate, antidementia, antiepileptic, antianxiety, and hypnotic sedative drugs. Accordingly, these data were included as well. In addition, in many countries, including the United States, Scr had been measured using the Jaffe method. However, Scr is measured using an enzymatic method in Japan. The Modification of Diet in Renal Disease (MDRD) equation based on Scr measured using the enzymatic method was published in 2006. In consideration of racial differences, the Japanese coefficient of 0.741 has been published by the Japan Society of Nephrology.

Male

$$\text{GFR} = 0.741 \times 175 \times (\text{Age})^{-0.203} \times (\text{Scr})^{-1.154} \quad (1)$$

Female

$$\text{GFR} = 0.741 \times 0.742 \times 175 \times (\text{Age})^{-0.203} \times (\text{Scr})^{-1.154} \quad (2)$$

In the present study, eGFR was calculated based on the MDRD equation as shown above.

2.3. Outcome Measure. The primary outcome of the present study is FIM-M efficiency. We compared the FIM-M efficiency between the polypharmacy and nonpolypharmacy groups to investigate the effect of drug number on FIM-M efficiency. ADL indicators such as the FIM and the Barthel index were used in the evaluation during the recovery period [15]. Given that the reliability of FIM has been previously confirmed [16], we used FIM to evaluate ADL in the present study. FIM is a scale for assessing disability based on five items associated with cognition and 13 items associated with motor function in daily life, with each item scoring from one (requiring maximum assistance) to seven (full independence). Thus, the highest possible total score is 126 and the lowest is 18, with higher scores indicating greater autonomy. FIM efficiency shows the improvement of rehabilitation per day. The FIM efficiency score was calculated as the FIM score at discharge minus the FIM score upon admission/length of stay.

The rehabilitation team in the convalescent rehabilitation ward of the Sagami Rehabilitation Hospital was composed of a physician, experienced nurses, physical therapist, occupational therapist, a speech-language-hearing therapist, and a pharmacist. The rehabilitation team discussed and evaluated the patients' FIM as a team. Drugs used during the observation period were changed to generic drugs or to drugs of the same type, or there were no drug changes. The same units of rehabilitation were carried out for all patients regardless of their FIM score, stroke severity, or length of stay.

2.4. Data Analysis. Results are presented as the mean ± standard deviation (SD). A normality test was performed to compare the data volume between the two groups. We used a Student's t-test for normally distributed data or a Mann–Whitney U-test for data that were not normally distributed. We used χ^2 test or Fisher's exact test to compare categorical data. Next, we adjusted for confounding variables and performed a multiple logistic regression analysis with the presence or absence of polypharmacy as a dependent variable to investigate the association of polypharmacy with patient background, FIM efficiency, laboratory data, and drugs used on admission. We chose significant factors as independent variables (age, diabetes mellitus, and FIM-M efficiency) on the basis of the univariate analysis results. Confirmation was achieved by a multiple logistic regression analysis when no multicollinearity existed between factors using Pearson or Spearman's rank-correlation coefficients. Results were considered significant at $p < 0.05$. All statistical analysis was performed using JMP® Pro (version 12, SAS Institute Inc., Cary, NC, USA).

2.5. Ethics Regulation. The present study was conducted with the approval of the Sagami Rehabilitation Hospital ethics committee. In addition, the present study was conducted with the approval of the School of Pharmacy, Nihon University Ethics Committee. This was a retrospective study using medical records, which complied with the Declaration of Helsinki and the "Ethical Guidelines for Clinical Research."

3. Results

3.1. Selection of Subjects. Figure 1 shows a flow chart of the selection of subjects who were discharged from the Sagami Rehabilitation Hospital between January 2013 and July 2014. According to a previous study [17], we defined an FIM-T of 110–126 points as mild, 80–109 points as moderate, and 18–79 points as severe. We excluded 22 patients with a mild FIM-T score upon admission, as it was difficult to ascertain their FIM efficiency because of the ceiling effect. In addition, 12 patients were excluded from the study because they were reported as having heart failure that may limit their movement according to the degree of severity as established by the New York Heart Association. Thirteen patients with depression and four patients with schizophrenia were also excluded because they were restricted in rehabilitation and their FIM could not improve because they were unable to complete routine rehabilitation [18, 19]. We also excluded 49 patients with matching FIM scores upon admission. Finally, a total of 144 patients were selected for the present study, 48 in the polypharmacy group and 96 in the nonpolypharmacy group. Furthermore, we surveyed patients with a CKD stage of 1–4.

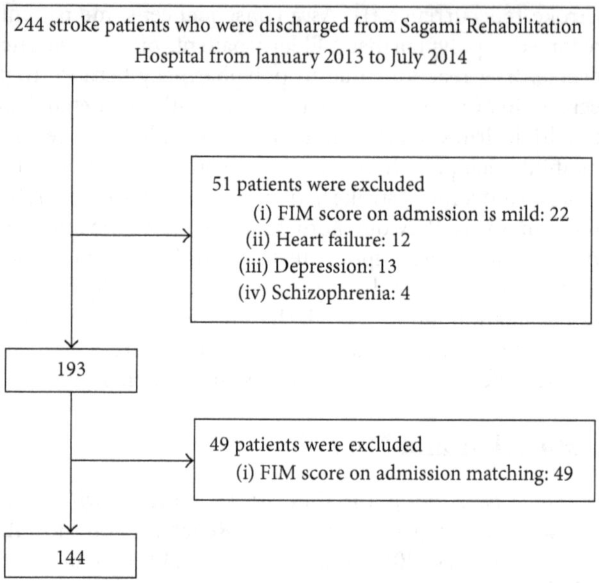

FIGURE 1: Flow chart of the subject selection process.

3.2. Comparison of Patient Background Characteristic Data. Patient background characteristic data for the polypharmacy and nonpolypharmacy groups are given in Table 1. The number of females was significantly higher in the polypharmacy group compared with that in the nonpolypharmacy group (60.4% versus 42.7%, $p = 0.045$). Similarly, the number of drugs upon admission, number of complications, and a medical history of diabetes mellitus and dementia were significantly higher in the polypharmacy group compared with those in the nonpolypharmacy group (drugs upon admission: 7.8±2.2 versus 3.4±1.2, $p \leq 0.0001$; number of complications: 3.8 ± 2.1 versus 2.7 ± 1.8, $p = 0.001$; diabetes mellitus: 41.7% versus 20.8%, $p = 0.008$; dementia: 25.0% versus 8.3%, $p = 0.006$). On the other hand, age, days from stroke onset to admission, length of stay, and a medical history of hypertension, dyslipidemia, cardiovascular disease, or epilepsy were not significantly different between the two groups.

3.3. Comparison of FIM Score upon Admission and at the Time of Discharge and FIM Efficiency. The FIM score upon admission and at the time of discharge and the FIM efficiency between the polypharmacy and nonpolypharmacy groups are given in Table 2. In the polypharmacy group, the FIM-T score at discharge was significantly lower compared with that in the nonpolypharmacy group (81.0 ± 29.6 points versus 90.5 ± 25.5 points, $p = 0.047$). Similarly, the FIM-C at discharge, FIM-T, and FIM-M efficiency in the polypharmacy group were significantly lower compared with those in the nonpolypharmacy group (FIM-C at discharge: 25.0 ± 7.7 points versus 28.1 ± 6.4 points, $p = 0.011$; FIM-T efficiency: 0.15 ± 0.14 versus 0.23 ± 0.17, $p = 0.007$; FIM-M efficiency: 0.13±0.12 versus 0.20±0.15, $p = 0.009$). In contrast, the FIM-T, FIM-M, and FIM-C upon admission, FIM-M at discharge, and FIM-C efficiency were not significantly different between the two groups.

3.4. Comparison of Laboratory Data. The laboratory data between the polypharmacy and nonpolypharmacy groups are given in Table 3. The FPG in the polypharmacy group was significantly higher compared with that in the nonpolypharmacy group (134.7 ± 39.0 mg/dL versus 119.8 ± 38.1 mg/dL, $p = 0.029$). On the other hand, the Alb, Scr, Ccr, eGFR, HbA1c, T-Cho, TLC, and WBC were not significantly different between the two groups.

3.5. Comparison of Oral Drugs Being Taken upon Admission. The number and type of drugs being taken upon admission between the polypharmacy and nonpolypharmacy groups are given in Table 4. The number of patients on antidiabetic drugs in the polypharmacy group was significantly higher compared with that in the nonpolypharmacy group (33.3% versus 9.4%, $p = 0.0003$). Similarly, the number of patients on antidementia and antianxiety drugs in the polypharmacy group was significantly higher compared with that in the nonpolypharmacy group (antidementia drug: 12.5% versus 2.1%, $p = 0.01$; antianxiety drug: 10.4% versus 0%, $p = 0.001$). On the other hand, the number of patients on antihypertensive, antihyperlipidemic, bisphosphonate, antiepileptic, and hypnotic sedative drugs was not significantly different between the two groups.

3.6. Multiple Logistic Regression Analysis. We evaluated all 144 patients using a multiple logistic regression analysis. Various factors associated with polypharmacy were used in

TABLE 1: Comparison of patient background characteristic data.

Characteristic	All patients (n = 144)	Polypharmacy group (n = 48)	Nonpolypharmacy group (n = 96)	p value
Gender, females n, (%)	70 (48.6)	29 (60.4)	41 (42.7)	0.0450
Age (y)	70.9 ± 10.2	72.7 ± 10.1	70.0 ± 10.2	0.1475
Body mass index (kg/m^2)	21.4 ± 3.8	21.8 ± 3.8	21.2 ± 3.8	0.3895
Days from stroke onset to admission (d)	44.3 ± 25.7	46.0 ± 18.0	43.1 ± 28.7	0.4542
Length of stay (d)	123.9 ± 46.6	123.7 ± 45.2	123.9 ± 47.5	0.9789
Number of drugs upon admission	4.9 ± 2.7	7.8 ± 2.2	3.4 ± 1.2	<0.0001
Number of complications	3.0 ± 2.0	3.8 ± 2.1	2.7 ± 1.8	0.0011
Medical history n, (%)				
Hypertension	119 (82.6)	40 (83.3)	79 (82.3)	0.8764
Diabetes mellitus	40 (27.8)	20 (41.7)	20 (20.8)	0.0085
Dyslipidemia	36 (25.0)	15 (31.2)	21 (21.9)	0.2207
Cardiovascular disease	40 (27.8)	15 (31.3)	25 (26.0)	0.5107
Dementia	20 (13.9)	12 (25.0)	8 (8.3)	0.0064
Epilepsy	16 (11.1)	7 (14.6)	9 (9.4)	0.3485

Mean ± SD.

TABLE 2: Comparison of FIM score upon admission and at the time of discharge and FIM efficiency.

Characteristic	All patients (n = 144)	Polypharmacy group (n = 48)	Nonpolypharmacy group (n = 96)	p value
FIM score on admission (points)				
Total	63.5 ± 23.4	61.7 ± 22.1	64.4 ± 24.1	0.5167
Motor	40.2 ± 18.0	39.7 ± 17.1	40.4 ± 18.5	0.8346
Cognitive	23.4 ± 7.6	22.0 ± 7.3	24.1 ± 7.8	0.1276
FIM score at discharge (points)				
Total	87.4 ± 27.2	81.0 ± 29.6	90.5 ± 25.5	0.0471
Motor	60.4 ± 21.6	56.2 ± 22.9	62.4 ± 20.7	0.1017
Cognitive	27.1 ± 6.9	25.0 ± 7.7	28.1 ± 6.4	0.0119
FIM efficiency (points/d)				
Total	0.21 ± 0.16	0.15 ± 0.14	0.23 ± 0.17	0.0070
Motor	0.18 ± 0.14	0.13 ± 0.12	0.20 ± 0.15	0.0095
Cognitive	0.03 ± 0.05	0.02 ± 0.04	0.03 ± 0.05	0.1590

Mean ± SD.

TABLE 3: Comparison of laboratory data.

Characteristic	All patients (n = 144)	Polypharmacy group (n = 48)	Nonpolypharmacy group (n = 96)	p value
Alb (g/dL)	3.8 ± 0.5	3.7 ± 0.5	3.8 ± 0.4	0.6261
Scr (mg/dL)	0.7 ± 0.3	0.7 ± 0.2	0.7 ± 0.3	0.8645
Ccr (mL/min)	52.0 ± 17.7	51.2 ± 19.6	52.4 ± 16.7	0.7503
eGFR (mL/min/1.73 m^2)	78.3 ± 31.5	75.2 ± 29.2	80.4 ± 32.5	0.2622
HbA1c (NGSP) (%)	6.1 ± 1.1	6.3 ± 1.2	5.9 ± 0.9	0.0923
FPG (mg/dL)	124.8 ± 38.9	134.7 ± 39.0	119.8 ± 38.1	0.0295
T-Cho (mg/dL)	175.6 ± 35.0	173.1 ± 39.5	177.0 ± 3.3	0.5463
TLC (×10^3/μL)	1.5 ± 0.6	1.5 ± 0.5	1.5 ± 0.6	0.9251
WBC (×10^3/μm)	6.3 ± 1.9	6.3 ± 1.7	6.4 ± 1.9	0.8085

Mean ± SD.

TABLE 4: Comparison of oral drugs being taken upon admission.

Characteristic	All patients (n = 144)	Polypharmacy group (n = 48)	Nonpolypharmacy group (n = 96)	p value
Drugs n, (%)				
Antihypertensive	101 (70.1)	35 (72.9)	66 (68.8)	0.6065
Antidiabetic	25 (17.4)	16 (33.3)	9 (9.4)	0.0003
Antidyslipidemic	47 (32.6)	18 (37.5)	29 (30.2)	0.3790
Bisphosphonate	3 (2.1)	2 (4.2)	1 (1.0)	0.2158
Antiepileptic	16 (11.1)	8 (16.7)	8 (8.3)	0.1336
Antidementia	8 (5.6)	6 (12.5)	2 (2.1)	0.0101
Antianxiety	5 (3.5)	5 (10.4)	0 (0)	0.0013
Hypnotic sedative	14 (9.7)	5 (10.4)	9 (9.4)	0.8423

Mean ± SD.

TABLE 5: Multiple logistic regression analysis of various factors associated with polypharmacy.

Factor	Adjusted odds ratio	95% CI	p value
Age	1.0424	1.0025–1.0871	0.0366
FIM-M efficiency	0.0078	0.0002–0.1717	0.0015
Diabetes mellitus	4.1131	1.7872–9.8729	0.0008

95% CI: 95% confidence interval (n = 144).

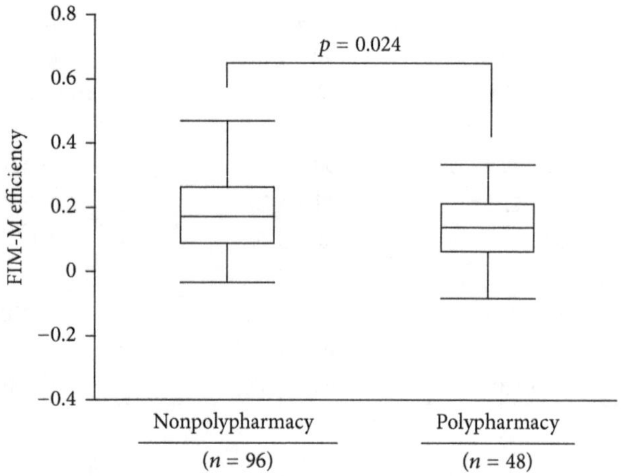

FIGURE 2: Effect of polypharmacy on FIM-M efficiency. We used the Mann–Whitney U-test to compare FIM-M efficiency between polypharmacy and nonpolypharmacy. Polypharmacy: six or more drugs; nonpolypharmacy: less than six drugs.

the analysis. Significant differences were observed in FIM-M efficiency, age, and the presence of diabetes mellitus (Table 5).

3.7. Effect of Polypharmacy on FIM-M Efficiency. We examined the effect of the presence or absence of polypharmacy on FIM-M efficiency. FIM-M efficiency was significantly lower in the polypharmacy group compared with the nonpolypharmacy group (0.13 ± 0.12 versus 0.20 ± 0.15, $p = 0.024$) (Figure 2).

4. Discussion

The most important finding of the present study was the positive association of polypharmacy with FIM-M efficiency, age, and diabetes mellitus. In addition, we revealed that when it comes to polypharmacy, it is difficult to obtain FIM-M efficiency when compared with nonpolypharmacy.

It is important to strictly manage blood pressure, lipids, and plasma glucose as a secondary preventive measure against stroke [1]. CKD is one risk factor of a stroke and its onset and progression is associated with lifestyle-related diseases such as hypertension, dyslipidemia, and diabetes mellitus [1]. Therefore, it is often the case that stroke patients with CKD are necessarily associated with polypharmacy. Adverse drug reactions or the risk of adverse drug interactions caused by polypharmacy has been reported globally and has become a major obstacle in the safe and reliable treatment of a stroke [20]. In particular in the convalescent rehabilitation ward, we cannot deny the possibility that the expression of adverse drug reactions affects FIM. Therefore, we examined the effect of polypharmacy on FIM.

We revealed that diabetes mellitus was the most common independent risk factor with approximately 4.1-fold increased risk of polypharmacy. The number of drugs used by patients with diabetes mellitus was approximately two agents larger than that used by patients without diabetes mellitus (6.3 ± 2.7 versus 4.4 ± 2.4, $p < 0.0001$). Even if the control of plasma glucose is improved with a monotherapy of an antidiabetic drug, sometimes the control deteriorates and the use of a multidrug combination is necessary. In addition, it is known that plasma glucose control deteriorates due to comorbidity or concomitant drugs. Oishi et al. [21] reported a change in the antidiabetic drugs prescribed from 2002 to 2011. While monotherapy accounted for 52.8% of the cases in 2002, it had significantly decreased to 35.9% by 2011. Subsequently, a combination therapy increased over time and a dual therapy was the most common treatment protocol by 2011, accounting for 33.3% of cases. A triple therapy accounted for 24.8% of cases, although this treatment protocol has seen a twofold increase compared to 2002. A quad combination therapy increased 14.8-fold from 2002 to 2011. Thus, combination therapies have the potential to be further increased because of the sodium-glucose transporter 2 inhibitors that are currently on the market. We believe that the trends of antidiabetic drugs are reflected as the factor of polypharmacy in patients with diabetes mellitus.

In the present study we revealed the possibility that the FIM-M efficiency was also associated with polypharmacy. In other words, the FIM-M efficiency with six or more drugs was significantly lower compared with less than six drugs. This finding suggested that, in regard to polypharmacy, it was difficult to obtain FIM-M efficiency. Thus, we consider it desirable to reduce the number of prescribed drugs to five or fewer drugs when possible.

The results of the univariate analysis demonstrated that the proportion of antidiabetic, antidementia, and antianxiety drugs in the polypharmacy group was significantly higher compared with those in the nonpolypharmacy group. Therefore, these drugs might be associated with FIM-M efficiency. In the relationship between antidiabetic drugs and FIM-M efficiency, maximum oxygen uptake of diabetic patients without an insulin treatment was 20% less than in healthy people [22]. In addition, a decrease in the muscle mass of the lower limbs or in muscle strength of elderly patients with type 2 diabetes mellitus was significantly greater compared with nondiabetic elderly patients [23]. Furthermore, in a previous study we revealed that when using sulfonylurea (SU) drugs, it was difficult to obtain FIM efficiency compared with using α-glucosidase inhibitor (α-GI) drugs [24]. Thus, we consider that it is difficult to obtain FIM efficiency because of diabetic patients' reduced ability to exercise, likely due to an insufficient supply of ATP caused by a failure of oxidative phosphorylation in their mitochondria [25]. In other words, as the average age of patients in the polypharmacy group was 74 years, the energy production required in order to exercise would have been decreased by a reduced incorporation of plasma glucose into the periphery due to their decrease in skeletal muscle. Therefore, we should further examine whether reinforcing muscular strength by resistance training or the administration of branched-chain amino acids would improve muscle-building or physical strength for patients who have a decreased muscle mass [26–28].

The reason why the use of antidementia drugs was significantly higher in the polypharmacy group was as follows. Dementia is a chronic disease that increases in prevalence as one ages, and there are some cases in which patients with dementia have a chronic disease in addition to dementia because they are elderly. Furthermore, in recent years, drugs with different mechanisms of action, such as memantine, are on the market and the usefulness of administering cholinesterase inhibitors in combination with memantine has been demonstrated in patients with moderate to severe Alzheimer's disease. Therefore, patients with these diseases have an especially high risk of polypharmacy. In the present study, the number of drugs upon admission in patients with Alzheimer's disease tends to be higher compared with patients without Alzheimer's disease (5.8 ± 2.8 versus 4.8 ± 2.6, $p = 0.070$). Alzheimer's disease often presents as recent memory impairment and behavioral psychological symptoms of dementia such as wandering, restlessness, and emotional instability. In Lewy body dementia, mental symptoms such as delusion and hallucinations are frequent. There are some cases where antipsychotic, antianxiety, and psychotropic drugs are administrated as supportive care for these symptoms. Thus, this factor has the potential to promote polypharmacy.

Associated with antidementia drugs and FIM-M efficiency are some cases in which patients with Alzheimer's disease forget to eat or do not feel hungry due to cognitive dysfunction. In addition, as the dementia progresses it is difficult to eat because of emotional instability resulting in malnutrition which caused the anorexia and weight loss [29]. Soysal et al. [30] reported that cholinesterase inhibitors were associated with weight loss and elderly patients with dementia often have protein energy malnutrition [31]. Therefore, we believe that it is difficult to obtain FIM-M efficiency because dementia patients are prevented from recovering their body's functions due to less motivation, decreased strength, and fatigue due to malnutrition. We consider it important to perform nutritional management in order to improve strength and motivation that will enhance the effects of rehabilitation and consequently improve motor function.

In the present study we identified that age is also likely to be a factor of polypharmacy with a risk of up to 1.04-fold imposed by age. Toba et al. [10] reported that the number of drugs taken increased with age, a finding supported in the present study.

The present study contains several limitations. First, it was a cross-sectional, single-center study with only a small number of patients undergoing analysis. Second, we hypothesized that side effects caused by renal dysfunction may be involved in rehabilitation outcome. However, there were no significant differences in renal function between polypharmacy group and nonpolypharmacy group. Thus, in present study, we were unable to confirm the association between polypharmacy and renal function. Third, the severity of the dementia was unclear. In general, the Hasegawa Dementia Scale-Revised (HDS-R) or Mini-Mental State Examination (MMSE) is used as an objective assessment scale for the severity of dementia. However, in the present study we could not analyze these data adequately and consider this factor to likely affect our results. However, we do believe that this influence on the results was small because the FIM-C scores on admission were not significantly different between the polypharmacy and nonpolypharmacy groups. Fourth, doses and types of drugs were not considered. We consider that this factor was likely to have affected the results of the present study because, especially for antidiabetic drugs, the frequency of hypoglycemia was different depending on the dose and type of drugs used. Thus, in the future, it is necessary to verify these points by a prospective cohort study.

5. Conclusion

Polypharmacy interferes with the rehabilitation of stroke patients with CKD. Pharmacists should make efforts to optimize prescriptions to be able to respond to the outcome of each individual patient, bearing in mind that each prescribed drug is necessary for the patient.

Competing Interests

The authors have no potential conflict of interests to declare with respect to the research, authorship, and/or publication of this article.

References

[1] The Japan Stroke Society, *Japanese Guidelines for the Management of Stroke*, 2015.

[2] T. Katsumata, "CKD and stroke," *Nosotchu*, vol. 36, no. 2, pp. 120–124, 2014.

[3] T. Ninomiya, Y. Kiyohara, M. Kubo et al., "Chronic kidney disease and cardiovascular disease in a general Japanese population: the Hisayama Study," *Kidney International*, vol. 68, no. 1, pp. 228–236, 2005.

[4] F. Irie, H. Iso, T. Sairenchi et al., "The relationships of proteinuria, serum creatinine, glomerular filtration rate with cardiovascular disease mortality in Japanese general population," *Kidney International*, vol. 69, no. 7, pp. 1264–1271, 2006.

[5] Y. Kokubo, S. Nakamura, T. Okamura et al., "Relationship between blood pressure category and incidence of stroke and myocardial infarction in an Urban Japanese population with and without chronic kidney disease: the suita study," *Stroke*, vol. 40, no. 8, pp. 2674–2679, 2009.

[6] T. Kitazono, Y. Kumai, H. Sugimori et al., "Impact of hypertension and chronic kidney disease on acute ischemic stroke; the Fukuoka Stroke Registry," *Japanese Journal of Stroke*, vol. 31, no. 6, pp. 564–569, 2009.

[7] E. Imai, M. Horio, K. Iseki et al., "Prevalence of chronic kidney disease (CKD) in the Japanese general population predicted by the MDRD equation modified by a Japanese coefficient," *Clinical and Experimental Nephrology*, vol. 11, no. 2, pp. 156–163, 2007.

[8] E. Imai, M. Horio, T. Watanabe et al., "Prevalence of chronic kidney disease in the Japanese general population," *Clinical and Experimental Nephrology*, vol. 13, no. 6, pp. 621–630, 2009.

[9] *Clinical Practice Guidebook for Diagnosis and Treatment of Chronic Kidney Disease*, 2012.

[10] K. Toba, M. Akishita, Y. Mizuno et al., "Adverse drug reaction in the elderly," *Japanese Journal of Geriatrics*, vol. 36, no. 3, pp. 181–185, 1999.

[11] M. Akishita, S. Teramoto, H. Arai et al., "Incidence of adverse drug reactions in geriatric wards of university hospitals," *Japanese Journal of Geriatrics*, vol. 41, no. 3, pp. 303–306, 2004.

[12] J. Senda, K. Ito, K. Hamada, T. Kotake, H. Kishimoto, and G. Sobue, "Investigation of inpatient rehabilitation outcomes in different ischemic stroke disease types : relationships with leukoaraiosis in MRI," *The Japanese Journal of Rehabilitation Medicine*, vol. 47, no. 8, pp. 559–568, 2010.

[13] W. Usui, S. Sonoda, T. Suzuki, S. Okamoto, T. Higashiguchi, and E. Saitoh, "Validating a Nutrition Support Team's (NST) effect in convalescent stroke rehabilitation using the functional independence measure," *The Japanese Journal of Rehabilitation Medicine*, vol. 45, no. 3, pp. 184–192, 2008.

[14] T. Kojima, M. Akishita, Y. Kameyama et al., "High risk of adverse drug reactions in elderly patients taking six or more drugs: analysis of inpatient database," *Geriatrics and Gerontology International*, vol. 12, no. 4, pp. 761–762, 2012.

[15] S. Saeki, "The knowledge of the rehabilitation necessary for clinical pathways for the local stroke network," *Japanese Journal of Stroke*, vol. 31, no. 6, pp. 497–501, 2009.

[16] K. J. Ottenbacher, Y. Hsu, C. V. Granger, and R. C. Fiedler, "The reliability of the functional independence measure: a quantitative review," *Archives of Physical Medicine and Rehabilitation*, vol. 77, no. 12, pp. 1226–1232, 1996.

[17] Y. Hirata, "Present conditions and future issues concerning a liaison critical path for stroke patient-from the standpoint of a convalescence rehabilitation hospital," *The Journal of Japan Society for Health Care Management*, vol. 9, pp. 409–414, 2008.

[18] A. Senzaki, M. Inamura, and T. Mamada, "Depression and dementia in elderly people," *Clinical Rehabilitation*, vol. 18, pp. 229–238, 2009.

[19] A. Senzaki, H. Takagi, H. Yamada, and M. Kamikozuru, "Rehabilitation for schizophrenic patients with spinal cord injury following suicidal jumping," *The Japanese Journal of Rehabilitation Medicine*, vol. 42, pp. 379–382, 2005.

[20] Y. Ogawa, M. Sakoh, K. Mihara, R. Ogawa, and H. Echizen, "Factors influencing the number of drugs among elderly patients hospitalized in a rehabilitation ward," *Journal of Pharmaceutical Health Care and Sciences*, vol. 42, pp. 56–62, 2016.

[21] M. Oishi, K. Yamazaki, F. Okuguchi, H. Sugimoto, A. Kanatsuka, and A. Kashiwagi, "Changes in oral antidiabetic prescriptions and improved glycemic control during the years 2002–2011 in Japan (JDDM32)," *Journal of Diabetes Investigation*, vol. 5, no. 5, pp. 581–587, 2014.

[22] H. M. De Feyter, N. M. A. Van den Broek, S. F. E. Praet, K. Nicolay, L. J. C. Van Loon, and J. J. Prompers, "Early or advanced stage type 2 diabetes is not accompanied by in vivo skeletal muscle mitochondrial dysfunction," *European Journal of Endocrinology*, vol. 158, no. 5, pp. 643–653, 2008.

[23] M. Leenders, L. B. Verdijk, L. van der Hoeven et al., "Patients with type 2 diabetes show a greater decline in muscle mass, muscle strength, and functional capacity with aging," *Journal of the American Medical Directors Association*, vol. 14, no. 8, pp. 585–592, 2013.

[24] E. Kose, M. Toyoshima, T. Tachi, H. Teramachi, T. Kawakubo, and H. Hayashi, "Effects of antidiabetes drugs on functional independence measure on a subacute rehabilitation ward for stroke patients," *Pharmazie*, vol. 70, no. 7, pp. 489–493, 2015.

[25] S. Kinugawa and H. Tsutsui, "Insulin resistance and exercise capacity: effect of intramyocellular lipid," *Cardioangiology*, vol. 71, pp. 424–429, 2012.

[26] R. J. F. Manders, S. F. E. Praet, R. C. R. Meex et al., "Protein hydrolysate/leucine co-ingestion reduces the prevalence of hyperglycemia in type 2 diabetic patients," *Diabetes Care*, vol. 29, no. 12, pp. 2721–2722, 2006.

[27] C. S. Katsanos, H. Kobayashi, M. Sheffield-Moore, A. Aarsland, and R. R. Wolfe, "A high proportion of leucine is required for optimal stimulation of the rate of muscle protein synthesis by essential amino acids in the elderly," *American Journal of Physiology-Endocrinology and Metabolism*, vol. 291, no. 2, pp. E381–E387, 2006.

[28] F. Yoshizawa, "The regulatory function of isoleucine in glucose metabolism and its clinical application," *Seikagaku*, vol. 86, no. 3, pp. 345–351, 2014.

[29] M. Kuzuya, "Nutrition," *Japanese Journal of Geriatrics*, vol. 50, no. 1, pp. 46–48, 2013.

[30] P. Soysal, A. T. Isik, B. Stubbs et al., "Acetylcholinesterase inhibitors are associated with weight loss in older people with dementia: a systematic review and meta-analysis," *Journal of Neurology, Neurosurgery & Psychiatry*, vol. 87, no. 12, pp. 1368–1374, 2016.

24

Osteosarcopenic Visceral Obesity and Osteosarcopenic Subcutaneous Obesity, Two New Phenotypes of Sarcopenia: Prevalence, Metabolic Profile, and Risk Factors

Simone Perna, Daniele Spadaccini, Mara Nichetti, Ilaria Avanzato, Milena Anna Faliva, and Mariangela Rondanelli

Department of Public Health, Experimental and Forensic Medicine, School of Medicine, Endocrinology and Nutrition Unit, University of Pavia, Pavia, Italy

Correspondence should be addressed to Simone Perna; simoneperna@hotmail.it

Academic Editor: Antonello Lorenzini

Background. The main criticism of the definition of "osteosarcopenic obesity" (OSO) is the lack of division between subcutaneous and visceral fat. This study describes the prevalence, metabolic profile, and risk factors of two new phenotypes of sarcopenia: osteosarcopenic visceral obesity (OSVAT) and osteosarcopenic subcutaneous obesity (OSSAT). *Methods.* A standardized geriatric assessment was performed by anthropometric and biochemical measures. Dual-energy X-ray absorptiometry (DXA) was used to assess body composition, visceral adipose tissue (VAT), subcutaneous adipose tissue (SAT), osteoporosis, and sarcopenia. *Results.* A sample of 801 subjects were assessed (247 men; 554 women). The prevalence of osteosarcopenic obesity (OSO) was 6.79%; OSSAT and OSOVAT were, respectively, 2.22% and 4.56%. OSVAT (versus the others) showed a higher level of inflammation (CRP and ESR, $p < 0.05$), bilirubin ($p < 0.05$), and risk of fractures (FRAX index over 15%, $p < 0.001$). Subjects with OSSAT did not show any significant risk factors associated to obesity. *Conclusions.* The osteosarcopenic visceral obesity phenotype (OSVAT) seems to be associated with a higher risk of fractures, inflammation, and a worse metabolic profile. These conditions in OSVAT cohort are associated with an increase of visceral adipose tissue, while patients with OSSAT seem to benefit related to the "obesity paradox."

1. Introduction

The main criticism of the definition of osteosarcopenic obesity or sarcopenic obesity is due to a lack of division between subcutaneous or visceral fat mass. Osteosarcopenic obesity (OSO) is a multifactorial syndrome that includes the following conditions: decrease of muscle mass and bone (osteopenia/osteoporosis and sarcopenia) and an increase of adiposity (obesity) [1]. Regarding the condition of adiposity, related to sarcopenia and osteoporosis, until now no study has considered the role of visceral fat.

Recent evidence by Dimitri et al. suggests that site-specific adiposity may exert differing effects on bone "with visceral fat acting as a pathogenic fat depot and subcutaneous fat exerting protective effects" [2]. For example, in the study performed by Perna et al., a positive association between adiposity and BMD was explained by biomechanical forces or by increased aromatization of androgens to weak estrogens in subcutaneous fat tissue [3].

The main risk factors associated with OSO are poor nutritional status, a high grade of inflammation, and fractures [4]. Recent findings suggest that the incidence of sarcopenia, sarcopenic obesity, and osteosarcopenic obesity was 31.5, 5.1, and 4.1%, respectively [5]. Recently, the prevalence of OSO was assessed as 19% in a study performed in Mexico. In addition, OSO is a common condition in middle-aged and older women, and it is independently associated with frailty and poor physical performance [6].

There are no other studies that have assessed the prevalence of OSO in a large population cohort and specifically

TABLE 1: Diagnostic criteria for osteosarcopenic obesity based on body composition (via dual-energy X-ray absorptiometry) [2, 3, 5].

Diagnostic criteria	*T*-score for BMD ≤ −1.0 SD at the hip femoral	SMI > 5.5 kg/h² for women and 7.23 kg/h² for men	Fat mass ≥ 38% for women and ≥28% for men	Visceral/subcutaneous fat ratio > 1
Osteopenia/osteoporosis	Yes	No	No	No
Sarcopenia	No	Yes	No	No
Visceral obesity	No	No	Yes	Yes
Subcutaneous obesity	No	No	Yes	No
Osteopenic sarcopenia	Yes	Yes	No	No
Osteopenic subcutaneous obesity	Yes	No	Yes	No
Osteopenic visceral obesity	Yes	No	Yes	Yes
Sarcopenic subcutaneous obesity	No	Yes	Yes	No
Sarcopenic visceral obesity	No	Yes	Yes	Yes
Osteosarcopenic subcutaneous obesity	Yes	Yes	Yes	No
Osteosarcopenic visceral obesity	Yes	Yes	Yes	Yes

BMD: bone mineral density; SMI: skeletal muscle index [5].

none in Europe. As shown recently, adiposity over 33% is negatively associated with bone mineral density (BMD) [7]. However, obesity has a role in overnutrition, as a mediator of the adverse effect in osteoporosis and sarcopenia pathogenesis [8].

In recent years, there has been increasing interest in the influence of visceral (VAT) and subcutaneous adipose tissue (SAT) on sarcopenic patient outcomes. Obesity has been identified as an adverse factor in sarcopenia [9]. As a matter of fact, no studies show the effects of visceral or subcutaneous fat as adverse prognostic factors in sarcopenic patients.

DXA quantification of fat distribution is a potentially valuable tool to diagnose these situations. To our knowledge, only one study has examined the relationship between visceral adipose tissue and muscle mass, reported to be a principal determinant of major morbidity in patients undergoing pancreaticoduodenectomy for cancer [10]. Most mechanisms of sarcopenia are also associated with visceral obesity, which may lead to a vicious cycle of intricate interactions among risk factors. Insulin resistance plays an important role in muscle fiber atrophy and mitochondrial dysfunction [11].

Also, intermuscular adipose tissue (IMAT) has been observed in the skeletal muscles of older adults with sarcopenia [12]. The relationship between the possible negative outcome associated with visceral adipose tissue and muscle mass is unclear.

This study describes for the first time in the literature two different phenotypes of sarcopenia: osteosarcopenic visceral obesity (OSVAT) and osteosarcopenic subcutaneous obesity (OSSAT), in addition to analyzing the prevalence, metabolic profile, and the risk factors.

2. Methods

2.1. Study Population. This cross-sectional study in elderly patients was performed in the city of Pavia (Italy). Inclusion criteria were (1) admission to the post-acute geriatric care unit for functional loss secondary to a nondisabling medical disease; (2) aged 65 years or older; (3) bedridden patients who were ambulatory prior to hospitalization; and (4) willingness to participate and to provide signed informed consent. At time of admission, the patients were not diagnosed with disabling diseases that could directly affect muscle weakness (such as neurological diseases, hip fractures, or amputations). However, participants with diabetes, metabolic disease, or neoplasia, as well as patients treated with steroids, or who were able to walk, were excluded.

Exclusion criteria were subjects affected by acute illness; severe liver (as defined by ESPEN guidelines) [13], heart (European Society of Cardiology proposed guidelines for the diagnosis) [14], or kidney dysfunction (acute kidney "risk, injury, failure" as defined by the newly developed RIFLE classification) [15]; or severe dementia (MMSE < 18 points) [15].

The stability of BMI is fundamental in our study because the body weight represents the primary difference between three groups; for this reason, we considered only people who had a stable clinical situation for the previous six months. The data were collected over a six-year period, from January 2011 to January 2017, in collaboration with the University of Pavia. All participants gave informed consent, and the research institute ethics committee approved the study.

2.2. Observed Variables. As suggested by Ilich et al. [5], there are two assessment steps for obtaining a more comprehensive diagnosis for OSO. This could be performed in any clinical setting with the DXA technology. Thus, the physical diagnosis would range from osteopenia, sarcopenia, and/or obesity to osteopenic obesity, sarcopenic obesity, osteopenic sarcopenia, and osteosarcopenic obesity (Table 1).

2.3. Diagnosis of Osteosarcopenic Visceral\Subcutaneous Obesity. Diagnostic criteria for osteosarcopenic obesity based on body composition (via dual-energy X-ray absorptiometry (DXA)) are shown in Table 1 [4, 5].

2.4. Body Composition Assessment. Body composition such as free fat mass (FFM), fat mass (FM), gynoid and android (subcutaneous or visceral) fat distribution was measured with dual-energy X-ray absorptiometry (DXA) using a Lunar Prodigy DXA (GE Medical Systems). The in vivo CVs were 0.89% and 0.48% for whole-body fat (fat mass) and FFM, respectively.

2.5. Diagnosis of Sarcopenia. The skeletal muscle index (SMI) was taken as the sum of the fat-free soft tissue mass of arms and the fat-free soft tissue mass of legs and dividing by height squared. Whole body and FFM were divided by height squared to obtain the FFM index (FFMI). FFM depletion was defined as having whole body FFMI below the 5th centile for age- and gender-matched healthy subjects [4, 5, 16]. Table 1 summarises the main phenotype of sarcopenia following the classification by Perna and Rondanelli and following the preexisting classification by Ilich et al. [4, 5].

2.6. Diagnosis of General Obesity. Obesity was diagnosed as fat mass over 38% in women and 27% in men. Taking into account that fat mass in normal weight subjects corresponds to 15% in men and 25% in women, ideal lean body mass was calculated in kilogram as the sum of 85% of ideal body weight in men or 75% in women plus 25% of excess weight, expressed as body weight exceeding a reference body weight corresponding to a BMI > 25 kg/m^2, considering that excess body weight includes not only fat mass but also a certain amount of muscle mass [5–19].

2.7. Diagnosis of Visceral or Subcutaneous Obesity. Abdominal subcutaneous fat (SAT) and visceral fat (VAT) were estimated within the android region. Fat mass data from DXA was transformed into X-ray computed tomography (CT) adipose tissue volume using a constant correction factor (0.94 g/cm^3). This gave the VAT/SAT ratio. Subjects with values over >1 were classified as having visceral obesity, and subjects with values under <1 were classified as having subcutaneous obesity.

2.8. Assessment of Bone Mineral Density. Bone mineral density (BMD) (g/cm^2) of the total hip was measured using DXA. BMD was labeled as normal when *T*-score > −1.0, osteopenic if *T*-score < −1.0, and osteoporosis when *T*-score ≤ −2.5 [19]. In addition, we evaluated the FRAX index that considers bone mineral density (BMD) at the femoral neck and the osteoporosis risk factors to calculate the fracture risk at 10 years [20].

2.9. Blood Sample Measurements. Fasting venous blood samples were drawn between 8 am and 10 am, with the subjects in a sitting position. Blood handling and collection were carried out under strictly standardized conditions. Folate and vitamin B12 were determined using an immunoassay, and high-performance liquid chromatography was used to measure total plasma homocysteine levels. Serum albumin was also analyzed using a nephelometric method, with a 2% coefficient of variation. Fasting blood total cholesterol and triglyceride levels were measured by automatic biochemical analyzer. High-sensitivity C-reactive protein (CRP), erythrocyte sedimentation rate (ESR), creatinine, azotemia, glycemia, and complete hemochrome were also assessed.

2.10. Assessment of Functional Performance. Handgrip strength was assessed using a Jamar dynamometer adhering to the standardized protocol recommended by the American Society of Hand Therapists. Dominant and nondominant handgrip strength was measured with a calibrated dynamometer (Baseline, Elmsford, NY, USA). The grip handle was adjusted to accommodate the size and comfort of the participant's hand, and the elbow was flexed to 90° to guarantee the strongest grip strength measurement. A weak handgrip was defined as <30 kg for men and <20 kg for women using the average value of the two handgrip measurements of the dominant hand [21–23].

2.11. Assessment of Hydration. All subjects underwent bioelectrical impedance vector analysis (BIVA) with a single-frequency bioimpedance analyzer (Model BIA 101, AKERN-RJL, Italy). Measurements were performed while the subjects lay comfortably, with the limbs abducted from the body. Body hydration was determined by injecting 800 μA and 50 kHz alternating sinusoidal current using a standard tetrapolar technique [24, 25].

2.12. Statistical Analysis. All analyses were performed using Statistical Package for the Social Sciences, version 22.0 (SPSS Inc., Chicago, IL, USA). Descriptive statistics representing raw data for each category and the full sample were provided, including means, standard deviations, and frequencies, where appropriate.

After the verification of the normal distribution of the continuous variables, data were analyzed and statistically compared between groups using one-way ANOVA. Variances were considered to be statistically significant for p value < 0.05.

Pearson's correlation analysis was used to compare the association between (OSVAT and OSSAT) versus other outcomes. The model was adjusted by the covariates of age and sex.

3. Results

3.1. Sample. As shown in Figure 1, we selected 1290 patients: 480 patients were lost because they were unable to be assessed with DXA. The sample of 801 subjects was categorized as follows: healthy (n = 41), with obesity (n = 57), with sarcopenia (n = 16), with osteopenia or osteoporosis only (n = 442), with sarcopenic (visceral or subcutaneous) obesity (n = 27), with osteopenic or osteoporosis and obesity (n = 63), with osteopenia or osteoporosis and sarcopenic (n = 90), and with osteosarcopenic obesity (n = 55).

3.2. Prevalence of Osteosarcopenic SAT and VAT. The prevalence of osteosarcopenic obesity was 6.86%, where the

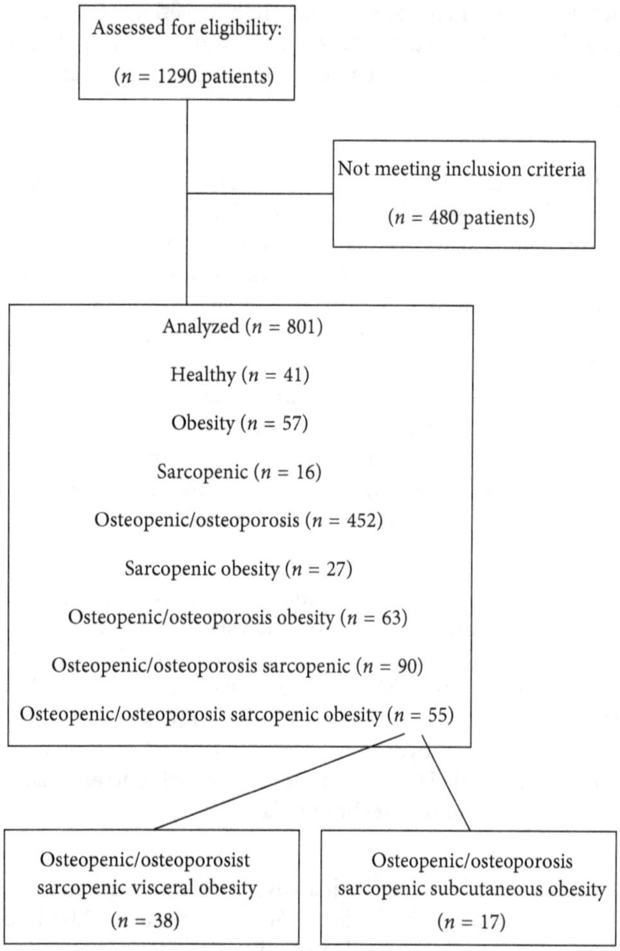

FIGURE 1: Flow diagram of the study.

OSOSAT and OSOVAT prevalence was, respectively, 2.10% and 4.70%.

It is interesting that those who were healthy (without sarcopenia, obesity, and osteopenia or osteoporosis) were only 5.5% of the sample.

The elderly with osteopenia and osteoporosis alone made up over 60% of the sample. This points the attention to this condition that involves 69% of women and 37% of men (without sarcopenia and obesity). In addition, sarcopenia is closely to osteoporosis and obesity.

3.3. Metabolic Profile of OS Visceral Obesity. Table 2 describes the characteristics of the sample. One-way ANOVA analysis of variance detected statistically significant differences between groups ($p < 0.05$) in hemoglobin, erythrocyte, iron, triglyceride, cholesterol, erythrocyte sedimentation rate, and FRAX index. As shown in Figure 2, OSVAT (versus the other cohorts) showed a higher level of inflammation (CRP > 2.34 mg/dl), higher risk of fracture (FRAX > 15%), and a reduction of glycemic control (glycemia > 112 mg/dl). In addition, VAT in OSVAT was significantly correlated to FRAX ($r = 0.316$; $p < 0.05$). We found that osteosarcopenic visceral obesity subjects had albumin values under the normal range (<4 gr\dl) and a higher level of azotemia (>40 mg\dl), glycemia (>110 mg\dl), and FRAX (15% of risk of fractures). Also, the level of strength was under the cut-off level of 20 kg for women.

3.4. Association between OSSAT\OSVAT with All Other Outcomes. Table 3 reports the results of Pearson's correlation analysis of VAT and SAT with other metabolic outcomes in the cohort of osteosarcopenic obesity women. VAT was significantly correlated to FRAX index ($r = 0.316$; $p < 0.05$) and to bilirubin ($r = 0.328$; $p < 0.05$). SAT was significantly correlated to platelet ($r = 0.290$; $p < 0.05$) and creatinine ($r = -0.299$; $p < 0.05$). No other correlations were observed.

4. Discussion

For the first time in the literature, this study describes two new phenotypes of sarcopenia: osteosarcopenic visceral obesity and osteosarcopenic subcutaneous obesity.

This study has been performed using dual-energy X-ray absorptiometry (DXA), with a new tool to quantify visceral adipose tissue (VAT) in the android region. In this way, the fat in the android region was categorized as visceral or subcutaneous. Using VAT, and in particular the VAT/SAT ratio with a cut-off ≥1 by DXA, we defined the visceral or subcutaneous phenotype.

An important finding of this study was the prevalence of OSVAT (4.56%) compared to OSSAT (2.22%). In general, the prevalence of OSO was 6.79%.

The main finding of this study is that VAT is deleterious for bones. In fact, the elderly patients with OSVAT had a higher risk of fractures, as suggested by a higher FRAX index.

The literature supports our results as regards the negative effects on bone of visceral adipose tissue. In particular, the negative effects are related to a proinflammatory state that promotes bone resorption [25–27].

Until now, there was great confusion in the literature of the effects on bone of obesity. We know that on one side obesity in elderly may be protective, following "obesity paradox," while on the other side fat heavily decreases osteoblastogenesis [27].

Similar findings were highlight by Ayça and Ilich et al. [28, 29], who showed that increased visceral fat and lower handgrip strength may be related to increased no-reflow rate.

In addition, we found differences on several metabolic outcome, such as hemoglobin, triglycerides, iron, calcium, and cholesterol (as indicators of nutritional status and mortality risk). Although OSVAT showed an impairment of nutritional status, as suggested by the level of albumin under the normal range with an increase of functional decline, with lower handgrip strength, this data did not differ from OSSAT.

Limitations to our study include small sample size of OSO and a majority of the sample being women. We could only study causation in the women in this study due to lack of men with these diagnoses. This study lays the foundations for the diagnostic values of these phenotypes of sarcopenia. We highlight that the current cut-point for visceral/subcutaneous obesity was defined using the VAT/SAT ratio. No study has assessed this specific cut-off.

TABLE 2: Characteristics and metabolic outcomes evaluated by ANOVA analysis.

Variables	Healthy ($n = 41$)	Obesity ($n = 57$)	Sarcopenic ($n = 16$)	Osteopenic/ osteoporosis ($n = 452$)	Sarcopenic obesity ($n = 27$)	Osteopenic/ osteoporosis obesity ($n = 63$)	Osteopenic/ osteoporosis sarcopenic ($n = 90$)	Osteosarcopenic subcutaneous obesity ($n = 17$)	Osteosarcopenic visceral obesity ($n = 38$)	p value
General data										
Age (years)	78.00 (9.25)	77.11 (7.88)	75.94 (7.41)	81.38 (7.19)	77.04 (9.59)	81.00 (2.65)	82.29 (7.00)	81.32 (4.32)	**82.43 (3.44)**	$p < \mathbf{0.001}$
Biochemical parameters										
WBC K/μL (4.00–10.00)	6.60 (1.85)	7.25 (2.29)	8.12 (2.74)	6.86 (3.42)	8.12 (2.34)	8.05 (2.31)	7.23 (2.56)	8.03 (2.18)	8.24 (1.34)	0.059
RBC M/μL (4.00–5.00)	4.32 (0.49)	4.30 (0.62)	3.97 (0.89)	4.21 (0.71)	4.33 (0.61)	4.05 (0.30)	4.12 (0.65)	4.16 (0.45)	4.15 (0.49)	0.545
Hb g/dl (12.0–16.0)	12.81 (1.77)	12.92 (1.60)	11.60 (2.04)	12.41 (1.69)	12.52 (1.44)	12.43 (1.53)	11.80 (1.87)	12.52 (1.31)	12.56 (1.41)	$p < \mathbf{0.001}$
Hct % (36.0–46.0)	38.74 (4.98)	38.91 (4.71)	35.38 (6.84)	37.91 (4.80)	39.46 (4.14)	38.10 (3.08)	36.23 (5.34)	38.08 (1.31)	37.95 (4.23)	$p < \mathbf{0.001}$
MCV fL (81.0–93.0)	88.93 (7.65)	88.56 (6.85)	91.83 (1.62)	91.47 (7.82)	87.95 (5.34)	91.90 (1.84)	81.17 (14.34)	90.06 (3.64)	84.867 ± 6.0335	0.103
PLT K/μL (140–450)	253.28 (99.03)	245.19 (87.80)	303.70 (88.56)	241.51 (99.03)	257.45 (79.50)	216.67 (61.01)	242.01 (82.83)	292.84 (101.03)	234.703 ± 71.5732	0.418
Lymph n K/μL (0.80–3.60)	1.73 (0.59)	1.98 (0.53)	1.46 (0.52)	1.78 (0.73)	2.12 (0.43)	1.75 (0.31)	1.71 (0.57)	2.10 (0.55)	1.72 (0.58)	0.289
Iron mcg/dl (45–145)	65.19 (32.29)	73.67 (26.63)	47.36 (25.06)	68.46 (34.28)	57.96 (26.90)	69.33 (34.27)	57.78 (32.01)	68.62 (37.12)	61.324 (25.41)	$p < \mathbf{0.001}$
Trg mmol/L (<200)	110.78 (43.59)	141.29 (68.36)	122.00 (38.55)	121.28 (60.56)	136.33 (42.81)	100.00 (19.98)	102.95 (38.29)	136.58 (46.91)	122.58 (47.19)	$p < \mathbf{0.05}$
Total Chol mmol/L (<200)	184.58 (41.04)	195.68 (44.50)	154.80 (32.59)	189.46 (43.10)	187.04 (45.07)	120.00 (33.18)	174.39 (45.46)	190.00 (37.59)	166.38 (48.56)	$p < \mathbf{0.001}$
Alb g/dl (4.02–4.76)	3.77 (0.54)	3.79 (0.46)	3.44 (0.60)	3.81 (2.99)	3.67 (0.53)	3.53 (0.42)	3.36 (0.57)	3.40 (0.35)	3.40 (0.53)	0.787
Creat mg/dl (0.57–1.11)	0.86 (0.28)	0.91 (0.28)	0.98 (0.50)	1.04 (2.61)	1.15 (0.67)	1.47 (0.55)	0.95 (0.62)	0.80 (0.18)	1.07 (0.70)	0.998
Azotemia mg/dl (14–40)	39.16 (13.10)	41.41 (16.90)	39.57 (16.39)	45.31 (22.94)	47.54 (24.17)	73.67 (31.90)	47.58 (34.35)	37.23 (12.66)	49.76 (24.84)	0.193
Na mmol/l (136–145)	139.11 (3.39)	139.06 (3.40)	138.27 (2.71)	139.28 (5.49)	139.82 (2.11)	141.67 (1.53)	138.72 (3.36)	138.87 (2.77)	138.85 (3.04)	0.867
K mmol/l (3.6–5.5)	4.14 (0.42)	4.19 (0.42)	4.19 (0.62)	4.19 (0.50)	4.30 (0.55)	4.33 (0.57)	4.20 (0.47)	4.50 (0.70)	4.00 (0.01)	0.948
Cl mmol/l (98–112)	102.84 (4.55)	103.63 (4.37)	101.93 (5.86)	104.19 (3.65)	104.32 (3.79)	105.33 (5.77)	103.68 (4.28)	104.43 (2.87)	103.38 (4.11)	0.164
Ca mmol/l (8.4–10.2)	9.01 (0.57)	9.18 (0.60)	9.12 (0.63)	10.97 (0.91)	9.43 (0.33)	8.97 (0.51)	8.92 (0.65)	8.97 (0.36)	9.05 (0.80)	$p < \mathbf{0.001}$
Uric acid mg/dl (2.6–6.0)	5.00 (1.69)	5.45 (1.60)	6.22 (2.69)	5.17 (2.17)	6.00 (1.70)	5.40 (0.35)	4.89 (2.04)	5.73 (1.77)	5.57 (1.97)	0.119
Bilirub mg/dl (0.30–1.20)	0.68 (0.33)	0.70 (0.40)	0.61 (0.51)	0.71 (0.58)	0.65 (0.37)	0.82 (0.07)	0.71 (1.53)	0.58 (0.38)	0.68 (0.34)	0.855
AST I.U./l (7–35)	17.33 (5.38)	21.60 (12.13)	23.13 (29.62)	19.79 (13.74)	19.00 (10.42)	14.67 (2.31)	21.79 (19.44)	20.29 (15.11)	21.94 (14.30)	0.702
ALT I.U./l (7–55)	14.65 (7.06)	21.32 (17.10)	18.20 (16.02)	17.51 (15.40)	19.22 (14.02)	10.33 (6.66)	18.51 (24.66)	17.00 (9.96)	23.73 (18.19)	0.577
gGT U/l (5–35)	25.26 (27.61)	27.83 (23.11)	29.50 (17.97)	31.37 (38.72)	27.88 (22.64)	29.67 (15.89)	41.80 (55.37)	48.47 (44.48)	44.00 ± 39.2776	0.144
GLIC mg/dl (70–110)	121.58 (68.94)	114.57 (33.91)	110.67 (34.92)	105.59 (35.11)	106.04 (28.64)	103.00 (33.45)	100.70 (48.08)	117.35 (35.55)	112.57 (37.06)	0.067
ESR mm/h (<15)	40.38 (28.12)	45.31 (26.38)	54.27 (38.95)	39.78 (29.16)	61.09 (30.48)	52.00 (28.69)	56.97 (33.44)	59.52 (28.83)	52.31 (28.55)	$p < \mathbf{0.001}$
CRP mg/dl (<0.50)	1.62 (2.66)	1.18 (2.73)	1.98 (3.02)	1.10 (2.24)	1.50 (2.24)	0.83 (0.97)	1.62 (2.57)	2.22 (4.22)	2.34 (3.59)	0.22
Folic acid ng/mL (4.6–18.7)	9.97 (15.35)	20.38 (76.10)	8.61 (11.96)	10.86 (23.44)	8.94 (8.81)	13.37 (7.58)	11.59 (18.87)	11.71 (11.84)	12.33 (18.44)	0.749
Vit B12 pg/mL (197–771)	457.42 (614.25)	429.17 (214.13)	630.00 (446.52)	512.04 (900.44)	830.50 (1455.45)	413.00 (202.30)	632.60 (1289.47)	544.92 (555.12)	625.57 (595.10)	0.803
Homoc micromol/l (5-12)	18.99 (7.99)	19.22 (7.16)	19.56 (5.95)	20.53 (11.12)	20.38 (12.12)	17.43 (2.47)	19.05 (8.56)	18.93 (8.98)	18.67 (5.22)	0.961
Nutritional assessment										
BMI kg/m^2 (18.5–24.9)	24.90 (2.81)	30.44 (4.28)	21.25 (2.89)	25.25 (4.76)	23.96 (2.89)	27.68 (3.99)	19.59 (2.60)	24.786 (2.44)	25.343 (3.24)	$p < \mathbf{0.001}$
Strength										
Handgrip dx kg (>20–>30)	22.14 (7.14)	17.71 (5.42)	17.64 (8.00)	16.51 (6.71)	17.47 (6.40)	22.67 (7.51)	16.02 (6.79)	14.00 (5.42)	18.06 (8.95)	$p < \mathbf{0.05}$
Risk of fractures										
Frax anca %	10.48 (0.97)	10.83 (1.10)	10.09 (0.72)	7.75 (1.37)	10.48 (1.26)	10.77 (2.67)	10.57 (3.48)	10.071 (2.66)	15.63 (4.40)	$p < \mathbf{0.001}$
Hdration										
TBW % (56–60)	54.76 (6.59)	48.43 (5.87)	60.08 (5.59)	52.26 (6.90)	52.66 (5.33)	50.71 (1.46)	58.44 (6.52)	48.73 (3.14)	51.42 (5.50)	$p < \mathbf{0.001}$
ECW % (42–50)	49.93 (5.78)	51.73 (4.39)	52.99 (5.50)	53.15 (6.97)	52.66 (3.57)	55.97 (4.49)	55.53 (7.91)	55.00 (3.51)	51.25 (1.51)	$p < \mathbf{0.05}$
ICW % (50–58)	50.05 (5.75)	48.29 (4.42)	46.57 (5.15)	46.77 (6.53)	47.52 (3.41)	44.03 (4.49)	44.54 (7.76)	45.00 (3.23)	48.75 (6.95)	$p < \mathbf{0.05}$

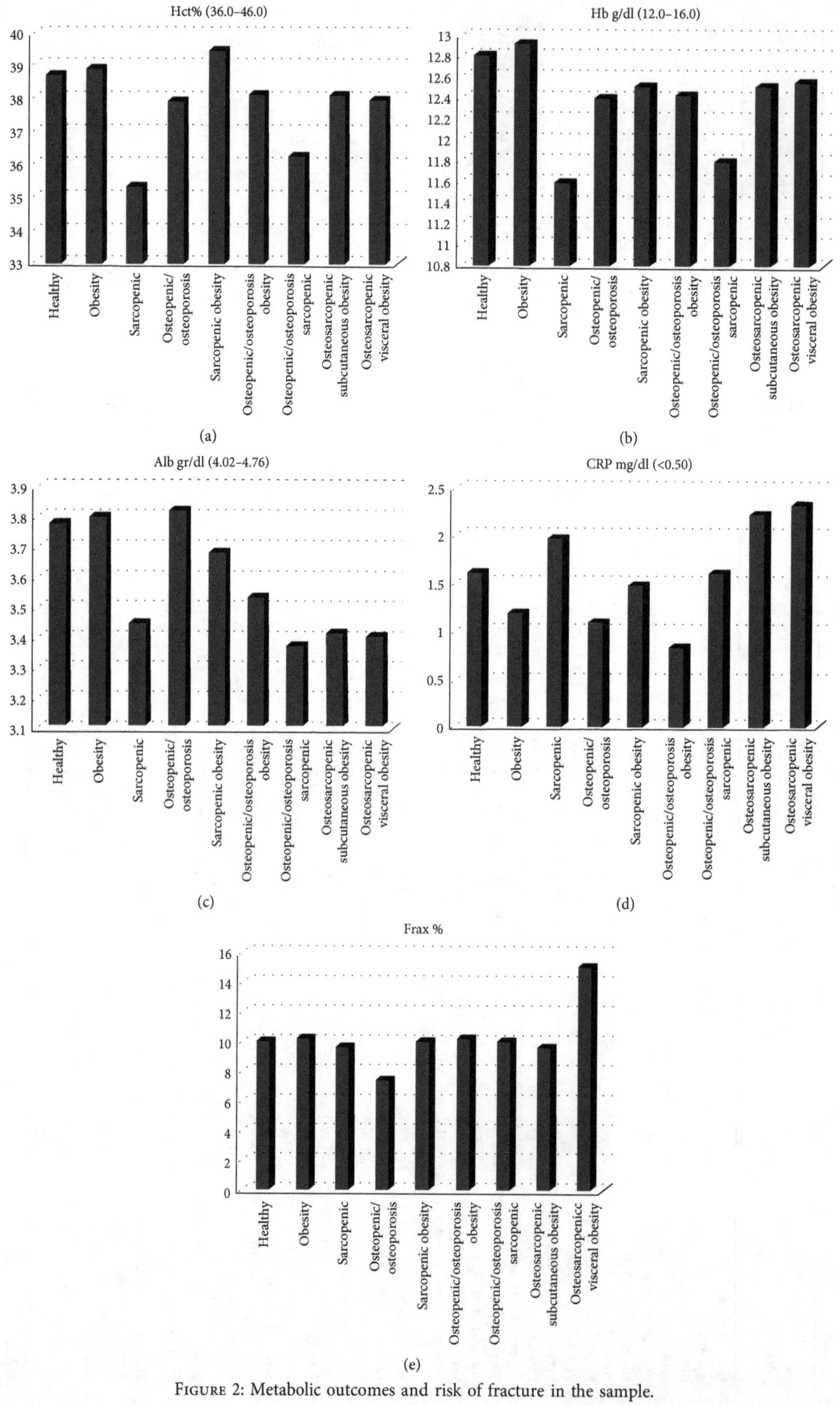

FIGURE 2: Metabolic outcomes and risk of fracture in the sample.

TABLE 3: Association between VAT and SAT with other outcomes in osteosarcopenic obesity cohort.

Variables	Visceral adipose tissue (r)	Subcutaneous adipose tissue (r)
WBC K/μL (4.00–10.00)	0.108 ($p = 0.442$)	0.051 ($p = 0.719$)
RBC M/μL (4.00–5.00)	0.087 ($p = 0.540$)	0.051 ($p = 0.719$)
Hb g/dl (12.0–16.0)	0.063 ($p = 0.642$)	0.003 ($p = 0.983$)
Hct % (36.0–46.0)	0.019 ($p = 0.896$)	0.020 ($p = 0.890$)
MCV fL (81.0–93.0)	−0.723 ($p = 0.123$)	−0.102 ($p = 0.722$)
PLT K/μL (140–450)	−0.155 ($p = 0.268$)	**0.296 ($p < 0.05$)**
Lymph n K/μL (0.80–3.60)	−0.115 ($p = 0.518$)	0.313 ($p = 0.069$)
Iron mcg/dl (45–145)	−0.058 ($p = 0.782$)	0.184 ($p = 0.200$)
Trg mmol/L (<200)	−0.155 ($p = 0.255$)	0.219 ($p = 0.222$)
Total Chol mmol/L (<200)	−0.236 ($p = .0.089$)	0.238 ($p = 0.092$)
Alb g/dl (4.02–4.76)	0.055 ($p = 0.692$)	0.699 ($p = 0.153$)
Creat mg/dl (0.57–1.11)	0.185 ($p = 0.189$)	**−0.299 ($p < 0.05$)**
Azotemia mg/dl (14–40)	0.190 ($p = 0.173$)	−0.237 ($p = 0.94$)
Na mmol/l (136–145)	−0.182 ($p = 0.192$)	0.186 ($p = 0.192$)
K mmol/l (3.6–5.5)	−0.574 ($p = 0.234$)	**0.960 ($p < 0.01$)**
Cl mmol/l (98–112)	0.087 ($p = 0.538$)	0.126 ($p = 0.384$)
Ca mmol/l (8.4–10.2)	−0.210 ($p = 0.130$)	−0.022 ($p = 0.978$)
Uric acid mg/dl (2.6–6.0)	−0.042 ($p = 0.765$)	−0.048 ($p = 0.742$)
Bilirub mg/dl (0.30–1.20)	**0.328 ($p < 0.05$)**	−0.108 ($p = 0.457$)
AST I.U./l (7–35)	0.076 ($p = 0.588$)	−0.170 ($p = 0.233$)
ALT I.U./l (7–55)	**0.340 ($p < 0.05$)**	−0.130 ($p = 0.363$)
gGT U/l (5–35)	−0.056 ($p = 0.696$)	0.124 ($p = 0.385$)
GLIC mg/dl (70–110)	0.049 ($0 = 0.730$)	0.101 ($p = 0.483$)
ESR mm/h (<15)	−0.053 ($p = 0.706$)	−0.031 ($p = 0.828$)
CRP mg/dl (<0.50)	0.047 ($p = 0.742$)	−0.050 ($p = 0.725$)
Folic acid ng/mL (4.6–18.7)	0.128 ($p = 0.471$)	0.032 ($p = 0.859$)
Vit B12 pg/mL (197–771)	0.001 ($p = 0.944$)	−0.065 ($p = 0.713$)
Homoc micromol/l (5–12)	−0.098 ($p = 0.588$)	−0.150 ($p = 0.413$)
BMI kg/m^2 (18.5–24.9)	**0.593 ($p < 0.001$)**	**0.387 ($p < 0.01$)**
FRAX anca %	**0.316 ($p < 0.05$)**	0.050 ($p = 0.750$)
Handgrip strength dx	0.335 ($p = 0.053$)	−0.079 ($p = 0.668$)
TBW % (56–60)	−0.180 ($p = 0.325$)	−0.185 ($p = 0.312$)
ECW % (42–50)	−0.274 ($p = 0.129$)	0.219 ($p = 0.228$)
ICW % (50–58)	−0.042 ($p = 0.767$)	0.031 ($p = 0.867$)

NS: not statistically significant.

5. Conclusion

Osteosarcopenic visceral obesity phenotype (OSVAT) seems to be closely linked to a higher risk of fractures, inflammation, and a worse metabolic profile. These conditions in the OSVAT cohorts are associated with an increase of visceral adipose tissue. It is important that patients with OSVAT must be assessed and identified in the clinical setting, because they are a cohort with a major exposure of risks. In contrast, the patients with OSSAT seem to be beneficiaries of the obesity paradox.

Consent

Participants in the cohorts included in this analysis provided informed consent at enrollment.

Conflicts of Interest

The authors declare that there are no conflicts of interest regarding the publication of this paper.

Authors' Contributions

Dr. Simone Perna and Dr. Mariangela Rondanelli wrote the paper and contributed to the conception or design of the work, data collection, data analysis, and interpretation, drafting the article, critical revision of the article, and final approval of the version to be published. Dr. Daniele Spadaccini, Dr. Ilaria Avanzato, Dr. Milena Anna Faliva, and Dr. Mara Nichetti contributed to the data collection.

References

[1] J. Z. Ilich, O. J. Kelly, J. E. Inglis, L. B. Panton, G. Duque, and M. J. Ormsbee, "Interrelationship among muscle, fat, and bone: connecting the dots on cellular, hormonal, and whole body levels," *Ageing Research Reviews*, vol. 15, pp. 51–60, 2014.

[2] P. Dimitri, N. Bishop, J. S. Walsh, and R. Eastell, "Obesity is a risk factor for fracture in children but is protective against fracture in adults: a paradox," *Bone*, vol. 50, no. 2, pp. 457–466, 2012.

[3] S. Perna, G. Peroni, M. A. Faliva et al., "Sarcopenia and sarcopenic obesity in comparison: prevalence, metabolic profile, and key differences. A cross-sectional study in Italian hospitalized elderly," *Aging Clinical and Experimental Research*, vol. 29, no. 6, p. 1249, 2017.

[4] P. JafariNasabian, J. E. Inglis, O. J. Kelly, and J. Z. Ilich, "Osteosarcopenic obesity in women: impact, prevalence, and management challenges," *International Journal Women's Health*, vol. 9, pp. 33–42, 2017.

[5] J. Z. Ilich, O. J. Kelly, and J. E. Inglis, "Osteosarcopenic obesity syndrome: what is it and how can it be identified and diagnosed?," *Current Gerontology and Geriatrics Research*, vol. 2016, Article ID 7325973, 7 pages, 2016.

[6] J. H. Chung, H. J. Hwang, H. Y. Shin, and C. H. Han, "Association between sarcopenic obesity and bone mineral density in middle-aged and elderly Korean," *Annals Nutrition Metabolism*, vol. 68, no. 2, pp. 77–84, 2016.

[7] C. Szlejf, L. Parra-Rodríguez, and O. Rosas-Carrasco, "Osteosarcopenic obesity: prevalence and relation with frailty and physical performance in middle-aged and older women," *Journal of the American Medical Directors*, vol. 18, no. 8, pp. 733.e1–733.e5, 2017.

[8] P. Y. Liu, J. Z. Ilich, K. Brummel-Smith, and S. Ghosh, "New insight into fat, muscle and bone relationship in women: determining the threshold at which body fat assumes negative relationship with bone mineral density," *International Journal of Preventive Medicine*, vol. 5, no. 11, pp. 1452–1463, 2014.

[9] M. Rondanelli, D. Guido, A. Opizzi, M. A. Faliva, S. Perna, and M. Grassi, "A path model of sarcopenia on bone mass loss in elderly subjects," *Journal of Nutrition Health and Aging*, vol. 18, no. 1, pp. 15–21, 2014.

[10] M. Sandini, D. P. Bernasconi, D. Fior et al., "A high visceral adipose tissue-to-skeletal muscle ratio as a determinant of major complications after pancreatoduodenectomy for cancer," *Nutrition*, vol. 32, no. 11, pp. 1231–1237, 2016.

[11] K. M. Choi, "Sarcopenia and sarcopenic obesity," *Korean journal of internal medicine*, vol. 31, no. 6, p. 1054, 2016.

[12] A. M. Abbatecola, G. Paolisso, P. Fattoretti et al., "Discovering pathways of sarcopenia in older adults: a role for insulin resistance on mitochondria dysfunction," *Journal of Nutrition Health and Aging*, vol. 15, no. 10, pp. 890–895, 2011.

[13] M. Plauth, E. Cabré, O. Riggio et al., "ESPEN guidelines on enteral nutrition: liver disease," *Clinical Nutrition*, vol. 25, no. 2, pp. 285–294, 2006.

[14] R. S. Vasan and D. Levy, "Defining diastolic heart failure a call for standardized diagnostic criteria," *Circulation*, vol. 101, no. 17, pp. 2118–2121, 2000.

[15] E. A. Hoste, G. Clermont, A. Kersten et al., "RIFLE criteria for acute kidney injury are associated with hospital mortality in critically ill patients: a cohort analysis," *Critical care*, vol. 10, no. 3, p. 73, 2006.

[16] R. N. Baumgartner, K. M. Koehler, D. Gallagher et al., "Epidemiology of sarcopenia among the elderly in New Mexico," *American Journal of Epidemiology*, vol. 147, no. 8, pp. 755–763, 1998.

[17] A. M. Joosen, A. H. Bakker, and K. R. Westerterp, "Metabolic efficiency and energy expenditure during short-term overfeeding," *Physiology Behavior*, vol. 85, no. 5, pp. 593–597, 2005.

[18] R. N. Baumgartner, S. J. Wayne, D. L. Waters, I. Janssen, D. Gallagher, and J. E. Morley, "Sarcopenic obesity predicts instrumental activities of daily living disability in the elderly," *Obesity Research*, vol. 12, no. 12, pp. 1995–2004, 2004.

[19] M. F. Folstein, S. E. Folstein, and P. R. McHugh, ""Mini-mental state": a practical method for grading the cognitive state of patients for the clinician," *Journal of Psychiatric Research*, vol. 12, no. 3, pp. 189–198, 1975.

[20] J. A. Kanis, A. Oden, H. Johansson, F. Borgström, O. Ström, and E. McCloskey, "FRAX® and its applications to clinical practice," *Bone*, vol. 44, no. 5, pp. 734–743, 2009.

[21] B. E. Klein, R. Klein, M. D. Knudtson, and K. E. Lee, "Frailty, morbidity and survival," *Archives of Gerontology and Geriatrics*, vol. 41, no. 2, pp. 141–149, 2005.

[22] D. B. Rolfson, S. R. Majumdar, R. T. Tsuyuki, A. Tahir, and K. Rockwood, "Validity and reliability of the Edmonton frail scale," *Age Ageing*, vol. 35, no. 5, pp. 526–529, 2006.

[23] V. Mathiowetz, C. Rennells, and L. Donahoe, "Effect of elbow position on grip and key pinch strength," *Journal of Hand Surgery American*, vol. 10, no. 5, pp. 694–697, 1985.

[24] F. Landi, R. Liperoti, A. Russo et al., "Sarcopenia as a risk factor for falls in elderly individuals: results from the il SIRENTE study," *Clinical Nutrition*, vol. 31, no. 5, pp. 652–658, 2012.

[25] C. T. Liu, K. E. Broe, Y. Zhou et al., "Visceral adipose tissue is associated with bone microarchitecture in the Framingham osteoporosis study," *Journal of Bone and Mineral Research*, vol. 32, no. 1, pp. 143–150, 2017.

[26] T. Lang, J. A. Cauley, F. Tylavsky et al., "Computed tomographic measurements of thigh muscle cross-sectional area and attenuation coefficient predict hip fracture: the health, aging, and body composition study," *Journal of Bone and Mineral Research*, vol. 25, no. 3, pp. 513–519, 2010.

[27] M. J. Ormsbee, C. M. Prado, J. Z. Ilich et al., "Osteosarcopenic obesity: the role of bone, muscle, and fat on health," *Journal of Cachexia, Sarcopenia and Muscle*, vol. 5, no. 3, pp. 183–192, 2014.

[28] B. Ayça, D. Kafadar, M. Avsar et al., "Lower muscle strength and increased visceral fat associated with no-reflow and high gensini score in STEMI," *Clinical and Applied Thrombosis/Hemostasis*, vol. 23, no. 4, pp. 367–373, 2015.

[29] J. Z. Ilich, J. E. Inglis, O. J. Kelly, and L. McGee, "Osteosarcopenic obesity is associated with reduced handgrip strength, walking abilities, and balance in postmenopausal women," *Osteoporosis International*, vol. 26, no. 11, pp. 2587–2595, 2015.

25

Effects of Long-Term Cultivation on Medium with Alpha-Ketoglutarate Supplementation on Metabolic Processes of *Saccharomyces cerevisiae*

Nadia Burdyliuk and Maria Bayliak

Department of Biochemistry and Biotechnology, Vasyl Stefanyk Precarpathian National University, 57 Shevchenko Str., Ivano-Frankivsk 76018, Ukraine

Correspondence should be addressed to Maria Bayliak; bayliak@ukr.net

Academic Editor: Arshad Jahangir

During last years, alpha-ketoglutarate (AKG), an important intermediate in the Krebs cycle, has been intensively studied as a dietary supplement with stress-protective and potential antiaging effects. Here, we examined the effects of exogenous AKG on metabolic processes and survival of yeast *Saccharomyces cerevisiae* during long-term cultivation. Growth on AKG had no effect on the total cell number but increased the number of reproductively active cells at the late days of cultivation (from day 7 to day 15). A gradual increase in levels of total protein, glycogen, and trehalose was found over 7-day cultivation with more pronounced effects in AKG-grown cells. In control cells, metabolic activity and the activities of superoxide dismutase and catalase decreased, whereas levels of carbonyl proteins and low-molecular-mass thiols increased during 7-day cultivation. This suggests development of oxidative stress in stationary phase cells. Meanwhile, stationary phase cells cultured on AKG possessed higher levels of low-molecular-mass thiols and lower levels of carbonyl proteins and α-dicarbonyl compounds when compared to control ones. Collectively, higher levels of storage carbohydrates and an activation of antioxidant defense with diminishing oxidative protein damage can prevent a loss of reproductive ability in yeast cells during long-term cultivation on AKG-supplemented medium.

1. Introduction

Alpha-ketoglutarate (AKG), an anion of alpha-ketoglutaric acid, is an important intermediate in the Krebs cycle, which couples amino acid metabolism with glucose oxidation. Studies on animal models have shown that dietary AKG supplementation confers many favorable effects on metabolism, stress resistance, and functional decline of various age-related processes [1–3]. The beneficial effects of AKG are mainly explained by its role as a precursor of certain amino acids such as glutamate, glutamine, leucine, and proline [1, 4]. In addition, AKG can inhibit protein catabolism and activate anabolic processes in animal tissues [5]. Furthermore, exogenous AKG can be involved in the Krebs cycle and thereby intensify mitochondrial respiration [6]. As a result, an increased generation of reactive oxygen species (ROS), by-products of respiratory metabolism, may occur and that leads to oxidative stress development [7]. Thus, the higher ROS levels were shown in nematode *Caenorhabditis elegans* grown on AKG-supplemented medium [8].

Previous studies suggest that exogenous AKG can induce oxidative stress of low intensity which is accompanied by an activation of defense systems. The mentioned stimulation of protective mechanisms was supposed to be responsible for higher tolerance of AKG-treated organisms to challenge strong oxidative or other kinds of stresses. It may also contribute to preventing functional decline with age [2, 3, 9]. In particular, the AKG-supplemented food prevents an age-related increase in free radical damage to biomolecules in aged mice [3] and increases stress resistance in *Drosophila melanogaster* flies [9]. Meanwhile, AKG affected differently oxidative stress parameters and levels of storage macromolecules in young and old *D. melanogaster* [2, 9]. We reported recently that growth on

AKG-supplemented medium increased resistance of exponentially growing yeast *Saccharomyces cerevisiae* to oxidative stress induced by hydrogen peroxide. Moreover, AKG-grown yeast cells showed higher activities of catalase and glutathione reductase and higher levels of thiol-containing compounds, indicating an activation of antioxidant system [10].

Since we already know that the functioning of antioxidant system is strongly connected with carbon/energetic metabolism and protein synthesis, this study aimed to examine effects of AKG on *S. cerevisiae* cells during long-term cultivation by analyzing various metabolic parameters and indicators of ROS homeostasis. Among metabolic parameters, the main focus was made on total metabolic activity and levels of protein and stored carbohydrates, glycogen, and trehalose, which play important roles in long-term yeast viability [11–14]. Prolonged cultivation leads to chronological aging of yeast cultures, which means a loss of reproductive ability that is followed by death of yeast cells [15, 16]. Based on data showing that AKG has antiaging effects in multicellular animals, we tested if AKG was able to slow down aging in *S. cerevisiae*. For this aim, the chronological lifespan of yeasts cultured with and without of AKG in the medium was determined by counting the number of reproductive active cells.

2. Materials and Methods

2.1. Reagents. Phenylmethylsulfonyl fluoride (PMSF), ethylenediamine-tetraacetic acid (EDTA), 2,4-dinitrophenylhydrazine (DNPH), 5,5′-dithiobis(2-nitrobenzoic acid) (DTNB), 2,3,5-triphenyltetrazolium chloride (TTC), Girard's reagent T, amyloglucosidase (#10115), trehalase (#T8778), peptone, and yeast extract were obtained from Sigma-Aldrich Corporation (USA); N,N,N′,N′-tetramethylethylenediamine (TEMED) and quercetin were from Reanal (Hungary); disodium salt of alpha-ketoglutaric acid (99% purity) was from Protista AB (Sweden); all reagents for determination of glucose and triacylglycerides (TAG), aspartate aminotransferase (AST), and alanine aminotransferase (ALT) activities were from PZ Cormay S.A. (Łomianki, Poland). All other reagents were obtained from local suppliers (Ukraine) and were of analytical grade.

2.2. Growth Conditions and Stationary Phase Survival. The *S. cerevisiae* strain YPH250 (wide type, *MAT***a** *trp1-Δ1 his3-Δ200 lys2-801 leu2-Δ1 ade2-101 ura3-52*) used in this study was kindly provided by Dr. Youshiharu Inoue (Kyoto University, Japan). Cells were grown at 28°C with agitation at 175 rpm in a liquid YPD medium containing 1% (w/v) yeast extract, 2% (w/v) peptone, 2% (w/v) glucose, and 10 mM disodium salt of α-ketoglutaric acid (AKG). The initial cell titre in the medium was about 0.3×10^6 cells/ml.

The viability of yeast cells was determined by colony-forming assay [15]. For that, aliquots (100 μl) were sampled from each of yeast cultures, serially diluted, and plated in triplicate on YPD medium with agar. The viability was assessed as an ability of an individual yeast cell to reproduce and form a colony (a colony-forming unit or CFU) on YPD agar. Cells were grown at 28°C for three days before colony counting. The total number of cells in yeast cultures was counted in a Goryaev chamber after 50-fold dilution under light microscope.

2.3. Preparation of Cell-Free Extracts and Assay of Enzyme Activities and Protein Concentration. The total number of cells in yeast cultures was counted at 18 h (late exponential phase), at 42 h (early stationary phase), and at day 7 (late stationary phase) of growth. After counting, cells from experimental cultures were collected by centrifugation at room temperature (5 min, 3000g) and washed with 50 mM potassium phosphate buffer (KPi, pH 7.0). The yeast pellets were weighed and resuspended in lysis buffer (50 mM KPi, 1 mM PMSF, and 0.5 mM EDTA). Cell extracts were prepared by vigorous vortexing yeast suspensions with glass beads (0.5 mm) as described earlier [17] and kept on ice for an immediate use. The biochemical parameters were measured with spectrophotometers Spekol-211 (Carl Zeiss, Jena, Germany) or SF-46 (LOMO, Leningrad, Russia).

The measurement of activities of superoxide dismutase (SOD, EC 1.15.1.1) and catalase (EC 1.11.1.6) was conducted as described earlier [17].

Activities of aspartate aminotransferase (ASAT, EC 2.6.1.1) and alanine aminotransferase (ALAT, EC 2.6.1.2) were measured by modified methods according to International Federation of Clinical Chemistry (IFCC) using Liquick Cor-ASAT and Liquick Cor-ALAT kits, respectively.

Soluble protein concentration was determined by the Coomassie brilliant blue G-250 dye-binding method [18] with bovine serum albumin as a standard.

2.4. Determination of Levels of Low-Molecular-Mass Thiols. To determine the levels of low-molecular-mass thiols (L-SH), aliquots of cell extracts were mixed with trichloroacetic acid to the final acid concentration of 10% and centrifuged (16,000g, 5 min, 21°C) to remove pelleted protein and the final supernatants were used for assays.

Free thiol-containing compounds were measured in the obtained protein-free supernatants as absorbance of thiol conjugates with 5,5′-dithiobis-2-nitrobenzoic acid (DTNB) at 412 nm [19]. Aliquots of supernatants (75 μl) were incubated with 20 μM DTNB in 50 mM KPi buffer (pH 8.0) in a final volume of 1.5 ml for 30 min. In blanks, supernatant was substituted for the respective volume of trichloroacetic acid solution. Absorption was read at 412 nm and a molar extinction coefficient of 14×10^3 $M^{-1}cm^{-1}$ was used to calculate the thiol level. Thiol levels were expressed as nanomoles of SH-groups per 10^8 cells.

2.5. Determination of α-Dicarbonyl Compounds and Carbonyl Proteins. The content of carbonyl groups in proteins (CP) was measured by determining the amount of 2,4-dinitrophenylhydrazone formed upon reaction with 2,4-DNPH as described previously [17]. Carbonyl content was calculated from absorbance of 2,4-dinitrophenylhydrazone measured at 370 nm using an extinction coefficient of 22 $mM^{-1}cm^{-1}$. The results are expressed in nanomoles per mg of protein.

α-Dicarbonyl compounds (DC) were measured by the Girard-T reaction [20]. The absorbance of the disubstituted compound, which is formed by binding of two Girard's reagent T molecules to dicarbonyl groups, was measured at a maximum absorption wavelength of 325 nm using an extinction coefficient of 18.8 $mM^{-1}cm^{-1}$ for glyoxal [16]. The results are expressed in nanomoles of glyoxal equivalents per mg of soluble protein.

2.6. Determination of Carbohydrate and Triacylglyceride Levels. For experiments, 2×10^8 cells from experimental cultures were harvested and washed twice with distilled water. The yeast pellets were resuspended in 50 mM Na-acetate buffer (pH 5.2) for carbohydrate measurement or in PBST buffer (10 mM Na_2HPO_4, 2 mM KH_2PO_4, 137 mM NaCl, 2,7 mM KCl, and 0.05% Triton X-100, pH 7.4) for triacylglyceride assay. The cell suspensions were vortexed for 7 min with glass beads (2 : 1, w/w, yeasts/beads) at room temperature and heated at 70°C for 5 min to inactivate endogenous enzymes. Cell debris was removed by centrifugation for 15 min at 16000g at room temperature. The cell extracts were used for the further assays.

The content of free intracellular glucose was measured by glucose oxidase assay using a diagnostic kit, Liquick Cor-glucose, following the manufacturer's instructions. The content of glycogen and trehalose in cell extracts was determined by measuring glucose released by amyloglucosidase or trehalase, respectively [21]. For that, 10 μl of the sample was incubated overnight with 10 μl (1 U/ml) amyloglucosidase or 10 μl (0.025 U/ml) trehalase with slight agitation at 37°C. The amount of glucose released from trehalose and glycogen was determined by Liquick Cor-glucose kit. The levels of trehalose and glycogen were calculated by subtraction of the amount of free intracellular glucose from the total glucose content in samples after overnight incubation with the enzymes. Standard glucose solutions in a concentration range from 2 to 20 μg/ml were used to calculate glucose content in yeast cell extracts. Results are expressed as μg glucose per 10^8 cells.

Triacylglyceride (TAG) levels were measured using a diagnostic kit, Liquick Cor-TG, following the manufacturer's instructions. Standard TAG solutions in the concentration range from 3 to 30 μg/ml were used for calculation of TAG content in yeast cell extracts. Results are expressed as μg TAG per 10^8 cells.

2.7. Determination of Metabolic Activity. To evaluate metabolic activity of the yeast, 2,3,5-triphenyltetrazolium chloride was used [16]. For experiments, 3×10^8 cells from experimental cultures were harvested and washed twice with distilled water. The yeast pellets were resuspended in 1 ml of 50 mM KPi (pH 7.0) and mixed with 0.35 ml of 0.5% 2,3,5-triphenyltetrazolium chloride (TTC). Metabolically active cells are able to reduce the dye to a water-insoluble red formazan that was extracted from the cells with ethanol/acetone mixture (2 : 1), and the absorbance of this solution was measured at 485 nm [22]. The results are expressed as OD_{485} units per 10^8 cells.

2.8. Statistical Analysis. Experimental data are expressed as the mean value of 4–8 independent experiments ± the standard error of the mean (SEM). Comparison between means was performed using a two-tailed Student's t-test or analysis of variance (ANOVA) followed by the Student-Newman-Keuls test.

3. Results

3.1. Alpha-Ketoglutarate Increases Reproductive Ability of Yeast Cells in Aged Cultures. Yeast cells were cultivated in rich YPD medium. In the YPD medium, yeast cells are actively budding and produce a large amount of young cells. Thus, the population always contains a mixture of young and old yeast cells. It causes troubles with an accurate estimation of maximal yeast lifespan. Furthermore, regrowth of yeast cells can be observed due to utilizing the nutrients released by dead cells after the culture reaches the maximum density [15]. Despite these limitations, the cultivation in YPD medium allows estimating reliably the effects of different supplements on aging rate of yeast populations [16, 23, 24]. In particular, we previously found the ability of *Rhodiola rosea* extract to increase yeast viability in the YPD medium under prolonged cultivation [24].

Earlier, we examined the effects of different AKG concentrations on yeast growth in the YPD medium and oxidative stress resistance of exponentially growing yeast cells [10]. We found that at the concentration of 10 mM AKG had no effect on yeast growth but it enhanced endogenous antioxidant defense and increased yeast resistance to oxidative stress. In addition, the medium supplemented with sodium chloride was used as an additional control to exclude effects of sodium ions. We did not found any effects of 20 mM NaCl on antioxidant defense system and yeast stress resistance. In this study, the total cell number and number of reproductively active cells were measured in yeast cultures grown on YPD medium supplemented with 10 mM AKG. In both control and AKG-supplemented cultures, the total cell number was changed in a similar way during cultivation (Figure 1(a)). At 18 h of growth, yeast cultures had the lowest cell number, which later increased approximately twice at 42 h ($P < 0.005$). Then, the number of cells increased slightly at day 3 ($P < 0.05$) and remained unchanged till day 11. By 16% and 13%, reductions in total cell number were observed at day 15 in the control and experimental cultures, respectively, compared with day 11 (Figure 1(a)). The number of reproductively active cells in yeast cultures was assessed by the ability of a cell to form a colony on YPD agar plates. As seen in Figure 1(b), colony-forming ability increased from day 1 to day 11 in both yeast cultures. It correlated to higher total cell number in these cultures (Figure 1(a)). However, total number of cells and number of reproductively active cells were coincided only at day 1. At further cultivation, the number of reproductive active cells was lower than the total cell number, suggesting a decrease in reproductive potential of yeast cultures with an age. Colony-forming abilities were similar in the control and AKG-supplemented cultures at days 1–3. However, AKG-supplemented cultures had by 25% and 35% more reproductively active cells at days 7 and 11

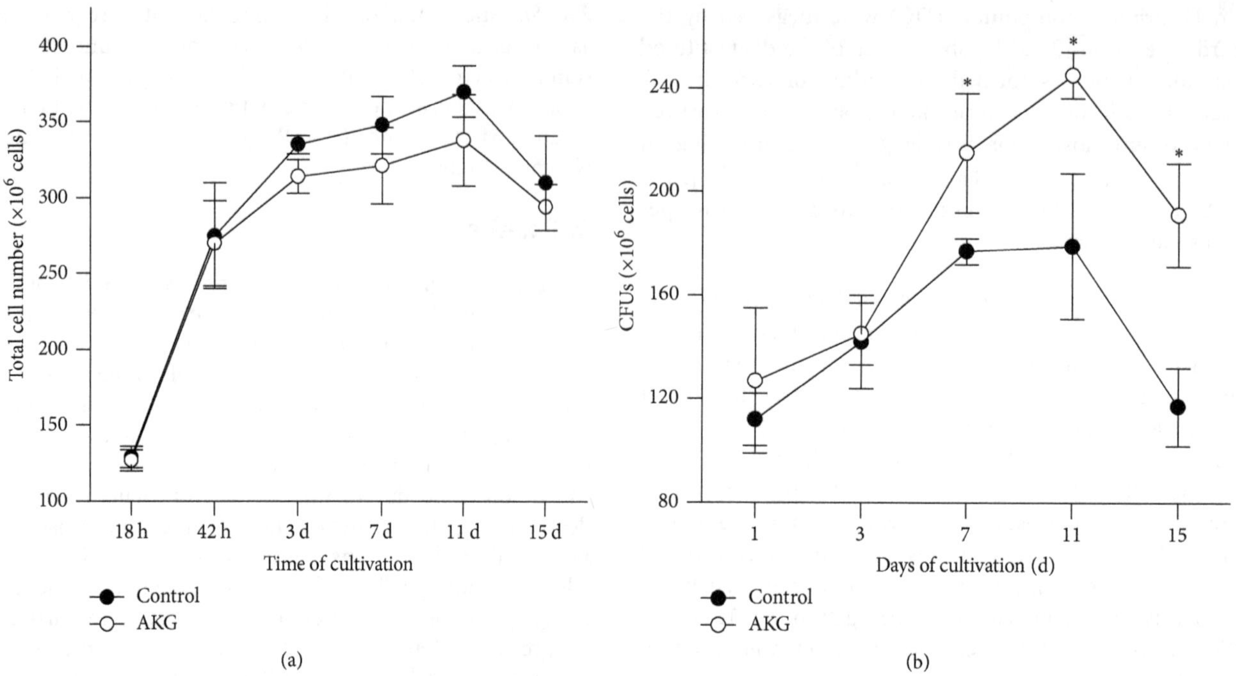

FIGURE 1: Effects of growth conditions on total cell number (a) and number of colony-forming units (CFUs) (b) in *S. cerevisiae* cultures. Yeast cells were grown during 7 days in the control medium or in the medium supplemented with 10 mM AKG. The starting cell concentration in the medium was about 0.3×10^6 cells/ml. Results are shown as means ± SEM ($n = 5$–7). *Significantly different from respective control values with $P < 0.05$ using Student's t-test.

TABLE 1: Wet biomass and levels of α-dicarbonyl compounds (DC) and triacylglycerides (TAG) in *S. cerevisiae* cells during prolonged cultivation in the control or 10 mM AKG-supplemented medium.

Parameter	Growth conditions					
	Control			10 mM AKG		
	18 h	42 h	7 d	18 h	42 h	7 d
Wet biomass (mg/10^8 cells)	6.90 ± 0.81	NS	NS	7.90 ± 0.27*	NS	NS
TAG, μg/10^8 cells	16.5 ± 1.1	15.2 ± 2.3	15.2 ± 1.6	15.6 ± 1.7	18.5 ± 3.1	16.7 ± 2.5
DC, nmol glyoxal equivalents/mg protein	NS	NS	7.01 ± 0.33	NS	NS	5.53 ± 0.38*

Results are shown as means ± SEM ($n = 6$–8). *Significantly different from respective control values with $P < 0.01$ using Student's t-test. NS: not studied.

compared to the control ones. At day 15, reproductive ability of yeast cells was markedly reduced in comparison with day 11, but the control cells demonstrated more substantial loss of ability to reproduce than AKG-grown ones. Upon the similar total cell number, AKG-supplemented cultures had by 60% higher number of reproductive cells at day 15 than the control ones.

3.2. Cultivation on AKG Increases Cell Biomass and Protein Level in Yeast Cells. Protective effects of AKG on yeast viability were observed already at day 7 of cultivation (Figure 1(b)). Therefore, we examined several biochemical parameters characterizing the intensity of metabolic processes in *S. cerevisiae* cells cultivated with and without 10 mM AKG during a 7-day period. The parameters were measured in cells collected at late exponential phase (18 h), early stationary phase (42 h), and late stationary phase of growth (7 d). In Figure 2, we show level of water-soluble protein and activities of two enzymes of amino acid metabolism, ALAT and ASAT. Level of water-soluble protein increased over a time of cultivation on both control and AKG-supplemented media (Figure 2(a)). As a result, control and AKG-cultivated cells had 60% and 43% higher protein levels, respectively, at day 7 compared with 18 h of growth. Meanwhile, the cultivation on AKG-supplemented medium promoted higher protein levels in yeast cells. In particular, AKG-grown cells displayed 31% and 19% higher protein levels at 18 h and day 7, respectively, compared to the control ones at the same time points. Notably, in parallel with an increased protein level at exponential phase, AKG-grown cells had 15% higher wet biomass than the control ones (Table 1).

The activities of ALAT were similar in the control and AKG-grown cells over the cultivation period (Figure 2(b)). Yeast cells demonstrated the highest ALAT activity at 18 h

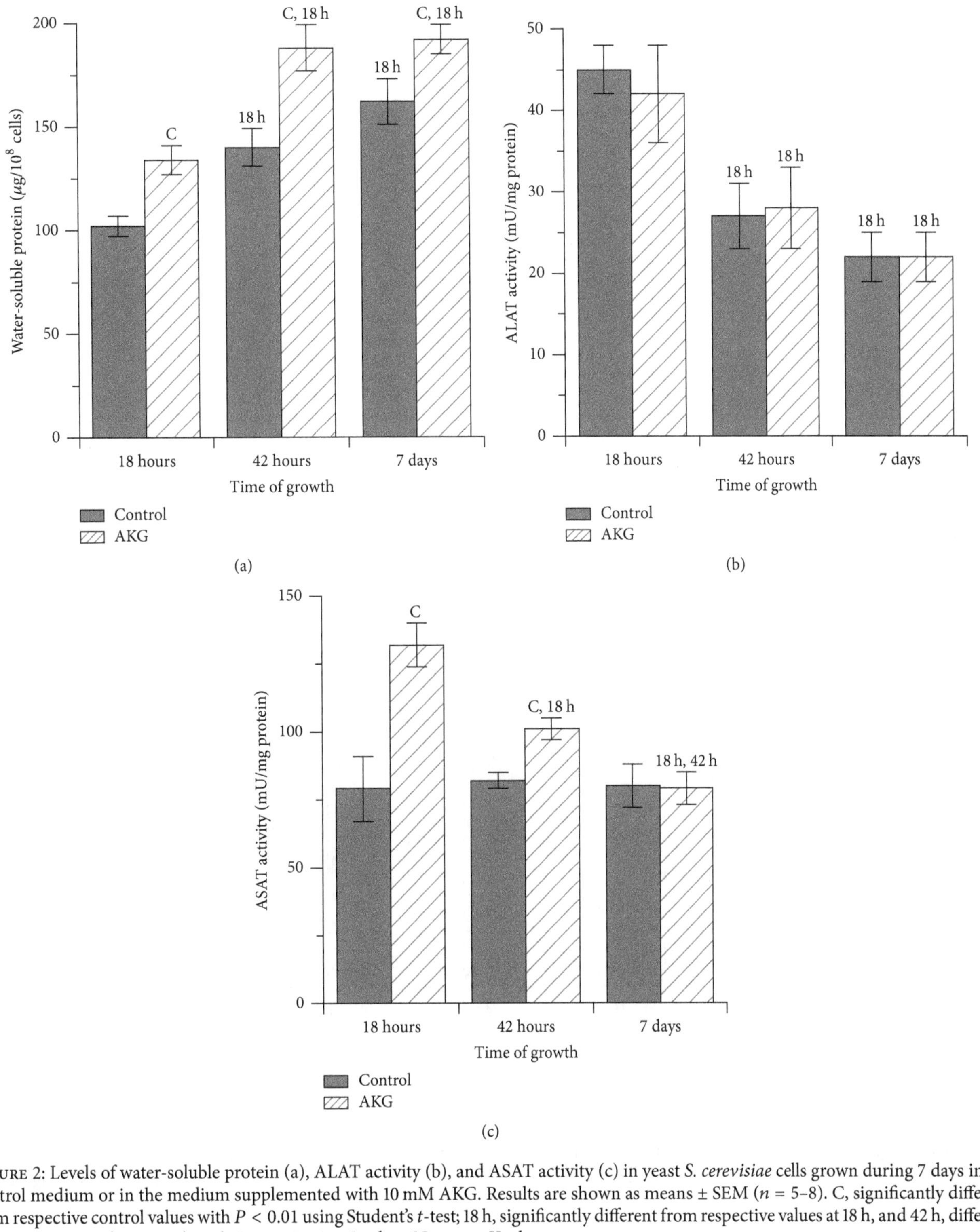

FIGURE 2: Levels of water-soluble protein (a), ALAT activity (b), and ASAT activity (c) in yeast *S. cerevisiae* cells grown during 7 days in the control medium or in the medium supplemented with 10 mM AKG. Results are shown as means ± SEM (n = 5–8). C, significantly different from respective control values with $P < 0.01$ using Student's t-test; 18 h, significantly different from respective values at 18 h, and 42 h, different from respective values at 42 h with $P < 0.05$ using Student-Newman-Keuls test.

of growth with further decreasing enzyme activity by ~40% and 50% at 42 h and day 7, respectively. The activity of ASAT showed different activity patterns in the control and AKG-cultivated cells (Figure 2(c)). At 18 h of growth, AKG-grown cells had 40% higher ASAT activity as compared to the control cells. The ASAT activity was unchanged in the control cells during next days of cultivation, whereas in AKG-grown cells, the activity demonstrated a time-dependent decrease, being 23% and 40% lower at 42 h and day 7, respectively, compared with the one at 18 h.

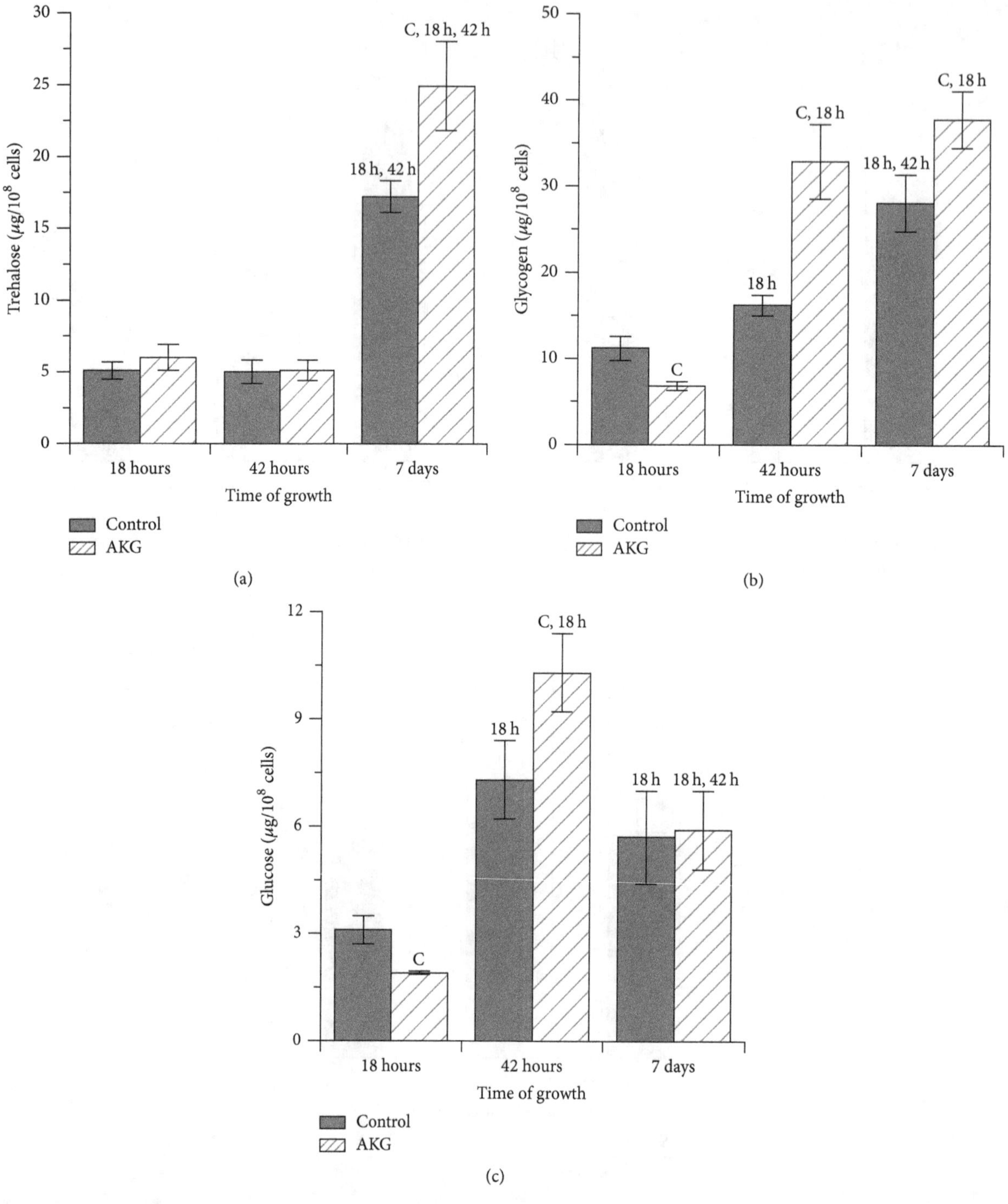

FIGURE 3: Levels of reserve carbohydrates, trehalose (a) and glycogen (b), and free glucose (c) in *S. cerevisiae* cells grown during 7 days in the control medium or in the medium supplemented with 10 mM AKG. Results are shown as means ± SEM ($n = 6$–8). Statistic as in Figure 2.

3.3. AKG Increases Levels of Storage Carbohydrates in Yeast Cells. In the control and AKG-supplemented cultures, content of storage carbohydrates, trehalose and glycogen, rose over experimental time (Figures 3(a) and 3(b)). Trehalose levels were similar at 18 h and 42 h of cultivation in both yeast cultures (Figure 3(a)). At day 7, 3.3-fold and 4.6-fold increases in trehalose level were observed in cells cultivated with and without AKG, respectively, when compared with the same yeast cultures at 18 h of cultivation. When comparing control and AKG-grown yeast cultures within day 7, in the supplemented yeasts, trehalose level was 1.4-fold higher. The level of glycogen was 40% lower in exponential phase cells grown with AKG supplementation compared to the control ones (Figure 3(b)). During next days of cultivation, glycogen seemed to be significantly accumulated in yeast cells from both cultures, but control cells showed less glycogen than

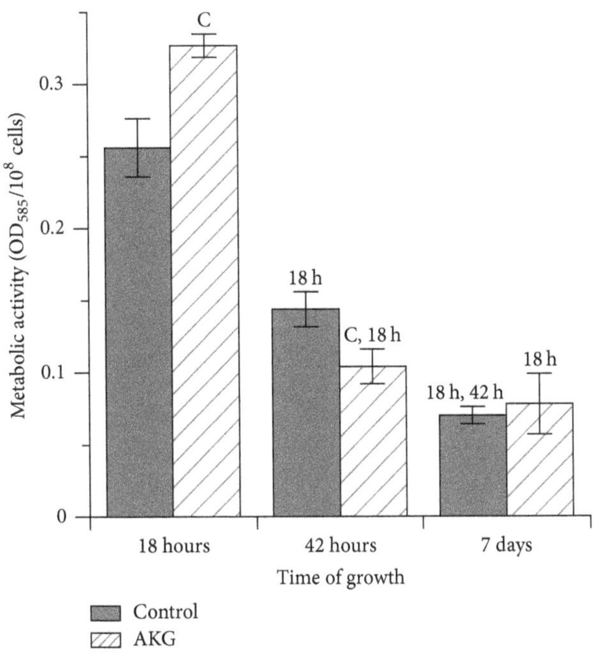

FIGURE 4: Metabolic activity of *S. cerevisiae* cells grown during 7 days in the control medium or in the medium supplemented with 10 mM AKG. Results are shown as means ± SEM (n = 5-6). Statistic as in Figure 2.

AKG-supplemented ones. Thus, glycogen levels were 1.4-fold and 2.5-fold higher in the control cells and 4.8-fold and 5.5-fold higher in AKG-cultivated cells at 42 h and day 7, respectively, as compared to values at 18 h of growth. A bell-shaped mode of glucose content was observed for yeast cells (Figure 3(c)). In both control and AKG-grown cells, glucose level was the lowest at 18 h and demonstrated a significant increase at 42 h (2.4-fold in the control and 5.5-fold in AKG-grown cells). Then, at day 7, in AKG-supplemented yeasts, glucose content became lower than that observed previously at 42 h of cultivation, but it was still higher than at 18 h, whereas for the control yeasts, the difference was not significant. It should be noted that AKG-grown cells displayed 39% lower and 40% higher free glucose level at 18 h and 42 h, respectively, than control cells at the same cultivation time. At day 7, there was no difference in glucose levels in cells from both cultures. The levels of TAG in yeast cells did not change regardless of cultivation period or AKG supplementation (Table 1).

3.4. Effect of AKG on Metabolic Activity and Parameters of ROS Homeostasis in Yeast Cells. The total metabolic activity of yeast cells decreased over time of cultivation in both the control and AKG-supplemented media (Figure 4). In cells cultivated with AKG supplementation, metabolic activity was 1.3-fold higher at exponential phase (18 h) and 28% lower when yeasts entered stationary phase (42 h) as compared to the control cells. At day 7 of cultivation, cells from both control and experimental cultures had similar levels of this parameter.

To investigate AKG influence on the antioxidant system of yeast cells, the activities of antioxidant enzymes and oxidative stress markers were estimated. Among known antioxidant enzymes, we tested superoxide dismutase (SOD), which catalyzes dismutation of superoxide anion radical ($O_2^{\bullet-}$) to hydrogen peroxide (H_2O_2), and catalase, which decomposes H_2O_2 to nontoxic water and oxygen [7]. The activities of SOD were similar in the control and AKG-grown cells at 18 h and at day 7 of cultivation (Figure 5(a)); only at 42 h, cells cultivated on AKG showed 55% higher SOD activity in comparison to the control ones. In the control yeast culture, SOD activity was the highest at 18 h and then decreased gradually with increasing age of yeast cultures. In AKG-grown cells, SOD activity reached maximal values at 42 h, where it was 2-fold higher than at 18 h, and at day 7 it decreased to the value close to that observed at 18 h. Regardless of medium type, catalase activity was the lowest at 18 h and the highest at 42 h of cultivation with a moderate decrease (~2-fold) at day 7 (Figure 5(b)). Significant difference in catalase activity between control and experimental cells was observed only at 18 h, where AKG-grown cells had 26% higher catalase activity than the control ones. The levels of oxidative stress markers, low-molecular-mass thiols (L-SH) (Figure 5(c)) and carbonyl proteins (CP) (Figure 5(d)), rose over a cultivation time in cells grown in medium with or without 10 mM AKG. At the same time, AKG-grown cells had 61%, 43%, and 29% higher L-SH levels at 18 h, 42 h, and day 7, respectively, as compared to the control cells at the same time points. The level of CP did not differ in cells from both cultures at 18 h (Figure 5(d)), but a significant increase in this parameter was observed in the control cells at next days of cultivation. Thus, the control cells had 63% and 74% higher CP level at 42 h and day 7, respectively, when compared with respective values at 18 h. At the same time, CP level in AKG-grown cells was only 31% and 37% higher at 42 h and day 7, respectively, as compared with 18 h. We also measured levels of α-dicarbonyl compounds (DC) in cells from 7-day cultures. These compounds together with ROS are intermediary products of nonenzymatic glycation/autoxidation of monosaccharides [16, 23]. Level of DC was 24% lower in cells grown in the presence of AKG compared with the control cells at day 7 of cultivation of yeast cultures (Table 1).

4. Discussion

Yeast *S. cerevisiae* is widely used to understand molecular mechanisms regulating metabolic processes in mammalian cells. It has been suggested that yeast culture at stationary phase is a good model to study aging of somatic cells in higher eukaryotic organisms, because at this stage yeasts become postmitotic cells and rely on mitochondrial respiration to maintain viability. In the yeast, process of entry into stationary phase is the best studied in glucose-containing liquid medium at 30°C and exhibits several distinct phases, including exponential phase, during which growth rates are maximal and cells use mainly glucose as carbon and energy source, and stationary phase, when all carbon energy sources are exhausted and cell number remains at relatively constant value [13, 15]. A variety of experimental data supports a key

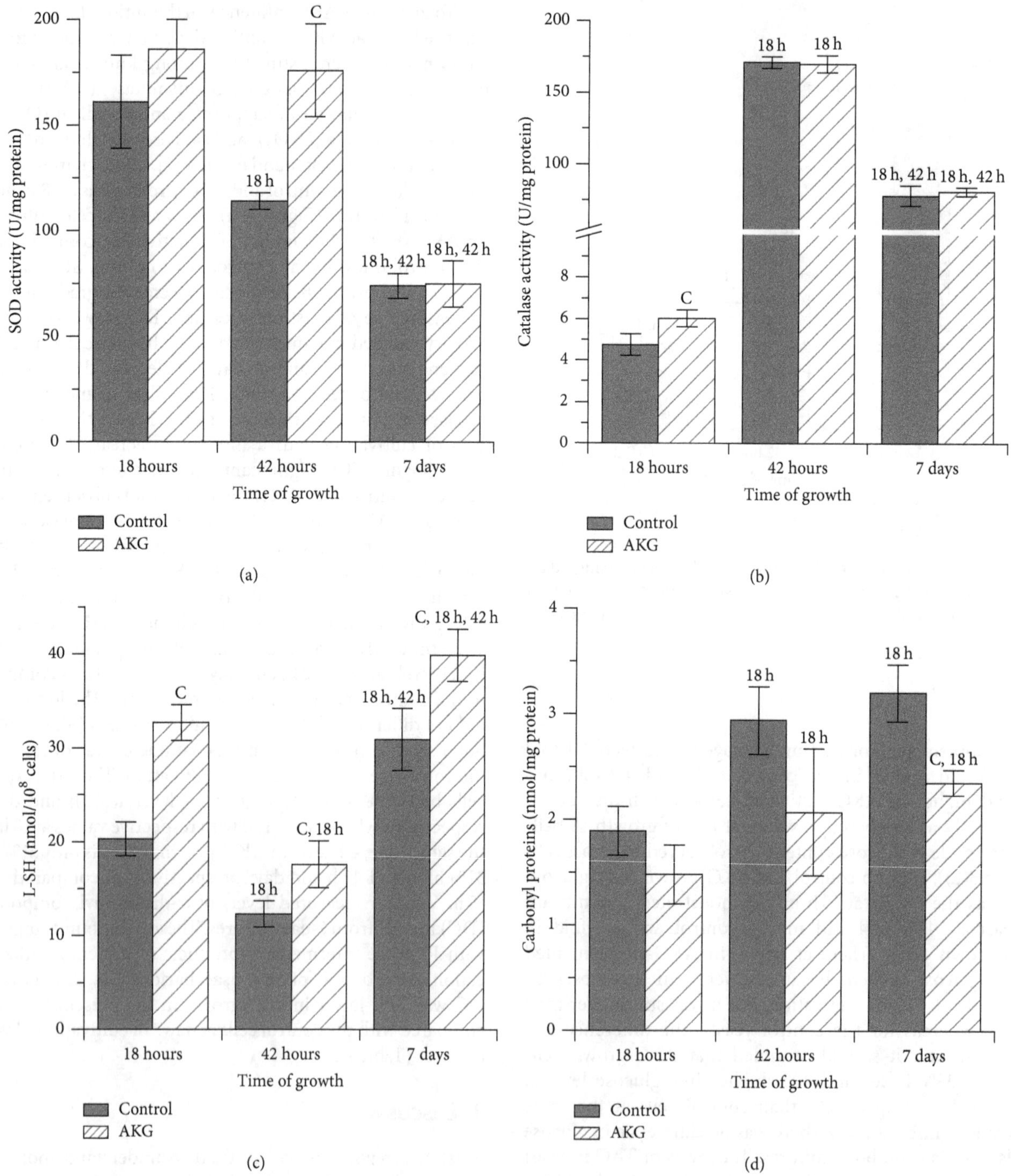

FIGURE 5: Activities of SOD (a) and catalase (b) and levels of low-molecular-mass thiols (c) and carbonyl proteins (d) in *S. cerevisiae* cells grown during 7 days in control medium or medium supplemented with 10 mM AKG. Results are shown as means ± SEM (n = 5–7). Statistic as in Figure 2.

role of antioxidant defense and stored carbohydrates in the extension of stationary phase yeast lifespan [11–16, 23–27].

Alpha-ketoglutarate (AKG) is an important intermediate of many metabolic processes combining catabolic and anabolic functions. Our previous results show that the supplementation with AKG did not affect growth of *S. cerevisiae* YPH250 strain (wild type) in glucose-containing medium starting from inoculation to 72 h of cultivation [10]. Here, we demonstrated that AKG supplementation had no effect on total cell number in YPH250 cultures during a 15-day cultivation period (Figure 1(a)). Meanwhile, total cell number was changed during yeast growth in accordance with features of typical growth pattern of *S. cerevisiae* in batch culture. The cell number was the lowest at 18 h and increased about twice at 42 h. Hence, 18 h of growth corresponded to a late exponential phase of growth curve. A true stationary phase was started at day 3, because no increase in cell number was observed anymore, and this phase lasted to day 11 (Figure 1(a)). At day 15, the total cell number phase decreased, indicating a phase of culture death. As the total cell number, the number of reproductively active cells in yeast culture also depended on time of cultivation (Figure 1(b)). At exponential phase of growth (day 1), almost all cells were able to proliferate and form colonies on YPD agar plates. The positive effects of AKG on proliferative ability were observed at days 7–15, when the control cells formed lower numbers of GFUs than AKG-grown ones. Thus, AKG increased the reproductive potential of aged yeast population. Mechanisms underlying protective AKG effects could be related with modulation of metabolic pathways, where this keto acid might be involved. Our results showed that AKG promoted different metabolic changes in exponential phase and stationary phase cells.

We show here that exponentially growing yeast cells had higher values of total metabolic activity (Figure 4), protein level (Figure 2(a)), and ASAT activity (Figure 2(b)) and lower levels of glycogen (Figure 3(b)) and free glucose (Figure 3(c)) in the AKG-supplemented medium than in the control one. These results let us suggest that exogenous AKG modifies protein/amino acid and glucose metabolism in exponential phase cells. The involvement of AKG in amino acid metabolism is well established; in particular AKG was found to serve as a precursor for the biosynthesis of such amino acids as glutamate, glutamine, leucine, and proline [1, 4, 9]. Obviously, an AKG-induced increase in amino acid levels could stimulate protein synthesis, leading to the higher levels of total protein seen in yeast cells (Figure 2(a)). In support of this finding, the ability of AKG to enhance protein synthesis due to increased production of amino acids was demonstrated in intestinal porcine epithelial cells [5]. The increased protein synthesis in AKG-grown cells can be a cause of higher biomass of these cells compared to the control ones (Table 1). In addition, AKG-supplemented cells had higher protein levels than control ones at stationary phase of growth. That may indicate that AKG prevented age-associated decrease in protein synthesis and/or increase in catabolism of proteins [11]. Moreover, some studies indicate that higher concentration of amino acids in the media can promote yeast growth and lifespan extension [28, 29]. Therefore, AKG-promoted synthesis of amino acids can be important for better yeast viability in our experiments.

Apart from involvement in protein/amino acid metabolism, AKG is a Krebs cycle intermediate. Previous studies show that the externally added AKG is actively utilized via the Krebs cycle, leading to increasing mitochondrial respiration and oxidative phosphorylation [6] and ATP production [30], as well as decreasing free glucose and TAG level [2, 4, 31]. These facts can explain lower glucose and glycogen levels in AKG-grown cells, since a more active Krebs cycle (due to increase of number of intermediates) requires more molecules of acetyl-CoA formed during aerobic glucose oxidation. However, it should be noted that the Krebs cycle and respiratory chain are poorly functioning in *S. cerevisiae* cells growing exponentially at high (2%) glucose levels. Glucose is preferentially metabolized via anaerobic glycolysis to form nonfermentable carbon compounds, particularly ethanol, and it exerts a strong catabolite repression with either enzymes required for respiration or enzymes of the Krebs cycle [11, 32]. After glucose is depleted, yeast cells reorganize their metabolism from fermentation to respiration in order to utilize other carbon sources presented in the medium such as ethanol. In our previous study, we showed that the glucose concentration at 18 h of growth in the media collected from control and AKG-grown *S. cerevisiae* cultures was lower than 0.2%. It means that cells were not under glucose repression and were able to obtain energy aerobically [10]. Our present data on the total metabolic activity (Figure 4) support an increase in metabolic rate in exponential phase yeast cells grown on AKG. Since method used for determination of metabolic activity reflects mainly functioning of mitochondria [22], it may be surmised that cells grown with addition of AKG to medium could respire more actively than their counterparts grown without AKG supplementation.

Since AKG can intensify mitochondrial respiration, it may lead to increased ROS production by mitochondria. In particular, the enhanced ROS level was found in *C. elegans* grown on AKG [8]. In the response to increased ROS levels, the antioxidant system can be activated [7]. In our previous study, we showed an activation of antioxidant enzymes, catalase and glutathione reductase, together with an enhanced level of low-molecular-mass thiols, which are represented mainly by glutathione [33], in AKG-grown yeast cells at exponential phase [10]. Here, the results on exponentially growing cells (Figure 5) confirmed our previous observations.

In stationary phase, both control and AKG-grown cells were characterized by higher levels and glucose, glycogen, and trehalose (Figure 3). It was quite expected, because many studies demonstrated increased gluconeogenesis and accumulation of reserve carbohydrates in stationary phase yeast cells [11, 14, 23]. Reserve carbohydrates not only serve as energy and carbon sources in starving cells but also have stress-protective functions, especially trehalose [11–14]. The supplementation of culture medium with AKG promoted higher values of reserve carbohydrates and glucose in stationary phase cells (Figure 3). This suggests that AKG may stimulate gluconeogenesis in yeast cells. This effect can be implemented via using of AKG for synthesis of glycogenic amino acids such as glutamine [1, 4] or via metabolizing AKG in Krebs cycle to oxaloacetate, a well-known precursor in glucose biogenesis. The increased activity of ASAT in early stationary phase cells grown on AKG (Figure 2(c)) can also contribute to oxaloacetate supply for gluconeogenesis as it was shown in starved animals [8]. In turn, the increased glucose level can be directed for synthesis of reserve carbohydrates.

Loss of yeast viability during stationary phase is accompanied by reduced total metabolic activity and accumulation of oxidatively damaged biomolecules [11, 13, 16, 25, 26]. At the same time, activation of antioxidant defense and accumulation of reserve carbohydrates are considered as beneficial events for yeast cells which allow them to remain viable in aged cultures during prolonged periods of nutrient depletion [11, 13, 14, 26, 27]. Our results are in a good agreement with literature data. In the control cells, decreased SOD activity and L-SH level and increased catalase activity and level of carbonyl proteins were observed at early stationary phase (42 h of growth), compared to 18 h of growth. These changes suggest the development of oxidative stress in yeast cells entering stationary phase, which is consistent with data of other authors [16, 25, 27]. In addition, cells in stationary phase decrease their metabolic activity to maintain viability during prolonged periods [11, 13, 23]. Our results are in line with this mechanism and confirmed a decrease in total metabolic activity in cells at stationary phase compared to yeasts at exponential phase (Figure 4). At the same time, it was found earlier that slowing metabolic activity is not always accompanied with decrease in ROS production; the ROS level may be even elevated [34], and stationary phase cells suffer from chronic oxidative stress [25]. As a result, oxidative modification of biomolecules may exceed the capacity of antioxidant system. In our case, an increase in level of oxidized proteins was observed in the control cells in both early and late stationary phase, despite higher values of catalase activity and L-SH-level in these cells in comparison with exponential phase cells. Moreover, the decreased SOD activity at 42 h and at day 7 comparatively with values at 18 h and a decrease in catalase activity at day 7 comparatively to 42 h could be caused by oxidative modification of these enzymes as it was reported earlier [17, 35].

In the case of AKG-supplemented cultures, the higher levels of L-SH and less oxidative damage to proteins were observed in stationary phase yeast cells compared to the control ones (Figures 5(c) and 5(d)). The activities of SOD and catalase in AKG-grown yeasts were similar to those in the control yeasts at day 7, but at 42 h SOD activity in AKG-grown yeasts was higher than that in control ones (Figure 5(a)). In addition, AKG-grown cells had lower level of α-dicarbonyl compounds (DC) than control ones at day 7 (Table 1). The α-dicarbonyl compounds together with ROS are intermediate products of nonenzymatic glycation/autoxidation of glucose, which participate in aging processes in yeasts [16]. Higher levels of glycation products are formed at high glucose levels in the medium (2% glucose), where glucose is mainly utilized via fermentation, and it shortens chronological yeast lifespan [16, 36]. However, caloric restriction or switch of glucose metabolism from fermentation to respiration may decrease glycation and extend yeast lifespan [36]. Since above we discussed that AKG may facilitate respiration metabolism in yeast cells when glucose is available at high concentrations, this may contribute to lower DC level in aged yeast cells. In addition, lower levels of oxidized proteins (CP) and DC in AKG-supplemented cells at late days of cultivation might be a result of increasing antioxidant potential of these cells at early cultivation period, compared with the control cells. In agreement with our data, an increased superoxide generation was found to act as a signal in young *C. elegans* animals to trigger changes of gene expression which prevent or attenuate the effects of subsequent aging [37]. Thus, we can assume that AKG-induced mild oxidative stress in exponentially growing cells may result in the adaptive induction of defense mechanisms. This adaptive response can provide sufficient protection against any subsequent strong oxidative or other stresses and prevent an age-related increase of free radical damage to biomolecules, thereby contributing to better yeast viability during prolonged cultivation.

5. Conclusions

Our results indicate that cultivation on AKG-supplemented medium modifies metabolic processes in yeast *S. cerevisiae* and prevents a loss of reproductive potential in aged cultures. The main metabolic effects of AKG included an increase in levels of total protein and reserve carbohydrates, glycogen and trehalose, as well as an enhancement of antioxidant defense with subsequent diminishing oxidative damage to proteins in yeast cells. These changes were supposed to contribute to better survival of AKG-supplemented cells under long-term cultivation in nutrient-deprived medium. Thus, our results extend knowledge on antiaging effects of AKG found previously in animals and suggest that AKG supplementation may also be beneficial at cellular level via increasing oxidative stress resistance and maintaining proliferative potential of cells.

Conflicts of Interest

The authors declare that there are no conflicts of interest.

Acknowledgments

The Authors are grateful to Dr. Y. Inoue for providing *S. cerevisiae* strain and are thankful to students L. Izerska and Kh. Hryshuk for technical assistance. They express their sincere gratitude to Dr. Olga I. Kubrak (Stockholm University) for English correction of the article.

References

[1] A. P. Harrison and S. G. Pierzynowski, "Biological effects of 2-oxoglutarate with particular emphasis on the regulation of protein, mineral and lipid absorption/metabolism, muscle performance, kidney function, bone formation and cancerogenesis, all viewed from a healthy ageing perspective state of the art—review article," *Journal of Physiology and Pharmacology*, vol. 59, supplement 1, pp. 91–106, 2008.

[2] M. M. Bayliak, M. P. Lylyk, H. V. Shmihel et al., "Dietary alpha-ketoglutarate promotes higher protein and lower triacylglyceride levels and induces oxidative stress in larvae and young adults but not in middle-aged *Drosophila melanogaster*," *Comparative Biochemistry and Physiology—Part A : Molecular and Integrative Physiology*, vol. 204, pp. 23–33, 2017.

[3] T. Niemiec, J. Sikorska, A. Harrison et al., "Alpha-ketoglutarate stabilizes redox homeostasis and improves arterial elasticity in aged mice," *Journal of Physiology and Pharmacology*, vol. 62, no. 1, pp. 37–43, 2011.

[4] B. D. Lambert, R. Filip, B. Stoll et al., "First-pass metabolism limits the intestinal absorption of enteral α-ketoglutarate in young pigs," *Journal of Nutrition*, vol. 136, no. 11, pp. 2779–2784, 2006.

[5] K. Yao, Y. Yin, X. Li et al., "Alpha-ketoglutarate inhibits glutamine degradation and enhances protein synthesis in intestinal porcine epithelial cells," *Amino Acids*, vol. 42, no. 6, pp. 2491–2500, 2012.

[6] N. M. Kurgalyuk and O. V. Goryn, "Effect of sodium α-ketoglutarate injected after the x-ray treatment on the respiration and oxidative phosphorylation of the liver's mitochondria," *Fiziolohichnyĭ zhurnal*, vol. 46, no. 5, pp. 63–70, 2000.

[7] V. I. Lushchak, "Free radicals, reactive oxygen species, oxidative stress and its classification," *Chemico-Biological Interactions*, vol. 224, pp. 164–175, 2014.

[8] R. M. Chin, X. Fu, M. Y. Pai et al., "The metabolite α-ketoglutarate extends lifespan by inhibiting ATP synthase and TOR," *Nature*, vol. 510, no. 7505, pp. 397–401, 2014.

[9] M. M. Bayliak, M. P. Lylyk, H. V. Shmihel et al., "Dietary alpha-ketoglutarate increases cold tolerance in *Drosophila melanogaster* and enhances protein pool and antioxidant defense in sex-specific manner," *Journal of Thermal Biology*, vol. 60, pp. 1–11, 2016.

[10] M. Bayliak, N. Burdyliuk, and V. Lushchak, "Growth on alpha-ketoglutarate increases oxidative stress resistance in the yeast *Saccharomyces cerevisiae*," *International Journal of Microbiology*, vol. 2017, Article ID 5792192, pp. 1–9, 2017.

[11] M. Werner-Washburne, E. L. Braun, M. E. Crawford, and V. M. Peck, "Stationary phase in *Saccharomyces cerevisiae*," *Molecular Microbiology*, vol. 19, no. 6, pp. 1159–1166, 1996.

[12] L. Shi, B. M. Sutter, X. Ye, and B. P. Tu, "Trehalose is a key determinant of the quiescent metabolic state that fuels cell cycle progression upon return to growth," *Molecular Biology of the Cell (MBoC)*, vol. 21, no. 12, pp. 1982–1990, 2010.

[13] H. M. Semchyshyn, M. M. Bayliak, and V. I. Lushchak, "Starvation in yeasts: biochemical aspects," in *Biology of Starvation in Humans and Other Organisms*, T. C. Merkin, Ed., pp. 103–150, Nova Science Publishers, 2011.

[14] L. Cao, Y. Tang, Z. Quan, Z. Zhang, S. G. Oliver, and N. Zhang, "Chronological lifespan in yeast is dependent on the accumulation of storage carbohydrates mediated by Yak1, Mck1 and Rim15 kinases," *PLoS Genetics*, vol. 12, no. 12, article e1006458, 2016.

[15] P. Fabrizio and V. D. Longo, "The chronological life span of *Saccharomyces cerevisiae*," in *Methods in Molecular Biology: Biological Aging: Methods and Protocols*, T. Tollefsbol, Ed., pp. 89–95, Humana Press, 2007.

[16] H. M. Semchyshyn, L. M. Lozinska, J. Miedzobrodzki, and V. I. Lushchak, "Fructose and glucose differentially affect aging and carbonyl/oxidative stress parameters in *Saccharomyces cerevisiae* cells," *Carbohydrate Research*, vol. 346, no. 7, pp. 933–938, 2011.

[17] V. Lushchak, H. Semchyshyn, S. Mandryk, and O. Lushchak, "Possible role of superoxide dismutases in the yeast *Saccharomyces cerevisiae* under respiratory conditions," *Archives of Biochemistry and Biophysics*, vol. 441, no. 1, pp. 35–40, 2005.

[18] M. M. Bradford, "A rapid and sensitive method for the quantitation of microgram quantities of protein utilizing the principle of protein dye binding," *Analytical Biochemistry*, vol. 72, no. 1-2, pp. 248–254, 1976.

[19] G. L. Ellman, "Tissue sulfhydryl groups," *Archives of Biochemistry and Biophysics*, vol. 82, no. 1, pp. 70–77, 1959.

[20] M. Sakai, M. Oimomi, and M. Kasuga, "Experimental studies on the role of fructose in the development of diabetic complications," *Kobe Journal of Medical Sciences*, vol. 48, no. 5-6, pp. 125–136, 2002.

[21] J. L. Parrou and J. François, "A simplified procedure for a rapid and reliable assay of both glycogen and trehalose in whole yeast cells," *Analytical Biochemistry*, vol. 248, no. 1, pp. 186–188, 1997.

[22] A. Conconi, P. Jager-Vottero, X. Zhang, B. C. Beard, and M. J. Smerdon, "Mitotic viability and metabolic competence in UV-irradiated yeast cells," *Mutation Research-DNA Repair*, vol. 459, no. 1, pp. 55–64, 2000.

[23] L. M. Lozinska and H. M. Semchyshyn, "Fructose as a factor of carbonyl and oxidative stress development and accelerated aging in the yeast *Saccharomyces cerevisiae*," *Ukrainian Biochemical Journal*, vol. 83, no. 4, pp. 67–76, 2011.

[24] M. M. Bayliak and V. I. Lushchak, "The golden root, *Rhodiola rosea*, prolongs lifespan but decreases oxidative stress resistance in yeast *Saccharomyces cerevisiae*," *Phytomedicine*, vol. 18, pp. 1262–1268, 2011.

[25] W. Jakubowski, T. Biliński, and G. Bartosz, "Oxidative stress during aging of stationary cultures of the yeast *Saccharomyces cerevisiae*," *Free Radical Biology & Medicine*, vol. 28, no. 5, pp. 659–664, 2000.

[26] A. B. Demir and A. Koc, "Assessment of chronological lifespan dependent molecular damages in yeast lacking mitochondrial antioxidant genes," *Biochemical and Biophysical Research Communications*, vol. 400, no. 1, pp. 106–110, 2010.

[27] V. Costa and P. Moradas-Ferreira, "Oxidative stress and signal transduction in *Saccharomyces cerevisiae*: insights into ageing, apoptosis and diseases," *Molecular Aspects of Medicine*, vol. 22, no. 4-5, pp. 217–246, 2001.

[28] A. L. Alvers, L. K. Fishwick, M. S. Wood et al., "Autophagy and amino acid homeostasis are required for chronological longevity in *Saccharomyces cerevisiae*," *Aging Cell*, vol. 8, no. 4, pp. 353–369, 2009.

[29] P. Gomes, B. Sampaio-Marques, P. Ludovico, F. Rodrigues, and C. Leão, "Low auxotrophy-complementing amino acid concentrations reduce yeast chronological life span," *Mechanisms of Ageing and Development*, vol. 128, no. 5-6, pp. 383–391, 2007.

[30] Y. Hou, K. Yao, L. Wang et al., "Effects of α-ketoglutarate on energy status in the intestinal mucosa of weaned piglets chronically challenged with lipopolysaccharide," *British Journal of Nutrition*, vol. 106, no. 3, pp. 357–363, 2011.

[31] R. P. Radzki, M. Bieńko, and S. G. Pierzynowski, "Effect of dietary alpha-ketoglutarate on blood lipid profile during hypercholesterolaemia in rats," *Scandinavian Journal of Clinical & Laboratory Investigation*, vol. 69, no. 2, pp. 175–180, 2009.

[32] J. M. Gancedo, "Yeast carbon catabolite repression," *Microbiology and Molecular Biology Reviews*, vol. 62, no. 2, pp. 334–361, 1998.

[33] V. I. Lushchak, "Glutathione homeostasis and functions: potential targets for medical interventions," *Journal of Amino Acids*, vol. 2012, Article ID 736837, pp. 1–26, 2012.

[34] J. M. Van Raamsdonk, Y. Meng, D. Camp et al., "Decreased energy metabolism extends life span in *Caenorhabditis elegans* without reducing oxidative damage," *Genetics*, vol. 185, no. 2, pp. 559–571, 2010.

[35] H. M. Semchyshyn and L. M. Lozinska, "Fructose protects baker's yeast against peroxide stress: potential role of catalase and superoxide dismutase," *FEMS Yeast Research*, vol. 12, no. 7, pp. 761–773, 2012.

Permissions

All chapters in this book were first published in JAR, by Hindawi Publishing Corporation; hereby published with permission under the Creative Commons Attribution License or equivalent. Every chapter published in this book has been scrutinized by our experts. Their significance has been extensively debated. The topics covered herein carry significant findings which will fuel the growth of the discipline. They may even be implemented as practical applications or may be referred to as a beginning point for another development.

The contributors of this book come from diverse backgrounds, making this book a truly international effort. This book will bring forth new frontiers with its revolutionizing research information and detailed analysis of the nascent developments around the world.

We would like to thank all the contributing authors for lending their expertise to make the book truly unique. They have played a crucial role in the development of this book. Without their invaluable contributions this book wouldn't have been possible. They have made vital efforts to compile up to date information on the varied aspects of this subject to make this book a valuable addition to the collection of many professionals and students.

This book was conceptualized with the vision of imparting up-to-date information and advanced data in this field. To ensure the same, a matchless editorial board was set up. Every individual on the board went through rigorous rounds of assessment to prove their worth. After which they invested a large part of their time researching and compiling the most relevant data for our readers.

The editorial board has been involved in producing this book since its inception. They have spent rigorous hours researching and exploring the diverse topics which have resulted in the successful publishing of this book. They have passed on their knowledge of decades through this book. To expedite this challenging task, the publisher supported the team at every step. A small team of assistant editors was also appointed to further simplify the editing procedure and attain best results for the readers.

Apart from the editorial board, the designing team has also invested a significant amount of their time in understanding the subject and creating the most relevant covers. They scrutinized every image to scout for the most suitable representation of the subject and create an appropriate cover for the book.

The publishing team has been an ardent support to the editorial, designing and production team. Their endless efforts to recruit the best for this project, has resulted in the accomplishment of this book. They are a veteran in the field of academics and their pool of knowledge is as vast as their experience in printing. Their expertise and guidance has proved useful at every step. Their uncompromising quality standards have made this book an exceptional effort. Their encouragement from time to time has been an inspiration for everyone.

The publisher and the editorial board hope that this book will prove to be a valuable piece of knowledge for researchers, students, practitioners and scholars across the globe.

List of Contributors

Ricardo Aurélio Carvalho Sampaio and Marco Carlos Uchida
School of Physical Education, State University of Campinas, 130883851 Campinas, Brazil

Hélio José Coelho Júnior
School of Physical Education, State University of Campinas, 130883851 Campinas, Brazil
Center of Health Sciences, University of Mogi das Cruzes, 08770-490 Mogi das Cruzes, Brazil

Samuel da Silva Aguiar
Center of Health Sciences, University of Mogi das Cruzes, 08770-490 Mogi das Cruzes, Brazil
Graduate Program on Physical Education, Catholic University of Brasilia, 71966-700 Brasilia, Brazil

Ricardo Yukio Asano
Center of Health Sciences, University of Mogi das Cruzes, 08770-490 Mogi das Cruzes, Brazil
School of Sciences and Letters of Braganca Paulista, SP, Brazil

Milton Rocha Moraes
Graduate Program on Physical Education, Catholic University of Brasilia, 71966-700 Brasilia, Brazil

Ivan de Oliveira Gonçalves
Community Center for Older People of Póa, Brazil

Nicole R. Fowler
Division of General Internal Medicine, Department of Medicine, School of Medicine, University of Pittsburgh, Pittsburgh, PA 15213, USA

Amber E. Barnato
Division of General Internal Medicine, Department of Medicine, School of Medicine, University of Pittsburgh, Pittsburgh, PA 15213, USA
Department of Health Policy and Management, Graduate School of Public Health, University of Pittsburgh, Pittsburgh, PA 15261, USA

Howard B. Degenholtz
Department of Health Policy and Management, Graduate School of Public Health, University of Pittsburgh, Pittsburgh, PA 15261, USA
Center for Bioethics and Health Law, University of Pittsburgh, Pittsburgh, PA 15260, USA

Angela M. Curcio
College of Medicine, Drexel University, Philadelphia, PA 19129, USA

James T. Becker
Department of Psychiatry, School of Medicine, University of Pittsburgh, Pittsburgh, PA 15213, USA

Lewis H. Kuller
Department of Epidemiology, Graduate School of Public Health, University of Pittsburgh, Pittsburgh, PA 15261, USA

Oscar L. Lopez
Department of Neurology, School of Medicine, University of Pittsburgh, Pittsburgh, PA 15213, USA

Kevin S. Heffernan
Human Performance Laboratory, Department of Exercise Science, Syracuse University, Syracuse, NY 13244, USA

Angela Chalé, Cynthia Hau, Gregory J. Cloutier, Edward M. Phillips, Kieran F. Reid, Jeffrey T. Kuvin and Roger A. Fielding
Nutrition, Exercise Physiology and Sarcopenia Laboratory, Jean Mayer USDA Human Nutrition Research Center on Aging at Tufts University, Boston, MA 02111, USA

Patrick Warner and Heather Nickerson
The Vascular Function Study Group, Division of Cardiology and the Molecular Cardiology Research Institute, Tufts Medical Center, Boston, MA 02111, USA

Prabhjot Singh
Disability Services, Queensland Department of Communities, Child Safety and Disability Services, Brisbane, QLD 4001, Australia

Adeel Khan and Roslyn Foskey
University of New England, Armidale, NSW, Australia

Rafat Hussain
School of Rural Medicine, University of New England, Armidale, NSW 2351, Australia

Lyn Irwin
Aged Care Standards and Accreditation Agency Ltd., Sydney, NSW2124, Australia

Maurits F. J. Vandewoude
Department of Geriatrics, ZNA St. Elisabeth Leopoldstraat 26, University of Antwerp, 2000 Antwerp, Belgium

Carolyn J. Alish, Abby C. Sauer and Refaat A. Hegazi
Scientific and Medical Affairs, Abbott Nutrition, Abbott Laboratories, 3300 Stelzer Road, Columbus, OH 43219, USA

I. Reuter and S. Mehnert
Department of Neurology, Justus-Liebig University, Klinikstraße 33, 35392 Giessen, Germany

G. Sammer
Department of Psychiatry, Cognitive Laboratory Justus-Liebig University, Am Steg 22, 35385 Giessen, Germany

M. Oechsner
Neurologisches Rehabilitation szentrum, HELIOS Klinik Zihlschlacht AG, Hauptstrße 2-4, 8588 Zihlschlacht, Switzerland

M. Engelhardt
Department of Orthopedic Surgery, Klinikum Osnabrück, Am Finkenhügel 1, 49076 Osnabrück, Germany

Eling D. de Bruin, Michéle Hubli, Pamela Hofer and Kurt Murer
Institute of Human Movement Sciences and Sport, ETH, 8093 Zurich, Switzerland

Peter Wolf
Sensory-Motor Systems Lab, ETH, Zurich, Switzerland

Wiebren Zijlstra
Center for Human Movement Sciences, University Medical Center Groningen, University of Groningen, Groningen, The Netherlands
Institut für Bewegungsund Sportgerontologie, Deutsche Sporthochschule Köln, Köln, Germany

P. K.-Y. Chang, S. Boridy, R. A. McKinney and D. Maysinger
Department of Pharmacology and Therapeutics, Faculty of Medicine, McGill University, 3655 Promenade Sir William Osler, Montreal, QC, Canada H3G 1Y6

Boon Peng Ng
Department of Economics, Wayne State University, 656WKirby St., 2074 FAB, Detroit, MI 48202, USA

Gail A. Jensen
Department of Economics and Institute of Gerontology, Wayne State University, 87 East Ferry St., Detroit, MI 48202, USA

Heather Fritz
Eugene Applebaum College of Pharmacy and Health Sciences and Institute of Gerontology, Wayne State University, 259 Mack Ave., Detroit, MI 48201, USA

Erin D. Bouldin
Health Services Research and Development Service, Department of Veterans Affairs, VA Puget Sound Health Care System, Seattle, WA 98101, USA
Department of Epidemiology, University of Washington, Seattle, WA 98195, USA

Gayle E. Reiber
Health Services Research and Development Service, Department of Veterans Affairs, VA Puget Sound Health Care System, Seattle, WA 98101, USA
Department of Epidemiology, University of Washington, Seattle, WA 98195, USA
Department of Health Services, University of Washington, Seattle, WA 98195, USA

Gina Rutherford and Philip Manning
Institute of Cellular Medicine, Newcastle University, Newcastle NE2 4HH, UK

Julia L. Newton
Newcastle Hospitals NHS Foundation Trust, UK
NIHR Biomedical Research Centre in Ageing and Age Related Disease, Newcastle University, Newcastle NE2 4HH, UK

Kaitlyn P. Roland and Kayla M. D. Cornett
Interdisciplinary Graduate Studies, Health and Exercise Sciences, University of British Columbia Okanagan, Kelowna, BC, Canada V1V 1V7

Olga Theou
Faculty of Geriatrics Medicine, Dalhousie University, Halifax, NS, Canada B3H 2E1

Jennifer M. Jakobi and Gareth R. Jones
School of Health and Exercise Sciences, Faculty of Health and Social Development, University of British Columbia Okanagan, 3333 University Way, Kelowna, BC, Canada V1V 1V7

Nina Hovanec
Health and Rehabilitation Sciences Graduate Program, Western University, London, ON, Canada N6G 1H1

Anuradha Sawant, Tom J. Overend and Anthony A. Vandervoort
School of Physical Therapy and Center for Physical Activity and Aging, Faculty of Health Sciences, Western University, London, ON, Canada N6G 1H1

Robert J. Petrella
Department of Family Medicine, Western University, London, ON, Canada N6G 1H1

Paule Denoël
Emergency Service, Europe Hospital, 1040 Brussels, Belgium

Jacques Vanderstraeten
Centre de Recherche en SantéEnvironnementale et en Santédu Travail, Ecole de Santé Publique, UniversitéLibre de Bruxelles, 1070 Brussels, Belgium

Pierre Mols
Emergency Service, Saint-Pierre University Hospital, Université Libre de Bruxelles, 1000 Brussels, Belgium

Thierry Pepersack
Department of Geriatrics, Erasme Hospital, Université Libre de Bruxelles, Lennik Street 808, 1070 Brussels, Belgium

Ryan T. Crews, Sai V. Yalla, Adam E. Fleischer and Stephanie C. Wu
Center for Lower Extremity Ambulatory Research (CLEAR), Dr. William M. Scholl College of Podiatric Medicine,
Rosalind Franklin University of Medicine and Science, 3333 Green Bay Road, North Chicago, IL 60064, USA

April B. C. G. Boessen, Renée Verwey, Saskia Duymelinck and Erik van Rossum
Centre of Expertise for Innovative Care and Technology (EIZT), Zuyd University of Applied Sciences, Heerlen, Netherlands

William Khalil El-Chaer and Otàvio Toledo Nóbrega
University of Brasília (UnB), 70910-900 Brasília, DF, Brazil

Clayton Franco Moraes
University of Brasília (UnB), 70910-900 Brasília, DF, Brazil
Catholic University of Brasília (UCB-DF), 71966-700 Brasília, DF, Brazil

Mohsen Bazargan, James Smith, David Martins and Hamed Yazdanshenas
Charles R. Drew University of Medicine and Science (CDU), Los Angeles, CA, USA
University of California, Los Angeles (UCLA), Los Angeles, CA, USA

Masoud Movassaghi
University of California, Los Angeles (UCLA), Los Angeles, CA, USA

Seyede Salehe Mortazavi
Mental Health Research Center, Tehran Institute of Psychiatry, School of Behavioral Sciences and Mental Health, Iran University of Medical Sciences, Tehran, Iran

Gail Orum
Keck Graduate Institute, School of Pharmacy, Claremont, CA, USA

Heather E. Cuevas, Alexa K. Stuifbergen and Catherine Ward
School of Nursing, e University of Texas at Austin, 1710 Red River, Austin, TX 78701, USA

Rachel Russell
School of Health Sciences, The University of Salford, Salford M6 6PU, UK

Marcus Ormerod
School of the Built Environment, The University of Salford, Salford M5 4WT, UK

Rita Newton
School of Health Sciences, The University of Manchester, Manchester M13 9PL, UK

Eiji Kose, Riku Maruyama and Hiroyuki Hayashi
Department of Pharmacotherapy, School of Pharmacy, Nihon University, Chiba, Japan

Susumu Okazoe
Department of Pharmacy, Sagami Rehabilitation Hospital, Kanagawa, Japan

Simone Perna, Daniele Spadaccini, Mara Nichetti, Ilaria Avanzato, Milena Anna Faliva and Mariangela Rondanelli
Department of Public Health, Experimental and Forensic Medicine, School of Medicine, Endocrinology and Nutrition Unit, University of Pavia, Pavia, Italy

Nadia Burdyliuk and Maria Bayliak
Department of Biochemistry and Biotechnology, Vasyl Stefanyk Precarpathian National University, 57 Shevchenko Str., Ivano-Frankivsk 76018, Ukraine

Index

R

S

T

V

www.ingramcontent.com/pod-product-compliance
Lightning Source LLC
LaVergne TN
LVHW060540210926
848485LV00005B/1231